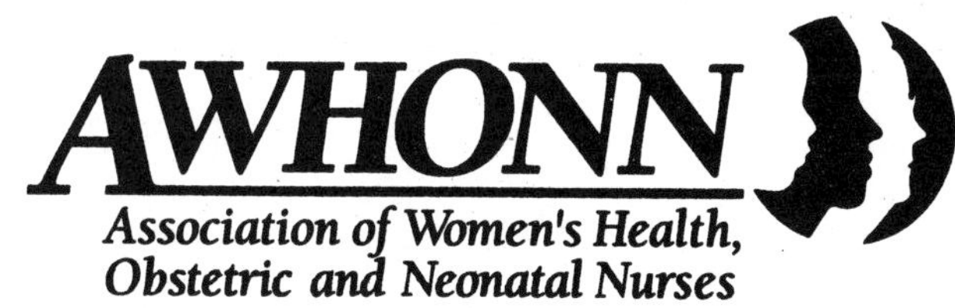

Perinatal Nursing

Kathleen Rice Simpson RNC, MSN
Perinatal Clinical Nurse Specialist
St. John's Mercy Medical Center
St. Louis, Missouri
Adjunct Clinical Instructor
Barnes College of Nursing
University of Missouri, St. Louis

Patricia A. Creehan RNC, MS, MA, ACCE
Perinatal Clinical Nurse Specialist
Palos Community Hospital
Palos Heights, Illinois

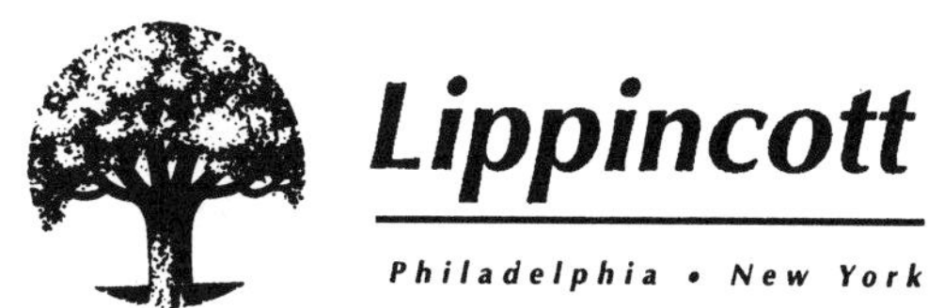

Acquisitions Editor: Jennifer E. Brogan
Coordinating Editorial Assistant: Danielle J. DiPalma
Senior Production Editor: Molly E. Dickmeyer
Design & Composition: Page Two Associates

 Printed in the United States of America. For information write Lippincott–Raven Publishers, 227 East Washington Square, Philadelphia, PA 19106.

Library of Congress Cataloging-in-Publications Data

AWHONN's Perinatal Nursing/ [edited by]Kathleen Rice Simpson,
Patricia A. Creehan. — 1st ed.
p. cm.
Includes bibliographical references and index.
ISBN 0-397-55134-7
1. Maternity nursing. I. Simpson, Kathleen Rice. II. Creehan, Patricia A. III. Association of Women's Health, Obstetric, and Neonatal Nurses.
[DNLM: 1. Maternal-Child Nursing. WY 157.3 A966 1996]
RG951.A985 1996
610.73'678—dc20
DNLM/DLC
for Library of Congress 96-44866
CIP

The material contained in this volume was submitted as previously unpublished material, except in the instances in which credit has been given to the source from which some of the illustrative material was derived.

Any procedure or practice described in this book should be applied by the healthcare practitioner under appropriate supervision in accordance with professional standards of care used with regard to the unique circumstances that apply in each practice situation. Care has been taken to confirm the accuracy of information presented and to describe generally accepted practices. However, the authors, editors, and publisher cannot accept any responsibility for errors or omissions or for any consequences from application of the information in this book and make no warranty, express or implied, with respect to the contents of the book.

The authors and publisher have exerted every effort to ensure that drug selection and dosage set forth in this text are in accordance with current recommendations and practice at the time of publication. However, in view of ongoing research, changes in government regulations, and the constant flow of information relating to drug therapy and drug reactions, the reader is urged to check the package insert for each drug for any change in indications and dosage and for added warnings and precautions. This is particularly important when the recommended agent is a new or infrequently employed drug.

Materials appearing in this book prepared by individuals as part of their official duties as U.S. Government employees are not covered by the above-mentioned copyright.

9 8 7 6 5 4

DEDICATIONS

To

the perinatal nurses at St. John's Mercy Medical Center in St. Louis, Missouri and
Palos Community Hospital in Palos Heights, Illinois

and

my parents William and Dorothy, my husband Dan, and my children
Daniel, Kate, Michael, John, and Elizabeth
KRS

my parents Raymond and Ruth
PAC

CONTRIBUTOR LIST

Cydney I. Afriat Menihan, CNM, MSN, RDMS
Clinical Teaching Associate
Brown University, School of Medicine
Nurse Midwife
Women and Infant's Hospital
Providence, RI
Chapter 9: Intrapartum Fetal Monitoring

Jean Bachman, DSN, RN
Associate Professor of Nursing
Barnes College of Nursing,
University of Missouri-St. Louis
St. Louis, MO
Chapter 8: Childbirth

Mary Lee Barron, RN-CS, MSN, FNP
Nurse Practitioner
Barnes Hospital
St. Louis, MO
Chapter 6: Antenatal Care and Risk Assessment Strategies

Linda Bertucci, CNM, MS, RNC
Assistant Clinical Professor
Department of OBGYN
University of Irvine, School of Medicine
Irvine, CA
Chapter 3: Collaborative Practice as a Systematic Method for Perinatal Care

Mary Ellen Burke, RN, MS
Perinatal Clinical Specialist
Division of Maternal/Fetal Medicine
Women and Infant's Hospital
Clinical Teaching Associate
Brown University, School of Medicine
Providence, RI
Chapter 7: Common Perinatal Complications

Bonnie Flood Chez, RNC, MSN
Director, Women's Center
University Community Hospital
Tampa, FL
Chapter 2: Professional and Legal Issues

Gwen Chute, RN, MS, IBCLC
Women's Health Educator and Lactation Consultant
Westmoreland Regional Hospital
Greensburg, PA
Chapter 15: Newborn Nutrition

Mary Coughlin, RN, BSN
Staff Nurse
Rush-Presbyterian -St. Lukes Medical Center
Assistant Education Coordinator
Rush Perinatal Center
Chicago, IL
Chapter 13: Newborn Adaptation to Extrauterine Life

Patricia A. Creehan, RNC, MS, MA, ACCE
Perinatal Clinical Nurse Specialist
Palos Community Hospital
Palos Heights, IL
Chapter 10: Pain Relief and Comfort Measures During Labor
Chapter 14: Newborn Physical Assessment

Jeanne Watson Driscoll, MS, RN, CS
Independent Practice
Clinical Nurse Specialist,
Psychiatric and Mental Health
Boston, MA
Chapter 4: Psychosocial Adaptation to Pregnancy and Postpartum

Mary Kay Fallon, RNC, MS, MAEd
Perinatal Nurse Coordinator
St. John's Mercy Medical Center
St. Louis, MO
Chapter 5: Physiologic Adaptation to Pregnancy

Joy Grohar, RNC, MS
President, Comprehensive Perinatal Consultants
Lockport, IL
Labor/Delivery Staff Nurse
Michael Reese Hospital Center
Chicago, IL
Chapter 11: Care of the Woman in the Postpartum Period

Jacqueline Jordan, RN, BSN, CCRN
Director of Quality Management
HOAG Memorial Hospital Presbyterian
Newport Beach, CA
Chapter 3: Collaborative Practice as a Systematic Method for Perinatal Care

Susan Kendig, RNC, MSN, WHCNP
Coordinator Women's Well, Perinatal Outreach
St. Mary's Health Center
St. Louis, MO
Chapter 6: Antenatal Care and Risk Assessment Strategies

Jo M. Kendrick, RNC, MSN
Obstetrics and Gynecology Nurse Practitioner
Universtiy of Tennessee Medical Center at Knoxville
Obstetrics and Gynecology
Knoxville, TN
Chapter 8, Childbirth

Karren Kowalski, PhD, RN, FAAN
Assistant Vice President and Administrator
Women's and Children's Hospital
Director of Patient Care Services
Associate Professor and Chairperson
Rush-Presbyterian St. Lukes Medical Center
Chicago, IL
Chapter 12: Pregnancy Loss and Bereavement

Marilyn Lowe, RNC, MSN
Perinatal Clinical Specialist
Nebraska Methodist Hospital Perinatal Center
Omaha, NE
Chapter 17: Discharge Planning

Alison Benzies Miklos, RNC, MSN
Neonatal Clinical Nurse Specialist
Christ Hospital and Medical Center
Oak Lawn, IL
Chapter 14: Newborn Physical Assessment

Diane C. Millea, RNC, MSN
Perinatal Clinical Specialist
Nebraska Methodist Hospital Perinatal Center
Omaha, NE
Chapter 17: Discharge Planning

Karen Sanders Moore, RNC, MSN, IBCLC
Perinatal Clinical Nurse Specialist
St. John's Mercy Medical Center
St. Louis, MO
Adjunct Faculty
Maryville University
St. Louis, MO
Chapter 15: Newborn Nutrition

Patricia Nash, RNC, MSN, IBCLC
Neonatal Nurse Practitioner
Cardinal Glennon Children's Hospital
St. Mary's Health Center
St. Louis, MO
Chapter 16: Common Neonatal Complications

Judith H. Poole, RNC, MN, FACCE
Coordinator of Perinatal Outreach Education
Carolinas Medical Center,
Department of Obstetrics and Gynecology
Charlotte, NC
Chapter 7: Common Perinatal Complications

Dawn E. Reimann, RNC, MS
Education Coordinator
Rush-Presbyterian-St. Lukes Medical Center
Chicago, IL
Chapter 13: Newborn Adaptation to Extrauterine Life

Linda J. Seibold, RN
Executive Vice President and Co-Founder
Healthy Homecomings Inc.
St. Louis, MO
Chapter 18: Perinatal Home Care Services

Kathleen Rice Simpson, RNC, MSN
Perinatal Clinical Nurse Specialist
St. John's Mercy Medical Center
St. Louis, MO
Adjunct Faculty
Barnes College of Nursing
University of Missouri–St. Louis
Chapter 1: Quality Care Issues: Service Excellence, Cost-Effective Practice, and Outcome Monitoring
Chapter 2: Professional and Legal Issues
Chapter 17: Discharge Planning
Chapter 18: Perinatal Home Care Services

Kim Stremsterfer, RN
President and Co-Founder
Healthy Homecomings Inc.
St. Louis, MO
Chapter 18: Perinatal Home Care Services

REVIEWER LIST

Cheryl Tatano Beck, DNSc, CNM, FAAN
Professor
University of Rhode Island, College of Nursing
Kingston, RI

Debi L. Bocar, RN, MS, MEd, IBCLC
Lactation Consultant
Breastfeeding Resource Center
Mercy Health Center
Oklahoma City, OK

Mary Ellen Burke, RN, MS
Perinatal Clinical Nurse Specialist
Division of Maternal/Fetal Medicine
Women and Infant's Hospital
Clinical Teaching Associate
Brown University School of Medicine
Providence, RI

Elaine M. Carty, RN, MSN, CNM
Associate Professor
School of Nursing
University of British Columbia
Vancouver, British Columbia, Canada

Elaine Cohen, EdD, RN
Assistant Vice President for Nursing
The General Hospital Center
Passaic, NJ

Margaret Comerford Freda, EdD, RN FAAN
Assistant Professor, Obstetrics and Gynecology
Director of Education and Community Affairs
Program to Reduce Obstetrical Problems and Prematurity (PROPP)
Albert Einstein College of Medicine
Bronx, NY

Nancy Jane Donoho, RNC, MSN
Maternal-Infant Clinical Nurse Specialist
Fort Sanders Health Systems
Knoxville, TN
Adjunct Instructor
Vanderbilt University
Nashville, TN

Deborah Eganhouse, RNC, MA
Perinatal Clinical Nurse Specialist
St. Luke's Hospital
Cedar Rapids, Iowa
Doctoral Candidate
University of Iowa, College of Nursing
Iowa City, Iowa

Maureen Giglio, RNC, BSN, FNP, IBCLC
Lactation Consultant
Palos Community Hospital
Palos Heights, IL
Family Nurse Practitioner/Lactation Consultation
Surburban Heights Medical Center
Chicago Heights, IL

Mary Gniady, RN, BSN, IBCLC, CCE
Lactation Consultant
Palos Community Hospital
Palos Heights, IL

Joan Harper, RNC, BS, FACCE
Director of Women's and Children's Education
Manager, Perinatal Center
St. John's Mercy Medical Center
St. Louis, MO

Mildred G. Harvey, RNC, MSN
Clinical Nurse Specialist for Obstetrics
Baptist Memorial Hospital East
Memphis, TN
Affiliate Faculty
University of Tennessee, College of Nursing
Memphis, TN
Senior Clinical Consultant
Harvey, Troiano Associates Inc.
Houston, TX

Barbara Heater, PhD, RN
Chairperson, Graduate Program
College of Nursing
South Dakota State University
Brookings, SD

Catherine Ingram Fogal, PhD, OGNP, FAAN
Associate Professor
University of North Carolina-Chapel Hill,
School of Nursing
Chapel Hill, NC

Jeanine Hummell, RNC, MSN
Director Maternal-Child Services
Shawnee Mission Medical Center
Shawnee Mission, KS

Jo M. Kendrick, RNC, MSN
Obstetrics and Gynecology Nurse Practitioner
University of Tennessee
Medical Center at Knoxville
Obstetrics and Gynecology
Knoxville, TN

Ermalym Kiehl, PhD, ARNP
Assistant Professor
University of Central Florida, School of Nursing
Orlando, FL

E. Jean Martin, MS, MSN, CNM
Associate Professor
Medical University of South Carolina
College of Nursing
Graduate Nursing Program
Charleston, SC

Mary Lou Moore, PhD, RNC, FACCE, FAAN
Research Assistant Professor
Wake Forest University
Bowman Gray Medical Center
Winston-Salem, NC

Nancy O'Brien-Abel, RNC, MN
Perinatal Clinical Nurse Specialist
Department of Obstetrics and Gynecology
Division of Perinatal Medicine
University of Washington School of Medicine
Seattle, WA

Judith H. Poole, RNC, MN, FACCE
Coordinator of Perinatal Outreach Education
Carolinas Medical Center
Department of Obstetrics and Gynecology
Charlotte, NC

Patsy L. Ruchala, DNSc, RN
Assistant Professor of Nursing
Coordinator, Perinatal Nursing Specialty
Saint Louis University, School of Nursing
St. Louis, MO

Patricia M. Sauer, RNC, MSN
Patient Care Administrator
Clinical Nurse Specialist
High Risk Obstetrics
Northside Hospital
Atlanta, GA

Francis Strodbeck, DNS, RNC, NNP
Director, Neonatal Nurse Practitioner Program
Rush-Presbyterian-St. Lukes Medical Center
Chicago, IL

Ellen Tappero, RNC, MN, NNP
Neonatal Nurse Practitioner
Luthern Medical Center
Wheat Ridge, CO

Carol Trotter, RNC, MPH, NNP
Director, Neonatal Nurse Practitioner Program
St. John's Mercy Medical Center
Department of Neonatology
St. Louis, MO

Sara Wheeler, RN, MSN
Certified Grief Counselor
Clinical Faculty
University of Illinois at Chicago-Urbana Regional Campus
Urbana, Illinois

Sue A. Woodson, RNC, MSN
Clinician IV
University of Virginia Medical Center
Charlottesville, VA

Marge Zerbe, RNC, BS
Perinatal Staff Nursing
Obstetrical Seminars and Consulting OBSC
Miami Valley Hospital
Dayton, OH

FOREWORD

The pace of changes in the delivery of healthcare is unprecedented. Not a day passes that one does not hear "managed care" and "healthcare reform" almost in the same breath. Nursing practice has to be responsive to the changes and meet the challenge to critically examine our traditional ways of meeting the needs of the childbearing woman. Nursing research has been an invaluable tool in assisting us to analyze current nursing practice and to validate more efficient and proficient ways of care giving.

The challenges will be ongoing as they have always been in performing assessments of both the mother and baby. Time with patients has been reduced significantly, and nurses have to be prepared to observe keenly the mother's emotional and physical health, implementing strategies to enable women to progress safely through pregnancy, labor, birth, and the postpartum period.

Much time and literature have been devoted to ensuring that perinatal nurses are prepared to meet the needs of the high-risk obstetrical patient. The body of knowledge combining technological advances with the art and science of nursing has facilitated nurses in establishing high standards of care when caring for mothers and infants at risk. With the changes taking place in the healthcare arena, there is a tremendous need for our specialty to move forward and be creative in developing new means of needs assessments, strategies to meet those needs within shortened time frames, and mechanisms to evaluate effectiveness and quality.

In Perinatal Nursing, editors Kathleen Simpson and Patricia Creehan have systematically presented a comprehensive resource for the perinatal nurse working in the low-risk setting. Recognizing there is much to be learned from nurses around the country, they have called upon experts from all areas of perinatal nursing to contribute knowledge and expertise.

This extensive, valuable source of information will greatly facilitate and enable nurses to glean ideas and information relevant to today's healthcare arena and to improve nursing practice in the perinatal setting.

Chee Hamilton Stanton, RN, MN, ACCE
1994 President, AWHONN

ACKNOWLEDGMENTS

The authors gratefully acknowledge Diana Intenzo, former Vice President, Nursing Division; Jennifer Brogan, Editor; Eleanor Faven, Senior Developmental Editor; and Danielle DiPalma, Editorial Assistant, at Lippincott–Raven Publishers, for their editorial assistance, advice, and enthusiasm. Thanks to Joan Podalak for her assistance in typing part of the manuscript. We would also like to thank Saundra Brenner, Jennifer Plaat, Mayris Woods, Kathy Alsup, and Tom Gann, medical librarians at St. John's Mercy Medical Center in St. Louis, Missouri, and Gail Lahti, medical librarian at Palos Community Hospital, Palos Heights Illinois who spent many hours locating resources and checking references. Their hard work and dediction to this project was invaluable. Special thanks to Jennifer Plaat.

INTRODUCTION TO PERINATAL NURSING

Much of the current literature related to perinatal nursing focuses on the childbearing woman at risk or at high risk for complications during pregnancy and birth. The body of high-risk and critical care knowledge in obstetrics is growing rapidly, as is the subspecialty in perinatal nursing. Less attention has been given to women who progress through the pregnancy, labor, birth, and postpartum period without complications, although these women comprise the majority of consumers of perinatal nursing care. Approximately 80-90% of childbearing women experience a low-risk pregnancy and birth. Many women in the United States and Canada give birth in the community hospital in an LDR/LDRP setting. One possible reason for the lack of attention in the literature to normal antepartum, intrapartum, postpartum, and newborn care is the assumption among caregivers that this area of nursing is devoted to routine practices. However, as length of stay (LOS) continues to decrease and cost-to-benefit analyses of practice are carefully scrutinized by multiple parties, challenges and opportunities exist for nurses caring for women and newborns experiencing childbirth without complications.

Over the last decade significant changes in the delivery of perinatal nursing care have occurred. Factors responsible for practice changes include fundamental restructuring of third-party reimbursement for perinatal services, a continued emphasis on cost reduction, rapidly decreasing length of hospitalization, consumer demands for less aseptic, more homelike childbirth setting, increased participation by women and their families in healthcare decision making, and increased use of technology. Expected skill levels for perinatal nurse providers of care during pregnancy and childbirth have also changed. Postpartum and newborn nurses no longer provide routine or custodial care. Critical assessment skills for identifying women and infants at risk are essential competencies for today's perinatal nurse. The ability to provide accurate, concise information on self-care, newborn care, and safety issues in a limited time period is a basic practice expectation. Current LOS includes precious few hours for supportive care and parent teaching. Nursing assessments, interventions, and evaluations provided over a 3- to 4-day period in the past must now be accomplished in several hours.

Efforts to improve quality of perinatal nursing care have resulted in an emphasis on the desires of childbearing women and families. Research suggests maternal satisfaction with childbirth and hospitalization is increased in the LDR/LDRP model. These positive responses to single-room care have resulted in the redesign of nursing care delivery models, in which nurses have expanded their skills to care for women and infants during all phases of the childbirth experience. Increased focus on the cost-to-benefit analysis of routine care has resulted in elimination of unnecessary procedures and long-term practices that are no longer useful. Clinical pathways have allowed perinatal nurses to streamline care and monitor outcomes systematically. Tracking clinical indicators and variances provide objective data for improving quality and for planning future care strategies.

In response to decreased LOS, perinatal nurses have expanded their practice to the home, where the majority of women who experience childbirth without complications are discharged 24 hours after birth. Changes in practice setting have been frustrating at times, as are all changes, but positive results have occurred. Benefits of perinatal homecare are a 1 to 2 hour period devoted to the women exclusively, in which questions can be answered, concerns addressed, and earlier teaching reinforced, in a convenient setting that may be more conducive to learning. Research on early discharge and perinatal homecare has shown that 24 hour LOSs are safe for appropriately screened women and infants. Maternal satisfaction and confidence in mothering abilities also appear to be positively influenced by shorter hospitalization.

The goal of this text is to provide readers with a comprehensive resource reflecting the current state of perinatal nursing practice. In the course of preparing the text, many regional differences were discovered, but practice similarities emerged. Efforts were made to reflect national practice as much as possible. Some areas of the country have been dealing with shortened LOS for many years, while others are just beginning to move in that direction. We can learn effective strategies to provide quality perinatal care from colleagues who have been working with less than 24 hour LOS successfully. Examples of medical record forms, assessment tools, quality improvement surveys, and clinical pathways/caremaps are included in an attempt to make the text as practical as possible. These are provided as suggestions and blueprints for individual perinatal centers desiring to develop similar tools.

Perinatal nurses are meeting the challenges as changes in perinatal healthcare delivery continue to evolve. This is an exciting time. We must be proactive in our involvement and provide meaningful input into the future course of care for healthy childbearing women and infants. We hope this text provides valuable suggestions for moving forward toward that goal.

Kathleen Rice Simpson
Patricia A. Creehan

CONTENTS

Appendix B:
Perinatal Unit Core Competencies
St. John's Mercy Medical Center, St. Louis, MO

Appendix C:
Daily Postpartum Assessments and Interventions
Initial Newborn Assessment
Palos Community Hospital, Palos Heights, IL

Appendix D:
Algorithm/Practice Parameter:
Management of Hyperbilirubinemia in the Healthy Term Infant
American Academy of Pediatrics Committee for Quality Improvement and Subcommittee on Hyperbilirubinemia. (1994). *Pediatrics*, 94(4), 563-565.
Reproduced with Permission

Appendix E:
Newborn Sepsis Algorithms
Diagnosis and Management of Asymptomatic Newborns
Diagnosis and Management of Symptomatic Newborns
Jeanne Fischesser, RNC, NNP
St. John's Mercy Medical Center, St. Louis, MO

Appendix F:
Algorithm: Nonreassuring Fetal Heart Rate Pattern
Meriter Health Services, Madison, Wisconsin

Appendix G:
Algorithm: Labor Dystocia
Meriter Health Services, Madison, Wisconsin

Appendix H:
Obstetric Prenatal Care Path
Antepartum Complications Care Path
Vaginal Birth Care Path
Cesarean Birth Care Path
Normal Newborn Care Path
Care Path Exception Log
St. John's Mercy Medical Center, St. Louis, MO

Appendix I:
Vaginal Delivery Clinical Path
Cesarean Birth Clincial Path
Normal Newborn Clinical Path
University Community Hospital, Tampa, FL

Appendix J:
Prenatal Care Pathway
Vaginal Delivery Care Pathway
Cesarean Section Care Pathway
Uncomplicated Newborn Care Pathway
Postpartum Home Visit
Anderson, S., Hoffstetter, S., Pimmel, K., Soehlke, M.J., & Tompkins, R.
St. Mary's Health Center, SSM Health Care System, St. Louis, MO.

Appendix K:
Normal Spontaneous Vaginal Delivery Multidisciplinary Action Plan (MAP)
Beth Isreal Medical Center, New York, NY

Appendix L:
The Laboring Patient Clinical Pathway
Newborn Baby Clincial Pathway
Fairview Health Systems, Edna, MN

Appendix M:
Vaginal Birth Clinical Map
Postpartum Clinical Map
University of Illinois at Chicago Medical Center, Department of Nursing, Parent Child Health Division, Chicago, IL

Appendix N:
Integrated Vaginal Birth Clinical Pathway
Integrated Cesarean Birth Clinical Pathway
Integrated Normal Newborn Clinical Pathway
Integrated Preterm Labor Clinical Pathway
Johnson, M.B., Dietz, R., Fey, S., Paulson, N., Clementson, G., Gaspar, D., & Storevik, W.
Sioux Valley Hospital, Sioux Falls, SD

Appendix O:
Newborn Clinical Path
The Family Birthplace, St. Joseph's Medical Center, Wichita, KS

Appendix P:
Family Focused Childbirth Care Paths:
Prenatal Period
Scheduled Cesarean Birth
Vaginal Birth
Cesarean Birth (Unscheduled)
St. John's Mercy Medical Center, St. Louis, MO

Appendix Q:
Maternal Confidence Scale
Bradley, C.F. (1993). Psychological consequences of intervention in the birth process. Canadian Journal of Behavior Science, 15(4), 422-438

Appendix R:
Satisfaction with Nursing Care
Bradley, C.F., Carty, E.M., & Hall, W.A. (1989). An evaluation of early postpartum discharge from a tertiary maternity hospital. Final report. School of Nursing, Universtiy of British Columbia, Vancouver, British Columbia, Canada.

Appendix S:
Acutely Ill Neonatal Transport Collaborative Carepath
Neonatal Return Collaborative Carepath
Loyola University Medical Center Perinatal Network
Loyola University of Chicago, Maywood, IL

PART

1

Foundations for Practice

Quality Care Issues: Service Excellence, Cost-Effective Practice, and Outcome Monitoring

Kathleen Rice Simpson

- **Current Issues**
- **Healthcare Policy Changes**
- **Service Excellence**
  - Patient Satisfaction
  - Identifying Realistic Goals for Patient Outcomes
- **Cost-Effective Practice**
  - Routine Laboratory Tests
  - Routine Medications and Products
  - Disposable Products
  - Standardized Prepackaged Kits
  - Practice Models
  - Documentation
  - Marketing Strategies
- **Outcome Monitoring**
  - The Joint Commission on Accreditation of Healthcare Organizations' (JCAHO) Indicator-Based Monitoring System
  - Clinical Pathways and Clinical Algorithms
- **Summary**

Perinatal nurses, like other healthcare providers, have focused on defining and measuring quality. This can be a complex process because providers, consumers, and third-party payors have varying expectations and definitions of quality. Quality of care, or the clinical aspects of care delivered, is frequently measured by patient outcomes, quality improvement processes, and clinical indicators. Quality of service, or the manner in which patient care is delivered, is typically measured by patient satisfaction surveys (Crain, 1993). Both aspects of quality are equally important and play a key role in evaluating total effectiveness of perinatal care delivery systems.

Frequently, quality of service is the single factor used by patients to judge the overall quality of care received (Crain, 1993). Quality care, as documented by both clinical outcomes and costs, is used by third-party payors to select institutional providers for healthcare plan members (Graham & DePorter, 1991; Holthof & Prins, 1993). The financial stability of healthcare institutions hinges on their ability to consistently provide high-quality care in a cost-effective manner. The purpose of this chapter is to provide an overview of current issues related to quality perinatal healthcare, including suggestions for service excellence, evaluating the costs-to-benefits ratio of routine practices, and outcome monitoring.

CURRENT ISSUES

Healthcare costs in the United States exceeded $910 billion in 1993, or over $3,300 per person, which accounted for 14.3% of the gross domestic product (GDP). Estimations for healthcare costs in 1994 are

$1 trillion (Fries et al., 1993). The United States spends far more GDP dollars on health care than other industrialized nations, yet available data do not suggest our system provides better care or has better patient outcomes. Infant mortality rates are frequently used as quality indicators of national healthcare services. Despite spending billions on prenatal care, preterm birth prevention programs, and "high-tech" neonatal services, the United States consistently ranks unfavorably compared with other developed countries. These dollars are not dispersed equally across populations. Access to care continues to be a problem for many Americans. Clearly there is a need for fundamental changes in the country's healthcare delivery system. The exact nature and scope of these changes remain controversial.

Various strategies and delivery models have shown promise in improving quality of care while decreasing or at least controlling costs. Managed-care programs have had some success for third-party payor groups and employers who use these healthcare reimbursement plans for employee participants, but additional data are needed to get a more accurate picture of the actual cost savings realized. Case management/clinical paths/clinical algorithms have been initiated recently by some healthcare institutions in an effort to manage patient care in a cost-effective manner. An analysis of nursing work-flow patterns is underway by nurse experts. Highly skilled nursing professionals spend much of their time on low-skill tasks such as clerical duties, housekeeping, and transportation (Curran, 1991). Conversely, healthcare institutions may have an excess of high-salaried administrators. For example, on an average day in 1968, U.S. hospitals employed 435,100 managers to assist with the care of 1,378,000 inpatients. By 1990, the average daily number of inpatients had fallen to 853,000, but the number of administrators had risen to 1,221,600 (Woolhandler, Himmelstein, & Lewontin, 1993). Programs to redesign management structures and provide unit-based personnel to assist with low-skill jobs are in progress in many healthcare institutions. These cost-avoidance methodologies also must be studied more closely to examine their impact on quality and savings. Efforts to sort various strategies in terms of actual effectiveness are underway by economic and healthcare experts, and a redefinition of quality care, as well as the setting in which that care is provided, is evolving.

HEALTHCARE POLICY CHANGES

While there is much concern among both healthcare providers and healthcare consumers that policy changes from proposed federal legislation will lead to decreased quality and quantity of care, opportunities exist to reexamine current practice, identify unnecessary services and procedures, and develop research-based, patient-care strategies that will ultimately lead to improved patient outcomes. By the mid-1990s, healthcare reform focused on developing a system to provide access to services for all Americans and a restructuring of reimbursement and third-party payor systems. Healthcare reform's initial goal is to provide universal access and insurance coverage, rather than stimulate comprehensive reform of healthcare delivery systems.

Previous reimbursement structures did not provide incentives to practice cost effectiveness. The traditional fee-for-service insurance plans paid 100% of billed charges. Certainly, nurses were rarely involved in the evaluation of patient care in terms of cost (Wilson, 1993). The 1990s have brought increased awareness of issues related to the costs of providing care. Quality improvement plans must now consider the cost-to-quality benefits of all patient-care strategies. Nurses are ideal to identify potentially unnecessary but costly practices, services, and products because they have the expertise to analyze the implications of proposed practice changes on patient outcomes. The increased emphasis on cost of care and it's relationship to quality of care is a reality. This is an opportunity for perinatal nurses to take a leadership role by active participation in the process, with retention of high-quality patient-care delivery systems as the ultimate goal.

SERVICE EXCELLENCE

Patient Satisfaction

It is not enough to provide excellent quality perinatal nursing care if childbearing women and their families don't perceive it as such. A key element in this process is understanding patient expectations of nursing care, because patients often describe quality care in terms different from those used by healthcare providers. While technical aspects of care are critically important in successful patient outcomes, psychosocial aspects of care may be what patients remember most when asked to rate satisfaction with nursing services. Listening to concerns, providing information, spending time, caring, empathetic attitudes, respect for privacy, and not keeping the patient waiting are issues patients feel are elements of quality nursing care (Messner, 1993). Patients' expectations of quality also include a nurse-patient relationship based on mutual trust and respect (Price, 1993). Family-centered perinatal care contributes to increased personal satisfaction from the childbirth experience, greater self-confidence in caring for the newborn, and a closer relationship with the newborn. Rooming-in positively affects satisfaction related to increased support and information provided by perinatal nurses and a more individualized approach to care (McKay & Phillips, 1984). Women who perceive nurses as answering their questions, providing personalized care, maintaining their personal privacy, and providing information in preparation for discharge have increased satisfaction with perinatal nursing services (Alexander, Sandridge, & Moore, 1993).

Nursing care is an important determinant of overall patient satisfaction with hospitalization. Satisfaction with nursing care is a crucial patient outcome associated with new and return business (Greeneich, 1993). A satisfied patient typically relates a positive experience to only one or two others, whereas a dissatisfied patient will share a negative experience with at least ten others (Masters & Masters, 1993). Childbearing women and families' intention to return to the institution for future health needs, as well as new patients attracted by the positive experiences of former patients, are critical to the economic well-being of healthcare institutions (Greeneich). Women make most family healthcare decisions and, if satisfied with their childbirth experience, will continue to use that healthcare institution for future family healthcare needs (Triolo, 1987). Therefore, it is vital for healthcare institutions to develop systems to determine patients' perceptions of quality nursing care and continually monitor patient satisfaction with these expectations.

One way for perinatal centers to gain insight into patients' expectations and perceptions of quality nursing care is to hold focus groups for women who have used the institution during childbirth. Valuable information solicited from previous patients can be useful in improving content validity of tools developed to measure patient satisfaction. Few questionnaires designed to measure patient satisfaction with sufficient validity and reliability have been reported in the literature, although work toward this process is evolving (Abramowitz, Cote, & Berry, 1987; Alexander et al., 1993; Carey & Seibert, 1993; Greeneich, 1993; Price, 1993). Instrument design in this area remains a challenge for institutions and nurse researchers because satisfaction with nursing care is a multidimensional concept. It is known that central to this concept is the incorporation of nurses' relationships with patients into the satisfaction model (Greeneich).

The Joint Commission on Accreditation of Healthcare Organizations (JCAHO) suggests inclusion of patient-satisfaction measures as part of a comprehensive quality assessment program (Joint Commission on Accreditation of Healthcare Organizations [JCAHO], 1995). As healthcare institutions are required to measure quality and evaluate quality-improvement strategies, patient-satisfaction instruments that are reliable and valid will become increasingly important. Perinatal centers desiring to maintain or increase their market share of births will need to be active participants in this process. The gap between care perinatal nurses provide and care desired by childbearing women can be minimized through the use of well-designed patient-satisfaction surveys (Alexander et al., 1993). It is not enough to collect patient-satisfaction data; there must be a method of reporting this information to both providers and consumers. Results can be used to heighten nurses' awareness of patient-satisfaction issues and modify practice to reflect the patient's expectations of quality nursing care. (See Appendix A for sample patient satisfaction tool.) Women planning births in Missouri have access to the *Buyer's Guide: Obstetrical Services* (Missouri Department of Health, 1994) that lists selected quality clinical indicators and levels of patient satisfaction for all perinatal centers in the state.

Identifying Realistic Goals for Patient Outcomes

An analysis of current patient-care-delivery methods must include institutional definitions of quality care and the desired patient outcomes. As length of stay (LOS) has decreased for perinatal services, it has become increasingly difficult for most perinatal centers to provide the scope of care traditionally offered to women during the childbirth process. No longer do we have the luxury of a 3- to 4-day stay to teach parents all they need to know about newborn care, breast or bottle feeding, and normal involution processes. Time for reassurance and supportive nursing care is minimized as women are discharged 8 to 24 hours after childbirth. New definitions of quality outcomes based on current LOSs must be developed by individual institutions. Clinical pathways and clinical algorithms are useful in defining quality parameters if clear expectations are listed with specific outcomes criteria. Variances can be tracked, and strategies to improve outcomes continually redesigned (Cohen, 1991).

Institutional definitions and evaluations of quality outcomes must incorporate both professional standards of care and JCAHO clinical indicators. (For a list of professional organizations that have developed standards related to perinatal nursing practice see Display 1.1.) The ultimate success of new strategies, for care that is both high quality and cost effective, is related to the ability to gain support from key persons in administrative, nursing, medical, and allied health disciplines within the institution. A multidisciplinary approach and follow-through is essential (Goode & Blegen, 1993). After quality outcomes goals are clearly defined and agreed upon by all members of the healthcare team, the processes to achieve those goals can be developed.

Decreasing LOSs have had an impact on redefining realistic patient-care outcomes. For example, how much information can be provided to and absorbed by new parents in a few hours during the postpartum period? Classic research by Rubin (1961) has suggested that women may not be able to assimilate parenting information in the immediate postpartum period. Yet, in the inpatient setting, perinatal nurses have few hours try to present this important content. Innovative programs to identify women early in pregnancy and encourage participation in parenting classes during the prenatal period have been developed to meet those needs. Surveys to elicit parent preferences for specific teaching needs during hospitalization have been used with success in some perinatal units (see Chapter 17, Discharge Planning). Core content can be defined by perinatal nurses to provide for all women after birth (i.e., safety issues and self-care needs). Women then select other parenting information as needed, resulting in individualized care and avoidance of repetitive or previously mastered material. Differences in parity, experience, and support systems available affect individual learning needs. Booklets and videotapes may be given to parents to use at home. Parent "warmlines" are useful to answer questions after discharge. Each perinatal center must develop strategies to meet the needs of the specific population served. Evaluation of the success of these strategies can be measured through patient-satisfaction surveys and by tracking perinatal readmissions.

Physiologic determinants of outcomes also must be adjusted based on LOS. Bowel and bladder function, lochia characteristics, perineal healing, lactation, and involution processes are not at the same levels 6 to 12 hours after birth as 3 to 4 days postpartum. Realistic, attainable goals must be identified for each physiologic care parameter and plans to achieve those goals clearly outlined. Clinical paths are ideal tools for this process if outcome criteria are listed for each goal (Goode & Blegen, 1993; Woodyard & Sheetz, 1993).

Sample clinical pathways will be included throughout this text to highlight the potential effectiveness of this patient care delivery method and provide blueprints to begin the development process. It is important to note that clinical pathways developed internally, designed to meet the needs of individual institutions and specific patient populations, are usually more successful than purchasing or adopting another institution's existing care pathways. Purchasing clinical pathways circumvents multidisciplinary collaboration in the development process, one of the critical elements for success (Goode & Blegen, 1993).

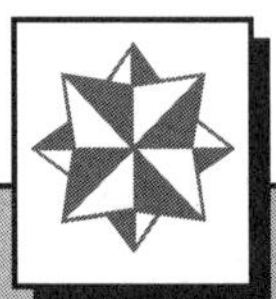

DISPLAY 1-1

Professional Organizations with National Standards Related to Perinatal Nursing Practice

AWHONN	Association of Women's Health, Obstetric, and Neonatal Nurses
ANA	American Nurses' Association
AACN	American Association of Critical Care Nurses
ACOG	American College of Obstetricians and Gynecologists
AAP	American Academy of Pediatrics
ASPAN	American Society of Postanesthesia Nurses
ASA	American Society of Anesthesiologists
AORN	Association of Operating Room Nurses
NANN	National Association of Neonatal Nurses

COST-EFFECTIVE PRACTICE

The combination of decreasing LOS and prospective payment has resulted in significant changes in delivery of perinatal services. In the early 1980s, the average LOS for a vaginal birth was 3 to 4 days with billed charges for most insured women reimbursed in full to the institutions. The current scenario is a 8 to 24 hour LOS after vaginal birth, with reimbursement under $1,000 for the care of both mother and infant, regardless of actual costs incurred. Therefore, perinatal centers must critically examine every aspect of care delivered and identify those practices and services that do not have a direct impact on an individual center's definition of quality care. The goal must be to improve or at least maintain quality, while decreasing costs.

Successful implementation of practice changes cannot occur in isolation. Collaboration with all members of the healthcare team is essential. Kiehl (1991) suggested the use of a multidisciplinary cost-management task force with clearly stated objectives: perinatal standards review, quality care continuance, cost reduction, medical staff input, and bedside care-providers' involvement. Information should be provided about the financial implications of changing LOS and reimbursement structures. Especially helpful is data related to differences in billed charges, actual costs, and reimbursement for routinely used products and services.

It is not common knowledge among nurses that billed charges have limited implication for reimbursement. Nurses who have been careful to ensure that patients were charged appropriately for all services and products used are surprised to learn the amount on the bill bears little resemblance to the amount actually paid. With reimbursement based on diagnosis-related groups (DRGs), groups of DRGs, or capitation, actual costs are the most important financial information to consider. Capitation, prospective payment to institutions based on number of covered lives and estimations of healthcare services used by members enrolled in the management care plan, is becoming more common in the United States. With a capitation contract, after agreement of a fixed reimbursement rate, the institution provides care for all plan members during a predetermined time period. Contracts are usually renegotiated on an annual basis. This type of reimbursement places more financial risk on the institution, especially if the number and acuity of patients requiring care are underestimated, or costs of care provided are not within budgeted projections. With capitated reimbursement, patient care is not viewed as an opportunity to generate income, but rather in terms of actual cost of care needed and delivered. Some institutions have changed the designation of department budgets from revenue centers to cost centers to highlight the necessary change in financial thinking in order to survive in a capitated healthcare system. Information provided by nurse managers can be the key to success for staff participation in changing long-standing practices. Staff nurses enjoy involvement in this process and can provide valuable input in the cost-to-quality benefit analysis of proposed practice changes (Graham & DePorter, 1991; Simpson, 1993; Takes, 1992).

Many practices and services currently provided are based on previous LOS. In identifying those potential practices and services to discontinue or use for a limited number of patients, it is helpful to analyze which are based on "reason" and which are based on long-standing "rituals" (Kiehl, 1991). Routine practices should be especially scrutinized. A systematic evaluation of all current services and products should begin with a review of routine or standing intrapartum, postpartum, and newborn nursery orders.

Routine Laboratory Tests

Most routine orders include admission laboratory tests such as complete blood counts (CBC), blood typing and screening, VDRL or RPR, urinalysis, etc. While these tests are necessary for thorough assessments in certain at-risk patient populations, they may not be necessary for low-risk women with prenatal care documentation. Two recent studies suggest intrapartum admission hemoglobin and hematocrit test results vary little from prenatal hemoglobin and hematocrit levels (Kiehl, 1991; Simpson, 1993). If blood tests are done during prenatal office visits, the results should be available to healthcare providers in the inpatient setting. It may be possible to eliminate routine admission tests if there is a system to ensure access to prenatal laboratory test data. Many perinatal units also routinely draw blood in anticipation of a possible cesarean birth for all women attempting a vaginal birth after a prior cesarean birth (VBAC). However, there is no evidence to suggest women who are appropriate candidates to attempt VBAC have a higher incidence of cesarean births than other laboring women. If institutional laboratory response time is sufficient, anticipatory blood tests can be eliminated and blood drawn only from those women who actually have a cesarean birth.

Routine postpartum CBC or hemoglobin and hematocrit orders are common practice in many perinatal units; however, decreased LOS has affected accuracy and clinical implications. True hemodynamic status is not reflected by hemoglobin and hematocrit results obtained before 24 to 48 hours after major blood loss. Variation in hematocrit and hemoglobin values from prenatal and postpartum laboratory data test is minimal for women with normal blood loss during the birth process (Simpson, 1993). When LOS was 3 or 4 days, postpartum hemoglobin and hematocrit provided more accurate information and results were used to make clinical decisions. In current practice, postpartum women are instructed to continue prenatal vitamins with iron, and women with very low hemoglobin and hematocrit levels are considered candidates for transfusion only if symptomatic. Even those who are symptomatic are rarely transfused. Frequently, because of LOS, tests results are not available on the medical record for physician review prior to discharge. This combination of factors suggests routine postpartum CBC or hemoglobin and hematocrit results rarely influence patient care management decisions.

Many newborn nurseries routinely measure blood glucose levels by Dextrostix or Chemstrips and hematocrit values via heel stick. The routine testing of all newborns for a particular disorder, before clinical manifestations are evident, should result in a positive benefit-cost ratio according to the Committee on Fetus and Newborn of the American Academy of Pediatrics (American Academy of Pediatrics [AAP], 1993).

> *There should be a high enough incidence of the disorder to justify screening for it unless the disorder, if left undetected and untreated, would result in such significant morbidity that even with a relatively low incidence the benefit-cost ratio of screening would be positive, i.e., phenylketonuria screening.* (AAP, 1993, pp. 474.)

The screening methodology should have high sensitivity and specificity to avoid reporting subjects as false-negative or false-positive. The methodology should be simple, cost effective, accurate, and reproducible. The disorder (i.e., hypoglycemia, anemia, or polycythemia) should be one in which early detection and early treatment will improve the outcome. Based on this criteria, universal screening of blood glucose for hypoglycemia and hematocrit for anemia and polycythemia is not warranted in most nurseries (AAP, 1993). Universal screening for selected infants at risk may be indicated. For further clarification, refer to the *Policy Statement on Routine Evaluation of Blood Pressure, Hematocrit, and Glucose in Newborns* (AAP, 1993). Individual units should adopt guidelines for selective screening for abnormal levels of glucose and hematocrit for newborns.

A final but significant variable in considering discontinuation of routine blood work is the impact of the needle-stick itself. Having blood drawn is not without patient discomfort. Elimination of opportunities for blood exposure for those performing these tests is an added incentive (Simpson, 1993). The cost of one needle-stick from a contaminated needle is conservatively estimated at between $600 and $1,200 (Armstrong, 1991; Dugger, 1992). If the contaminated needle involves a woman who is HIV positive, the costs would be much higher.

Significant savings can be realized by reevaluating the need for routine blood tests and using these assessment tools for selected patient populations. Institutions with many low-risk women and those with systems to ensure access to prenatal laboratory data by inpatient providers have the potential for greatest cost savings in this area. Before considering elimination of this practice, it may be helpful to randomly select a number of medical records and compare variations in hematocrit and hemoglobin results from the prenatal period, intrapartum admission, and postpartum stay for women with documentation of normal blood loss at delivery. This data will be invaluable in gaining multidisciplinary support for proposed changes in practice.

Routine Medications and Products

Standardization of routine medications results in cost savings by decreasing nursing time spent counting multiple narcotics and substituting generic brands for name brands. Medical record audits can identify commonly ordered medications for pain relief. Institutions still using breast cream, may consider discontinuing this practice after review of current literature. Epifoam, benzocaine sprays, and premoistened witch hazel pads (Tucks) may not be necessary for all episiotomies; only patients with hemorrhoids are candidates for related preparations. Eliminating prompts from postpartum order records is one way to discourage routine ordering of all possible medications and products for all patients. A system to ensure crediting and returning unopened medications to the pharmacy is important. Two recent studies indicated significant savings after standardizing and reducing the number of commonly prescribed medications (Kiehl, 1991; Simpson, 1993).

Sizes and amounts of commonly used products may be based on previous LOS. Most perinatal centers can no longer afford to provide women with a week's supply of products to use after discharge. If the multidisciplinary task force decides that it is not a goal to continue this practice, consideration should be given to downsizing commonly supplied products. A 2-ounce tube of A & D ointment or petroleum jelly ($2.10) for circumcision care may have been appropriate in the past; however, single-use foil packets of a generic substitute ($0.04) are more cost effective. Instead of placing a package of 28 brand-name, disposable diapers in every bassinet and giving the extras to take home, consider buying generic diapers in packages of 60 or more and placing only those needed in the bassinet. Pacifiers ($1.00) are not recommended in the first few days of life, especially for breastfeeding infants; therefore, nurseries need not provide pacifiers for every infant. A generic baby bath soap ($0.38) can be used instead of the more common brand-name soap ($2.30). A warm washcloth ($0.02) can be substituted for a disposable heel warmer ($0.75 to $1.75) in preparing newborns for heel sticks. Admission maternity kits many times have many more peripads than would normally be used during current LOS. Consider reevaluating the contents so kit supplies reflect expected usage during actual hospitalization. Disposable ice peripads ($1.12) are much more expensive than chipped-ice-filled zip-lock plastic bags ($0.02) for episiotomy discomfort. Patients report that the real ice is colder than the chemical "ice" and, therefore, provides better perineal pain relief (Simpson, 1993). Breast pads may be reserved for mothers whose milk comes in while hospitalized, instead of providing a box of breast pads ($2.50) to every breastfeeding mother. Simple, routine practices frequently offer the greatest potential for savings but are often the practices easiest to overlook, when attempting to identify cost-saving opportunities.

Disposable Products

The use of disposable products has increased dramatically. The impact of these disposable products has been an increase in both product costs and disposal costs. Expenditures for biohazardous waste disposal are significant due to blood and body-fluid contamination of products used in perinatal services, especially during labor and delivery. Reducing the size and number of disposable sterile drapes used for vaginal births is possible, based on physician or nurse-midwife practices. Standard vaginal supply packs may contain sterile drapes rarely used by most practitioners in the more homelike LDR/LDRP setting. Significant cost savings can be realized by reevaluating the contents of vaginal supply packs (Kiehl, 1991; Simpson, 1993). Disposable vacuum-extractor suction kits ($21.50) are much more expensive than reusable vacuum extractor suction equipment ($290) that can be used for hundreds of births, when sterilized appropriately.

Reusable impervious gowns for both physicians and circulating nurses are also more cost effective. Reusable gowns ($11.00) can be washed 100 times, according to most manufacturers, before affecting permeability, while disposable gowns ($2.00 to $10.00) are designed for single use. If disposable scrub suits are used for support persons attending vaginal births, consider using cloth scrubs or eliminating the use of scrubs entirely for this group. Scrub use by support persons attending vaginal births is no longer current practice in most perinatal centers. Cloth scrubs can be worn by support persons attending cesarean births. Hospital-provided and hospital-laundered scrubs for healthcare providers are very expensive. Consider converting to nurse-purchased and nurse-laundered scrubs. A sterile reusable impervious gown can be worn by nurses attending cesarean births. Multiple studies have suggested that hospital-provided scrubs do not have an impact on nosocomial infection rates. To gain support for this practice change, provide key decision makers with a thorough review of current, related literature and names of other perinatal centers that no longer provide staff scrubs and report no increase in infection rates.

Most disposable products have added convenience, and decreased risk of nosocomial infection. One way to reduce the financial and environmental implication of usage is to consider recycling clean plastics and paper. If this is not feasible, careful segregation of wastes so only items that meet the biohazardous criteria are labeled as such can decrease biohazardous waste disposal costs.

Standardized Prepackaged Kits

Use of kits, such as those for intravenous (IV) starts, catheterization, and admission can be a timesaving device for nurses; however, review of practice discovered many times kits are opened for one item. (Simpson, 1993). For example, a catheterization kit ($2.15) may be opened to empty the bladder at birth when a single catheter ($0.35) will suffice. Additional IV start kits ($0.95) sometimes are used to get more tape ($0.02). An admission kit ($12.80) may be opened to get additional peripads ($1.85) or a sanitary belt ($0.26). Stocking single items in each room, and increasing staff awareness of the cost implications of opening kits unnecessarily, can change practice (Simpson). Vendors charge more for customizing kits for individual institutions. Savings can be realized by having hospital volunteers pack selected types of kits such as those used for admission.

Practice Models

Perinatal units still using traditional care models with separate labor, delivery, recovery, postpartum, and newborn nursery units may need to reevaluate practice settings and work-flow designs, based on current LOS. Time and costs spent transporting patients, providing comprehensive reports to multiple caregivers, and supplying housekeeping services can be decreased by delivery systems allowing labor, birth, recovery, and postpartum periods to occur in the same room with care provided by the same nurse. Eliminating costs associated with traditional models can also result in increased quality due to improved continuity of care and avoidance of patient inconvenience. Family-centered perinatal care positively affects patient satisfaction with nursing care (Alexander et al., 1993). Fluctuations in census and acuity frequently cause difficulty in predicting staffing needs; however, perinatal units can no longer afford to staff for "what if." Crosstraining and on-call or paid-on-standby systems are cost effective and can increase flexibility in meeting dynamic staffing requirements for quality care delivery. These practice models have the potential to avoid costly overstaffing while allowing units to effectively handle unexpected variances in census and acuity. Tracking time and costs related to transfer and reports can provide valuable data to support care-delivery-model changes.

Documentation

Rising acuity in the inpatient clinical setting, increased nurse-patient ratios, rigorous reimbursement criteria, and legal scrutiny have placed more emphasis on the importance of thorough, comprehensive, user-friendly, nursing documentation tools. As labor costs continue to rise, the issue of quantity of nursing time spent on "paperwork" versus direct care takes on a new meaning. In order to reduce human resource consumption, healthcare institutions must evaluate new methods of charting, such as bedside computer terminals and multidisciplinary documentation tools. Avoiding duplication of documentation is essential. For example, examine frequency of noting basic information in medical records used for one perinatal unit admission. Age, obstetrical history, birth plan, attendance at prenatal classes, infant feeding choice, etc., can be charted on the admission record only, rather than being copied on all subsequent medical records. Eliminating areas of duplicate documentation not only saves time but can improve patient satisfaction. If the labor nurse, postpartum nurse, and nursery nurse all ask the woman her age, how many times she has been pregnant, if she is planning to formula feed or breast feed, etc., the woman may wonder if there is lack of communication among care providers. Well-designed flowsheets, computer programs, and charting by exception are cost-effective methods of documentation presently in use in many perinatal centers. Clinical pathways that serve as documentation tools are especially useful. Examples of medical records are included in Appendix C and examples of clinical pathways are included in Appendices H through O.

Marketing Strategies

In some highly competitive markets, perinatal centers have provided expensive incentives to attract or maintain their share of births. However, as more women enroll in managed-care plans, choice of childbirth institution will be limited. Providing steak dinners for new parents, beepers for support persons, gift baskets on discharge, etc., are very costly and may no longer be financially feasible or directly affect institution selection. As participation in managed-care plans increases and institutional networks develop in each market area, perinatal centers should consider eliminating frills that do not have a direct impact on quality outcomes.

OUTCOME MONITORING

Outcome monitoring is not new to the nursing profession. One of the earliest proponents of outcome evaluation was Florence Nightingale, who used morbidity and mortality statistics to demonstrate effects of substandard care during the Crimean War (Marek,

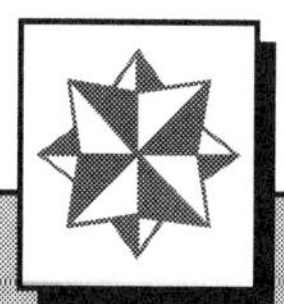

DISPLAY 1-2

IMSystem Performance Measures

- **Focus:** Preoperative patient evaluation, intraoperative and postoperative monitoring, and timely clinical intervention.

  Numerator: Patients developing a central nervous system (CNS) complication within 2 postprocedure days of procedures involving anesthesia* administration.

- **Focus:** Preoperative patient evaluation, appropriate surgical preparation, intraoperative and postoperative monitoring, and timely clinical intervention.

  Numerator: Patients developing a peripheral neurological deficit within 2 postprocedure days of procedures involving anesthesia* administration.

- **Focus:** Preoperative patient evaluation, intraoperative and postoperative monitoring, and timely clinical intervention.

  Numerator: Patients developing an acute myocardial infarction within 2 postprocedure days of procedures involving anesthesia* administration.

- **Focus:** Preoperative patient evaluation, intraoperative and postoperative monitoring, and timely clinical intervention.

  Numerator: Patients with a cardiac arrest within 2 postprocedure days of procedures involving anesthesia* administration.

- **Focus:** Preoperative patient evaluation, intraoperative and postoperative monitoring, and timely clinical intervention.

  Numerator: Intrahospital mortality to patients within 2 postprocedure days of procedures involving anesthesia* administration.

- **Focus:** Prenatal patient evaluation, education, and treatment selection.

  Numerator: Patients delivered by cesarean section.

  Denominator: All deliveries.

- **Focus:** Prenatal patient evaluation, education, and treatment selection.

  Numerator: Patients with vaginal birth after cesarean section (VBAC).

  Denominator: Patients delivered with a history of previous cesarean section.

- **Focus:** Prenatal patient evaluation, intrapartum monitoring, and clinical intervention.

  Numerator: Live-born infants with a birthweight less than 2,500 grams.

  Denominator: All live births.

- **Focus:** Prenatal patient evaluation, intrapartum monitoring, and clinical intervention.

  Numerator: Live-born infants with a birthweight greater than or equal to 2,500 grams, who have at least one of the following: an Apgar score of less than four at 5 minutes, a requirement for admission to the neonatal intensive care unit within 1 day of delivery for greater than 24 hours, a clinically apparent seizure, or significant birth trauma.

  Denominator: All live-born infants with a birthweight greater than 2,500 grams.

DISPLAY 1-2 (cont.)

- **Focus:** Prenatal patient evaluation, intrapartum monitoring, neonatal patient evaluation, and clinical intervention.
  Numerator: Live-born infants with a birthweight greater than 1,000 grams and less than 2,500 grams who have an Apgar score of less than four at 5 minutes.
  Denominator: All live-born infants with a birthweight greater than 1,000 grams and less than 2,500 grams.
- **Focus:** Surveillance and prevention of surgical site infection.
  Numerator: Selected inpatient and outpatient surgical procedures complicated by a surgical site infection.
  Denominator: Number of selected inpatient and outpatient surgical procedures.
- **Focus:** Surveillance and prevention of ventilator-associated pneumonia.
  Numerator: Ventilated inpatients who develop pneumonia
  Denominator: Inpatient ventilator days.
- **Focus:** Surveillance and prevention of primary bloodstream infection.
  Numerator: Inpatients with a central or umbilical line who develop primary blood stream infection.
  Denominator: Inpatient central or umbilical line days.

* For the indicators related to perioperative care, the population of interest includes all patients undergoing procedures involving anesthesia and an inpatient stay.

[1] An Indicator Statement (as contrasted with a numerator) is used when the measure is a continuous variable.

From Joint Commission on Accreditation of Healthcare Organizations. (1996). 1996 Accreditation manual for hospitals. Standards, 1. Oakbrook Terrace, IL: Author. Reprinted with permission.

1989). While methods of data collection and analysis in the 1990s are much more sophisticated, the goals remain the same: measurement and evaluation of patient outcomes related to the nursing care provided.

The Joint Commission on Accrediation of Healthcare Organizations' (JCAHO) Indicator Measurement Monitoring System

The JCAHO developed an indicator measurement system (IMSystem) (Display 1-2) that healthcare institutions had the option to use on a voluntary basis beginning in 1994. The IMSystem will be a mandatory part of the accreditation process sometime after 1996. A clinical indicator is a quantitative measure of an aspect of patient care that can be used as a guide to monitor and evaluate the quality and appropriateness of healthcare delivery. Healthcare institutions can use indicators to continuously monitor, evaluate, and improve care. Implementation of clinical indicators as monitoring tools enhances accreditation evaluation because they are based on measures and measurement processes that are consistent and uniformly applied across all organizations (JCAHO, 1996). The IMSystem will allow healthcare institutions to compare performance data with others and provide a national performance database as a resource for health services research. Because it can take months to institute a successful data collection system, the JCAHO recommends beginning this process as soon as possible even though it is optional. Early participation in the indicator monitoring system can assist healthcare institutions to implement an effective system before it is required and used in the survey and accreditation process (JCAHO, 1995). In 1994 some healthcare institutions initiated data collection and submission to the IMSystem, and thus received comparative performance feedback from the JCAHO. An important benefit from participation in the process is the ability to provide comparative performance data to potential and current patients, providers, third-party payors, and others who want to make informed healthcare decisions (JCAHO, 1995).

Clinical Pathways and Clinical Algorithms

In addition to outlining important patient care activities with specific time frames, care paths can be used to track, measure, and evaluate patient outcomes. When designed based on professional standards of care and practice guidelines, this care delivery system has the potential to improve quality by reducing variances in clinical processes. Variance tracking can provide an important database for continuous quality improvement. Necessary changes in practice can be identified and modifications made. A primary focus of clinical pathways is on reducing diagnostic tests and therapeutic measures that are not of value, while improving those that do add value (Goode & Blegen, 1993). In addition to improving quality perinatal care delivery, clinical pathways (see Appendices H to O) have been shown to reduce costs (Weilitz & Potter, 1993). For a more in-depth discussion, see Chapter 4.

When variances in patient care continually occur with use of a particular clinical pathway, use of a clinical algorithm can be helpful in guiding healthcare providers through the "if, then" decision-making process (Schriefer, 1994). For example, clinical algorithms developed, based on published standards and practice guidelines, can be used to plan a sequence of care in the case of a nonreassuring fetal heart rate (FHR) pattern during labor or to ensure an adequate trial of labor when dystocia is suspected, thus avoiding an unnecessary cesarean birth. Algorithms are also used to ensure patients meet criteria for induction of labor or repeat cesarean birth. Appendices D, E, F, and G are sample clinical algorithms. Use of algorithms in selected patients can be effective in improving outcomes by providing individualized care within the clinical pathway model. Clinical pathways work best for the relatively routine, high-volume procedures such as uncomplicated vaginal or cesarean births and full-term newborn care, for which the plan of care is similar (Schriefer). Clinical algorithms are more useful for patients who require complex decision-making processes and when practice among providers varies, such as with preterm-labor management, pregnancy-induced hypertension, preeclampsia, nonreassuring FHR patterns, inadequate labor progress, or newborn hyperbilirubinemia (Schriefer). If data indicate frequent variance from expected progression on a clinical pathway, development of an algorithm specific to the variance can make the pathway more useful in guiding quality-care decisions.

SUMMARY

Balancing the cost/quality equation continues to be one of the biggest challenges for healthcare institutions as the healthcare reform process unfolds. In order for institutions providing perinatal services to survive, financially sound, proactive measures that continually monitor quality care and patient outcomes are critical. Determining patient expectations of care and improving satisfaction with nursing care delivery are also essential. While suggestions presented here for improving care and reducing costs may not be applicable for all perinatal units, this chapter can serve as a basis for discussion and the development of strategies specific to individual institutions. Perinatal nurses have an opportunity to take a leadership role in ensuring that financial solutions to clinical situations have a quality-care focus. Participation in financial aspects of quality patient-care delivery and development of quality-care strategies must be components of perinatal nursing practice.

References

Abramowitz, S., Cote, A.A., & Berry, E. (1987). Analyzing patient satisfaction: A multianalytic approach. Quality Review Bulletin, 13(4), 122-130.

Alexander, L., Sandridge, J., & Moore, L. (1993). Patient satisfaction: An outcome measure for maternity services. Journal of Perinatal and Neonatal Nursing, 7(2), 28-39.

American Academy of Pediatrics: Committee on Fetus and Newborn. (1993). Routine evaluation of blood pressure, hematocrit, and glucose in newborns. Pediatrics, 92 (3), 474-476.

Armstrong, S.E. (1991). The cost of needle-stick injuries: The impact of safer medical devices. Nursing Economics, 9(2), 426-430, 433.

Carey, R.G., & Seibert, J.H. (1993). A patient survey system to measure quality improvement: Questionnaire reliability and validity. Medical Care, 31(9), 834-845.

Cohen, E.L. (1991). Nursing case management: Does it pay? Journal of Nursing Administration, 21(4), 20-25.

Crain, C.A. (1993). Service excellence. Nursing matters, St. Louis, MO: St. John's Mercy Medical Center.

Curran, C.R. (1991). Changing the way we do business. Nursing Economics, 9(5), 296-316.

Dugger, B. (1992). Introducing products to prevent needlesticks. Nursing Management, 23(10), 62-66.

Fries, J.F., Koop, C.E., Beadle, C.E., Cooper, P.P., England, M.J., Greaves, R.F., Sokolov, J.J., & Wright, D. (1993). Reducing health care costs by reducing the need and demand for medical services: The health project consortium. New England Journal of Medicine, 329(5), 321-325.

Goode, C.J., & Blegen, M.A. (1993). Developing a caremap for patients with a cesarean birth: A multidisciplinary process. Journal of Perinatal and Neonatal Nursing, 7(2), 46-52.

Graham, R.G., & DePorter, J.G. (1991). Managing nursing quality. Topics in Health Care Financing, 18(2), 46-49.

Greeneich, D. (1993). The link between new and return business and quality of care: Patient satisfaction. Advances in Nursing Science, 16(1), 62-72.

Holthof, B., & Prins, P. (1993). Comparing hospital perinatal mortality rates: A quality improvement instrument. Medical Care, 31(9), 801-807.

Joint Commission on Accreditation of Healthcare Organizations. (1995). Accreditation manual for hospitals. Standards, 1. Oakbrook Terrace, IL: Author.

Joint Commission on Accreditation of Healthcare Organizations. (1996). Accreditation manual for hospitals. Standards, 1. Oakbrook Terrace, IL: Author.

Kiehl, E.M. (1991). A strategy for budgeting obstetrical costs. Nursing Management, 22(10), 50-52, 54.

Marek, K. (1989). Outcome measurement in nursing. Journal of Nursing Quality Assurance 4(1), 1-9.

Masters, M.L., & Masters, R.J. (1993). Building TQM into nursing management. Nursing Economics, 11(5), 274-278.

McKay, S., & Phillips, C. (1984). Family centered maternity care: Implementation strategies. Rockville, MD: Aspen Publishing.

Messner, R.L. (1993). What patients really want from their nurses. American Journal of Nursing, 93(8), 38-41.

Missouri Department of Health. (1994). Buyer's guide: Obstetrical services. Jefferson City, MO: Author.

Price, P.J. (1993). Parents' perceptions of the meaning of quality nursing care. Advances in Nursing Science, 16(1), 33-41.

Rubin, R. (1961) Puerperal change. Nursing Outlook 9, 753-755.

Schriefer, J. (1994). The synergy of pathways and algorithms: Two tools work better than one. Journal on Quality Improvement, 20(9), 485-499.

Simpson, K.R. (1993). Meeting the challenge of the 1990s: Strategies to provide quality perinatal services in an era of decreasing reimbursement. Journal of Perinatal and Neonatal Nursing, 7(2), 1-9.

Takes, K.L. (1992). Cost-effective practice: Do OR nurses care? Nursing Management, 23(4), OR Ambulatory Surgery Ed), 96Q-R, 96 V-X.

Triolo, P.K. (1987). Marketing women's health care. Journal of Nursing Administration, 17(11), 9-15.

Weilitz, P.B., & Potter, P.A. (1993). A managed care system: Financial and clinical evaluation. Journal of Nursing Administration, 23(11), 51-57.

Wilson, A.A. (1993). The cost and quality of patient outcomes: A look at managed competition. Nursing Administration Quarterly, 17(4), 11-16.

Woodyard, L.W., & Sheetz, J.E. (1993). Critical pathway patient outcomes: The missing standard. Journal of Nursing Care Quality, 8(1), 51-57.

Woolhandler, S., Himmelstein, D.V., & Lewontin, J.P. (1993). Administrative costs in U.S. hospitals. New England Journal of Medicine, 329(6), 400-403.

Professional and Legal Issues

Kathleen Rice Simpson
Bonnie Flood Chez

When Florence Nightingale founded the nursing profession in the 1850s, she was motivated by courage, compassion, and the desire to make a difference. These goals and ambitions remain the foundation for contemporary professional nursing practice. She and her fellow nursing pioneers went to the Crimean War zone armed with practice guidelines and protocols with the belief that researched-based interventions provided with a systematic approach to specific clinical situations could improve patient outcomes, increase trauma survival rates, and address the psychosocial needs of injured soldiers. That success solidified her role in founding the profession of nursing as it is known today (Donahue, 1985). After the war, she returned to England to continue the tasks of educating nurses and developing practice guidelines and quality improvement measures. These activities helped to identify nursing practice as a separate but collaborative healthcare profession.

Over the years, various regulatory agencies, federal and state legislatures, accrediting bodies, and professional organizations have developed practice guidelines and standards for licensure, credentialing, and certification for nurses. The intention is to provide for the public welfare, assuring patients and their family members that nursing care will be given by competent nursing professionals. As the body of medical and nursing knowledge has expanded, the subspecialty of perinatal nursing has emerged, benefitting from an increased research database and improved technologies. This chapter provides an overview of professional and legal issues related to perinatal nursing practice in the 1990s.

PROFESSIONAL ISSUES

Definitions of Perinatal Nursing Practice

The American Nurses' Association (ANA) defines maternal health nursing as a "specialized area of nursing focused on the health needs of women, their partners, and their families throughout their reproductive and childbearing years" (American Nurses' Association [ANA], 1983). The *Standards for the Nursing Care of Women and Newborns* from the Nurses' Association of the American College of Obstetricians and Gynecologists (NAACOG), now known as the Association of Women's Health, Obstetric, and Neonatal Nurses (AWHONN), states that "the nature of obstetric, gynecologic, and neonatal nursing practice addresses healthcare needs of women and infants in a holistic approach designed to meet physical, psychological, and spiritual needs of individuals and families." (Nurses' Association of the American College of Obstetricians and Gynecologists [NAACOG], 1991, pp. 3). Perinatal nursing is unique among nursing specialties because nurses caring for pregnant women always have a minimum nurse-patient ratio of 1:2. The woman and her fetus are considered together; any therapy will affect two individuals, each with potentially different outcomes (Poole, 1992).

Licensure

Nursing licensure in the United States is governed by nurse practice acts enacted by state legislatures. The legal basis for licensure is government's power to protect the public's health, safety, and welfare. Licensure sets the standards for entry into practice, defines a scope of practice, and allows for disciplinary action (Northrop & Kelly, 1987). State boards of nursing develop nurse practice acts, defining the practice of nursing for individual states. Nurses should be aware of the specific wording of the nurse practice act of their respective states. Educational criteria identifies individuals qualified to write national licensure examinations. Standardization of licensure examinations has improved the quality of this process and facilitated licensure reciprocity between states. The development of the National Council of State Boards Licensing Exam (NCLEX) with standard minimum passing scores ensures that nurses practicing in all areas of the country have met the same stringent educational criteria before entering into clinical practice.

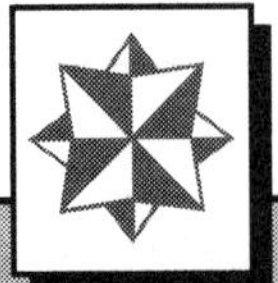

DISPLAY 2-1

Examples of Certification Options for Perinatal Nurses

- American Nurses' Credentialing Center (ANCC)
  - *Perinatal Nurse*
- American Society for Psychoprophylaxis in Obstetrics, Inc. (ASPO)
  - *ASPO Certified Childbirth Educator*
- Council of Childbirth Educators
  - *Certified Childbirth Educator*
- International Childbirth Education Association
  - *Internationally Certified Childbirth Educator*
- National Certification Corporation for the Obstetric, Gynecologic, and Neonatal Nursing Specialties
  - *Ambulatory Women's Health Care Nurse*
  - *Women's Health Care Nurse Practitioner*
  - *Reproductive Endocrinology/Infertility Nurse*
  - *Maternal Newborn Nurse*
  - *Inpatient Obstetric Nurse*
  - *High-Risk Obstetric Nurse*
  - *Low-Risk Neonatal Nurse*
  - *Neonatal Intensive Care Nurse*
  - *Neonatal Nurse Practitioner*
- International Board of Lactation Consultant Examiners
  - *International Board Certified Lactation Consultant*

Certification

Certification is a process by which a nongovernmental agency or association certifies that an individual licensed to practice a profession has met certain predetermined standards specified by that profession for a specialty practice (ANA, 1979). The certification process validates an individual registered nurse's qualifications and special knowledge in a defined clinical area of nursing (American Nurses Credentialing Center [ANCC], 1994). Certification indicates to the public and healthcare community that an individual has demonstrated commitment to quality nursing care and to increased knowledge and expertise (National Certification Corporation for the Obstetric, Gynecologic, and Neonatal Nursing Specialties [NCC], 1994). Although each specialty group has its own objectives for certification, the following goals generally are included: assessment of special knowledge, promotion of excellence in practice, encouragement of professional growth, standardization of qualifications necessary for specialty practice, and advancement of specialty knowledge and standards.

Perinatal nurses have many avenues available for seeking certification. Examples of nationally recognized certification programs are included in Display 2-1; the list is not all inclusive. Some healthcare institutions have developed credentialing and/or certification programs for their own employees, specific to an area of practice, such as mother-baby nursing; labor, and delivery room (LDR) nursing; labor, delivery, recovery, and postpartum (LDRP) nursing; electronic fetal monitoring (EFM); childbirth education; lactation consulting; and grief counseling. These programs may be a requirement for employment and are generally nontransferable to other institutions.

Certification has recently been available from academic institutions and private organizations for additional areas of perinatal nursing practice. For example, the University of Texas Medical Branch and Vanderbilt University offer a course and examination leading to certification in high-risk and critical-care obstetric nursing. The Doulas of North America (DONA) provides course work and examination leading to certification as a professional labor support provider (LSP).

Several companies in different areas of the country offer EFM certification. The Electronic Fetal Monitoring Certification Corporation (EFMCC) provides an examination as "a measurement of EFM knowledge." The Professional Education Center has developed a course and certification examination in advanced fetal monitoring designed to "confirm knowledge in advanced EFM concepts and document demonstrated proficiency in interpretation." Educational Resources, Inc. offers an independent study course using videotapes and examination "intended to solely test special fetal heart rate (FHR) knowledge."

The fees, prerequisites, certification examinations, and continuing education requirements for certification and recertification vary depending on the certification body. Generally, a specific number of clinical hours in the specialty practice area combined with designated years of experience are examination prerequisites, although sometimes academic preparation at the baccalaureate level is needed. Some certification companies require nurses to complete a company-sponsored course as well. Most certification processes involve a written examination. Recertification usually requires continued practice in the specialty area, continuing education hours and/or reexamination, and an additional fee.

Issues Related to Certification

The many options for certification within the perinatal nursing specialty can cause confusion for nurses desiring a credential to validate and document their level of knowledge and expertise in a specific area of practice. Controversy continues to exist concerning nonnursing bodies providing certification for nurses and offering the same certification to both nurses and other healthcare providers. Questions related to the validity and reliability of items used in these various certification examinations have not been adequately addressed. National recognition and acceptance of the certification credential may be limited if it is obtained through a company or institution that is not sponsored or endorsed by a national professional organization. Certification processes developed by an individual or small group of individuals may reflect regional practice. In addition, these individuals may lack experience in item writing and examination development and may not have the personnel or financial resources for adequate psychometric evaluation of results. Advantages of certification in a finite area of practice such as EFM are unclear because it is difficult to isolate EFM from other perinatal nursing practices. Knowledge of the physiologic basis for FHR monitoring, interpretation of FHR patterns, and appropriate nursing interventions are integral components of expected antepartum and intrapartum nursing practice and should be evaluated as such (Afriat, Simpson, Chez, & Miller, 1994).

Considerable time and expense is involved in the certification/recertification process, including the examination fees, preparation for the examination, and continuing education requirements, so the importance of these issues should not be minimized (Simpson,

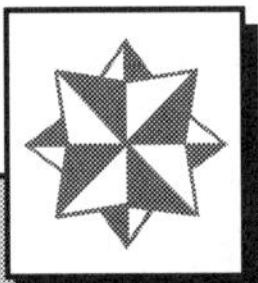

DISPLAY 2-2

Suggestions for Evaluating Certification Programs

- Who is the sponsoring organization of the certification program?
- What is the program's philosophy of certification? How is certification defined by the organization?
- What are the entry requirements?
- What are the objectives of the program?
- How much time does the certification program take?
- How long has the certification program been established?
- How many nurses have been certified by the organization since the program began?
- Is the same certification offered to healthcare providers/educators who are not nurses?
- If a course is required, what does the curriculum include? How many hours of continuing education are given? What organization approves the continuing education?
- Can the educational portion be taken for college credit?
- Who are the faculty, and what are their credentials?
- Is the content outline of the examination available to the candidates?
- Are recognized review courses offered?
- Who provides the review courses?
- What materials are needed to prepare for examination?
- Is there a method for determining validity and reliability of test items?
- What is the mechanism for psychometric evaluation of examination results?
- Who is responsible for item development and what are their credentials?
- What is the reputation of the certification program among the healthcare/nursing community?
- Is the certification credential recognized nationally? Internationally?

Adapted from Nichols F.H. (1993). Issues in perinatal education. AWHONN'S Clinical Issues in Perinatal and Women's Health Nursing, 4(1), 55-59.

1990). It is not within the scope of this chapter to discuss all of the areas of controversy; however, Display 2-2 contains general questions which may be useful to the candidate for certification. After careful analysis, nurses should choose the program that best meets their needs and resources, while recognizing the program's strength and weaknesses (Nichols, 1993).

LEGAL ISSUES

Nursing Accountability

The perinatal nurse is responsible for decisions and actions within the domain of nursing practice. Important aspects of this responsibility are the promotion of a safe and therapeutic environment for both the recipients and providers of nursing care; acquisition of specialized knowledge and skills and additional formal education to provide specialized care; and demonstration and validation of competence in nursing practice. Legal accountability extends to nurse practice acts, parameters of professional practice established by professional organizations, institutional standards, and legislative changes that affect practice and policies, procedures, and protocols within the practice environment (NAACOG, 1991). Perinatal nurses must have a knowledge of physician-prescribed medical and surgical interventions, drug action and interaction, normal and abnormal laboratory values, and physical examination and assessment (Poole, 1992). Competency in a variety of technical skills and critical thinking in emergency situations are requisite. All nurses are responsible and accountable for their actions; therefore, perinatal nurses must recognize the limits of their knowledge and capabilities and act within those limitations. Potential liability exists for failure to exercise independent judgment in implementing orders or procedures (Northrop & Kelly, 1987; Poole).

Professional Liability

In many activities of daily life, for example driving a car, the law requires exercising reasonable care for the safety of others. Failure to exercise reasonable care is negligence. Harm caused to others because of negligence is the basis for liability. Negligence by a professional (i.e., a nurse, a physician, or an attorney) is malpractice. Thus, medical malpractice is medical negligence. To be found guilty of professional negligence, a series of facts first must be established.

1. That the nurse had a responsibility to the patient (**duty**)
2. That the nurse failed to carry out that responsibility (**breach of duty**) by deviating from a standard of care
3. That an injury was sustained by the patient (**damages**)
4. That there was a causal relationship between the patient's injury and the nurse's breach of duty (**proximate cause**)

Establishing the duty of a nurse to a patient is generally not an area of dispute in the institutional setting. The nurse is an employee of the institution that accepts the patient into its care. Therefore a relationship exists until it is terminated either by the completion of care or patient request to voluntarily withdraw from care.

In contrast, establishing adherence to or violation of professional standards of care may involve differences of opinion. This is because there may be equivalently reasonable interpretations or courses of action to meet a given generic standard. For example, the *NAACOG Standards for the Nursing Care of Women and Newborns* states, "It is important to those agencies or individuals who may consult this manual to recognize that the standards set forth are presented as recommendations and general guidelines rather than as a body of rigid rules. The standards are intended to be adapted to many different situations, taking into account the needs and resources particular to the locality, institution, or type of practice setting" (NAACOG, 1991, pp. ii). As such, standards serve as a frame of reference for institutions to use in developing more specific policies, procedures, and protocols.

In the legal sense, the professional standard of care requires that the nurse possess and exercise that degree of knowledge, care, and skill that other nurses would ordinarily exercise under the same or similar circumstances. That is, the nurse should act in a way that is acceptable to professional nursing peers or to reasonably prudent nurses. This broad requirement provides room for debate about what is "acceptable" or reasonably prudent behavior in any given clinical situation. Standards of care violations frequently cited in perinatal litigation are listed in Display 2-3. This list is not necessarily all inclusive or limited to all potential areas of litigation.

Injury and Legal Causation

In addition to showing that a nurse deviated from the standard of care, the claimant must also prove that an injury occurred and that the injury was caused by the professional's negligence. Referred to as causation, this is often the most difficult entity for the claimant to prove. This is especially true in obstetric malpractice cases where it may be difficult to show, for example, that earlier recognition and intervention for a nonreassuring electronic fetal heart tracing that was present on admission would have led to a better outcome.

Strategies to Decrease Professional Liability

Standards of Care and Practice Guidelines

A number of governmental agencies, accreditation bodies, and professional organizations have published practice guidelines and standards of care applicable to perinatal nursing practice, including individual state nurse practice acts and the Joint Commission on Accreditation of Healthcare Organizations (JCAHO) (Display 1-1). While some standards of care are broad (ANA, JCAHO), others are more inclusive and specific (the Association of Women's Health, Obstetric, and Neonatal Nurses [AWHONN], the American Association of Critical Care Nurses [AACN], the National Association of Neonatal Nurses [NANN], the Association of Operating Room Nurses [AORN], the American Society of Postanesthesia Nurses [ASPAN], the American College of Obstetricians and Gynecologists [ACOG], the American Academy of

Pediatrics [AAP], and the American Society of Anesthesiologists [ASA]). In addition, institutions have written policies and procedures based on national standards of care governing clinical practice. The goal of all standards of care and practice guidelines is the provision of safe, therapeutic, quality care by competent healthcare providers. Adherence to established standards of care and practice guidelines can decrease the likelihood of nurses being involved in situations resulting in professional liability.

Institutional Policies and Procedures

Debate exists concerning the development of unit-specific policies and procedures. The questions of which policies and procedures should be included in unit manuals, and how specific they should be are frequently asked. One approach is to identify routine unit practices and provide references to published standards, guidelines, and perinatal nursing texts for specifics, as opposed to the more traditional method of listing multiple steps in an all-inclusive policy or procedure manual (Adels & Pringle, 1992). For example, a policy concerning labor induction/augmentation may reference *Cervical Ripening and Induction and Augmentation of Labor* (AWHONN, 1993) and *Guidelines for Perinatal Care* (ACOG & AAP, 1992, pp. 79-80); the procedure for amnioinfusion may reference *Fetal Monitoring* (Tucker, 1992, pp. 120-122). Advocates of this approach cite the elimination of lengthy policy and procedure manuals, cost savings related to decreased nonproductive time spent writing and revising these manuals, standardization of perinatal nursing practice, and improvement of overall quality of care as benefits. Nursing staff awareness of and adherence to national standards is an added advantage. Policies, procedures, and protocols should be reviewed on an annual basis or more frequently as advances in practice, new technologies, and research are identified (NAACOG, 1991).

Documentation

Of all strategies to decease liability, accurate and thorough documentation is the easiest to accomplish, yet the most common missing piece. The nurse providing care is in control of the information included in the nursing portions of the medical record. Frequently, in issues of litigation, the nurse cannot recall the specific patient or incident and, therefore, must rely

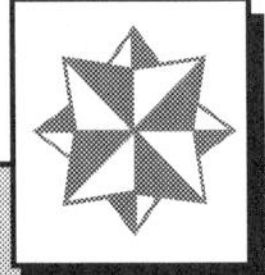

DISPLAY 2-3

Violations of Standards of Care Frequently Cited in Perinatal Litigation

Failure to:

- Have in place adequate policies, procedures, and protocols governing the care and treatment of perinatal patients.
- Adhere to established hospital policies, procedures, protocols, or JCAHO standards.
- Properly evaluate and/or diagnose a condition.
- Adequately monitor (mother, fetus, newborn).
- Interpret data.
- Timely report changes in the patient condition or critical clinical event.
- Recognize that care being provided is inappropriate and act accordingly.
- Use lines of authority/responsibility (chain of command).
- Mobilize emergency resources in a timely fashion.
- Provide sufficient documentation.
- Resuscitate properly.
- Timely transfer.
- Witness informed consent or ensure that it is obtained.
- Carry out medical orders.

on written nurses notes. Lack of documentation (presumed lack of care) may be difficult to defend. In emergent situations, documentation directly on the FHR strip can assist the nurse in constructing notes after patient stabilization. Retrospective charting is better than no documentation. However, late entries following a "bad" outcome are often areas of controversy in litigation, especially if they are written days after the event. Flow sheets are useful tools in prompting appropriate notations, especially in the labor and delivery setting. Development of institutional or unit-specific medical records is preferrable to purchasing standard forms in many cases. Avoid using forms with preprinted times. These types of forms lead to inherently inaccurate documentation. Vital signs and other maternal/fetal assessments and/or emergencies do not occur at predetermined 15-minute intervals. For the women with a reassuring FHR pattern, a few minutes may not make a difference; however, in emergencies an accurate account is critical in recording sequential appropriate interventions.

Incident Management

An incident can be defined as any happening that is not consistent with the routine care of a particular patient. Many adverse perinatal outcomes that result in litigation derive from perinatal incidents that are unexpected and/or the result of an emergency occurrence.

Emergency occurrences can be categorized as actual, evolving, or perceived. Actual emergencies may include maternal hemorrhage, prolapsed cord, amniotic fluid embolism, shoulder dystocia, or neonatal asphyxia. Evolving emergencies are those that develop gradually and go unrecognized until an acute situation occurs. Examples include fetal stress progressing to severe stress, severe preeclampsia converting to overt eclampsia, or an unrecognized malpresentation going to precipitous delivery without appropriate preparation. Finally, perceived emergencies are the "near misses" that have the potential to result in adverse outcomes. These may include insufficient resources, inadequate communication, professional knowledge deficits, or ineffective lines of authority and responsibility.

Incident management, therefore, plays an important role in reducing institutional liability. The goal is to obtain an accurate, valid account of what happened (or what might have happened) from those individuals who possess first-hand knowledge. This process requires time, extensive communication, and a systematic framework. Generally, incident management is a retrospective process that includes the examination of all of the events surrounding the incident. Key factors in the review include the following:

- What happened?
- What were the contributing factors?
- Was it preventable or nonpreventable?
- How was it handled?
- Were sufficient resources available?
- Was there the opportunity to handle it better?
- Is there a need for remedial action?
- What is the appropriate follow-up?
- What is the required documentation?

Validation of Core Competencies

The JCAHO has published standards regarding development and validation of core competencies in nursing practice, including both general nursing units and specialty units (JCAHO, 1995). Institutions must identify core competencies that are specific to each nursing unit and develop processes to validate the nursing staff's level of competence. The JCAHO guidelines specify the identification of both beginner and expert levels of practice. Validation only on the basis of skill checklists is not enough to meet this standard. A system to validate the knowledge base that is required for clinical practice must also be developed and implemented. Completion of written self-assessment tools, computer-simulated examinations, oral or written case presentations, peer and manager reviews, and medical-record audits examining individual practice are additional methods of validating core competencies. The critical issue is to incorporate both the expected skills verification and the requisite knowledge-base evaluation into the competency validation process.

Validation of core competencies and documentation of that process should be done at the completion of the unit orientation, at specific time intervals during the first year, and on an annual basis thereafter. Nurses who are expected to provide care in areas that deliver services secondary to their primary area of expertise must also meet minimum competency requirements in those areas (JCAHO, 1995). This standard is especially important for perinatal nurses who may be routinely expected to provide care for a variety of patients of different acuity levels in multiple settings, including women during the antepartum, intrapartum, and postpartum periods and infants in the newborn nursery, intermediate care nursery, and neonatal intensive care nursery. Perinatal units can refer to the *Standards for the Nursing Care of Women and Newborns* (NAACOG, 1991) and the *Accreditation Manual for Hospitals* (JCAHO, 1995) for lists of nursing practices that may reflect the expected practice in each institution. (See Appendix B for example of core competencies for perinatal units.)

Continuing Education

The dynamic nature of perinatal nursing practice makes it imperative that nurses keep abreast of advancements in knowledge and new technologies. Current financial climate in most healthcare settings has placed restraints on institutions' continuing education budgets. Limited institutional funding for continuing education does not relieve the perinatal nurse of responsibility to maintain a research-based practice. Perinatal nurses are responsible for obtaining new knowledge and maintaining competence in their practice. They must have an awareness of changing practices and professional and ethical issues, seek new knowledge and clinical skills by attending in-service education and/or professional continuing education programs, be cognizant of pertinent research data and professional literature, and incorporate newly acquired knowledge and skills into practice (NAACOG, 1991).

Subscribing to professional nursing journals, attending continuing education offerings, and belonging to professional nursing organizations are methods to obtain knowledge of new practice guidelines and research in the field. Journal clubs, organized by nurses in specialty practice areas, that meet on a regular basis to review the latest articles in perinatal nursing and medical journals are one way to ensure currency in practice. It is important to note that publication processes often delay the dissemination of articles and research reports by up to one year or more, so current articles usually report on studies that were completed during the previous year. Innovative programs are available to provide current information such as computer-assisted instructional programs (CAIs), video tape

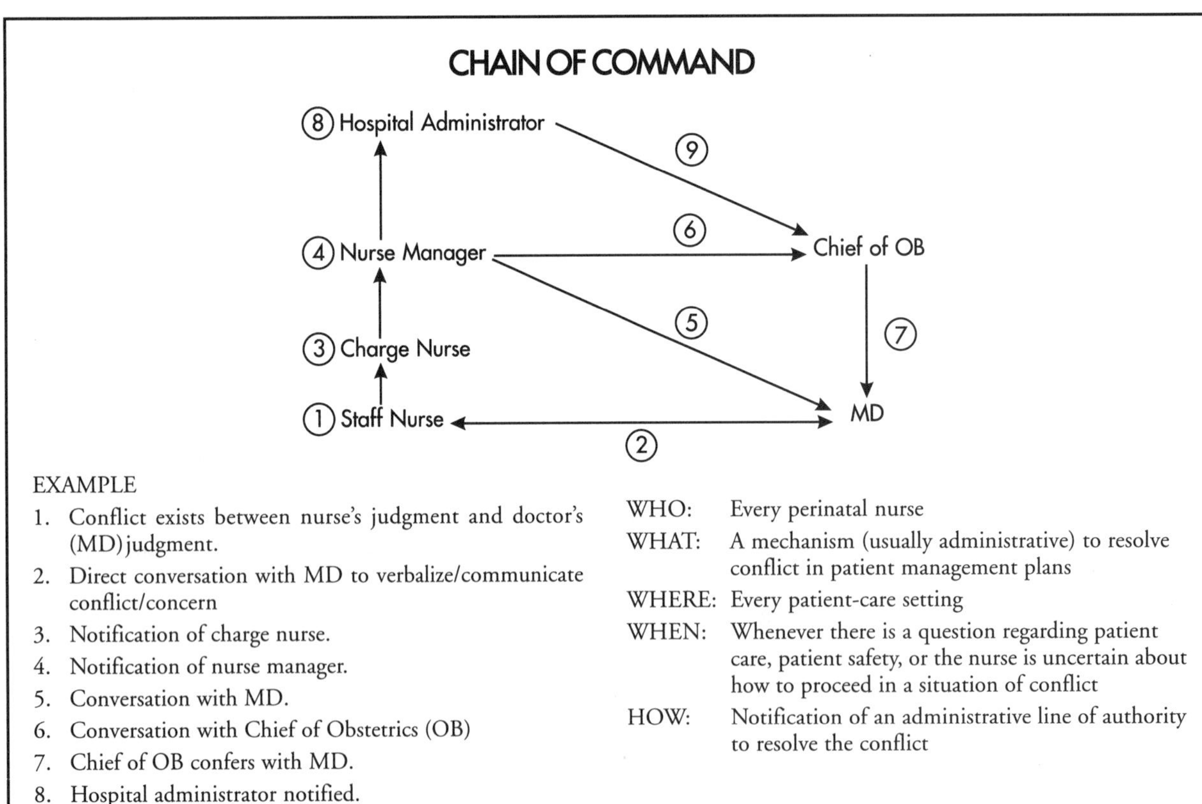

EXAMPLE

1. Conflict exists between nurse's judgment and doctor's (MD) judgment.
2. Direct conversation with MD to verbalize/communicate conflict/concern
3. Notification of charge nurse.
4. Notification of nurse manager.
5. Conversation with MD.
6. Conversation with Chief of Obstetrics (OB)
7. Chief of OB confers with MD.
8. Hospital administrator notified.
9. Hospital administrator confirms resolution of conflict.

WHO: Every perinatal nurse
WHAT: A mechanism (usually administrative) to resolve conflict in patient management plans
WHERE: Every patient-care setting
WHEN: Whenever there is a question regarding patient care, patient safety, or the nurse is uncertain about how to proceed in a situation of conflict
HOW: Notification of an administrative line of authority to resolve the conflict

Figure 2-1. Each perinatal care setting should have its own administrative chain of command to assist in conflict resolution in the management of patients. Such a chain of command is illustrated here.

From Chez, B.F., Harvey, C.J., Murray, M.L. (1990). Critical Concepts in Fetal Heart Rate Monitoring. (pp. 32). Reprinted with permission.

series and teleconferences. Institutions can purchase these resources as one approach to offer quality programs to a large number of nurses at a relatively low cost per staff member. CAIs and video tapes can become part of a unit's lending library allowing staff members to borrow resources for home use at their convenience. Continuing education may also be obtained through self-study programs. A variety of perinatal and neonatal nursing educational resources are available through AWHONN, NCC, Mosby, J.B. Lippincott, the March of Dimes, and Williams & Wilkins.

Attendance at perinatal nursing conferences and workshops is a common method of assimilating new information. Not only is the course content useful to practice, but conference attendance provides opportunities to talk with professional colleagues from other institutions and other areas of the country. Regional differences in practice can be identified, and those differences that may be an improvement for individual institutions may be promoted and implemented as a result of national conference participation. Some institutions elect to bring a nurse speaker on site for the benefit of all staff rather than send several nurses to a national perinatal conference as a more cost-effective method of providing continuing education. There are merits to this approach; however, the collaboration and sharing with colleagues from other areas of the country is limited. Informal telephone networks with nursing colleagues can be used to overcome this limitation.

Conflict Resolution and Nurse/Physician Relationships

No group of individuals can be together in an organization and always have the same expectations, mutual goals, and identical perspectives. Conflict is an inevitable result when reality does not meet with individual expectations. While individual expectations may differ, usually there exists among caregivers a basic commitment to quality and to the best possible outcomes for both mother and newborn. In theory, discussions between professional colleagues are based on mutual respect. When involved in a clinical or administrative situation that can potentially cause conflict, it is helpful to consider that both parties probably have the best interests of the patient in mind, although there may be very different approaches proposed to achieve that goal. At times, clinical practice issues arise when the "way we've always done it" conflicts with a new or an alternate approach.

Classic principles of conflict resolution can be used to successfully resolve the inevitable differences of opinion that occur in everyday clinical practice. If the conflict is not related to an emergent patient situation (i.e., there is at least some time for discussion), effective communication techniques can enhance the chances of conflict resolution to the satisfaction of both parties. Taking time to really listen and analyze the other opinion, before insisting that your way is the only "right" one, is an effective approach. Other successful strategies include a calm and collected attitude and careful consideration of the goal to be accomplished and why. Selecting the best time and place for interaction is also essential. Ideally the setting will not allow opportunity for patients, family members, or other colleagues to overhear the discussion. The use of positive, nonverbal gestures such as direct eye contact and a comfortable stance, convey a willingness to listen rather than, indicating an attack on the colleague involved in the conflict. Phrases such as, "I have a different perspective" are usually more helpful in conflict resolution than, "You are wrong." The focus of the discussion should remain on the issue, preferably on the potential impact on patient care. If the conversation deteriorates or the colleague becomes verbally abusive, ending the discussion until a later time and/or bringing in an objective third party may be helpful.

Chain of Command

Some issues of conflict in the clinical setting cannot be solved at the lowest level and do not allow the luxury of time. If, after careful deliberation, the issue is determined to be a matter of maternal/fetal well-being or there is potential for the clinical situation to deteriorate rapidly, the nurse must initiate an appropriate course of action. An example is (but not limited to) failure of the physician to respond to a nonreassuring FHR pattern or deteriorating maternal condition. Decisive, timely nursing intervention may be necessary to avoid a potentially adverse outcome. Knowledge and the use of the chain of command is one way to attempt to resolve differences of opinion in clinical practice settings. An example of chain of command is given in Figure 2-1. If discussions with the physician or nurse-midwife do not result in care appropriate for the clinical practice situation, the primary-care nurse has the responsibility to use the perinatal unit institutional chain of command to avoid harm to the mother and/or newborn. Failure to do so increases the likelihood of professional nursing liability should the situation result in litigation at a later date.

Professional Liability Insurance

Perinatal nurses continue to ask the question, "Should I carry my own liability insurance?" The question is an important one, in light of increased litigation surrounding adverse perinatal outcomes. However, the prevalence of litigation has little to do with the decision-making that the individual nurse must go through. There are multiple factors for the perinatal nurse to consider.

All perinatal nurses engaged in the practice of nursing should be insured against liabilities to third parties arising out of their professional practice. The means by which a professional nurse elects to insure professional practice should be based on an informed decision. Insurance options available to nurses include reliance on the employer-provided insurance or purchase of self-insurance as an independent practitioner or as part of a group when there is no employer-provided insurance. Either option fulfills the expectation that there exists a financial responsibility for professional practice.

The issue for nurses is the dilemma of whether or not to purchase individual coverage, in addition to employer-provided coverage. The nurse is an employee of the institution. Therefore, an institutional liability policy will cover the nurse for acts that are within the scope of employment. The nurse should assess his or her clinical practice against the established policies and procedures of the institution. The nurse is covered by the employer's policy whenever the nurse is acting within the employer's direction and control and within the stated scope of practice.

A fear among nurses is that the employer will attempt to recover partial damages from the nurse should the nurse be found negligent in a malpractice action. This process is referred to as Indemnification and Contribution. While there is limited data on separate suits against nurses in this regard, that is not to say that it has not been attempted. However, it is important to recognize that there are valid reasons why healthcare institutions would not or should not sue nurses. Among these reasons, the nurse is an employee of the institution and since the nurse is acting under the institution's power and control, it is responsible for all actions of the nurse. Another reason is that it makes for very poor public relations when an institution sues its own employees. Finally, if a nurse has no personal insurance policy to recover from, it may not be worth it from a financial standpoint.

An additional concern among nurses is the loss of personal assets if they are not separately insured. Unfortunately, there is scant data on the liability of uninsured nurses. However, in many states there are laws protecting money and property that are jointly held. Further, an uninsured nurse is an unlikely financial "deep pocket" for any claimant.

A final consideration for nurses is that the purchase of individual/personal coverage may make it more likely for a nurse to become involved as an individual in a malpractice action. This is primarily due to the fact that the nurse with significant coverage is viewed as a financial deep pocket, separate and distinct from the employer. Further, where both the employer and the nurse have policies, which policy is the "primary" coverage will depend on the nature and language of the policies and pro-rated contributions may result if the nurse is determined to be negligent in a malpractice action.

SUMMARY

As knowledge and technologic advances continue in the fields of perinatology and neonatology, responsibilities and opportunities for perinatal nurses are evolving. Keeping current with changes in practice and developing new research-based knowledge is critically important for perinatal nurses, to insure provision of quality care for childbearing women and newborns and to avoid professional liability.

References

Adels, N., & Pringle, S. (1992). Stop re-inventing the wheel: Textbooks as procedure manuals. Nursing Management, 23(5), 74-75.

Afriat, C.I., Simpson, K.R., Chez, B.F., & Miller, L.A. (1994). Electronic fetal monitoring competency–to validate or not to validate: The opinions of experts. Journal of Perinatal and Neonatal Nursing, 8, 1-16.

American Academy of Pediatrics, & American College of Obstetricians and Gynecologists. (1992). Guidelines for perinatal care (3rd ed.). Washington, DC: Author.

American Nurses' Association. (1979). The study of credentialing in nursing: A new approach (Vol. 1). The Report of the Committee, Kansas City, MO: Author.

American Nurses' Association. (1983). Standards of maternal and child health nursing practice. Kansas City, MO: Author.

American Nurses' Credentialing Center. (1994). Nurses Credentialing Center certification catalog, Washington, DC: Author.

Association of Women's Health, Obstetric, and Neonatal Nurses. (1993). Cervical ripening and induction and augmentation of labor: Practice resource. Washington, DC: Author.

Donahue, M.P. (1985). Nursing, the finest art: An illustrated history. St. Louis, MO: C.V. Mosby.

Joint Commission on Accreditation of Healthcare Organizations. (1995). Accreditation manual for hospitals: Standards, 1. Chicago: Author.

National Certification Corporation for the Obstetric, Gynecologic, and Neonatal Nursing Specialties (NCC). (1994). Certification program. Chicago: Author.

Nichols, F.H. (1993). Issues in perinatal education. AWHONN's Clinical Issues in Perinatal and Women's Health Nursing 4(1), 55-59.

Northrop, C.E., & Kelly, M.E. (1987). Legal issues in nursing. St. Louis, MO: C.V. Mosby.

Nurses Association of the American College of Obstetricians and Gynecologists. (1991). Standards for the nursing care of women and newborns (4th ed.). Washington, DC: Author.

Poole, J.H. (1992). Legal and professional issues in critical care obstetrics. Critical Care Nursing Clinics of North America 4,(4), 687-690.

Simpson, K.R. (1990). A specialty certification incentive program: Costs versus benefits. Journal of Nursing Staff Development, 6(4), 181-185.

Tucker, S. (1992). Fetal monitoring (2nd ed.). St. Louis, MO: Mosby-Year Book.

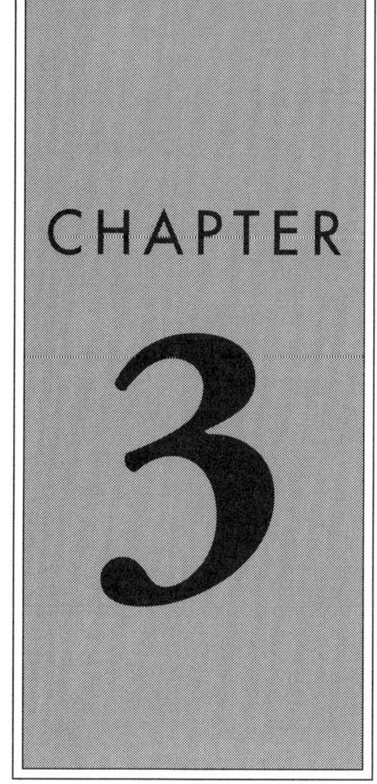

Collaborative Practice as a Systematic Method for Perinatal Care

Linda Bertucci
Jacqueline Jordan

Delivery methods, universal access, shifting reimbursement patterns, limited resources, and an increased emphasis on quality outcomes by both consumers and payors are significant driving forces behind changes in health care today. Uncontrolled rising costs have resulted in a shift from expensive inpatient stays to lower-cost outpatient procedures and homecare, a renewed focus on health maintenance and prevention, and a trend away from fee-for-service reimbursement to payment based on case rates and capitation. Payors (i.e., the government, employers, and insurance companies) have begun to limit their subsidies and shift the burden of costs to individuals and providers. Hospital net revenues are adversely affected by declining inpatient volume, rising costs, shortened lengths of stay (LOS), lower revenues per procedure, and payor restrictions. For a hospital or a healthcare system to remain competitive in this rapidly changing arena, the challenge is to provide high-quality care at low cost. This can be accomplished by adopting a systematic method to improve the quality of patient care, prospectively define and measure outcomes, and streamline systems to increase efficiency and reduce waste. It is important that quality outcomes are then communicated to payors and consumers of health care. Various models of case management and use of clinical pathways have been identified in a number of perinatal centers involved in efforts to increase quality while decreasing costs; however, few institutions report meaningful success or satisfaction with use of one model in isolation.

Successful implementation of a collaborative-practice model that incorporates four current concepts of health care is discussed in this chapter. First, a description of collaborative practice, its members, and their roles is given. The model is then discussed and strategies for development, implementation, and evaluation are given. While all components may not be applicable for individual institutions, the model can serve as a basis for discussion and initiation of strategies appropriate for any perinatal center.

COLLABORATIVE PRACTICE AS A MODEL OF CARE

Four concepts in healthcare practice have emerged in the 1990s: managed care, case management, collaborative care, and continuous quality improvement. A description of each follows.

Managed care is a system that provides a generalized structure and focus when managing the use, cost, quality, and effectiveness of health care services (Cohen & Cesta, 1993). Tools such as clinical pathways and variance records are used to monitor patient care at the unit level.

Case management is a process model that organizes the various components and services used in delivering patient care (Cohen & Cesta, 1993). The care manager coordinates management of specific patient populations across an episode of care. For the obstetrical population, this concept can be expanded beyond the previous narrow focus of the inpatient setting to encompass continuous care delivered in the physician's office, the hospital, and the home.

Collaborative care is a model which uses an interdisciplinary approach to manage continuity of care. Interdisciplinary group practices (core groups) are responsible for allocating resources, managing care across the continuum, and improving clinical outcomes. The purpose of interdisciplinary groups is to integrate care practices into a comprehensive approach to meet patient needs. Development of a common purpose is a prerequisite to collaboration (Nugent, 1992), With the development of cohesion in the interdisciplinary group, issues of ambiguity, confusion, and fragmentation of care can be resolved. Shared decision making fosters the common purpose of achieving desired clinical outcomes.

Continuous quality improvement techniques have been shown to raise performance standards and reduce variation, thereby increasing consistency of the standard or outcome desired (Leebow, 1991). The process of continuous quality improvement, which includes the application of the scientific method to improve systems, can be used to analyze patient satisfaction, outcome criteria, practice patterns, and staff satisfaction.

Many hospitals have embraced parts of managed care and case management philosophy, but they never seem to be able to bring all of the pieces together effectively to make it work. For example, significant time can be spent on educating staff and designing tools. When tools such as clinical pathways are implemented, staff go to great lengths to collect data about variances from the pathway. Often, the data collected is so voluminous and detailed that it becomes overwhelming. A common result of this approach is that the information collected is never used to make improvements. Furthermore, data collection systems can be cumbersome and can greatly impede ability to improve patient care. Feedback mechanisms for each group practice are needed to monitor progress and evaluate outcomes.

The challenge in a collaborative-practice model is to implement a system that integrates all four components in a comprehensive and cost-effective manner.

What Is a Collaborative-Practice Model?

Collaborative practice is a systematic method of healthcare delivery that links quality clinical practice with efficiency and cost-effective strengths. A model of collaborative practice should be systematic, patient centered, interdisciplinary, and outcome focused. A care manager is responsible for coordination of care across an episode of illness for a specific population of patients.

A collaborative practice model must be comprehensive so that the changes will improve the quality of care, reduce costs, streamline systems, and increase patient satisfaction. It places the patient as the focus of attention, with team members working toward a common, defined goal in an outcome-based model. Patient focus has the benefit of breaking down interdepartmental and interdisciplinary barriers as the core members use change and continuous quality improvement theory to coordinate the patient's care episode.

Goals of Collaborative Practice

The goals of Collaborative Practice are to improve both the quality of care and the patient's perception of the healthcare experience in a cost-effective manner. This is accomplished by defining outcomes of care and by reducing performance variability through appropriate resource utilization. The result is care that is consistent and replicable, in a defined population, over time. These outcomes are dynamic, not static, and are refined and monitored periodically.

Clinical Pathways and Variance Records

Primary tools used to facilitate the transition of the patient from one phase of care to another are the clinical pathway and variance record. The clinical pathway is used to chart the patient's episode of care and identify all the components of care. The clinical pathway describes management protocols (e.g., induction of labor, epidural management, newborn care), nursing diagnoses (both potential and actual), intermediate interventions that must be achieved during the hospital stay, and discharge criteria. The variance record is used to monitor patient, system, and practitioner deviations from the clinical pathway that may alter the expected outcome.

The clinical pathway is based on information from past medical records, current literature, and the clinical expertise of the core team members. Pathway components include medications, consultations, activities, tests, treatments, nutrition, teaching, protocols, and discharge planning. The clinical pathway includes all expected components of the patient's episode of illness, from admission to discharge. It is intended to facilitate the patient's transition through the hospital in an efficient and timely manner. Progress is monitored hourly, daily, or weekly, as needed. Concurrent monitoring by staff and the care manager allows for continuous, timely quality improvement.

Variances from the pathway are identified by the medical, nursing, and ancillary staff on a daily basis and documented on the variance record. A variance, which can be either positive or negative, is categorized as applying to the patient, system, or practitioner. For instance, a patient-related variance is an unexpected complication, such as a wound dehiscence. An example of a system-related variance is when laboratory results are delayed because of a computer backlog at peak operating times. A practitioner-related variance might include delay of initiation of a therapy. Examples are oxytocin administration delay, potentially increasing length of labor, or ambulation delay after cesarean birth, resulting in slow return of bowel sounds. At the end of each month, the care manager prepares aggregates of the variances and identifies any patterns or trends to be analyzed by the Collaborative Practice Team for possible opportunities to improve care.

Variance analysis leads to identification and description of problems for analysis and resolution. Thus, patterns and trends are evaluated on a global scale, with application to a population of patients as opposed to a single individual or episode. This provides the basis for modification of the clinical pathway to achieve better outcomes. For example, one outcome is LOS, an indication of resource consumption that is measured in minutes, hours, days, or visits. LOS reduction is an effective means of maximizing reimbursment, so identification and resolution of variances that can increase LOS are critically important to success.

Benefits of Collaborative Practice

The Collaborative Practice model improves patient care and, therefore, benefits patients, team members, and the medical center.

Patients benefit by knowing what is going to happen to them. The clinical pathway is a useful tool for helping patients understand what to expect during the hospital stay and what their role is in the recovery process. Patients who understand the pre- and postoperative procedures and are educated about their recovery process are less anxious. When patients are motivated, they participate more actively in their recovery and recover faster. Frequent contact and communication build rapport and an environment of trust and support.

Caregivers benefit by predefined expectations that help to organize and direct workload. The continuous quality improvement process can be used to identify and implement system solutions. Contributions made to improve systems are rewarding and enhance job satisfaction. Systems changes have a wide application to a large population of patients and increase daily job efficiency.

As Collaborative Practice team members work together, they are challenged to develop creative solutions to enhance the quality of patient care. Mutual respect develops across disciplines when ideas are successfully implemented, and measures of success validate the positive impact on changing practice patterns.

Institutional benefits of Collaborative Practice include shortened LOS, decreased cost per case, increased systems efficiencies, and improved patient care. Cases with revenues that in the recent past were less than costs now break even or show a profit (e.g., scheduled inductions). Payors are interested in outcome quality measures. This enables the hospital to contract with more payors and to increase patient volume. Both the hospital and physician benefit by improved relationships accruing from increased patient volume for individual practices.

MEMBERS OF THE COLLABORATIVE GROUP PRACTICE AND THEIR ROLES

Important components of a collaborative practice model are the coordination of disciplines and development of a team atmosphere. Central to the process is the care manager.

The Nurse Care Manager

The registered nurse care manager is responsible for managing a predefined population of patients. Prerequisites are the ability to envision a patient's episode of illness, knowledge to comprehend the components of care needed, and skill to move the patient along the continuum by achieving predetermined outcomes by discharge. The care manager must be able to evaluate, prioritize, and communicate daily activities, tests, and assessments that are needed to ensure patient progression as planned.

The care manager is a professional nurse who plans, manages, coordinates, implements, and evaluates the ongoing care of a specific patient case type. The case type equates, for the most part, to a diagnosis-related-group (DRG) code (e.g., vaginal birth without complications, cesarean birth without complications, ectopic pregnancy, normal newborn, and neonatal sepsis). The care manager is responsible for developing the collaborative group practice. The care manager then acts in collaboration with members of the healthcare team, patient, and patient's family as the pivotal person responsible for coordination of delivery of effective, efficient, and appropriate care during an entire episode of hospitalization. The care manager is accountable to the quality improvement committee for ongoing monitoring and evaluation of patient outcomes. Key characteristics that contribute to the success of the care manager are advanced education, management experience, clinical expertise, and group facilitation skills. A job description is given in Display 3-1.

Collaborative Practice Team

A multidisciplinary team of caregivers works with the care manager to define and monitor safe, effective care for the patient population defined. (Caregiver may be defined as any person who may come in contact directly or indirectly with the patient.) Caregivers include, but are not limited to, the physician, bedside nurse, registered dietician, respiratory care technician, central supply technician, and business office representative. The Collaborative Practice team includes core members, who meet on a regular basis to define and monitor goals, and ad hoc members, who participate as needed when a problem is defined.

The group's goal is to continually evaluate and improve the quality of patient care. The team may meet monthly or bi-monthly, based on the ongoing needs of the patient population. Activities include the following:

- review cases and analyze trended variances
- evaluate achievement of specific outcomes
- identify opportunities for improvement
- identify case–related learning needs
- share new clinical information

Collaborative Practice Council

To ensure continued evolution of the role of care manager and implementation and expansion of Collaborative Practice teams, an internal support system may be formed. This group, the Collaborative Practice Council, comprises care managers, the director of quality improvement, utilization management coordinators, and other ad hoc members (e.g., representatives from infection control, quality improvement, and social service). The purpose of the council is to disseminate information, establish standards, promote professional practice, provide peer consultation and ongoing education. The council operates under a set of by-laws providing for the election of a chairperson and co-chairperson, defining common goals and setting annual objectives.

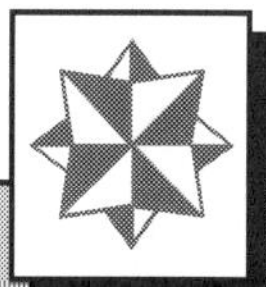

DISPLAY 3-1

Care Manager in a Collaborative Practice Model

Job Description

Nursing Process

Assessment: Conducts and/or reviews each patient's comprehensive healthcare assessment and history in their caseload upon or prior to admission. Analyzes assessment data and formulates appropriate clinical pathways in an ongoing and systematic manner.

Planning: Uses and initiates appropriate clinical maps for patients to facilitate achievement of expected outcomes in collaboration with the caregivers to determine estimated length of stay and expected outcomes.

Implementation: Monitors patient progress and conducts periodic reassessment of changes in health status, based on established procedures, protocols, and standards.

Evaluation: Analyzes patterns of variances from standardized clinical maps and implements strategies to resolve them for both individual patients and case types.

Leadership and Coordination

Communication: Facilitates communication among members of the healthcare team. Communicates appropriate information to members of the healthcare team and Collaborative Practice members.

Working Relationships: Works collaboratively with members of the healthcare team involved in the case-managed population.

Leadership: Coordinates and conducts the Collaborative Practice meetings. Develops and implements effective communication to all members of the Collaborative Group Practice, in their absence.

Coordination: Manages each patient's transition through the system and transfers accountability to the appropriate person or agency upon discharge.

Consultation: Serves as resource for other personnel in assessing patient and family status, in planning nursing care, participating in the development of hospital procedures, protocols, standards, and regulations appropriate to type managed.

Standards: Develops and reviews standardized clinical maps for standardized outcomes for each case type.

Clinical Skills

Knowledge Base: Uses a broad knowledge base to examine patient issues and anticipate potential issues over the entire episode of care.

Competency: Demonstrates competency in professional patient-care management, in keeping with approved standards of care.

Fiscal Responsibility

Financial Management: Establishes and monitors Collaborative Practice costs per case type. Participates in the collection and analysis of financial data for each patient.

Utilization Management: Assesses appropriateness of acute hospitalization, as related to intensity of service and severity of illness, for their caseload.

DISPLAY 3-1 (cont.)

Data Analysis: Evaluates and analyzes trends and collaborates closely with physicians to establish guidelines to improve the delivery of care and prevent adverse outcomes.

Patient Education

Patient/Family: Works collaboratively with the caregivers, to enhance quality of patient education which includes family members and support persons. Provides resources and support as needed.

Discharge Planning: Initiates, coordinates, and facilitates the preadmission, admission, hospitalization, discharge, and follow-up care for their caseload.

Professionalism

Professional Development: Demonstrates self-directed learning and accountability for own professional practice.

Staff Education: Educates other staff about Collaborative Practice and the unique needs of the caseload. Facilitates and coordinates patient care conference for their caseload. Works with core group members to enhance staff education as it relates to Collaborative Practice issues identified via variances and trends.

Case Review: Collaborates with other care managers regarding patient-care issues and opportunities for resolution.

Research Utilization: Identifies problems that influence patient-care delivery/nursing practice and uses current nursing research for problem resolution.

Quality Management

Group Practice: Reviews, in collaboration with the Group Practice team, practice patterns and patterns of variances for targeted populations of patients.

Medical Committees/Physician Participation: Provides guidance and direction in initiating and implementing change, through medical committees and physician participation, to improve quality of care and affect appropriate allocation of resources and LOS.

From Saddleback Memorial Medical Center, Laguna Hills, CA. Reprinted with permission.

THE SADDLEBACK MEMORIAL MEDICAL CENTER (SMMC) MODEL OF PERINATAL COLLABORATIVE PRACTICE

Collaborative Practice was implemented at SMMC as a competitive healthcare strategy for the 1990s. SMMC, an affiliate of Memorial Health Services, Inc., is a 221-bed, private, tertiary care, not-for-profit corporation in southern California.

Included under Patient Care Services at SMMC is the Family Birth Center, a Level III perinatal unit. The Family Birth Center has 24 private labor, delivery, recovery, and postpartum (LDRP) suites, plus related surgical suites and nurseries. The restricted surgical suite consists of two operating rooms and a semirestricted recovery room with two monitored beds. The observation nursery is a semirestricted eight-bed unit in which normal newborns may be observed when they are not rooming-in. Two additional licensed beds are for boarders or extended-care infants. The Infant Special Care Unit (ISCU) consists of 19 tertiary care licensed beds.

Prior to the implementation of Collaborative Practice, healthcare team members frequently worked in isolation, with differing time frames and outcome measures, resulting in duplication, miscommunication, and a general lack of cohesiveness common in many units. Therefore, SMMC developed a Collaborative Practice Program to streamline treatment for specific patient populations.

SMMC's vision is to be the dominant, operationally excellent, fiscally sound provider of comprehensive, high-quality, acute healthcare services in the area. The six values identified in SMMC's vision statement are service, integrity, compassion, innovation, collaboration, and fiscal responsibility.

A conscious decision was made to design a system that would improve healthcare delivery, create positive change that was long lasting, and improve the financial bottom line for the hospital. Once that was accomplished, an additional goal was to advertise SMMC's success and use results to aggressively pursue contracts and actively market services.

Development of the Program

Collaborative Practice was first applied to the care of complex cardiac surgery patients. Success, as measured by a shorter LOS with fewer complications or readmissions, provided the springboard for development in other areas. Translating this benefit to the perinatal population, however, provided obstacles in the initial stages. Questions were raised about the incremental benefits in a well population that already enjoyed a short LOS and few complications. The ideas for a perinatal program received a boost when problems began to be identified in this patient population, one of which was the staff's inability to consistently meet educational needs for our patients and to prepare them for self-care at home. Collaborative Practice was implemented as a potential means of resolving these problems. The program developed in three phases: (1) the start-up phase, which lasted about 3 months of the first year, (2) the implementation phase, which comprised 3 to 6 months, and (3) the analysis phase of 6 to 12 months, during which data were collected and the impact on quality quantified.

Start-Up Phase

Case-Type Selection

Selection of case types that would benefit from Collaborative Practice and case management was based on the following criteria and populations: High volume (normal vaginal birth), problem prone (newborn), obstetrical high risk (preterm labor), and high cost (cesarean birth). The first three patient populations developed were women scheduled for an induction of labor, women scheduled for a cesarean birth, and newborns of these mothers. All were problem-prone or high cost and had similarities in their care. Clinical pathways for cesarean birth and surgical patients were fairly straightforward because of their predictability in terms of preoperative work up, scheduled procedure, and a postoperative recovery phase.

Core Group Member Identification

The qualified candidate for care manager at SMMC had to meet the following criteria:

- A registered nurse with a current license in the State of California
- Qualifications and expectations that meet the Clinical III or IV job description
- Certification in specialty area (preferred)
- A minimum of 2 years' clinical experience documented in the clinical area relevant to the patient case load the care manager is expected to oversee
- Excellent verbal and written communication skills
- Demonstrated ability to negotiate and affect desired patient outcomes in collaboration with other members of the healthcare team
- Recent completion of the Core Curriculum for the care manager
- Employment by the SMMC for at least 6 months prior to advancement to care manager status.

Physician groups were approached to determine interest, receptivity, and openness to a new approach to patient care. A program outline, sample clinical pathways, and brief overview of benefits to be realized from implementation of collaborative practice were developed. The success of other group practices was used to illustrate the potential of Collaborative Practice when meeting with obstetricians and pediatricians in their offices. Several physician groups volunteered to participate.

Other healthcare personnel were recruited as part of the core group (Figure 3-1). Priority was given to disciplines with interactions with the majority of targeted patients during their hospital stay. Membership included representatives from pharmacy, laboratory, home health, food and nutrition, newborn nursing, labor and delivery, mother-baby nursing, and medicine. Ad-hoc members included personnel from social service, anesthesia, and quality improvement.

Clinical Pathway Development

Initial clinical pathways were based on individual physician group practice patterns as determined through retrospective chart audits of LOS, laboratory orders, fluid management, pain management, sequencing of medical intervention, length of time in the operating

SADDLEBACK MEMORIAL MEDICAL CENTER

Collaborative Practice Core Group Members

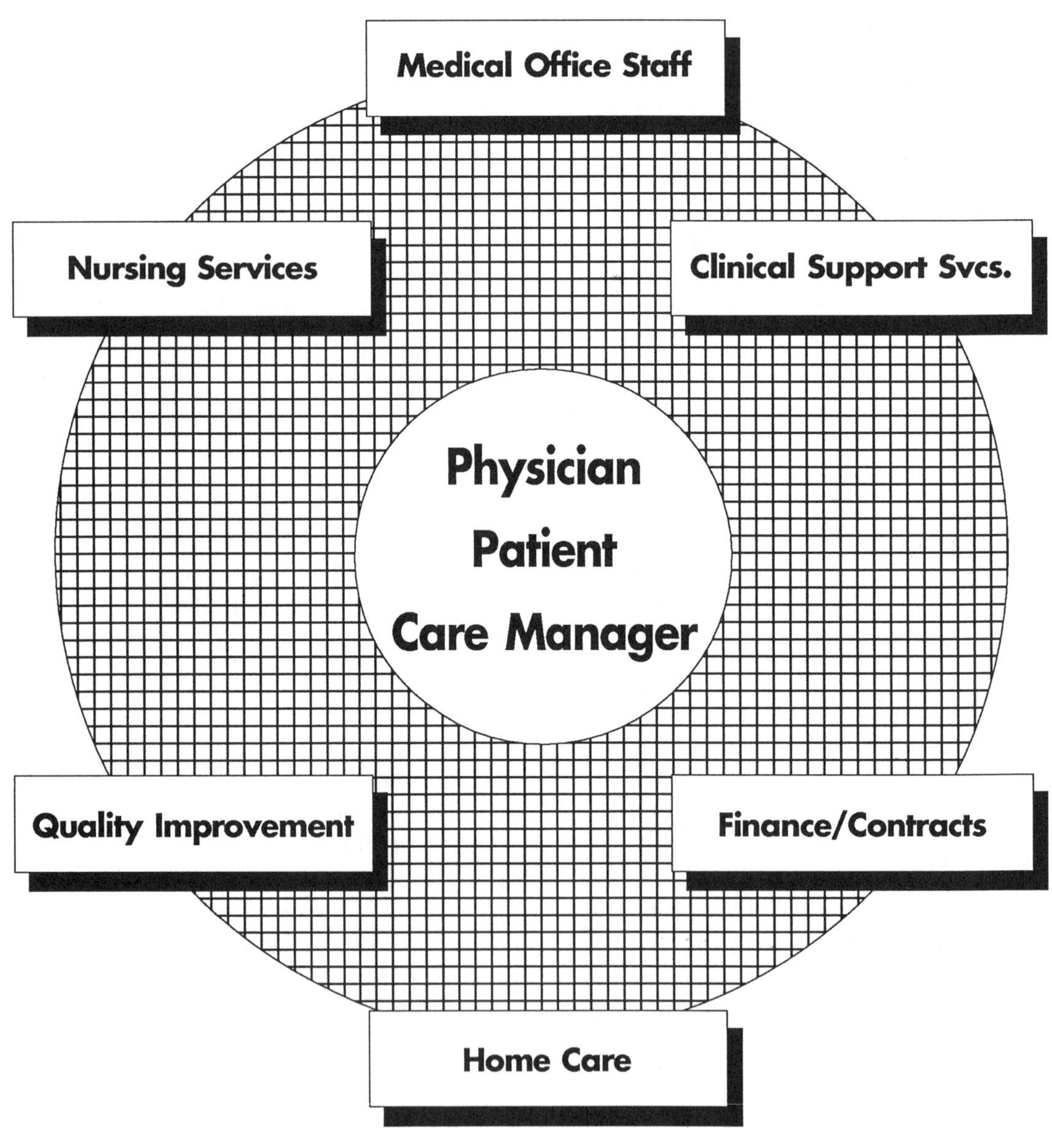

Figure 3-1.

Copyright Saddleback Memorial Medical Center, 1992, Collaborative Practice. Reprinted with permission.

room, length of labor induction, ambulation, nutrition, education, cesarean rate, and morbidity. Each medical practice group was shown its statistics in comparison with the other groups. Each physician group identified goals and the components to be incorporated into their clinical pathways to modify their practice to achieve certain patient outcomes.

A draft of the clinical pathway was developed for each group and distributed to the Collaborative Practice core group for their input. For example, the physician group may have identified the need for results of preoperative laboratory tests to be available and on the chart prior to beginning the prescribed treatment. Laboratory staff and the core group mutually agreed that the most cost-effective and timely way to achieve this was to see the woman the day before the procedure to obtain the blood samples and to review results. To accomplish this, laboratory tests were incorporated into the preoperative teaching phase of the clinical pathway. This achieved the physicians' goal of having the laboratory results available prior to the procedure, improved use of laboratory personnel during-down time, and was convenient for pregnant women by incorporating laboratory testing into their prenatal visit.

Implementation Phase

Education

During the implementation phase, core team members, other staff, patients, and families were educated about the program. Systematic methods and tools were developed for group practices to use in the design and development of clinical pathways. Successful practice ideas from the literature were encouraged, when appropriate. Formation of group practices, with representatives from all disciplines, resulted in increased staff participation in problem solving. Group practices also provided a forum for greater collaboration and sharing of ideas. Tools were developed to monitor and evaluate outcomes of care. Emphasis was placed on the importance of variance analysis and feedback from customers to identify and implement ways to improve. Communication of results achieved were reported regularly to medical staff committees and the hospital board.

Formal education of staff was accomplished through a series of inservices that described and elaborated key components of Collaborative Practice. Education for patients and family members was incorporated into preoperative teaching and daily bedside visits. Informal education occured at frequent bedside discussions of clinical pathways and patient progress. Open dialogue encouraged patients and staff to contribute their creative ideas to improve and modify the plan of care.

Implementation of Clinical Pathways

The first clinical pathways implemented were scheduled induction of labor, scheduled cesarean birth, and the normal newborn. By using discreet, identifiable groups to begin the process, there was an ability to test the tools, minimize variability, and work out any problems.

Women who were scheduled for induction and cesarean birth were identified from the schedule book prior to the procedure. Physician groups that had agreed to participate were called, and preoperative appointments were scheduled with their patients. Women were asked to report to the care manager's office at the appointed time. The purpose of the initial meeting was to establish rapport, review the components of the clinical pathway, obtain patient input, and identify the patient's educational needs. Emphasis was placed on outcome criteria to be achieved prior to discharge. Laboratory personnel were available during this initial session to obtain blood samples. Follow-up support systems were discussed and reinforced with handouts and videotapes the family could take home. The woman's concerns and questions were addressed before leaving, including appointment time for the scheduled procedure.

After seeing the woman, a portfolio was compiled, including the labor induction or cesarean birth clinical pathway, newborn clinical pathway, physician prenatal record, laboratory results, obstetrical assessment sheet, and suspended physician orders. (Examples of three clinical pathways—vaginal induction, cesarean birth and neonatal care—appear in Chapter Appendix 3-1, 3-2, and 3-3. The portfolio was placed in the front of the woman's chart for easy access and use during the hospital stay. Initially, the portfolio was not a permanent part of the chart, but it has since become integrated into the medical record.

Patients were followed by the care manager on a daily basis. Progress was assessed against the criteria established in the clinical pathway, and variance from the pathway was documented on the variance record for future analysis. All members of the healthcare team were encouraged to chart on the pathway and provide positive and negative feedback. By evaluating patient progress on a daily basis, there were opportunities to identify problems proactively and to intervene to minimize variance.

Evaluation Phase

After the pathway had been in use for about 3 months, there was enough variance information to identify patterns and trends. Volume statistics and quality indicators were used to evaluate the program's impact. Data were tabulated, analyzed, and presented to the group practice for evaluation. Opportunities for improvement were identified, and steps were initiated to resolve problems. Progress continues to be reported formally to the appropriate hospital committees (i.e., Obstetrics and Pediatrics).

Analysis of the Program's Impact

Volume Statistics. Volume statistics were used to quantify and describe the patient population being studied. Elements of data collection included LOS, case type, payor mix, average age, and total number of cases. These statistics are useful for determining the number of patients in the Collaborative Practice program at any given time and to help to determine the financial and clinical impact of the program.

Indicators. The most useful indicators were found to be those identified through variance analysis of our own case types because they are pertinent to the actual patient population (American Hospital Association, 1991). Using this technique, quality indicators were identified for the Perinatal Group Practice, and data were analyzed and presented to the medical committee for approval. Indicators for women with cesarean births that were tracked monthly include hemorrhage, infection, neonatal admission to the ISCU, length of time for bowel sounds to return, readmissions, and mortality.

Thresholds. To monitor the ongoing care patients were to receive, numerical thresholds were established as a measure to evaluate how consistently predicted clinical outcomes were met or exceeded. When available, thresholds were based on national statistics and/or American College of Obstetricians and Gynecologists (ACOG) criteria. When thresholds were not standardized in the literature, 6 to 12 months of hospital data were collected to establish an internal threshold.

Opportunities for Improvement

An opportunity for improvement (OFI) is a tool for problem identification, analysis, action, and evaluation. It (1) identifies the team members responsible for resolution of the problem, (2) summarizes the problem, and (3) outlines the action to be taken, the outcome expected, and to whom it should be reported. It is based on the ten-step monitoring and evaluation process from the Joint Commission on Accreditation of Healthcare Organizations (JCAHO) (Joint Commission on Accreditation of Healthcare Organizations,' 1991). The written tool was developed by SMMC's quality improvement department as a mechanism to reinforce the JCAHO process, document interdisciplinary resolution of problems, and provide periodic evaluation of systems improvement.

An example of an OFI applied to Perinatal Group Practice is postoperative gas formation and pain. Women with cesarean births had an increased LOS related to gas formation, delayed bowel sounds, and delay in feeding. From a literature review, we identified rocking chair therapy as a possible intervention for these women. The study showed mothers who rocked, ate a low-fiber diet, and were given simethicone, ambulated earlier, had a shorter LOS, and used fewer medications than mothers who did not have the intervention (Thomas, Ptak, Giddings, Moore, & Opperman, 1990). To implement these changes, several systems required modification. These included changing medical orders (e.g., diet, activity, and medication); placing rocking chairs in the patient's rooms; and patient, staff, and physician education. The changes were implemented and the results evaluated after 90 days. The outcome of the implementation of rocking-chair therapy was earlier ambulation and decreased gas formation which resulted in a decreased LOS. Results were reported with semiannual statistics to the quality improvement committee, and the original OFI was completed.

Reporting

The variance data are collected daily, tabulated monthly, and reported quarterly to Obstetrics and Pediatrics committees and semiannually to the Quality Improvement Committee and the hospital Board. Standardized forms are used to report data to committees. During the formal presentation of these data, statistics are reviewed and possible changes in practice patterns are identified. Responses to new interventions reported and new practice approaches identified in the literature are explored for possible future implementation. For example, initially all women with cesarean births received incentive spirometer treatments postsurgery. After reviewing our variance report, which was negative for respiratory complications, we reviewed the literature for randomized trials of incentive spirometry use. There was no literature support for this therapy in healthy patients undergoing abdominal surgery. Because our respiratory complication rate was 0%, this information was presented to committee with a recommendation to discontinue incentive spirometry treatment for routine patients. There have been no adverse outcomes related to this practice change.

ADVICE FOR SETTING UP A COLLABORATIVE PRACTICE

After meeting successful implementation in SMMC's inpatient setting, development of programs for outpatient care will be SMMC's next logical step. Another future consideration is to place care managers in the community setting, increasing effectiveness in improving access to care as well as making an impact on healthcare promotion and prevention.

The SMMC model has been offered as an example of Collaborative Practice for Perinatal Care. The model is still developing. In fact, it is hoped that the SMMC model will give an impetus to other hospitals to set up Collaborative Practice as a cost-effective yet patient-safe method of perinatal care. The accompanying display (3-2) outlines strategies for success.

Needs Identification and a Forward Look

The key to starting Collaborative Practice in the perinatal area involves both an identified need for change and a willingness to apply a new perspective to improve patient care.

As described earlier, the situation providing the impetus to try Collaborative Practice at SMMC was patient and staff dissatisfaction with postpartum patient education. The goal was to teach new mothers newborn care prior to discharge from the hospital. This goal was not consistently achieved. When this issue was brought to the Collaborative Group Practice meeting, members were asked to offer a free flow of ideas. It was one of the nonnursing members who pointed out the obvious: There was not enough time in a 12-hour postpartum stay to teach the woman about newborn care. This insight allowed the group to shift focus and formulate new goals.

The current goal of postpartum teaching prior to discharge is to begin teaching newborn care skills. Other goals were identified which extended education into the patient's home. These goals were achieved through the development of a Newborn Care Video parents take home, a Mother's Helper Program, a Visiting Nurse Program, and a Newborn Care Class in which siblings can participate.

The enthusiasm generated by solving one of the major problem-prone activities in the unit led to active staff and patient participation as Collaborative Practice was expanded.

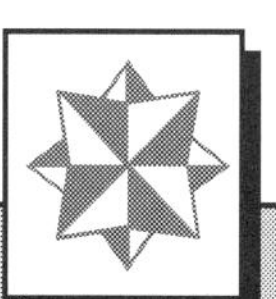

DISPLAY 3-2

Strategies for Success of a Collaborative Group Practice

- Identify a significant high-risk, high-volume, and/or high-cost patient population.
- Solicit volunteers from every area that interfaces with the identified population to participate.
- Talk informally with individuals prior to meetings, to introduce the concepts and elicit spontaneous ideas.
- Consider problems as opportunities to try new ideas. Encourage members to offer ideas freely without regard to cost, previous failure, or obstacles.
- Identify suggestions that solve a piece of the problem. The whole puzzle does not have to be solved at once.
- Do not be afraid to try and fail. Failure may generate a whole new set of solutions.
- Give credit to both individuals and the group as a whole for their ideas.
- Celebrate your successes.

Development of Clinical Pathways

How These Tools Will Be Used

Before beginning development of critical pathways, key decisions must be made related to how these tools will be used. An important issue is whether or not the clinical pathway will replace routine or standing orders. If the clinical pathway will serve the dual purpose of a documentation tool, design must be flexible enough to allow notation of individual clinical situations and include space for dates, times, and provider signatures. A potential benefit of this approach is reduction in nursing time spent on documentation.

A clear definition of what constitutes a variance must be developed. Variances are most useful when they provide clues that the patient is not meeting critical criteria along the pathway, and they allow methods for timely identification and early intervention. The clinical pathway should be written in such a way that individual clinical situations that are within normal parameters do not result in a variance report. For example, educational opportunities may not occur as planned for a variety of reasons. The woman may be too fatigued to discuss details of infant care within the specific time frames of the clinical pathway. There should be enough flexibility to allow this teaching to be incorporated at another, more appropriate time during the hospitalization. However, deviations from essential clinical criteria should be noted and addressed in a timely manner. Examples include maternal temperature over 100.4° F, excessive postpartum bleeding, difficulty in resuming bladder function, delay in return of bowel sounds, and problems in establishing breastfeeding. In addition to deciding variance definition, identification of who will be responsible for variance interventions and tracking this data must be agreed upon by the group. Ideally a care manager will coordinate variance reports and data analysis. One of the most commonly reported frustrations with clinical pathways is the increased paperwork generated and increased time spent by nurse managers manually recording variances. Careful thought should be given to the role of the person responsible for this activity and how the information will be used to enhance quality practice.

Using Routine Orders

The actual development of clinical pathways for perinatal services is not as complex as for medical conditions or surgical procedures in other areas of specialty practice because many perinatal units have routine intrapartum and postpartum orders. These routine orders can provide the framework for initial discussion about clinical pathway development. For example, routine labor admission assessments, laboratory data, intravenous fluids, oral nutrition, methods of fetal monitoring, criteria for ambulation, labor induction/augmentation protocols, anesthesia protocols, immediate postpartum recovery criteria, etc., are frequently already in place. Routine postpartum orders for episiotomy care, incision care, diet advances, ambulation, breast care, medications, and laboratory data are also useful.

Using Protocol and Standards of Care

Tools that may help in developing outcome criteria include national standards from the *Accreditation Manual* (JCAHO, 1995), ACOG Technical Bulletins, *Guidelines for Perinatal Care* (American College of Obstetricians and Gynecologists & American Academy of Pediatrics [ACOG & AAP], 1992), *Practice Resources and Clinical Commentaries* (Association of Women's Health, Obstetric, and Neonatal Nurses [AWHONN]), and risk management protocols.

Most units have a standardized protocol for teaching maternal self-care and infant care. Educational needs can be reevaluated, based on current LOS, and a core list of important issues to be reviewed with the new mother can then be integrated into the clinical pathway at appropriate time frames. For example, it is essential to encourage the initial feeding immediately after birth if the mother has chosen to breastfeed and both mother and newborn are stable. The first ambulation to the bathroom after birth is an appropriate time to begin discussion of pericare and normal lochia characteristics. The newborn's bath at the mother's bedside is an opportunity to begin teaching bathing and infant-safety issues. Planning educational components of postpartum care across the hospitalization period avoids the rushed experience of discharge teaching immediately before mother and newborn are ready to leave for home. The woman and her family members have a chance to integrate some of the new knowledge, and there are real opportunities for follow-up questions and discussions of specific concerns.

Standards of care for vital sign frequency, maternal/fetal assessments, and nurse-patient ratios for common clinical situations are published by professional organizations (see Chapter 2 for examples). Incorporation of established routine orders and professional standards of care into clinical pathways can greatly facilitate the development process.

If individual physician groups have their own routine or standing orders, medical record audits and careful evaluation of patient outcomes for each group can be used to identify "best practice" routines. Data related to outcomes of individual group routine orders can be presented at physician meetings without identifying names. Since the common goal is quality outcome-based practice, most physicians are interested in routines that have demonstrated effectiveness in providing optimal outcomes. In SMMC's experience, the "best practice" routines were quickly adopted by the other physician groups.

Determination of appropriate LOS is usually not the issue for clinical pathways in perinatal services. Increasingly, third-party payors have influenced LOS by prospective payment to institutions, based on prenegotiated LOSs for each DRG. Each contract is different, but generally LOS is predetermined for women experiencing an uncomplicated childbirth and for healthy full-term newborns. When complications occur, recertification for additional LOS usually is required for reimbursement by third-party payors.

Drafting Tools

A multidisciplinary core group can use these tools to draft clinical pathways for the most common high-volume groups such as vaginal birth without complications, scheduled cesarean birth, and the healthy newborn. The key to success is participation by all care providers including physicians, nurses, anesthesia personnel, dietary staff, social workers, and home health caregivers. Representatives from these areas can work together to develop a draft which can be distributed to all potential providers for input. It is important that core group members include direct-care providers as well as administrators. Bedside nurses have a unique perspective and can provide keen insight as to appropriate interventions, realistic time frames, and achievable outcomes. Modifications can be made after suggestions from noncommittee members are reviewed.

After successful implementation of the initial clinical pathways, attention can be directed to development of clinical pathways or clinical algorithms for common complications such as pregnancy-induced hypertension, preterm labor, and neonatal sepsis, etc. The same process of group collaboration can be used.

SUMMARY

Collaborative Practice is a proactive, systematic approach to patient care that reduces performance variability, promotes consistency and continuity, and reduces risk of patient complications through ongoing monitoring and evaluation. The ongoing effectiveness of perinatal Collaborative Practice is monitored through the core group and the respective medical committees. Collaborative Practice is effective in the perinatal arena even though LOS is measured in hours and patients are generally healthy. The focus on increasing patient satisfaction, systems improvements, and continuously looking for new ways to improve clinical outcomes results in a responsive environment that delivers a high-quality, comprehensive, and cost-effective perinatal care.

References

American Academy of Pediatrics. American College of Obstetricians and Gynecologists (1992). Guidelines for perinatal care (3rd ed.). Washington, DC: Author.

American Hospital Association. (1991). Practice pattern analysis: A tool for continuous improvement of patient care quality. Chicago: Author.

Cohen, E.L., & Cesta, T.G. (1993). Nursing case management: From concept to evaluation. St. Louis, MO: Mosby.

Joint Commission on Accreditation of Healthcare Organizations. (1991). What is quality improvement? In An introduction to quality improvement in health care (pp. 13-38). Chicago: Author.

Joint Commission on Accreditation of Healthcare Organizations. (1995). Accreditation manual for hospitals. Chicago: Author.

Leebow, W. (1991). The quality quest: A briefing for health care professionals. Chicago: American Hospital Association.

Nugent, K.E. (1992). The clinical nurse specialist as case manager in a collaborative practice model: Bridging the gap between quality and cost of care. Clinical Nurse Specialist, 6(2), 106-111.

Thomas, L., Ptak, H., Giddings, L.S., Moore, L., & Oppermann, C. (1990). The effects of rocking, diet modifications, and antiflatulent medication on post cesarean section gas pain. The Journal of Perinatal and Neonatal Nursing, 4(3), 12-24.

APPENDIX 3-1. Vaginal Induction

DISCHARGE OUTCOMES:

	Yes	No
1. Ambulate without assistance.	☐	☐
2. Temperature < 100°.	☐	☐
3. BP < 90 diastolic and < 140 systolic.	☐	☐
4. Hgb > 9.0.	☐	☐
5. Patient voids > 100cc without difficulty.	☐	☐
6. Menstrual flow moderate without clots.	☐	☐
7. No CVA tenderness.	☐	☐
8. Negative Homan's sign.	☐	☐
9. Incision dry and healing.	☐	☐
10. Patient reports pain control w/oral analgesia.	☐	☐
11. Fundus firm, less than +2U.	☐	☐
12. D/C booklet/video received.	☐	☐
13. Patient demonstrates ability to care for baby.	☐	☐
14. MD DC order.	☐	☐

* Comment in Nursing Notes for outcomes not met.

Patient Signature ____________ Date ________ Date of D/C ________

SADDLEBACK MEMORIAL MEDICAL CENTER

PERINATAL CLINICAL PATHWAY

INDUCTION OF LABOR

PHYSICIAN: ______________________

PATIENT ADDRESSOGRAPH

DATE: / HOSPITAL AREA: / DILATION:	O.P. / LDRP	ADM 4 HRS. / LDRP / 0-4 cm	8 HRS. / LDRP / 5-10 cm	12 HRS. / LDRP / DELIVERY	16 HRS. / LDRP	28 HRS. / LDRP-11:00 A.M.
CONSULTS	Care Manager or Clin III		Anesthesia			
ACTIVITY		Ambulate Rocking chair	Bed	Ambulate 2-4° delivery Breast feeds < 2°		Shower
TREATMENTS	CBC Hold clot	AROM Telemetry Dip UA - send if +	Epidural Datascope: q 5 min. X 30 minutes q 30 min until delivery Cooling measures	Delivery VS 15 min x 4 then VS q 8° DC datascope/Epi Icepack	Jacuzzi DC IV	H&H Jacuzzi
MEDICATIONS	Prostin gel	Pain meds prn Pit/active management		Pain/sleep meds prn	Stool softener Pain meds prn	DC meds Rubella vaccine Rho Gam
FLUIDS/ NUTRITION	NPO after midnight	Ice chips IV LR	IV Ice chips	Regular diet	Regular diet	
TEACHING	Anesthesia/Analgesia	Review breathing & pain control options; sibling visitation		Discharge packet Video, booklet	Infant feeding: Breast Bottle	Baby care Self care Activity
REFERRALS/ OTHER	OSCAR orders entered	OSCAR orders Admission Assessment Sign Circ. Consent Sign Tubal Consent	Assess need for Social Service referral	Activate post-partum orders		RN home visit OB appt. 6 weeks Lactation specialist Peds appointment Home helper New babies class
NSG. PROTOCOL		___ Pitocin Protocol - - - - - - - - ___ Epidural Protocol - - - - - - - -	- - - - - - - -	- - - - - - - -		
R.N. SIGNATURE	A.M. ______ P.M. ______	A.M. ______ P.M. ______	A.M. ______ P.M. ______	A.M. ______ P.M. ______	A.M. ______ P.M. ______	A.M. ______ P.M. ______

PERINATAL COLLABORATIVE PRACTICE

indction.lh 2/94

APPENDIX 3-2. Cesarean Section

DISCHARGE OUTCOMES:

	Yes	No
1. Ambulate without assistance.	☐	☐
2. Temperature: < 100°.	☐	☐
3. BP: < 90 diastolic; < 140 systolic.	☐	☐
4. Hgb: > 9.0.	☐	☐
5. Voids > 100cc without difficulty.	☐	☐
6. Flow moderate without clots.	☐	☐
7. No CVA tenderness.	☐	☐
8. Homan's sign.	☐	☐
9. Incision dry and healing.	☐	☐
10. Patient reports pain control with oral analgesia.	☐	☐
11. Fundus firm, less than +2U.	☐	☐
12. Parents demonstrate ability to care for infant.	☐	☐
13. M.D. D/C order.	☐	☐

* Comment in Nursing Notes for outcomes not met.

Patient Signature ______ Date ______ Date of D/C ______

SADDLEBACK MEMORIAL MEDICAL CENTER

PERINATAL CLINICAL PATHWAY

CESAREAN SECTION

DRG: ________

PHYSICIAN: ______________________

PT. ADDRESSOGRAPH

DATE: HOSPITAL AREA:	OP LDRP	DOS OR/LDRP	PO 1 LDRP	PO 2 LDRP	PO 3 LDRP
CONSULTS	CNS	Consent C/S Consent TL Consent for Circumcision			
ACTIVITY		Dangle at 6° Ambulate by 12° Turn q 2° Breast feeding	Ambulate Rocker 4 x 15 minutes Shower --->\ Breast feeding --->	---> ---> ---> --->	---> ---> ---> --->
TESTS	CBC T&S Dip UA - send if +	Bowel sounds Rho Gam studies (if indicated)	BS in 4 quadrants	Hbg/Hct Pass flatus	BM
TREATMENTS		Foley cath IV LR Abd. clipper Dressing check Incentive spirometry	Dressing removed Foley dc'd	Incision check Sign Birth Certificate	Staples dc'd Steri-strips applied
MEDICATIONS		Mylicon Benadryl as indicated	Mylicon Anaprox prn Rho Gam (if indicated)	---> --->	---> ---> Rubella vaccine
FLUIDS/ NUTRITION	NPO after midnight	Advance if + B.S. Warm Cl Liq P.O. I&O	Low fiber diet if + B.S.	Low fiber diet	Low fiber diet
TEACHING	Ambulate Incentive Spirometry VBAC Brochure Anesthesia questions Car seat	Infant feeding	Discharge packet, Video, Booklet	--->	---> Self care Activity
REFERRALS/OTHER	OSCAR orders entered	Activate OSCAR orders	Activate post-partum orders		Referral to: RN home visit OB appt. - 6 weeks Lactation specialist Pediatrician appt. Home helper New babies class
NSG. PROTOCOL		___ Epidural Protocol ________________ ___ Intraspinal Protocol ________________			
RN SIGNATURE	A.M. ________ P.M. ________	A.M. ________ P.M. ________	A.M. ________ P.M. ________	A.M. ________ P.M. ________	A.M. ________ P.M. ________

PERINATAL COLLABORATIVE PRACTICE

PS-SMMC.01 2/94

APPENDIX 3-3. Normal Newborn

DISCHARGE OUTCOMES:

		Yes	No
1.	Feeding: q 2-4° br/form.	☐	☐
2.	Void: X1.	☐	☐
3.	Stool: X1.	☐	☐
4.	Cord dry or clamp intact, no redness or induration.	☐	☐
5.	Temperature: > 98 and < 100°F.	☐	☐
6.	Heart rate: 100 - 180.	☐	☐
7.	Respirations: 30 - 60.	☐	☐
8.	D/C weight w/n 10% of birth weight.	☐	☐
9.	Blood pressure: mean > 40.	☐	☐
10.	Newborn screen drawn.	☐	☐
11.	MD exam w/n 24 hours of D/C.	☐	☐
12.	Maternal HbSAG documented on chart. Pediatrician notified if +; neonate vac. if + or if HbSAG unobtainable.	☐	☐
13.	Circumcision: no active bleeding.	☐	☐
14.	No jaundice if D/C < 24 hours.	☐	☐
15.	Birth certificate signed.	☐	☐
16.	ID bands verified and removed.	☐	☐
17.	MD D/C order.	☐	☐

* Comment in Nursing Notes for outcomes not met.

Patient Signature ________ Date ________ Date of D/C ________

SADDLEBACK MEMORIAL MEDICAL CENTER

PERINATAL CLINICAL PATHWAY

NORMAL NEWBORN

DRG: ________

PHYSICIAN: ________________________

PATIENT ADDRESSOGRAPH

DATE: / HOSPITAL AREA:	0-4 HRS. / LDRP	8 HRS. / LDRP	12 HRS. / LDRP	16 HRS. / LDRP	20 HRS. / LDRP	24 HRS. / LDRP-11:00 A.M.
CONSULTS	Pediatrician notified Circumcision consent signed, on newborn chart					
ACTIVITY	Footprints				Photo	
TESTS	NB admission completed Document B.G. & Hct if indicated				Weigh NB screen BP	
TREATMENTS	V.S q hour x 4 Bath Cord care				Circumcision Circumcision observation x 2° Remove cord clamp or instruct mother to see Pediatrician Cord care	
MEDICATIONS	Erythromycin Vitamin K *HBIG/Heptavax after bath if indicated					
FLUIDS/ NUTRITION	Feed q 2-4°	Feed q 2-4°	Feed q 2-4°	Feed q 2-4°	Feed q 2-4°	Feed q 2-4°
TEACHING	Mom bath demo Cord care Diaper change Temperature	Feeding video	Discharge instructions Infant care video Discharge booklet			Circumcision care
REFERRALS/ OTHER	OSCAR orders activated				Birth Certificate	Pediatrician appt. Lactation consult Home helper Comp. home visit
R.N. SIGNATURE	A.M. ______ P.M. ______	A.M. ______ P.M. ______	A.M. ______ P.M. ______	A.M. ______ P.M. ______	A.M. ______ P.M. ______	A.M. ______ P.M. ______

newborn.lb 12/93

PART 2

Antepartum

Physiologic Changes of Pregnancy

Mary Kay Fallon

Pregnancy is a dynamic state. The body and its respective systems undergo dramatic changes to meet the demands of the developing fetus.

Maternal adaptations are attributed to significant hormonal changes and mechanical pressures exerted from the growing fetus and enlarging uterus. These changes protect the woman's normal physiologic functioning and facilitate fetal development. Physiologic changes in pregnancy affect normal physical findings and laboratory values. An understanding of normal physiologic changes of pregnancy is essential to recognize normal or potentially abnormal responses. It is important to realize that values and physical findings considered normal in the nonpregnant woman may not be useful in assessing women during pregnancy.

The following review of normal physiologic changes during pregnancy will serve as a baseline of information to guide the healthcare provider in conducting an accurate and thorough assessment of the pregnant woman.

CARDIOVASCULAR SYSTEM

The cardiovascular system undergoes the most profound changes during pregnancy (Brinkman, 1993; Harvey & Moretti, 1993) (Table 4-1). These changes are necessary in order to support the additional maternal and fetal circulatory requirements and include both anatomic and hemodynamic alterations. Changes occurring in the cardiovascular system have an impact on all organ systems.

Heart

The growing uterus exerts pressure on the diaphragm, displacing the heart upwardly and to the left. The heart enlarges due to increases in blood volume and cardiac output during pregnancy. The left ventricle is slightly enlarged due to increased blood volume. Cardiac volume increases approximately 10–20% (75 ml) (Hume & Killam, 1990).

Heart rate increases 10–20 beats/min at term. In the twin pregnancies, maternal heart rate increases as much as 40% above nonpregnant levels at term (Elkayam & Gleicher, 1990). Immediately after birth, as the uterus contracts it shunts blood into the systemic circulation increasing venous return to the heart. This results in an autotransfusion of approximately 1,000 ml. (Harvey & Moretti, 1993). Cardiac output increases from the release of obstructed venous return to the heart and the mobilization of intracellular fluid. Heart rate slows, but the woman is able to maintain an adequate cardiac output due to the increase in stroke volume (Cruikshank & Hays, 1991). By 6 weeks postpartum, heart rate returns to a prepregnant rate.

A systolic murmur may be heard in approximately 90% of pregnant women although there are no characteristic changes in the electrocardiogram (Gibbs, 1981). Physical symptoms may occur during pregnancy in response to normal cardiovascular changes. Some women report palpitations, light headedness, or a decreased tolerance for activity. Dependent edema may also be present and worsen as pregnancy progresses.

Blood Volume

To support maternal and fetal circulation, blood volume increases approximately 45% (1,450–1,750 ml) by 32 weeks of gestation. This increase begins in the first trimester, reaches a peak in the third trimester, and returns to a prepregnant volume 2 to 3 weeks postpartum. Blood volume is greater in multiple

TABLE 4-1. Cardiovascular Changes During Pregnancy

Parameter	Change
Heart Rate	Increases 15% (10–20 bpm)
Blood Volume	Increases 45% (1,450–1,750 ml)
Plasma Volume	Increases 45% (1,200–1,300 ml)
Red Cell Mass	Increases 20%–30% (250–450 ml)
Cardiac Output	Increases 30%–50% (6.2±1.0 L/min)
Stroke Volume	Increases 50%
Systemic Vascular Resistance	Decreases 21%
Colloid Oncotic Pressure	Decreases 20% (23 mmHg)

gestations (2,000–2,500 ml) and increases according to number of fetuses (Lee & Cotton, 1991).

Alterations in blood volume are necessary to provide adequate blood flow to the uterus, fetus, and changing maternal tissues and to accommodate blood loss at delivery. This increase in blood volume results from increases in plasma volume and red cell mass.

Plasma volume increases approximately 45% (1,200–1,300 ml) by term. Red cell mass increases 20–30% (250–450 ml). The rapid increase in plasma volume and later rise in red blood cell (RBC) volume results in hemodilution. This is often referred to as the "physiologic anemia of pregnancy" (Drummond, 1992) although this is not a true pathologic state. This hemodilution is believed to reduce the risk of thrombus formation by decreasing blood viscosity and enhancing uteroplacental circulation. Even with an increased RBC production, hemoglobin values decrease during pregnancy (12–16 g/dl blood) and the hematocrit values decrease as well (37–47%). This decrease is more obvious during the second trimester when the rapid increase in blood volume occurs (Klein, 1995).

Increased levels of estrogen and progesterone cause increases in both plasma renin activity and aldosterone levels. These increases cause tubular reabsorption of sodium and an increase in total body water (Davison, 1985). Total body water increases by six to eight liters, of which four to six are extracellular (Fuschino, 1992). Progesterone produces venous wall relaxation to accommodate the increase in blood volume.

After childbirth, the contracted uterus shunts blood from uterine vessels into the systemic circulation, causing an autotransfusion of approximately 1,000 ml. The rise in cardiac output is accompanied by a reflex decrease in heart rate, and therefore, stroke volume is greatly increased and persists for 1 to 2 weeks following the birth (Cruikshank & Hays, 1991). Average blood loss at birth ranges from 500–600 ml for a vaginal birth to 800–1,200 ml for a cesarean birth or vaginal birth of multiples (Fuschino, 1992). Blood loss during birth accompanied by the postpartum diuresis reduces the plasma volume within 5 days postpartum (Metcalfe, McAnulty, & Ueland, 1981) and returns to prepregnant levels 2 to 3 weeks postpartum.

Cardiac Output

Cardiac output increases 30–50% during pregnancy and reaches a volume of 6–7 L/min (Harvey, 1992). This increase begins in the first trimester, peaks in the second trimester, and remains at this level until term. In early pregnancy, the increase in cardiac output is primarily due to an increase in stroke volume. Stroke volume is determined by preload and afterload volumes and contractility. As pregnancy progresses, the increase in cardiac output results from an increase in heart rate. Changes in cardiac output during the intrapartum period are dependent upon maternal position, type of anesthesia, and method of delivery.

Maternal position can greatly influence cardiac output. Changes can be most dramatic during the third trimester. In the supine position, pressure exerted on the inferior vena cava from the gravid uterus decreases venous return and, therefore, results in decreased cardiac output. This position may also lead to supine hypotension with diaphoresis and possible syncope. Changing from the supine position to the lateral position can increase cardiac output 25–30% (Harvey, 1991), with a resultant increase in uterine and renal blood flow. It is important to note that recent studies demonstrate not only left, as previously believed, but both right and left lateral positions optimize cardiac output (Clark et al., 1991). Cardiac output is optimized in the lateral position, somewhat decreased in the sitting position, and markedly decreased in the supine position (Clark et al., 1991).

Cardiac output rises progressively during labor (Drummond, 1992) (Table 4-2). Uterine contractions create a rise in intrauterine pressure forcing blood into the systemic circulation, resulting in an autotransfusion and subsequent 10–25% transitory rise in cardiac output (Mangano, 1993).

Epidural anesthesia causes a decrease in venous return, resulting in decreased cardiac output. This decrease may be reversed or prevented with an intravenous fluid bolus before epidural placement. A well-managed epidural decreases pain, anxiety, and bearing-down efforts and prevents a rapid rise in cardiac output (Clark, 1981). General anesthesia decreases

TABLE 4-2. Intrapartum Increases in Cardiac Output

Labor Phase/Stage	Increase Above Prelabor Values
Latent Phase	15%
Active Phase	30%
Second Stage	45%
Immediately After Birth	65%

cardiac output, whereas local or paracervical anesthesia demonstrates a rise in cardiac output (Harvey, 1991).

Cardiac output increases significantly during the bearing-down efforts of a vaginal birth, while a cesarean birth may eliminate the increase in cardiac output, which occurs during second stage Valsalva's maneuver.

Immediately after birth, there is a dramatic increase in cardiac output. Pressure exerted by the fetus and placenta no longer exist after birth allowing improved blood flow from the lower extremities to the heart. In order to prevent hemorrhage, uterine vessels constrict after delivery of the placenta, shunting blood from uterine to systemic circulation. This autotransfusion of approximately 1,000 ml of blood maintains cardiac output even with a decrease in heart rate. Cardiac output progressively decreases and returns to nonpregnant levels by 6 weeks postpartum (Fuschino, 1992).

Distribution of Blood Flow

The majority of increased cardiac output and blood volume during pregnancy is distributed to the uterus, kidneys, breasts, and skin. The uterus accommodates one third of the additional blood volume at term (approximately 500 ml/min). The kidneys receive approximately 400 ml/min, a 30% increase. Glandular growth, distended veins, and engorgement reflect increased blood flow to the breast. Hyperemia of the cervix and vagina is also evident. Blood flow to the maternal skin increases to accommodate the additional heat loss requirements created by the active metabolism of the fetus (Metcalfe, Stock, & Barron, 1988).

Systemic Vascular Resistance

Systemic vascular resistance (SVR) decreases during pregnancy. The uteroplacental vascular system is a low-resistance network using a large percentage of maternal cardiac output. Progesterone produces relaxation of smooth muscle and vasodilation. Uterine vascular resistance also decreases during pregnancy and thus enhances increased uterine blood flow. Systemic vascular resistance decreases in early pregnancy, with a gradual increase by term. Mean SVR approximates nonpregnant values at term (Clark et al., 1989).

Blood Pressure

Blood pressure gradually decreases approximately 5–10 mmHg in the first trimester as a result of peripheral vasodilation. Change in blood pressure reflects a decrease in SVR and an increase in blood volume. Blood pressure reaches its lowest point in the second trimester and returns to prepregnant levels by the third trimester. Systolic pressure may decrease 10–15 mmHg while diastolic pressure drops 20–25 mmHg (Cugini et al., 1992). Pulse pressure (difference between systolic and diastolic pressure) widens slightly during the first two trimesters and returns to prepregnant values at term.

Maternal position influences blood pressure. Blood pressure is highest in the sitting position, lowest in the left lateral position, and intermediate in the supine position. Blood pressure increases during contractions and returns to baseline after contractions (Blackburn & Loper, 1992).

Renin, an enzyme produced in the kidneys, increases during pregnancy. Renin acts on its substrate angiotensinogen in the liver to form angiotensin I then angiotensin II that acts as a vasoconstrictor. During pregnancy, levels of angiotensin I and II increase; however, the pregnant woman is resistant to the pressor effects of angiotensin II. Women with preeclampsia lose this decreased sensitivity to angiotensin and blood pressure rises (Whalley, Everett, Gant, Cox, & MacDonald, 1983). Blood pressure does not change after birth or during the postpartum period unless significant blood loss occurs.

Hematologic Changes

To meet additional oxygen requirements of pregnancy, RBC volume increases 18–30%. Plasma volume increases to a greater degree than erythrocyte increase; therefore, the hematocrit decreases approximately 7%. Normal hematocrit values for pregnancy range between 37–47% (Klein, 1995).

Hemoglobin levels during pregnancy range between 12–16 g/dl (Klein, 1995). With the increase in the number of RBCs, the need for iron for the production of hemoglobin also increases. Gastrointestinal absorption of iron is increased during pregnancy, and additional iron supplementation is necessary. If iron stores are initially low and supplemental iron is not added to enhance the diet, iron deficiency anemia may result (Mashburn, Graves, & Gillmor-Kahn, 1992). The fetus uses iron from maternal stores if iron is not readily available.

Leukocyte production is equal to or slightly greater than blood volume. An average white cell count in the third trimester is 5,000–12,000/mm^3. Labor and early postpartum levels may reach 25,000/mm^3 or greater, without presence of infection (Cruikshank & Hays, 1991).

Coagulation and fibrinolytic systems undergo major changes during pregnancy. Pregnancy is considered a hypercoagulable state due to the increased levels of several essential coagulation factors. Increases occur in factor I (fibrinogen); in factors V, VII, VIII, IX, X, XII; and in prothrombin time during pregnancy (Sisson, 1992). (See Table 4-3 for summary of changes in clotting factors during pregnancy.) These changes occur to support the pregnancy and to accommodate blood loss at birth. Bleeding time, clotting time, and platelets remain unchanged despite an increase in clotting factors. Platelet counts range between 140,000–400,000. These changes and venous stasis place the pregnant woman at increased risk for venous thrombosis.

Following delivery, coagulation is initiated to prevent hemorrhage. Fibrinogen decreases as fibrin clots form, and platelets decrease to enhance clot formation.

Women with normal cardiovascular functioning should be able to accommodate the dramatic cardiovascular changes associated with pregnancy. Women with previous cardiovascular disease are at increased risk for complications during pregnancy and during the postpartum period, mainly due to alterations in volume and cardiac output.

RESPIRATORY SYSTEM

Changes in the respiratory system are required to accommodate increased maternal-fetal oxygenation requirements.

Structural Changes

Pressure from the uterus shifts the diaphragm upward 4 cm, decreasing the length of the lungs. To adjust to this decrease in length, the anteroposterior diameter of the chest enlarges by 2 cm. Increased pressure from the uterus widens the substernal angle 50%, which then causes lower ribs to flare out. Circumference of the thoracic cage may increase 5–7 cm, compensating for the decrease in lung length (Klein, 1995). Many of these changes are probably caused by hormonal influence since they occur before pressure is exerted from the growing uterus.

Breathing is more diaphragmatic than costal during pregnancy. These structural changes occur so that lung volume is not affected during pregnancy. (See Table 4-4 for changes in respiratory function during pregnancy.)

Lung Volume

Most changes are created by the rise in diaphragm and changes in the chest wall. Tidal volume (amount of air inspired and expired with normal breath) increases 30–40% from 500 to 700 ml. Vital capacity (maximum amount of air that can be forcibly expired after maximum inspiration) and inspiratory reserve volume (maximum amount of air that can be inspired at end of normal inspiration) remain unchanged. Expiratory reserve volume (maximal amount of air that can be expired from resting expiratory level) falls 20% (Moore, 1991).

The increase in tidal volume is responsible for the increase in respiratory minute volume (Cruikshank & Hays, 1991). The volume of the lungs is decreased due to the elevated diaphragm, which reduces total lung volume (amount of air in lungs at maximal inspiration) and residual volume (amount of air in lungs after maximum expiration) 5% and 20% respectively. Functional residual capacity (FRC) (amount of air remaining in the lungs at resting expiratory level, permitting air for gas exchange between breaths) is reduced by 20%, (Ueland, 1986).

TABLE 4-3. Clotting Factors During Pregnancy

Parameter	Change
Fibrin	Increases 40% at term
Plasma Fibrinogen	Increases 50% 300–600 mg/dl
Clotting Time	Unchanged
Coagulation Factors V, VII, VIII, IX, X, XII	Increases
Coagulation Factors XI, XIII	Decreases Slightly
Prothrombin Time	Increases Slightly or Unchanged
Platelets	Unchanged 140,000–440,000

TABLE 4-4. Respiratory Changes During Pregnancy

Parameter	Change
Tidal Volume	Increases 30–40%, from 500–700 ml.
Vital Capacity	Unchanged
Inspiratory Reserve Volume	Unchanged
Expiratory Reserve Volume	Decreases 20%
Respiratory Rate	Unchanged or slight increase
Functional Residual Capacity	Decreases 20%
Total Lung Volume	Decreases 5%
Residual Volume	Decreases 20%
Minute Ventilation	Increases 40%
pH	Slight increase to 7.40–7.45
Oxygen Consumption	Increases 15–20%
PaO_2	104–108 mmHg
$PaCO_2$	27–32 mmHg

Ventilation

Minute ventilation (amount of air inspired in 1 minute) increases 40% during late pregnancy and reaches 6.5–10 L/min at term. Minute ventilation is the product of the respiratory rate and the tidal volume. In pregnancy, the increase in minute ventilation is due to an increase in tidal volume since the respiratory rate remains unchanged for increases only slightly (Geiger-Bronsky, 1992). During labor, tidal volume can reach 40 L/min.

Oxygenation

Oxygen consumption increases 15–20% during pregnancy and may increase 300% during labor (Martin, 1992). This leads to increased alveolar and arterial PO_2 levels. Normal range for PaO_2 levels in late pregnancy is 104–108 mmHg.

$PaCO_2$ levels range from 27–32 mmHg in the second half of pregnancy, as compared to nonpregnant levels of 40 mmHg. The lower maternal $PaCO_2$ levels permit transfer of CO_2 from the fetus to the mother. During pregnancy, increased renal excretion of bicarbonate causes a slight increase in pH. This increase in pH facilitates the removal of fetal carbon dioxide. The acid-base status during pregnancy reflects a compensated respiratory alkalosis.

Circulating hemoglobin increases 20%. Maternal hemoglobin has a decreased affinity for oxygen while fetal hemoglobin has an increased affinity for oxygen. Oxygen consumption increases as pregnancy advances and is greater in multiple gestation. Fifty percent of oxygen is distributed to reproductive tissues and the fetus, and can reach 250–750 ml/min during labor. Oxygen consumption and respiratory rate increase during labor.

Most authors cite no change in respiratory rate during pregnancy (Cruikshank & Hays, 1991; Hume & Killam, 1990; Moore, 1991) while others report only a slight increase (Brinkman, 1989; Klein, 1995; Harvey & Moretti, 1993). Sixty to seventy percent of women report feeling shortness of breath at some time during their pregnancy (Thappa & Sicilian, 1992). The exact cause of this dyspnea is unclear but includes theories on hyperventilation, the effects of progesterone, increased oxygen consumption, and decreased $PaCO_2$ levels. Symptoms of nasal stuffiness and epistaxis may also be common for pregnant women and are related to vascular congestion resulting from increased levels of estrogen.

RENAL SYSTEM

Changes in renal function occur to accommodate the increased metabolic and circulatory requirements of pregnancy. The renal system excretes both maternal and fetal waste products. Pressure placed on the renal system and the relaxation effect of progesterone help the renal system accommodate to cardiovascular changes of pregnancy.

Structural Changes

The renal system undergoes both structural and functional changes during pregnancy. Kidneys enlarge 1–1.5 cm in length due to increased renal vascular and interstitial volume (Cunningham, MacDonald, Gant, Leveno, & Gilstrap, 1993). Relaxing effects of progesterone on smooth muscle are probably responsible for the dilation of the renal calyces, pelves, and ureters. Later in the gestation, the growing uterus places pressure on the ureters and bladder. The ureters become dilated and elongated. Dilation of the right side is more pronounced than that on the left due to the cushioning which occurs on the left side (Beydoun, 1985).

After 4 months of pregnancy, hyperemia of pelvic organs and hyperplasia of all muscles and connective tissues elevate the bladder and cause thickening of the interuretic margin (Kincaid-Smith & Fairley, 1993). The bladder is pushed forward and upward. Pressure placed on the bladder changes it from a convex to a concave organ, and retention capacity is decreased. Pressure on the renal system can impair drainage of blood and lymph, which increases risk of infection and trauma during pregnancy. The urethra also increases in length.

Renal Blood Flow and Glomerular Filtration Rate

Blood flow through the kidneys increases 25–50% during pregnancy. Glomerular filtration rate (GFR) increases approximately 50% by the second trimester. Renal plasma flow (RPF) increases 25–50% throughout early pregnancy and reaches 60–80% by midpregnancy (Davison, 1985). Urinary frequency is experienced by many women during pregnancy. GFR and RPF begin to rise after 12 weeks of gestation and continue rising until term. Women lying in the supine position can have a decrease in GFR and RPF in late pregnancy.

Many of the changes occurring in the renal system are thought to be related to the growth hormone effect of placental lactogen. Increased blood volume and cardiac output, with a lowered peripheral vascular resistance in the kidneys, accommodates the increased blood flow.

The increase in GFR is greater than the increase in RPF, which allows a greater proportion of plasma to be filtered; therefore, serum protein concentration in plasma is lowered approximately 1 g/L. This decreases the plasma oncotic pressure approximately 20%. Decreased colloid oncotic pressure facilitates the increased filtration of plasma by the kidneys.

With an increased GFR and RPF, the renal clearance of many substances is elevated during pregnancy with a related decrease in serum levels. Amino acids, glucose, proteins, electrolytes, and vitamins are excreted. (See Table 4-5 for changes in both the blood and urine.)

Serum urea and creatinine levels decline due to increased GFR. Blood urea nitrogen levels fall 25%. Serum uric acid levels decrease and rise again after 24 weeks.

Fluid and Electrolyte Balance

Potassium excretion is decreased to meet maternal-fetal growth demands. Kidneys play a significant role in the regulation of sodium content in the body. Intake or loss of sodium is compensated by changes in tubular reabsorption to keep sodium levels carefully balanced. Tubular reabsorption adjusts to changes in the filtered load of sodium. During pregnancy, there is a tendency for sodium depletion, making sodium regulation more difficult. As blood volume increases, sodium retention gradually occurs, which is necessary to maintain serum electrolyte balance.

Additional sodium is required during pregnancy to meet the need for increased intravascular and extracellular fluid volumes and to maintain a normal isotonic state. Increased GFR in pregnancy is accompanied by an increase in tubular reabsorption of sodium to prevent depletion. An increase in aldosterone levels is the primary factor in preventing sodium diureses. Plasma aldosterone levels increase to 200–700 mg/L as compared to 100–200 mg/l in nonpregnancy.

Renal sodium is the primary determinant of volume homeostasis. The filtered load of sodium increases from nonpregnant levels of 20,000 mEq/d to approximately 30,000 mEq/d during pregnancy (Davison, 1985). These changes are accompanied by increases in tubular reabsorption of sodium in order to avoid sodium depletion. An additional 2–6 mEq of sodium are reabsorbed each day for fetal and maternal stores. A gradual increase to 900 mEq of sodium is normally retained during pregnancy to meet fetal needs (Klein, 1995). Increases in GFR, increases in antidiuretic hormone, decreases in plasma albumin, elevated progesterone levels, and decreased vascular resistance all contribute to sodium excretion during pregnancy. Increases in aldosterone, estrogen, cortisol, prolactin, and placental lactogen all contribute to sodium reabsorption (Harvey & Moretti, 1993). Calcium and phosphorus are also excreted, creating an increased need for calcium during pregnancy.

TABLE 4-5. Laboratory Mean Values During Pregnancy: Renal Function

	Nonpregnant	Pregnant	
BLOOD			
Serum Creatinine	0.6–1.2 mg/dl	Decreases to	
		First Trimester	0.73 mg/dl
		Second Trimester	0.58 mg/dl
		Third Trimester	0.53 mg/dl
Blood Urea Nitrogen	8–20 mg/dl	Decreases to	
		First Trimester	11 mg/dl
		Second Trimester	9 mg/dl
		Third Trimester	10 mg/dl
Uric Acid	4.5–5.8 mg/dl	Decreases to	
		First Trimester	3.1mg/dl
		Second Trimester	2.0–3.0 mg/dl
		Increases to	
		Term	4.5–5.8 mg/dl
URINE			
Creatinine Clearance	90–130 ml/min/1.73m^2	Increases to 150–200 ml/min/1.73m^2	
Urea		Increases	
Uric Acid	250–750 mg/24 hr	Increases	
Glucose	60–115 mg/dl	Increases	

Glycosuria

There is no glomerular tubular balancing mechanism for glucose and amino acids. Renal tubules are unable to absorb the increased glucose load filtered by the glomeruli; therefore, glycosuria during pregnancy is common. Excess glucose is excreted in the urine and is not considered pathogenic during pregnancy. Clinical management of the woman with diabetes requires serum glucose evaluation rather than urine glucose evaluation during pregnancy.

Proteinuria

There may be an increase in excreted protein during pregnancy due to the increased GFR, but this increase should not be considered abnormal until it reaches amounts greater than 250 mg/dl. Levels higher than 250 mg/dl may indicate renal disease, preeclampsia, or urinary tract infection (Harvey, 1991).

GASTROINTESTINAL SYSTEM

Nutritional requirements during pregnancy increase, and changes in the gastrointestinal system occur to meet these demands. The alimentary tract is altered both physiologically and anatomically during pregnancy. Gastrointestinal tone and motility of the stomach are decreased during pregnancy due to the relaxing effect of progesterone on smooth muscle (Harvey & Moretti, 1993). Nausea and vomiting during early pregnancy is a common complaint and affects 50–80% of women (Anderson, Fullerton, & Newman, 1993). Several theories as to the cause of nausea and vomiting have been proposed, including relaxation of the smooth muscle of the stomach, elevated levels of steroid hormones and human chorionic gonadotropin (hCG) (Cruikshank & Hays, 1991; Key, 1989; Taylor & Pernoll, 1991), and emotional tension (Taylor & Pernoll, 1991). Soules et al. (1980) found no relationship between the levels of hCG and 17-hydroxyprogesterone and the incidence or severity of nausea and vomiting in pregnant women or women with molar pregnancies. In pregnancies where chorionic gonadotropins were unusually elevated, nausea and vomiting were likely to be more frequent and severe (Key).

Treatment is supportive and involves instructing the woman to avoid foods that trigger nausea and to eat smaller meals more frequently. Hyperemesis gravidarum is a more pronounced form of nausea and vomiting and is associated with weight loss, electrolyte imbalance, ketonemia, and dehydration. Any underlying illness should be ruled out and hospitalization for fluid and electrolyte replacement may be necessary.

Many of the common discomforts of pregnancy can be attributed to the gastrointestinal system. Sensitivity to taste and smell can also lead to gastrointestinal discomfort. Ptyalism may increase or become excessive. Hyperemia and softening of the gums may cause them to bleed easily.

Stomach

The stomach is displaced by the gravid uterus. Tone and motility of the stomach are decreased. Relaxation of the esophageal sphincter permits reflux of gastric contents into the esophagus causing pyrosis (heartburn). Gastric reflux is more common in later pregnancy. This regurgitation is due to displacement of the stomach, relaxation of the esophageal sphincter, and delayed gastric emptying time (Harvey & Moretti, 1993). Increased estrogen production causes decreased secretion of hydrochloric acid; therefore peptic ulcer formation during pregnancy is uncommon (Klein, 1995).

Gastric motility and emptying time are reduced due to hormonal and mechanical factors. Reduced motility, mechanical obstruction by the uterus, and increased water absorption from the colon causes feces to become hard and dry, making constipation a common problem. Hemorrhoids may develop from constipation and increased pressure exerted on the vessels below the level of the uterus (Neeson, 1990). Straining during bowel movements causes increased venous pressure to rectal vessels, and hemorrhoids may develop or worsen.

Small and Large Intestines

The intestines are also pushed upward and laterally. The appendix is displaced superiorly. Increased progesterone levels during pregnancy relax gastrointestinal tract tone, decreasing intestinal motility, which allows increased absorption from the colon. Absorption of nutrients from the small bowel, with the exception of iron, is unchanged during pregnancy (Cruikshank & Hays, 1991).

Liver

Liver size and morphology apparently do not change during pregnancy, but liver function is altered. (Cunningham et al., 1993). Hepatic blood flow is unchanged (Cruikshank & Hays, 1991). Liver function test values during pregnancy would be suggestive of hepatic disease in the nonpregnant patient.

Serum concentration of many proteins produced by the liver increases during pregnancy in response to estrogen. Fibrinogen levels increase by 50% by the end of the second trimester. Serum levels of bilirubin, aspartate aminotransferase (AST), and alanine aminotransferase (ALT) are unchanged in normal pregnancy (Cruikshank & Hays, 1991) (Table 4-6). Plasma albumin activity decreases to 3.0 g/dl compared to 4.3 g/dl in the nonpregnant woman (Cunningham et al., 1993). Such a decrease, in nonpregnant patients, could be indicative of liver disease. Serum alkaline phosphatase activity and serum cholesterol concentration can double due to the increased placental alkaline phosphatase isozymes (Moore, 1991).

TABLE 4-6. Liver Function During Pregnancy

Parameter	Normal Range	Change
Bilirubin	0.1–1.2 mg/dl	Unchanged
AST (SGOT) Aspartate Aminotransferase	0–35 IV/L	Unchanged
ALT (SGPT) Alanine Aminotransferase	0–35 IV/L	Unchanged
5-Nucleotidase		Unchanged
Prothrombin Time	11–15 seconds	Unchanged or slight increase

Gallbladder

Gallbladder function is altered during pregnancy. Elevated progesterone levels cause the gallbladder to be hypotonic and distended. Gallbladder smooth muscle contraction is impaired and may lead to stasis. Emptying time is slow after 12 weeks of gestation. In the second and third trimesters, fasting and residual volumes are twice as great as in the nonpregnant woman and the rate the gallbladder empties is much slower (Cruikshank & Hays, 1991). Hypercholesterolemia may follow and predispose the pregnant woman to gallstone formation (Hume & Killam, 1990).

ENDOCRINE SYSTEM

Thyroid Gland

Increased vascularity and hyperplasia of glandular tissue during pregnancy results in increased gland size and activity. Thyroxine increases until 6–12 weeks postpartum. Thyroid stimulating hormone (TSH) decreases. These changes may be due to hCG. Increases in the amount of iodine in the blood is found in the form of total thyroxine (T_4). The increase in serum protein-bound iodine (PBI) increases from a nonpregnant level of 5–12 μg/dl to 9–16 μg/dl during pregnancy (Brinkman, 1993).

The thyroid gland produces and releases more hormone. Although elevations in thyroid hormone are produced, the pregnant woman remains euthyroid (Smith, 1990).

Hyperthyroidism during pregnancy is rare. Poor metabolic control during pregnancy can result in preterm labor, fetal loss, or thyroid crisis, necessitating early recognition and treatment. Hypothyroidism has been associated with spontaneous abortion.

Parathyroid Glands

Size and concentration of parathyroid gland and hormone increase during pregnancy. Levels peak between 15–35 weeks and return to normal after birth.

Regulation of calcium is closely interrelated to magnesium, phosphate, parathyroid hormone, vitamin D, and calcitonin. Any alteration in one is likely to alter the others. Increases in calcium or magnesium suppress parathyroid hormone levels, while decreases in plasma calcium or magnesium stimulate the release of parathyroid hormone (Cunningham et al., 1993).

Pituitary Gland

The anterior pituitary enlarges somewhat and returns to its usual size after delivery. There is no significant change in the posterior lobe.

Follicle-stimulating hormone (FSH) stimulates ovum growth, and luteinizing hormone (LH) affects ovulation. Thyrotropin and adrenotropin alter metabolism to support the pregnancy. Prolactin is responsible for initial milk production for lactation.

The posterior pituitary secretes oxytocin, influencing contractility of the uterus, and stimulates milk ejection from the breasts. Vasopressin causes vasoconstriction, which increases blood pressure. Vasopressin has an antidiuretic role in the regulation of water balance. Secretion of vasopressin is controlled by changes in plasma osmolarity and blood volume.

Adrenal Glands

Few structural changes occur in the adrenal glands during pregnancy. Increased amounts of circulating cortisol lowers renal excretion. Circulating cortisol levels regulate carbohydrate and protein metabolism. Adrenals secrete increased levels of aldosterone as early as 15 weeks of gestation (Cunningham et al., 1993), to accommodate increased sodium excretion. If sodium excretion is restricted, aldosterone secretion is elevated even further.

HORMONAL CHANGES DURING PREGNANCY

Human Chorionic Gonadotropin

The trophoblast secretes hCG in early pregnancy, which stimulates progesterone and estrogen production by the corpus luteum until the developed placenta assumes this role. Human chorionic gonadotropin levels in multiple gestations are more than twice as high as in singleton pregnancies (Yen, 1989).

Human Placental Lactogen

Human placental lactogen (hPL), also known as human chorionic somatomammotropin, is produced by the syncytiotrophoblast of the placenta. Unlike hCG levels, serum hPL levels rise concomitantly with placental growth. Human placental lactogen is an antagonist of insulin (Yen, 1989). Human placental lactogen increases the amount of free fatty acids available for metabolic needs, and decreases maternal metabolism of glucose.

Estrogen

Estrogens are steroid hormones secreted by the ovaries in early pregnancy. By 7 weeks gestation, more than half of the estrogen is secreted by the placenta. Estriol is the primary estrogen produced by the placenta during pregnancy.

Progesterone

Initially produced by the corpus luteum and then by the placenta, progesterone plays a crucial role in maintaining the pregnancy. Major roles of progesterone include maintaining the endometrium, inhibiting uterine contractility, and aiding in the development of the acini and lobules of the breasts for lactation.

Relaxin

Relaxin is detectable by the first missed menstrual period and inhibits uterine activity, diminishes the strength of uterine contractions, softens the cervix, and has a long-term effect of remodeling collagen. Relaxin is secreted primarily by the corpus luteum and, in small amounts, by the placenta and decidua.

Prostaglandins

Prostaglandins are lipid substances and are found in high concentrations in the female reproductive tract and in the decidua during pregnancy. The exact function of prostaglandins during pregnancy is unknown. Prostaglandins affect smooth muscle contractility and some are potent vasodilators. Prostaglandins play an important role in the mechanism of labor. Increased levels of circulating prostaglandins may lead to vasodilation (Elkayam & Gleicher, 1990). The interplay between thromboxane and prostacyclin in believed to contribute to hypertensive disorders in pregnancy (Walsh, 1985).

Prolactin

During pregnancy there is a marked increase of prolactin. Serum prolactin concentration begins to rise in the first trimester to ten times the nonpregnant concentration at term (Yen, 1989). Prolactin is released from the anterior pituitary and is responsible for initial lactation. There is, however, a decrease in prolactin levels initially after delivery even in breastfeeding women. Prolactin can be found in fetal plasma and amniotic fluid (Cunningham et al., 1993).

NEUROLOGICAL SYSTEM

In general, there are no nervous system changes during pregnancy. Several discomforts reported by pregnant women are associated with the nervous system. Mild frontal headaches may occur in the first and second trimesters and may be caused by tension or may be related to hormonal changes since no other cause can be found. Severe headache, especially after 20 weeks of gestation may be associated with preeclampsia. This type of headache is a result of edema from vasoconstriction. Dizziness may result from vasomotor instability, postural hypotension, or hypoglycemia, especially after prolonged periods of sitting or standing. Hypotension may result from transient oligemia. Paresthesia of the lower extremities can occur due to pressure from the gravid uterus, interfering with circulation. Excessive hyperventilation, resulting in lower PCO_2 levels, creates a tingling sensation in the hands (Harvey, 1991).

INTEGUMENTARY SYSTEM

Increases in estrogen and progesterone may cause an increase in melanocyte-stimulating hormone, causing hyperpigmentation in the integumentary system. Blood flow to the skin increases three to four times above prepregnant levels. Skin changes include feelings of warmth, vascular spider nevi, increased nail growth, and palmar erythema.

Vascular spider nevi appear on the face, neck, chest, arms, and legs. These are small bright-red elevations of the skin radiating from a central body. Spider nevi are related to increased subcutaneous blood flow and increased estrogen levels in the tissues (Cunningham et al., 1993). During pregnancy, the numbers of hairs in the growth phase remain stable. After delivery, the proportion of hairs which enter the resting phase doubles so women experience an increase in hair loss 2 to 4 months after delivery (Cruikshank & Hays, 1991).

Striae gravidarum, or stretch marks, may occur on the skin of the breasts, hips, and upper thighs and are usually most pronounced on the abdomen. Striae result from the normal stretching of the skin and softening and relaxing of the dermal collagenous and elastic tissues during the last months of pregnancy and occur in about half of pregnant women (Cunningham et al., 1993).

Pigmentation becomes darker over the nipples and areola. The linea alba becomes the linea nigra and divides the abdomen longitudinally from the sternum to the symphysis.

Melasma (previously referred to as chloasma), or the "mask of pregnancy," appears as irregularly shaped brown blotches on the face, with a mask-like distribution on the cheekbone and forehead and around the eyes. Chloasma is due to elevated serum levels of sex steroids. Estrogen and progesterone also stimulate melanin deposits. Chloasma disappears after pregnancy but may reappear with excessive sun exposure or with oral contraceptive use (Cruikshank & Hays, 1991).

REPRODUCTIVE SYSTEM

Uterus

Before pregnancy, the uterus is a small semisolid pear-shaped organ and weighs 70 g (Neeson, 1990). During pregnancy, the uterus becomes globular and increases in length. At term the uterus weighs approximately 1,000–1,200 g due to the hypertrophy of the myometrial cells. One sixth of the total maternal blood volume is contained within the vascular system of the uterus. During the first few months of pregnancy, the wall of the uterus thickens in response to elevated estrogen and progesterone levels. The myometrial hypertrophy ends by the fifth month and the muscle wall thins, allowing palpation of the fetus. The size and number of blood vessels and lymphatics increase.

Placental blood flow is essential for adequate fetal growth and survival. By term, the blood flow from the uterine and ovarian arteries to the uterus is approximately 500 ml/min, 80% of which is directed to the placental bed. Maternal position, maternal arterial pressure, and uterine contractility influence uterine blood flow.

Cervix

The cervix undergoes changes characterized by increased vascularity, softening, and dilation (Resnik, 1989). Estrogen stimulates glandular tissue of the cervix, which increases the number of cells. Endocervical glands, which occupy half the mass of the cervix at term, secrete a thick tenacious mucus that forms the mucous plug and prevents bacteria and other substances from entering and ascending the uterus. This mucous plug is expelled when labor begins and is known as bloody show. Increased vascularity causes a softening and bluish discoloration of the cervix known as Chadwick's sign (Resnik). Hyperactive glandular tissue also causes an increase in the normal mucous production during pregnancy.

Ovaries

Ovulation ceases during pregnancy. Cells that line the follicles, known as thecal cells, become active in hormone production and serve as the interstitial glands of pregnancy. The corpus luteum persists and secretes hormones until the tenth to twelfth week. It secretes progesterone, which maintains the endometrium until adequate progesterone is secreted by the placenta.

Vagina

Vaginal epithelium undergoes hypertrophy, increased vascularization, and hyperplasia during pregnancy in response to estrogen levels. Loosening of the connective tissue and thickening of the mucosa increases vaginal secretions. These secretions are thick, white, and acidic and play a role in preventing infection. By the end of pregnancy, the vaginal wall and perineal body become relaxed enough to permit stretching of the tissues and accommodate the birth of the infant.

Breasts

Breasts increase in size and nodularity to prepare for lactation. Nipples become more erect and veins are more prominent. There is increased pigmentation of the areola. Montgomery's follicles, the sebaceous glands located in the areola, hypertrophy. Striae may develop as the breasts enlarge. Colostrum, a yellow secretion rich in antibodies, may leak from the nipples during the last trimester of pregnancy. Feelings of fullness, tingling, and increased sensitivity begin in the first few weeks of gestation.

MUSCULOSKELETAL SYSTEM

Early in pregnancy the ligaments of the pregnant woman soften from the effects of progesterone and relaxin (Hume & Killam, 1990). This softening especially occurs in the sacroiliac, sacrococcygeal, and pubic joints of the pelvis to facilitate delivery.

Center of gravity changes with advancing pregnancy due to the increase in weight gain, fluid retention, lordosis, and the mobilization of ligaments. In order to accommodate the increased weight of the uterus, the lumbodorsal spinal curve is accentuated and the woman's posture changes. The rectus abdominis muscle may separate from pressure exerted by the growing uterus, producing a diastasis recti.

Calcium intake should be increased to 1.5 g/day in the last trimester and during lactation. If calcium intake is insufficient, fetal needs will be met through demineralization of the maternal skeleton (Taylor & Pernoll, 1991). Increased parathyroid hormone levels enhance gastrointestinal absorption and decrease renal excretion of calcium. In normal pregnancy, there is no loss of bone density (Hume & Killam, 1990).

METABOLIC CHANGES

In normal pregnancies, profound metabolic changes occur to provide development and growth of the fetus.

Weight Gain

There has been increased awareness about the relationship between maternal weight gain and weight of the newborn. Prenatal care, socioeconomic factors, and adequate nutrition have an impact on pregnancy outcome. A nutritional assessment should be made at the initial prenatal visit, with referral to a registered dietitian as needed. If the woman is unable to financially meet her nutritional needs, a referral to the Women, Infants and Children (WIC) program is indicated. Table 4-7 outlines the approximate weight gain distribution that occurs during pregnancy. The woman's prepregnancy height and weight will determine her actual caloric intake. On average, the increased demands of pregnancy require an additional 300 kcal per day. Women who are pregnant with twins or higher order multiples will need an additional 300 kcal per fetus per day. Weight gain guidelines, as recommended by the American College of Obstetricians and Gynecologists, are outlined in Chapter 6. Note the differences in suggested weight gain based on prepregnancy weight. Those patients who are underweight prior to pregnancy are encouraged to gain more weight as compared with those patients who are overweight before conception.

TABLE 4-7. Weight Increase Distribution During Pregnancy

Source	Pounds
Fetus, Placenta, Amniotic Fluid	11
Uterus, Breasts	2
Blood Volume	4
Maternal Stores	5
Tissue, Fluid	3

Pancreas

Early in pregnancy, the effects of estrogen and progesterone most likely induce a state of hyperinsulinemia. These hormones stimulate β-cell hyperplasia, increasing insulin production (Hollingsworth, 1985). As pregnancy advances, increased tissue resistance is observed with continued hyperinsulinemia. Insulin antagonism is mainly caused by hPL secretion by the placenta. This glycoprotein and other placental hormones (progesterone, cortisol, prolactin) oppose the action of insulin and promote maternal lipolysis (Mandeville, 1991). During the latter half of pregnancy, maternal carbohydrate metabolism is stressed by rising hormone levels (Hollingsworth).

The National Diabetes Data Group defines gestational diabetes as carbohydrate intolerance, with onset or diagnosis during pregnancy. Up to 40% of women with gestational diabetes mellitus (GDM) will develop Type 1 or Type 2 diabetes within 10 years of the pregnancy. All women should be screened for diabetes between 24 and 28 weeks gestation, when the diabetogenic effect of pregnancy is detectable. Selective screening may miss many women with GDM. A fasting glucose of 135 mg/dl or above is considered a positive screen (Arias, 1993).

In early pregnancy, Type 1 diabetics may require less insulin as the hyperinsulinemic effects are exerted. In later pregnancy, Type 2 diabetics may require exogenous insulin to maintain optimal glucose levels. GDM usually does not present in the first trimester because the insulin antagonism is not signficant until approximately 26 weeks gestation.

Maternal morbidity is not increased in patients with GDM; however, there is an increase in maternal morbidity for Type 1 and Type 2 diabetics (Mandeville, 1992). Hypertensive disease is increased among advanced diabetic classifications (Mandeville, 1991). The incidence of diabetic ketoacidosis (DKA) is increased during pregnancy due to the accelerated fat breakdown enhancing the formation of ketones (Mandeville). Treatment goals during pregnancy focus on achieving and maintaining euglycemia and avoiding hypoglycemia. Antenatal testing provides insight into fetal well-being.

Nutrient Metabolism

Fats are stored in the early months of pregnancy, while later in pregnancy there is fat mobilization that correlates with the increased utilization of glucose and amino acids by the fetus (Kalkhoff, Kissebah, & Kim, 1979). Fats are more completely absorbed during pregnancy, while the demand for carbohydrates increases. In the second half of pregnancy, plasma lipids increase but triglycerides, cholesterol, and lipoproteins decrease soon after the birth (Moore, 1991). The ratio of low-density proteins (LDL) to high-density proteins (HDL) increases during pregnancy.

SUMMARY

Significant physical, metabolic, and structural changes occur from conception until weeks into the postpartum period. A thorough knowledge and understanding of these changes facilitates assessment of normal pregnancy progression. Recognition of variations from normal may result in early identification of risk factors and potential complications, so prompt management can be initiated to ensure optimal outcomes for both mother and fetus.

REFERENCES

American College of Obstetricians and Gynecologists. (1993). Nutrition during pregnancy. ACOG Technical Bulletin 179, 1-7. Washington DC: Author.

Arias, F. (1993). Practical guide to high-risk pregnancy and delivery (2nd ed.). St. Louis, MO: Mosby.

Beydoun, S. (1985). The physiology of the renal tract in pregnancy. Clinical Obstetrics and Gynecology, 28(2), 249-256.

Blackburn, S., Loper, D. (Eds.). (1992). The cardiovascular system. In Maternal, fetal and neonatal physiology: A clinical perspective. Philadelphia: W.B. Saunders.

Brinkman, C.R. (1993). Biologic adaptation to pregnancy. In R.K. Creasy, & R. Resnik. (Eds.), Maternal-fetal medicine: Principle and practice (2nd ed.). Philadelphia: W.B. Saunders.

Clark, R.B. (1981). Conduction anesthesia. Clinical Obstetrics and Gynecology, 24(2), 601-617.

Clark, S.L., Cotton, D.B., Lee, W., Bishop, C., Hill, T., Southwick, J., Pivarnik, J., Spillman, T., DeVore, G. R., Phelan, J., Hankins, G. D., Benedetti, T.J., & Trolley, D. (1989). Central hemodynamic assessment of normal term pregnancy. American Journal of Obstetrics and Gynecology, 161(6, Pt. 1), 1439-1442.

Clark, S.L., Cotton, D.B., Pivarnik, J.M., Lee, W., Hankins, G.D., Benedetti, T.J., & Phelan, J.P. (1991). Position change and central hemodynamic profile during normal third-trimester pregnancy and post partum. American Journal of Obstetrics and Gynecology, 164(3), 883-887.

Cruikshank, D.P., & Hays, P.M. (1991). Maternal physiology in pregnancy. In S.G. Gabbe, J.R. Niebyl, & J.L. Simpson. (Eds.), Obstetrics: Normal and problem pregnancies (2nd ed.). New York: Churchill Livingstone.

Cugini, P., DiPalma, L., Battisti, P., Leone, G., Pachi, A., Paesano, R., Masella, C., Stirati, G., Pierucci, A., Rocca, R., & Morabito, S. (1992). Describing and interpreting 24 hour blood pressure patterns in physiologic pregnancy. American Journal of Obstetrics and Gynecology, 166 (1, Pt. 1). 54-60.

Cunningham, F.G., MacDonald, P.C., Gant, N.F., Leveno, K.J., & Gilstrap, L.C. (1993). Maternal adaptations to pregnancy. In Williams obstetrics (19th ed.). Norwalk, CT: Appleton & Lange.

Davison, J.M. (1985). The physiology of the renal tract in pregnancy. Clinical Obstetrics and Gynecology, 28(2), 257-265.

Davison, J.M. (1987). Kidney function in pregnant women. American Journal of Kidney Diseases, 9(4), 248-252.

Drummond, S.B. (1992). Cardiac disease in pregnancy: Intrapartum considerations. Critical Care Nursing Clinics of North America, 4(4), 659-665.

Elkayam, U., & Gleicher, N. (1982). Cardiovascular physiology of pregnancy. In U. Elkyam, & N. Gleicher (Eds.), Cardiac problems in pregnancy. New York: Alan Liss.

Fuschino, W. (1992). Physiologic changes of pregnancy: Impact on critical care. Critical Care Nursing Clinics of North America, 4(4), 691-701.

Geiger-Bronsky, M.J. (1992) Asthma and pregnancy: Opportunities for enhancing outcomes. Journal of Perinatal Neonatal Nursing, 6(2), 35-45.

Gibbs, C.P. (1981). Maternal physiology. Clinical Obstetrics and Gynecology, 24(2), 525-543.

Harvey, M. (1991). Physiologic changes of pregnancy. In C. Harvey (Ed.), Critical care obstetrical nursing. Gaithersburg, MD: Aspen.

Harvey, M. (1992). Critical care for the maternity patient. American Journal of Maternal Child Nursing, 17(6), 296-309.

Harvey, M., & Moretti, M.L. (1993). Maternal adaptations to pregnancy. In R. Knuppel & J. Drukker (Eds.), High-risk pregnancy: A team approach (2nd ed.). Philadelphia: W.B. Saunders.

Hollingsworth, D.R. (1985). Maternal metabolism in normal and pregnancy complicated by diabetes mellitus. Clinical Obstetrics and Gynecology, 28(3) 457-472.

Hume, R.F., & Killam, A.P. (1990). Maternal physiology. In J.R. Scott, P.J. DiSaia, C.B. Hammond, & W. Spellacy (Eds.), Danforth's Obstetrics and Gynecology (6th ed.). Philadelphia: J.B. Lippincott.

Kalkhoff, R.K., Kissebah, A.H., & Kim, H.J. (1979). Carbohydrate and lipid metabolism during normal pregnancy: Relationship to gestation hormone action. In I.R. Merkatz, & P.A. Adam (Eds.), The diabetic pregnancy: A perinatal perspective. New York: Grune & Stratton.

Key, T.C. (1989). Gastrointestinal diseases. In R.K. Creasey & R. Resnik (Eds.), Maternal-fetal medicine: Principles and practice (2nd ed.). Philadelphia: W.B. Saunders.

Kincaid-Smith, P. S., & Fairley, K.F. (1993). The kidney and hypertension in pregnancy. New York: Churchill Livingstone.

Klein, P.M. (1995). Anatomy and physiology of pregnancy. In I. Bobak, D. Lowdermilk, & Jensen, M. (Eds.), Maternal nursing (4th ed.). St. Louis, MO: Mosby

Lee, W., & Cotton, D. (1991). Cardiorespiratory changes during pregnancy. In S. Clark, D. Cotton, G. Hankins, & J.P. Phelan (Eds.), Critical care obstetrics. Boston: Blackwell Scientific Publications.

Mandeville, L.K. (1991). Diabetes mellitus in pregnancy. In C. Harvey (Ed.), Critical care obstetrical nursing. Gaithersburg, MD: Aspen.

Mandeville, L.K. (1992). Diabetes mellitus in pregnancy. In L.K. Mandeville, & N.H. Troiano (Eds.), High-risk intrapartum nursing. Philadelphia: J.B. Lippincott.

Mangano, D.T. (1993). Anesthesia for the pregnant cardiac patient. In S.M. Shnider, & G. Levinson (Eds.), Anesthesia for obstetrics (3rd ed.). Baltimore: Williams & Wilkins.

Martin, J.M. (1992). Invasive hemodynamic monitoring in pregnancy. Critical Care Nursing Clinics of North America, 4(4), 652-657.

Mashburn, J., Graves, B.W., & Gillmor-Kahn, M. (1992). Hematocrit values during pregnancy in a nurse-midwifery caseload. Journal of Nurse-Midwifery, 37(6) 404-410.

Metcalfe, J., McAnulty, J.H., & Ueland, K. (1981). Cardiovascular physiology. Clinical Obstetrics and Gynecology, 24(3) 693-710.

Metcalfe, J., Stock, M.K., & Barron, D.H. (1988). Maternal physiology during gestation. In E. Knobil, & J.D. Neil (Eds.), The physiology of reproduction (Vol. 2). New York: Raven Press.

Moore, P. J. (1991). Maternal physiology during pregnancy. In Pernoll, M.L., Current obstetrics and gynecologic diagnosis and treatment (7th ed.). Norwalk, CT: Appleton & Lange.

National Diabetes Data Group. (1979). Classification and diagnosis of diabetes mellitus and other categories of glucose intolerance. Diabetes, 28(12), 1039-1057.

Neeson, J.D. (1990). Physiologic adaptations in pregnancy. In K.P. May & L.R. Mahlmeister (Eds.), Comprehensive maternity nursing: Nursing process and the childbearing family (2nd ed.). Philadelphia: J.B. Lippincott.

Newman, V., Fullerton, J.T., & Anderson, P.O. (1993). Clinical advances in the management of severe nausea and vomiting during pregnancy. JOGNN, 22(6) 483-490.

Resnik, R. (1989). Anatomic alterations in the reproductive tract. In R. Creasy & R. Resnik (Eds.), Maternal-fetal medicine: Principles and practice (2nd ed.). Philadelphia: W.B. Saunders.

Sisson, M. (1992). Disseminated intravascular coagulation. In L.K. Mandeville, & N.H. Troiano (Eds.), High-risk intrapartum nursing. Philadelphia: J.B. Lippincott.

Smith, J.E. (1990). Pregnancy complicated by thyroid disease. Journal of Nurse-Midwifery, 35(3), 143-149.

Soules, M.R., Hughes, C.L., Garcia, J.A., Livengood, C.H., Prystowsky, M.R., & Alexander, E. (1980). Nausea and vomiting of pregnancy: Role of human chorionic-gonadotropin and 17-hydroxyprogesterone. Obstetrics and Gynecology, 55(6), 696-700.

Taylor, C.M., & Pernoll, M.L. (1991). Normal pregnancy and prenatal care. In M.L. Pernoll Current obstetrics and gynecologic diagnosis and treatment (7th ed.). Norwalk, CT: Appleton & Lange.

Thappa, V., & Sicilian, L. (1992). Respiratory changes in pregnancy: Distinguishing between physiologic alterations and true disease. Consultant, 32(6) 136-140.

Ueland, K. (1986) Physiologic adaptations to pregnancy. In R. Knuppel & J. Drukker (Eds.), High-risk pregnancy: A team approach. Philadelphia: Saunders.

Walsh, S. (1985). Preeclampsia: An imbalance in placental protacyclin and thromboxane production. American Journal of Obstetrics and Gynecology, 152 (3), 335-340

Whalley, P. J., Everett, R.B., Gant, N.F., Cox, K., & MacDonald, P. C. (1983). Pressor responsiveness to angiotensin II in hospitalized primigravid women with pregnancy-induced hypertension. American Journal of Obstetrics and Gynecology, 145(4), 481-483.

Yen, S.S. (1989). Endocrine and other evaluations of the fetal environment. In R. Creasy & R. Resnik (Eds.), Maternal-fetal medicine: Principles and practice (2nd ed.). Philadelphia: W.B. Saunders.

Psychosocial Adaptation to Pregnancy and Postpartum

Jeanne Watson Driscoll

The goal of psychosocial care is the integration and normalization of the pregnancy and postpartum experience. It is hoped that with caring concern, the emotional development of the new family will be encouraged, supported, and valued. Many changes occur during pregnancy and postpartum. The woman experiences changes in physiology, body size, body shape, relationships, roles, and responsibilities. The partner also undergoes changes in roles, relationships, responsibilities, and coping strategies. All in all, the pregnancy and postpartum period is a time of increased vulnerability that also offers the potential for psychological growth (Flagler & Nicoll, 1990).

Although family development is an ongoing process that occurs during pregnancy and postpartum, it is not the focus of this chapter; rather this chapter focuses on the psychosocial aspects of the woman as she progresses through the normal process of pregnancy and postpartum. The purpose here is to provide the perinatal nurse with an overview of these normal psychosocial experiences so that she or he can provide comprehensive care to the woman and her family. Certainly it is by knowledge of normal experiences that the nurse is able to recognize deviations that may require referrals to multidisciplinary colleagues for collaborative, quality, holistic care.

As the woman moves through her pregnancy, the perinatal nurse provides anticipatory education and guidance regarding the physiological, psychological and spiritual journey. One cannot stress enough the significance of the role the nurse plays as confidant, information provider, and supporter.

ASPECTS OF PSYCHOSOCIAL NURSING CARE

Each woman is unique. To her pregnancy she brings experiences, relationships, and realities as she perceives them. It is this unique experiential history that makes her who she is. It is this identity of self that forms the foundation for her development of the maternal self and adaptation to the maternal role.

Psychosocial Assessment

The perinatal nurse plays an important role in the woman's psychosocial adaptation. A psychosocial relationship develops based on trust, mutuality, security, validation, and support. The nurse's knowledge of normal developmental and psychosocial processes allows for rapid identification of problems or alterations in the experience. Critical to the adaptation process are the concepts of care and communication. It is important for the woman to feel herself "heard" and validated. The perinatal nurse needs to be actively involved in the interaction, clarifying communications frequently and avoiding assumptive thinking. For instance, some people commonly say "you know what I mean." If the nurse does not understand what the woman is saying, her response should be, "No, I don't know what you mean. Help me understand what you are saying/feeling." This communication strategy places the responsibility onto the woman to describe her experience in her words and her reality.

The nurse needs to establish an atmosphere in which the woman can freely ask questions and engage in discussions about things that concern her. The most difficult aspect of the interaction may be that the nurse will, at times, have to sit with the woman as she "bares her soul," while the nurse knows there is no magic to make the woman feel better. It is important to validate the woman's uncertainties without paternalism, indifference, or judgment. Nursing actions should be directed at supporting the woman, by facilitating the woman's personal exploration of the uncertainties in order to understand and attach meaning to the situation (Sorenson, 1990).

Because there are transference issues in any relationship, the nurse's self-awareness is a necessity. If the nurse is unaware of his or her own issues, they may be projected onto the woman. The result may be that the woman will not feel safe. Such projections can lead to misinformation, lack of concern and validity, and disconnected relationships. If the nurse finds that she or he is reacting to something that has been said, it is imperative that the reactions be processed through self-inquiry or with consultation. For example, the fact that a nurse has been pregnant does not mean that she knows how every pregnant woman feels. It merely means that the nurse knows what she personally felt. A situation when projection may occur is during the admission of a 16-year-old primipara when the admitting nurse has a daughter of the same age. Self-awareness is especially important because many healthcare providers are the same age as their patients and at similar stages in development. Healthy, clear boundaries are necessary for the development of a therapeutic relationship.

Emphasis of the psychosocial assessment is on normalcy, health, universality, strengths, and developmental concepts, rather than on the formulation of a psychiatric diagnosis. The physiological aspects of pregnancy often get more attention than the psychosocial aspects, but pregnancy and postpartum are holistic experiences. The mind, body, and soul are affected by these major changes and transitions. The perinatal nurse can use the holistic model to provide total care for this woman.

Psychosocial assessment is dynamic and ongoing. The process includes the pregnant woman, her family, and the nurse. The focus of the assessment is to gather biopsychosocial-spiritual data. It is from these data that nursing diagnoses can be identified, care plans developed in collaboration with the woman and her family, and strategies developed, implemented, and evaluated.

Because the psychosocial assessment is an ongoing process, assessment is made at every visit. Key elements to be included in a psychosocial assessment are listed in Display 5-1.

The style of obtaining information is derived from the interviewing skills of the clinician. It may be helpful to use "permission-giving statements"; for example, "Many woman have told me they have some periods when they cry. Has this happened to you?" This allows the woman to hear that the nurse is open to her worries and concerns and that she does not have to be "fine." The timing and location of the interview are also important. If there is limited time for interaction and more time is necessary for disclosure and discussion, make another appointment. This strategy validates the woman's issues and demonstrates the nurses' caring and concern.

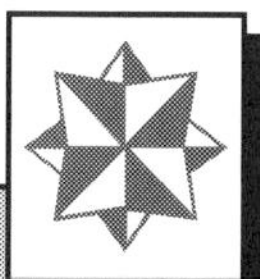

DISPLAY 5-1

Elements of a Psychosocial Assessment

- Family and social history
- Psychiatric history
- Mental status
- Self-concept/self-esteem
- Support systems
- Stressors: personal and occupational
- Coping strategies
- Spirituality: faith/beliefs
- Neurovegetative signs
  - sleep patterns
  - appetite
  - energy/motivation
  - mood state
  - sexual desire
- Knowledge of the pregnancy experience

Collaborative Care and Referral

A critical aspect of holistic-care planning is the coordination of the multidisciplinary team to provide care for this woman and her family. Often women present with issues, needs, and/or concerns that are beyond the realm of the perinatal nurse. These issues may require collaboration with the members of the psychiatric/mental health specialties, nutrition services, social services, or community agencies.

It has been demonstrated that there is a strong correlation between the onset of mood and anxiety disorders prior to pregnancy and their exacerbation in the postpartum period (Whiffin, 1988). All too often, when women talk about mood swings and increased anxiety during pregnancy, the reports of these uncomfortable symptoms are devalued with statements such as, "It's just due to your hormones. It will go away after you have the baby." This type of paternalistic remark denigrates the woman's feelings of importance and may silence her. It is important for perinatal healthcare providers to be aware that a woman with previous mood and anxiety disorders is at high risk for reoccurrence of these disorders during pregnancy and postpartum (Hamilton, Parry, & Blumenthal, 1988). A history of mood and anxiety disorders mandates coordination of the woman's care in a holistic manner, involving mind, body, and soul. If the perinatal nurse is vigilant about the adaptation and attainment processes during pregnancy, referrals to multidisciplinary colleagues can be made as appropriate to facilitate this woman's journey to motherhood.

The perinatal nurse should be aware of community mental health resources. This may require developing a resource list, talking with providers, and developing referral relationships.

ADAPTATIONS DURING PREGNANCY

In the following sections, the psychosocial aspects of pregnancy are presented. Ongoing assessment of anxiety levels and need for information and support is mandatory. Offering anticipatory guidance about physiologic and psychological changes during pregnancy supports the woman as she moves through these periods of uncertainty (Sorenson, 1990).

Reva Rubin, in her classic work (1984), described tasks that a woman needs to accomplish during her pregnancy. These tasks include the following: ensuring a safe passage for herself and her child; ensuring social acceptance of child by significant others; increasing affinal ties in the construction of the image and identity of the "I" and the "you"; and exploring the meaning of the transitive act of giving/receiving. The perinatal nurse plays a significant role in the promotion of attainment of these tasks in addition to the establishment of a strong professional relationship of care and concern.

First Trimester

A myriad of physiologic symptoms occur in the first trimester, and it is a time of strange feelings and secrets. The woman may know that she is pregnant as a result of a home pregnancy test, or she may deny the possibility until she requests a pregnancy test. Often the nurse calls the woman to tell her the test is positive. Therefore psychosocial assessment begins at this initial nurse-patient contact. What was her response to the news that she is pregnant: shock, disbelief, joy, anticipation, denial, fear? Major areas of assessment are listed in Display 5-2.

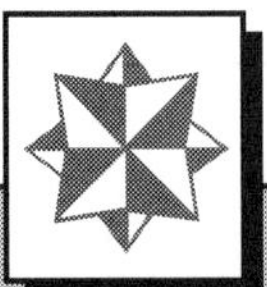

DISPLAY 5-2

Assessment Issues in the First Trimester

- Anxiety levels
- Meaning of the pregnancy (personal)
- Physical concerns/issues
- Partner/significant other's response
- Concerns regarding pregnancy/ postpartum experience
- Relationship with family
- Support systems
- Coping strategies
- Neurovegetative signs
  - sleep patterns
  - appetite
  - energy/motivation
  - mood state
- Spirituality: beliefs/values

"The task of the first trimester is progressive movement of the woman from a state of conflict and ambivalence to one of acceptance of the pregnancy, the child, and the motherhood role" (Lederman, 1990, p. 281). The nurse promotes this transition through concern, care, and support. Many women share that they are not sure what to feel. Moods can range from high to low, calm to panic, happy to sad, and acceptance to denial. She may feel a bit detached, emotionally labile, nauseous, fatigued, anxious, and concerned.

Often, women describe the feelings of the first trimester as "like being on a roller coaster." Ambivalence is high. "This is what I thought I wanted, why do I feel so confused and sick!" Anticipatory guidance will help the woman resolve some of these feelings. If this is her first pregnancy, she will need consistent information and support. If the woman has a history of pregnancy, how did she cope? Has she had any abortions? Were they spontaneous or elective? What was her response at that time? Does she have live children? Has she had a stillborn infant? It is the woman's history that will affect this pregnancy experience.

Today, with regular use of amniocentesis, the woman may delay attachment to the pregnancy until results of an amniocentesis are available, usually at about 20 weeks of pregnancy. So for almost 20 weeks, she may remain disconnected from her feelings and emotions in an effort to protect herself from potential pain and disappointment. If she has a history of miscarriage, she may be afraid to become attached to the pregnancy until she passes the "critical week" when she lost the other pregnancy. It is not uncommon for women with histories of loss to delay attachment until they see a live baby at birth.

Developing a therapeutic relationship with the woman takes work. Key aspects of this relationship include the development of trust, confidence, mutuality, active listening, and empowerment. Pregnancy is a time of emotional changes and she will need a "safe place" to share her thoughts and concerns. Suggest that she begin a journal of her pregnancy experiences as a place to share personal thoughts. What about the father of the baby? What are his thoughts? How does she think he is doing with this new information? Meeting with the woman's partner/significant other provides additional information to help the nurse with the complete family assessment. Ascertain any misconceptions, needs for information, and feelings about the pregnancy. What is his availability? What about other support people? Does the woman have a best friend/confidant or can she talk with other women who have experienced pregnancy and birth? What about her concepts of spirituality; is her faith or belief system helpful to her?

The woman needs validation and support. A major nursing role is to "listen" to the woman's experience. What does it feel like for her? All too often, she feels as though the people in the physician's office care only about the urine samples, her vital signs, and weight status. She is nervous and will do well with permission to feel, anticipatory information, and support as she moves through this first trimester.

Role of the Nurse

In summary, the role of the nurse during the first trimester includes the following:

- begin psychosocial assessment at initial contact; assess the woman's response to pregnancy
- promote the woman's accomplishment of the first task of pregnancy by showing concern and giving care and support
- give anticipatory guidance related to the experiences of the first trimester

- continue to make assessments by interviewing the partner/significant other
- validate the woman's concerns and support her emotional state

Second Trimester

As she moves into the second trimester, the pregnant woman begins to feel fetus activity. She may have seen an image of the fetus via ultrasound, but now she feels the baby move. "This phase is characterized by fantasy and exploration, and a growing definition and identity of the motherhood role" (Lederman, 1990, p. 281). What are her fantasies? Who does she imagine her baby looks like? What does she think it will be like to have a baby? It is by asking these types of questions that role development may be facilitated. Building on prior assessments, Display 5-3 contains issues critical to the second trimester.

The woman will be dealing with issues related to body changes. She begins to wear maternity clothes and people ask her about her pregnancy; it is no longer a secret. She may need to do some grief work and talk about the loss of her body shape and size. Again, the perinatal nurse must exercise caution and not project personal feelings onto the woman. For example, the perinatal nurse may say, "You must be excited about feeling the baby move." However, in reality, the woman may feel as though there is an alien inside; it is more frightening than exciting. Now she knows that the nurse thinks that she should be excited, so she better not reveal how she really feels. She's afraid the nurse may think something is wrong with her if she is not excited. She is vulnerable and needs to feel safe and confident that her feelings will be heard in a nonjudgmental way.

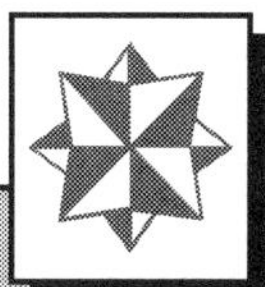

DISPLAY 5-3

Assessment Issues in the Second Trimester

- Anxiety levels
- Feelings/perceptions re: fetal movements
- Feelings about body changes/body image
- Attachment to fetus
- Neurovegetative signs
  - sleep patterns
  - appetite
  - energy/motivation
  - mood state
- Relationship with partner/significant other
- Relationship with work/family
- Knowledge of the process of pregnancy experience
- Spirituality: faith/beliefs

Pregnant women have increased vulnerability to emotional nuances in relationships. They perceive from the nurse's looks, innuendos, and responses whether or not they are being valued. Women have been socialized to be other-centered, so she may need help focusing on her needs, wants, and concerns (Miller, 1986). It is hard to share the feelings that may not seem "nice." If the nurse reacts negatively to the woman's feelings, it will close the door to the woman's development of trust, mutuality, and confidence in her own feelings as valid and real. Permission-giving statements should be used, such as, "In my clinical practice, women have shared with me that they are not too excited about the changes in their body. How do you feel about this?" This allows her to know that you have heard some negative things and that maybe it is safe for her to disclose her real feelings, contrary to what she has been told she should feel.

Although the second trimester is often thought to be a time of tranquility and quiescence, the pregnant woman may be experiencing increased anxiety as the baby makes his/her presence known. She begins to feel better physiologically and her focus may shift from her self-concern to baby-concern. The woman is more aware of her changing body size and her perception of her body space. She may be more anxious about these changes. She may begin to have some fears/phobias about something happening. If the nurse feels that the woman's anxieties and concerns are getting in the way of her healthy day-to-day functioning, a referral to a psychiatric/mental health care provider may be necessary. This lets the woman know that her concerns and fears are valued and that the goal is to provide holistic care.

The pregnant woman may tell you that she is having weird, at times frightening, dreams about "strangers" entering her life. When one stops to think about it, there is a "stranger" in her life. A woman's perception of her unborn child develops through watching images during ultrasound examinations and/or the personal characteristics the woman imagines in response to fetal movements. For example, many women describe, in detail, attributes of their baby based on ultrasound images or cycles of fetal activity. If fetal sex is known as a result of ultrasonography or genetic testing, more gender-specific traits can be imagined. It is not unusual for women to report, "He's a wild one," or "She likes to keep me up at night." Encourage her to share her perceptions and dreams with her partner or another significant person in her life. Tell the woman that it often helps to just talk about them. Let her know that some women find it worthwhile to write about their dreams and feelings in a journal during pregnancy. Benefits of keeping a journal include the woman's ability to review entries at a later date and analyze the development of her impressions as the pregnancy progresses.

Anticipatory information and education about the childbirth experience begin to be of importance now. It is time to register for prepared childbirth classes. Attending these classes appeals to the cognitive side of the process because she is becoming informed about her body and the upcoming labor and birth. Sometimes, a secondary gain of childbirth classes is development of new friendships among the participants based on shared experiences. These relationships often carry over into the postpartum period and beyond.

Role of the Nurse

In summary, the role of the nurse during the second trimester includes the following:

- continue ongoing psychosocial assessments of the woman, her partner/significant other
- encourage verbalization regarding grief process (body image, etc.)
- maintain a nonjudgmental attitude
- refer to psychiatric-care provider if anxieties seem greater than normal
- encourage the woman to share dreams, thoughts, and feelings with a close friend or her partner or keep a personal journal
- provide anticipatory guidance regarding normal changes and concerns
- provide information regarding childbirth classes for the woman and her partner

Third Trimester

During the third trimester, frequency of visits to healthcare providers increases. The woman may begin to ask more questions and verbalize increased concerns about what will happen during labor and birth.

The major issues of the third trimester are birth preparation and the baby's well-being. She may begin to experience an approach-avoidance conflict related to childbirth and the possible consequences that may evolve such as pain and loss of control (Rofe, Blittner, & Lewin, 1993). See Display 5-4 for assessment issues pertinent to this trimester.

During this trimester, some women experience physical discomforts because of body size and physiologic changes. They worry about what will happen when they go into labor. Role responsibilities are changing. The woman may be leaving work to begin maternity leave, a role change that may affect daily interaction with adults and potentially her identity. She may begin to talk about her fear of losing control during labor and birth: "What if I scream?...How will I know when I am in labor?...I won't leave the house!...What if my water breaks in the mall?" Her anxieties begin to rise. Ongoing assessment of her anxiety level is necessary. It is important to validate her concerns and support her normalcy. If the nurse feels that the woman's mood is more intense than usual, referral may be necessary for evaluation by the psychiatric/mental health team.

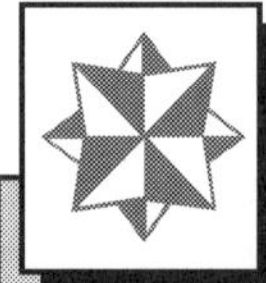

DISPLAY 5-4

Assessment Issues in the Third Trimester

- Anxiety levels
- Physical concerns
- Attachment to the fetus
- Body image/self-concept
- Expectations of self and partner re: labor and birth
- Neurovegetative signs
  - sleep patterns
  - appetite
  - energy/motivation
  - mood state
- Relationship with partner/significant other
- Relationship with family/work
- Spirituality: faith/beliefs

Her dreams may begin to include fears of being stuck or trapped, fears of some harm happening to her or the baby, and concerns for survival. It is not uncommon at this time for the woman to experience increased anxiety secondary to hearing other women's stories of their birth experiences. She worries about her performance and about the "awful" things that might happen. Again, she needs to have a safe place to share her concerns and worries.

It is important to discuss and plan for the postpartum experience. What about support? Who is going to help her? What are her expectations of the experience? If there are other children, who will take care of them and help her after she gets home with the new baby? Assist the woman to develop lists of things to do and people she needs to contact and enlist support from prior to birth. If she will be breastfeeding, encourage her to attend breastfeeding support groups prior to birth, to facilitate and promote relationship and resource development.

Role of the Nurse

The role of the perinatal nurse continues to be one of assessment, information, and support. In summary, the role of the nurse in the third trimester includes the following:

- continue ongoing psychosocial assessment of the woman, her partner/significant other
- support and reinforce information obtained in childbirth education classes
- facilitate verbalization of concerns related to employment status, role changes
- encourage sharing of feelings and concerns with partner/significant other
- provide anticipatory education regarding the postpartum experience
- facilitate planning for help at home after the birth
- encourage her to obtain information about new mothers' support groups, breastfeeding support groups

ADAPTATIONS DURING LABOR AND BIRTH

The labor and birth experience is a critical turning point. She makes the major physical and psychological transition . . . birth! The onset of labor can be a scary experience, especially when she realizes that there is no way back! Often she calls with the first twinges, "What should I do?" She needs a lot of support and gentle guidance. She is concerned about her well-being, that of her baby, and her partner. She is afraid that she will "lose it" and she wants to "be a good patient." Her sense of reality is intense.

If she is having her baby in the hospital or birth center, it is important that the perinatal nurse orient the woman and her partner to the unit and talk with them about their hopes and desires for this birth experience. The establishment of an empathic, therapeutic relationship is necessary to provide the woman with the connection and concern that she needs to proceed in the labor experience. Anticipatory guidance and information sharing need to be ongoing, as she may lose sense of time due to the crisis of labor. Continual assessment of her psychosocial ability to stay focused and connected to the experience is important. Pay close attention to the interaction between the laboring woman and her support person so that you will be available as needed to support them both.

Each woman will labor and birth in a unique way, therefore nursing care should be individualized rather than routine. Similarly, there is no behavior or response that one would expect to see after the birth. Some women will be jubilant and excited, want to hold their baby, count fingers and toes, and breastfeed, etc. Other women need to go into themselves to regroup on an intrapersonal level. There is no one right way! One woman, after a precipitous birth experience, when asked if she wanted to hold her new baby, said, "Not yet, give me some time to get myself together . . . I can't believe this is over." With all the pressure about "bonding," it is important for the nurse to support the individual new mother's request at this time. This is the beginning of the conflicts of new motherhood: do I take care of myself or do I put the baby first? "The urgings to parent and to achieve intimacy with the newborn while at the same time struggling with loss of control and autonomy, represents one of the most important foci around which adult growth takes place" (Cohen, 1988, p. 61). The psychosocial assessment issues of this experience are listed in Display 5-5.

Role of the Nurse

The role of the nurse during adaptation to the labor and birth experience is intense and critical. The woman may be scared, vulnerable, and/or excited. She may even regress in response to the stress of the situation. The role of the nurse during labor and birth includes the following:

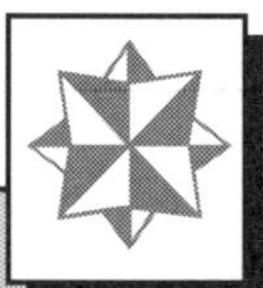

DISPLAY 5-5

Assessment Issues During Labor and Birth

- Anxiety levels
- Coping strategies
- Adjustment to the environment
- Relationship with partner/significant other
- Assess ability to focus and work with process
- Mood state
- Spirituality: faith/beliefs

- establish an empathic relationship based on trust
- orient the laboring woman and her support person to the unit or birth center
- facilitate the interaction between the woman and her labor suport person
- ongoing psychosocial assessment
- anticipatory guidance regarding labor experience
- encourage attachment to the baby after it is born, in relation to the new mother's needs

ADAPTATIONS IN THE POSTPARTUM PERIOD

The birth occurs. The family has a new member. The new mother begins her physiological recovery, relationship development with the "real" baby, and psychological adaptation to motherhood.

During this early postpartum period it is important for the perinatal nurse to observe the maternal-newborn attachment process and identify behavior patterns that may indicate the need for further follow-up care. It is critical to differentiate behaviors related to maternal exhaustion or discomfort from real problems with attachment. For example, the woman who asks that her baby spend the night in the nursery so she can get some rest is probably physically exhausted from the labor and birth, and the woman who doesn't want to hold her baby after a cesarean birth may be having significant incisional pain. Each woman is unique and responds to her newborn in her own way. A series of interactions are necessary for accurate assessment of maternal-newborn attachment. Nursing assessment should also focus on maternal confidence in basic newborn care skills such as comforting strategies, formula or breast feeding, bathing and diapering. Encouragement and reinforcement may be necessary as the new mother tries to learn all she needs to know about newborn care in the very short time she is hospitalized.

The new mother will need time to share her labor and birth experience (Rubin, 1984). This is often done by calling all of her friends on the phone or by meeting other new mothers in the perinatal unit and chatting. She is putting meaning into the experience by verbalizing her reality. This integration of the childbirth experience into her self-system is a major issue of the early postpartum experience (Rubin). There is the need to talk about and process reality versus fantasy. There is an element of loss as she begins to mourn the imagined childbirth experience (Driscoll, 1990). The perinatal nurse plays a significant role in the validation and clarification of the experience for this woman by listening and supporting her evolving maternicity.

Today, with the reality of shortened postpartum lengths of stay, the new mother has to move quickly from self-concern to other-concern: her newborn. In view of this, it is important that her physical and psychological needs be met so that she will be better able to focus on her newborn's care. She may become intensely focused on the cognitive learning needs related to newborn feeding and physical care. The new mother may verbalize anxiety and concern. If so, she needs to be heard and her concerns must be validated. The newly evolving relationship with the newborn is based on connection and care. If she has difficulty with these beginning skills, it may alter her self-esteem and maternal development (Driscoll, 1993). The woman brings with her many performance expectations that need to be discussed and clarified. Mercer (1986) described maternal role attainment as a process that takes a period of about 10 months to develop. During this postpartum phase, the new mother attaches to her newborn, gains competence as a mother, and expresses gratification in the mother-infant interaction. This adaptation can be delayed or altered if the woman's health and mental status is less than optimal. The reality of the current healthcare delivery system is that much of the work of the postpartum maternal adjustment and role attainment is done after discharge. Referral to community resources and discharge planning are imperative in the total care plan.

Emotionally, these early days can be disconcerting. It is supposed to be such an exciting time, but in reality she may be experiencing alternating periods of crying and joy, irritability, anxiety, headaches, confusion, forgetfulness, depersonalization, and fatigue. She may have the "baby blues." It has been estimated that between 70–80% of new mothers experience this transitory mood disorder. Unfortunately, this phenomenon occurs so frequently that it is often considered normal and therefore does not get the attention that it deserves. It is felt that this disorder is related to the normal physiologic and psychosocial changes that occur in the process of becoming a new mother. There is a rapid drop in pregnancy hormones following delivery of the placenta, which may alter biochemical neurotransmitters in the brain (Hansen, 1990). This transitory mood disorder can greatly affect the new mother and her family, especially if they are unaware of the possibility or what to do about it. Assessment issues relevant to the postpartum experience are listed in Display 5-6.

Women and their families need information about normal mood changes after childbirth. They should be aware that often with a lot of support, reassurance, rest, and good nutrition, these labile moods usually balance out, and the woman will begin to feel better and feel more organized and confident. However, if the moods do not stabilize by about 21 days, referral should be made to the psychiatric/mental health team specialists in postpartum mood and anxiety disorders.

A recent study of first-time mothers surveyed during the postpartum period revealed a 63% incidence of depressive disorders of early onset and lengthy duration (McIntosh, 1993). The majority of affected women reported they did not seek help because they felt their depression was secondary to the stress of becoming a mother; therefore they thought it was a "normal" reaction. An additional reason women cited for not talking to a professional healthcare provider about their feelings was the fear that they would be labeled as mentally ill and considered an unfit mother (McIntosh). Perinatal nurses must be proactive in identifying women with depressive disorders during the postpartum period to facilitate early intervention and referral to psychiatric-mental health specialists.

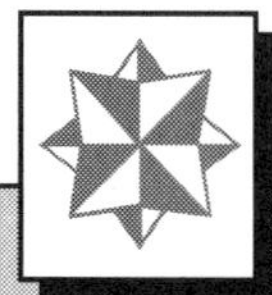

DISPLAY 5-6

Assessment Issues During the Postpartum Period

- Anxiety levels
- Perceptions of the birth experience
- Maternal–newborn attachment
- Relationship with partner/significant other
- Neurovegetative signs
  - sleep patterns
  - appetite
  - energy/motivation
  - mood state
  - pain levels
- Coping strategies
- Support systems
- Knowledge of postpartum process after discharge
- Spirituality: faith/beliefs

Postpartum Depression

Postpartum depression (PPD) is a mood disorder that is estimated to affect from 3–30% of women (Ugarriza, 1992). Symptoms of postpartum depression may include anxiety, irritability, fatigue, a demoralizing sense of failure, feelings of guilt, sleep disorders, appetite changes, suicide ideation, and excessive concerns about the baby. Treatment for postpartum depression and related mood and anxiety disorders may include antidepressant agents, antianxiety agents, psychotherapy, counseling, and support groups. With appropriate intervention, prospects for recovery are excellent.

Postpartum Psychosis

The most serious psychiatric disorder that can occur after the birth of a baby is postpartum psychosis. This is an organic psychosis that affects between 1 and 2 women per one thousand births. This disorder is a psychiatric emergency. The woman can demonstrate symptoms of psychosis within 1 to 2 days after the birth of her baby. The signs and symptoms of psychosis are sleep disturbances, confusion, agitation, irritability, hallucinations, delusions, and potential for suicide/infanticide. Hospitalization is mandatory. With aggressive treatment most women recover from this disorder (Hamilton & Harburger, 1992).

It can not be stressed enough that women and their families need anticipatory information about postpartum mood disorders so that prompt identification and early treatment can be initiated. A heightened awareness among perinatal healthcare providers of the incidence of postpartum mood disorders, and knowledge of common signs and symptoms and the prospects for recovery, can contribute to successful outcomes for affected women.

Discharge planning has become a critical issue in this time of shortened length of stay. Prior to discharge from the hospital, the woman should be given a list of telephone numbers of her care providers as well as any emergency services that she may need. It is important to go over the key support people with the new mother and her partner during discharge teaching.

Role of the Nurse

The role of the perinatal nurse during the postpartum experience is changing continually in response to current lengths of stay. Hospitals are developing home-discharge programs, private home health agencies are being established, and the majority of postpartum care occurs in the community. The role of the nurse during the postpartum period includes the following:

- continue ongoing psychosocial assessment of woman, partner/significant other
- assess and facilitate maternal attachment
- encourage verbalization of birth experience to promote integration
- assess and facilitate family development
- assess support systems and networks in the family and community
- provide education about normal postpartum emotional adjustments and provide anticipatory guidance regarding postpartum mood and anxiety disorders

SUMMARY

Psychosocial adaptation to pregnancy and postpartum is a dynamic process. The nurse plays a significant role in the promotion and facilitation of this experience in a healthy way. It is a time when the woman is open to great psychological growth and relies on the healthcare team for information and support. The nurse needs to be aware of the normal process in order to identify, those that are abnormal. It is helpful in the assessment of mood and emotional state to remember three words: frequency, duration, and intensity. If the woman describes to you that she is having difficulty functioning in her activities of daily living and having a tough time coping due to emotional and mood changes, referral is necessary. The referral process needs to be managed in an empowering, supportive way. Letting her know that she is valued and her concerns and feelings are important is a way for the perinatal nurse to give the woman the message that she deserves good care. Appropriate healthcare provider attitudes support the referral process.

In closing, it is important to reinforce the concept that due to the rapid changes in the healthcare delivery system and decreasing lengths of stay, it will be imperative for the perinatal nurse to actively pursue, nurture, and promote collaborative relationships with colleagues in the community. It is this active communication and relational approach to the care of this new mother and her family that will promote, facilitate, and encourage healthy maternal and paternal psychosocial adaptation and adjustment.

REFERENCES:

Cohen, R.L. (1988). Psychiatric consultation in childbirth settings. New York: Plenum.

Driscoll, J.W. (1990). Maternal parenthood and the grief process. Journal of Perinatal and Neonatal Nursing, 4(2), 1-10.

Driscoll, J.W. (1993). The transition to parenthood. In C.S. Fawcett, Family psychiatric nursing (pp. 97-108). St. Louis, MO: C.V. Mosby.

Flagler, S., & Nicoll, L. (1990). A framework for the psychological aspects of pregnancy. NAACOG's Clinical Issues in Perinatal and Women's Health Nursing, 1(3), 267-279.

Hamilton, J.A., & Harburger, P.N. (Eds.). (1992). Postpartum psychiatric illness: A picture puzzle. Philadelphia: University of Pennsylvania.

Hamilton, J.A., Parry, B.L., & Blumenthal, S.J. (1988). The menstrual cycle in context: Affective syndrome associated with reproductive hormonal changes. Journal of Clinical Psychiatry, 49(12), 474-480.

Hansen, C.H. (1990). Baby blues: Identification and intervention. NAACOG's Clinical Issues in Perinatal and Women's Health Nursing, 1(3), 369-374.

Lederman, R.P. (1990). Anxiety and stress in pregnancy: Significance and nursing assessment. NAACOG'S Clinical Issues in Perinatal and Women's Health Nursing, 1(3), 279-288.

McIntosh, J. (1993). Postpartum depression: Women's help seeking behavior and perceptions of cause. Journal of Advanced Nursing, 18(2), 178-184.

Mercer, R.T. (1986). First-time motherhood: Experiences from teens to forties. New York: Springer-Verlag.

Miller, J.B. (1986). Toward a new psychology of women (2nd ed.). Boston: Beacon.

Rofe, Y., Blittner, M., & Lewin, I. (1993). Emotional experiences during the three trimesters of pregnancy. Journal of Clinical Psychology, 49, 3-12.

Rubin, R. (1984). Maternal identity and the maternal experience. New York: Springer-Verlag.

Sorenson, D.L.S. (1990). Uncertainty in pregnancy. NAACOG's Clinical Issues in Perinatal and Women's Health Nursing, 1(3), 289-296.

Ugarriza, D.N. (1992). Postpartum Affective Disorders: Incidence and treatment. Journal of Psychosocial Nursing and Mental Health Services, 30(5), 29-32.

Whiffen, V. (1988). Vulnerability to postpartum depression: A prospective multivariate study. Journal of Abnormal Psychology, 97, 467-474.

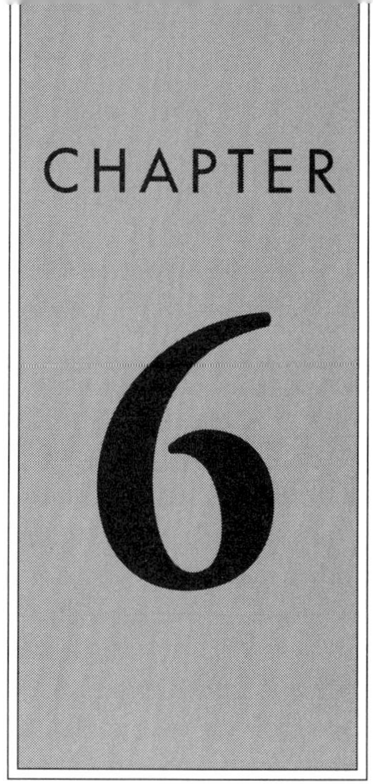

Antenatal Care and Risk Assessment Strategies

Susan Kendig
Mary Lee Barron

Quality prenatal care includes education and support for the pregnant woman, ongoing maternal-fetal assessment, preparation for parenting, and promotion of a positive physical and emotional family experience. The goals of prenatal care are the following:

- maintenance of maternal-fetal health
- accurate determination of gestational age
- ongoing risk assessment and risk-appropriate intervention
- woman/family education about pregnancy, birth, and parenting
- rapport with the childbearing family
- referral to appropriate resources.

BIRTH IN THE UNITED STATES

As the 21st century approaches, an examination of natality trends in the United States over the past several decades provides a basis for understanding current challenges and goals of prenatal care. Important trends to examine are the effect of the post-war "baby-boom" on age distribution of women of childbearing age and patterns of childbearing among women of various ages including the rise in the pregnancy rate of adolescents and unmarried women. Studies have shown that prenatal care has the greatest impact on those women who are at highest risk of poor pregnancy outcome such as adolescents and unmarried and minority women (Horton, 1995).

Birth Rate Trends

Since the baby boom of the late 1940s, 1950s and early 1960s, the birth rate in the U.S. has steadily declined. A reversal of that trend occurred between 1986 and 1990, when the annual number of births in the U.S. actually increased overall by 11% (National Center for Health Statistics [NCHS], 1993b). In 1990, there were approximately 4,065,000 births in the U.S.; the highest number since the baby boom years (NCHS, 1993b). However, since the peak in 1990, birth rates are again declining (by 2% in 1991 and by 2.5% in 1992) (NCHS, 1994). In 1993, the last year for which data are available, there were approximately 4,039,000 births (Centers for Disease Control and Prevention [CDC], 1995b).

Although the overall birth rate has declined, the number of births to women between ages 35 and 44 has continued to increase because as the population ages, there are more women in that age group (NCHS, 1993b). Birth rates for adolescents aged 15 to 17 and 18 to 19 increased between 1980 to 1991 (NCHS, 1993b), associated in part, to the growing proportion of teenagers who are sexually active (Children's Defense Fund, 1994). However, in 1992, the birth rate among U.S. teenagers aged 15 to 17 years decreased by 2% to 37.8 per 1,000 live births (NCHS, 1994), a reversal of the trend from 1986 to 1991 when births in this age group increased overall by 27%. In 1992 approximately 13% of infants were born to women under 20 years of age (NCHS, 1994). The number of births to unmarried women in 1991 was the highest ever reported in the U.S., a 4% increase over 1990 (NCHS, 1993b). This increase was 6% for African American women and 2% for Caucasian women, representing a percentage of all births to unmarried African American women of 67.9% and a percentage of all births to unmarried Caucasian women of 21.8% (NCHS, 1993b).

Social Trends

Social trends to consider related to U.S. natality statistics include decreased family size and an increased number of women in the work force. Family size, roles, and living environments have been affected by recent economic and technological changes. Factors influencing family dynamics include high divorce rates, increased age at first marriage, increased number of female-headed households, and an increased number of women of childbearing age who live alone. In addition, consideration must be given to recent data on chemical dependency, homelessness, and poverty. Growth in illicit drug use among women of childbearing age and their partners has contributed to epidemics of AIDS, and other sexually transmitted diseases. Socioeconomic factors, such as an increase in the poverty rate and a decline in healthcare insurance coverage, have created barriers to prenatal care and affected pregnancy outcomes (March of Dimes, 1993). Nearly one third of births in the United States are subsidized by Medicaid (Carpenter, 1995); however due to differences in state eligibility requirements, many poor women still do not receive prenatal care.

Infant Mortality

The infant mortality rate refers to the number of deaths in children younger than 1 year of age per 1,000 live births. Although incidence of infant deaths during the first year of life has decreased dramatically since the turn of the century, rate of decline has been slower in

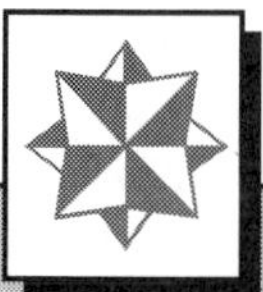

DISPLAY 6-1

Preterm Delivery and Neonatal Mortality and Morbidity

- 10% of all births account for 75% of perinatal deaths not due to congenital malformations
- 85% of neonatal deaths between 22 and 37 weeks are associated with preterm infants
- Preterm infants are 40 times more likely to die in the neonatal period than those with normal birth weights
- Low-birth-weight infants < 1,500 g have 3.2 hospital admissions during the first year of life
- Low-birth-weight infants > 1500 g are 200 times more likely to die during the first year of life than infants born weighing more than 2500 g.
- Neurodevelopmental handicaps—cerebral palsy, seizure disorders, and mental retardation—are 10 times more common in < 1,500 g versus> 2,500 g infants

Adapted from Morrison, J.C. (1990). Preterm birth: A puzzle worth solving. Obstetrics and Gynecology, 76 (1 Suppl.)., 58-128 and American College of Obstetricians and Gynecologists (1995b). Preterm labor. ACOG Technical Bulletin No. 206, Washington, DC: Author.

recent years. In 1991, the United States ranked twenty second among developed countries in infant mortality, and 39 countries had infant mortality rates lower than that of African Americans (NCHS, 1993a). The U.S. African American infant mortality rate (17.6) remains at 2.2 times the rate for Caucasian infants (7.5) (Children's Defense Fund, 1994).

Preterm birth, before 37 completed weeks' gestation, continues to be a significant cause of perinatal mortality and morbidity. During the last 20 years, advances in neonatal intensive care have improved outcomes for small neonates. Advances in perinatal care have allowed for increased lengths of gestation in women at risk for preterm birth. In spite of technological advances, the incidence of preterm birth of appropriate for gestational age infants has not declined over the past 40 years (American College of Obstetricians and Gynecologists [ACOG], 1995b). Preterm birth has become the single most common cause of poor birth outcome (Display 6-1), with 10% of all births contributing to at least 75% of perinatal morbidity and mortality (ACOG; Morrison, 1990). The highest percentage of perinatal mortality is related to preterm birth before 28 weeks' gestation (ACOG). Approximately 80% of preterm births occur after 32 weeks' gestation. Live-born infants of gestational age above 32 weeks have a risk in mortality similar to term infants and have only a mildly increased risk of serious morbidity when compared with term infants (Kiely, 1991). Interestingly, studies of the effect of prenatal care alone tend to show that the largest improvement in mortality occurs in term newborns, not those that are born preterm (Tyson, Guzick, & Rosenfeld, 1990).

Maternal Mortality

Numerous definitions of maternal death by professional organizations, individual states, government agencies, and the World Health Organization (WHO) have contributed to inconsistencies and inaccuracies in reporting maternal mortality statistics. The Centers for Disease Control and Prevention (CDC) estimates there is approximately 37% underreporting of maternal deaths in the United States (Atrash, Rowley, & Hogue, 1992). The CDC's definitions of maternal deaths are as follows:

- **Pregnancy-associated maternal death**—the death of any woman from any cause, while she is pregnant or within 1 calendar year of termination of pregnancy, regardless of duration and site of pregnancy;
- **Pregnancy-related maternal death**—the death of any woman resulting from complications of the pregnancy itself, the chain of events initiated by the pregnancy that led to the death, or aggravation of an unrelated condition by the physiologic or pharmacologic effects of the pregnancy that subsequently caused death (Ellerbrock, Atrash, Hogue, & Smith, 1988).

Maternal mortality has decreased at a slower rate during recent years than in the past years (Atrash, Rowley, & Hogue, 1992). From 1975 to 1981 the maternal mortality rate (MMR) decreased 34% from 12.8 to 8.5 per 100,000 live births; however, from 1982 to 1988, the MMR actually increased 6% from 7.9 to 8.4 (Atrash et al.). From 1975 through 1988, African American women had a MMR three to four times that of Caucasian women (Atrash et al., 1992). By 1990 the MMR had decreased slightly to 8.2. In 1991, the last year for which data are available, the MMR was 7.9, the same as it had been in 1982 (CDC, 1995a; NCHS, 1993a). Although the overall MMR has decreased 98% since 1940 when there were 363.9 deaths per 100,000 live births, maternal mortality during pregnancy and childbirth remains a significant problem, especially for women in minority groups (CDC, 1995a).

MMRs have traditionally been reported as rate per 100,000 live births, but this statistical methodology does not result in a true rate. While all maternal deaths, regardless of outcomes, are included in the numerator, only live births are included in the denominator. These data actually reflect a maternal mortality ratio. In 1988 the CDC proposed the following statistical measures of pregnancy-related mortality to facilitate comparisons and identify groups at special risk: (1) pregnancy mortality ratio—the number of pregnancy-related deaths per 100,000 live births; (2) pregnancy mortality rate—the number of pregnancy-related deaths per 100,000 reported pregnancies; and (3) outcome-specific pregnancy mortality rate—the number of deaths related to a specific outcome per 100,000 pregnancies that resulted in the same outcome (Ellerbrock, Atrash, Hogue, & Smith, 1988). Outcome-specific pregnancy mortality rates can be used to determine risk associated with specific pregnancy outcomes (live birth, stillbirth, ectopic pregnancy, molar pregnancy, abortion, and undelivered). While these data will improve accuracy, data on number of actual pregnancies are difficult to obtain. Legal abortions are reported in the United States, but spontaneous abortions may not be reported, especially if they occur early in gestation. When comparing across countries, it will be important to clarify the denominator (i.e., live births or all reported pregnancies).

ACCESS TO PRENATAL CARE

Many women in the United States receive little or no prenatal care even though there has been social support for the importance of prenatal care since the early 1900s. In 1992, 16% of all pregnant women in the United States received late or no prenatal care (defined as beginning care after the fifth month of pregnancy or beginning earlier but receiving fewer than half of the visits recommended by the American Academy of Pediatrics [AAP] and the American College of Obstetricians [ACOG] (1992) in *Guidelines for Perinatal Care* [Horton, 1995; March of Dimes, 1993]). Only 78% of pregnant women began care in the first trimester in 1992 (Givens & Moore, 1995). Women beginning care in the third trimester and women receiving no prenatal care are at increased risk of poor pregnancy outcomes. Regular prenatal care is associated with reduced infant mortality and favorable outcomes on measures of child health such as birth weight.

Many programs have been developed in an effort to improve birth outcomes in the United States. Most have focused on the antepartum period, with emphasis on increasing use of prenatal care. Opportunities for intervention before pregnancy have received less attention. Because many women become pregnant unintentionally, education about preconception health should be a component of care for all women of childbearing age (ACOG, 1995a). Information can be provided during routine healthcare visits, following discussion of family planning methods. Identification of medical complications that increase risks to both the woman and fetus allow opportunity for early intervention. Women with preexisting conditions such as diabetes, phenylketonuria, seizure disorders, or infectious diseases can especially benefit from preconception health counseling (ACOG). All women need information about the use of folic acid to prevent neural tube defects, the importance of avoiding certain prescription medications, and strategies to promote dietary and lifestyle changes before they become pregnant (ACOG). Family planning services and school-based nurses are in strategic positions to promote the importance of a planned pregnancy and early comprehensive prenatal care (Jamieson & Buescher, 1992). In a recent study of factors in the use of prenatal services by low-income African American women, an unanticipated finding was that many women delayed care because they were not aware of the pregnancy (Burks, 1992). Additionally, seeking early and frequent care was determined by the presence of known risk factors or symptoms (Burks).

Factors that Influence the Decision to Seek Prenatal Care

Relatively little is known about factors that influence pregnant women's decisions about initiating and continuing prenatal care. Key demographic factors associated with insufficient prenatal care include poverty, being unmarried, age under 20, higher parity, and having less than a high school education. In one study, ethnicity was not a significant predictor of the woman's decision to initiate prenatal care when other demographic variables were controlled (Goldenburg, Patterson, & Freese, 1992); however in the United States, African American and Hispanic women generally receive prenatal care later than Caucasian women. According to the most recent data, the percentage of African American women (39.4%) who did not receive prenatal care in the first trimester during 1990 was nearly twice that of Caucasian women (20.8%) (CDC, 1995a). Reasons for this disparity are unclear. The CDC suggests that differences in pregnancy-related morbidity, access to and use of healthcare services, and content and quality of prenatal care may be possible explanations. It is often difficult or impossible to separate the effects of poverty, marital status, or other socioeconomic factors from the decision to seek prenatal care (Goldenberg et al., 1992; March of Dimes, 1993). Variables that influence use of prenatal care and are associated with the previously mentioned demographic variables have been identified in a number of studies and include the following: an unintended pregnancy, little perceived value attached to prenatal care, a tenuous connection to the healthcare system, negative experiences with healthcare providers, financial difficulties, and ambivalence or fear regarding the pregnancy (Goldenberg et al.; Harvey & Faber, 1992; March of Dimes).

Trends in Provider Selection

In the recent past, the focus of prenatal care concerned collection and evaluation of laboratory values and physical measurements. This approach did not address what women may need in terms of health education, counseling, and social support (McClanahan, 1992). The majority of preterm birth prevention programs incorporating risk assessment, patient education, and frequent provider visits, have shown promise in reducing preterm births when compared with standard prenatal care programs (Morrison, 1990). Minimal progress in the decline of the infant mortality rate in the United States in recent years has stimulated a shift in focus from "high-tech" care to primary prevention. High-quality prenatal care (a multidisciplinary effort), including financial access to such care for poor women, is recognized as a key strategy for improving birth outcome (Handler & Rosenberg, 1992).

Advanced practice nurses (APNs) such as women's health nurse practitioners (WHNPs), family nurse practitioners (FNPs), and certified nurse-midwives (CNMs) are becoming more involved in providing primary care. APNs can provide many primary-care services as competently and more cost effectively than physicians (Brown & Grimes, 1993; Wilson, 1989). A recent study comparing adherence to ACOG guidelines for prenatal care among obstetricians, family physicians and certified nurse midwives found the CNMs' standards of practice most closely matched that recommended by ACOG (AAP & ACOG, 1992) in *Guidelines for Perinatal Care* (Baldwin, Raine, Jenkins, Hart, & Rosenblatt, 1994). Not only are APNs competent to perform physical assessments, but they also focus on psychosocial support, counseling, and education; this focus has been shown to have a positive effect on pregnancy outcome (McClanahan, 1992).

Perinatal clinical nurse specialists (CNSs) practice in an advanced role, primarily in the inpatient setting. Major functions of the CNS are consultation, patient and staff education, research, and coordination and delivery of nursing care to families requiring intensive nursing support. The perinatal nurse practitioner (PNNP) is a new role for advanced practice nurses in the perinatal specialty. PNNPs practice collaboratively with perinatalogists and obstetricians in the care of high-risk pregnant women in both acute-care and ambulatory care settings.

Rural areas, underserved by physicians, are the testing grounds for new models that allow nurses to function independently. Rural hospitals are relying more heavily on outpatient services for revenue, and APNs are viewed as the most economic providers of such care. Direct reimbursement for services and legal authority to write prescriptions are necessary for independent practice. Presently, 44 states have some type of prescriptive authority (Pearson, 1994). Reimbursement issues are more complex even though the U.S. Congress approved direct reimbursement for nurse practitioners in rural areas, and Medicaid reimbursement for certified nurse-midwives and pediatric and family nurse practitioners. Reimbursement administration varies from state to state.

Because there is an overlap between nursing and medical practice, conflict is likely. Consumers need to know more about nursing care and choices of healthcare providers. Information necessary to make a choice between a nurse practitioner, nurse-midwife, a family practice physician, and an obstetrician for safe, affordable primary care has not been widely available to the general public (Haller, 1992). If APNs are more accessible as providers, women enrolled in Medicaid programs may be able to initiate prenatal care earlier and, therefore, may have less risk for poor pregnancy outcome. Additionally, there are subgroups (i.e., adolescents and women with medical complications) that especially benefit from comprehensive care. A combined medical and nursing team approach could be used for providing prenatal care, with other professionals (e.g., social workers, nutritionists, etc.) consulted as needed. Collaboration complements the expertise of nurses and physicians. The woman benefits by receiving higher quality and more individualized care.

THE EFFECTS OF PRENATAL CARE ON BIRTH OUTCOME

Early, adequate prenatal care has long been associated with improved pregnancy outcomes. Continued contact with the pregnant woman, via comprehensive prenatal care, provides an ideal opportunity for the healthcare provider to assess for and identify potential problems that may place the woman and fetus at risk. Risk-appropriate prenatal care further enhances the possibility of a positive pregnancy outcome among women who are at increased medical or social risk (ACOG, 1995b; Chasnoff, 1989; Finnegan, 1990; McAnarney & Hendee, 1989).

More data are needed about which components of prenatal care are protective against adverse maternal-infant outcomes. A recent study examining the relationship of prenatal care and the risk of having a second preterm or low-birth-weight infant suggests the lack of scientific knowledge of causal factors for preterm birth and low-birth-weight infants contributes to the inability to design prenatal care programs that are more effective in preventing poor outcomes (Raine, Powell, & Krohn, 1994). Until the underlying pathophysiology of preterm birth and the risks related to socioeconomic and lifestyle factors are fully understood, prenatal care should be directed towards early identification, education, and intervention, with frequent contact between the pregnant woman and her primary healthcare provider.

Identification of Potential Problems

Birth defects, low birth weight/prematurity, and Sudden Infant Death Syndrome (SIDS) account for over one half of all infant deaths in the United States (March of Dimes, 1993). Lack of adequate prenatal care has been associated with an increased incidence of prematurity and low birth weight (ACOG, 1995b). These factors have also been closely associated with infant mortality (Carpenter, 1995; Children's Defense Fund, 1994).

Low-birth weight infants born to mothers who have received adequate prenatal care exhibit less respiratory distress and intraventricular hemorrhage and have significantly better perinatal survival experiences. National goals established for the year 2000 underscore the importance of prenatal care. Healthcare professionals must be diligent in efforts to remove barriers to accessing and using prenatal care services in order to achieve the national goal of 90% of all pregnant women being enrolled in early prenatal care by the year 2000 (Arnold & Grad, 1992).

Definition of Adequate Prenatal Care

General guidelines for prenatal care have been established (AAP & ACOG, 1992); however, these recommendations are not consistently followed by all healthcare providers (Baldwin et al., 1994). Traditionally, prenatal care has been evaluated using the number of prenatal visits, gestational age at entry into prenatal care, or a combination of these factors. If the number of prenatal visits is used as the sole evaluation criteria, women who deliver premature infants and, therefore, have less prenatal visits are misclassified. Lack of differentiation between women who seek prenatal care late in pregnancy and those women who have one or two early visits and then lose contact with the healthcare system further complicates the evaluation of adequate prenatal care and reporting of vital statistics.

Adequate prenatal care is a comprehensive process in which problems associated with pregnancy are identified and treated. Additionally, education and support arc provided. Three basic components of adequate prenatal care have been identified: early and continuing risk assessments, health promotion, and medical and psychosocial interventions with follow up (Expert Panel on the Content of Prenatal Care,

1989). Comprehensive services include health education, nutrition education, the Women, Infants and Children's (WIC) program, social services assessment, medical risk assessment, and referral as appropriate.

PRENATAL RISK ASSESSMENT

The goal of risk assessment is to identify women and fetuses at risk for developing antepartum, intrapartum, postpartum, or neonatal complications in order to promote risk-appropriate care, thus enhancing perinatal outcome. Despite advances in perinatal technology, the underlying causes of preterm labor and intrauterine growth restriction are not fully understood. Because of these limitations, a perfect risk-assessment system has not been identified (Edenfield, Thomas, Thompson, & Marcotte, 1995; Enkins, 1994; York & Brooten, 1992). However, a large body of knowledge regarding risk factors associated with prematurity and low birth weight has developed. These factors include demographic, medical, obstetric, sociocultural, lifestyle, and environmental risks. It is important to note that many risk factors have been identified in studies of women who develop complications of pregnancy or deliver preterm; however, no firm cause-and-effect relationship between some of the commonly associated risk factors and poor outcome has been established (Enkins). For example, marital status or low income does not cause poor pregnancy outcomes; however, many women who are unmarried or live in poverty do experience complications of pregnancy. Risk-assessment tools may be helpful in distinguishing between women at high and low risk. Unfortunately, the predictive value of these tools is limited. A significant number of problems occur in women not identified as high-risk. Approximately one third of the potential complications of pregnancy occur during the intrapartum period and are not predictable by current risk-assessment systems (AAP & ACOG, 1992; Auman & Baird, 1993;). However, many identified risk factors respond to interventions. It is imperative, therefore, that early and ongoing risk assessment be an integral part of prenatal care (York & Brooten). The nurse's knowledge of prenatal risk assessment allows for anticipatory planning, individualized education, and appropriate referral. The nurse's role in prenatal care is discussed within these parameters.

Initial Prenatal Visit

Antepartum assessment begins with the first prenatal visit. Generally, a woman with an uncomplicated pregnancy should be examined approximately every 4 weeks for the first 28 weeks of pregnancy, every 2–3 weeks until 36 weeks gestation, and weekly thereafter. Women with medical or obstetric problems may require closer surveillance. Intervals between visits are determined by the nature and severity of the problem (AAP & ACOG, 1992).

The initial prenatal visit is of vital importance and requires careful attention to detail. The nurse should practice within the framework of professional standards, such as *NAACOG Standards for the Nursing Care of Women and Newborns* (1991), and *Guidelines for Perinatal Care* (AAP & ACOG, 1992) that provide guidelines for practice in the ambulatory care setting. During the first prenatal visit, baseline health data are obtained and assessed, a patient-centered relationship is established, and the plan of care is initiated. Risk assessment during the initial prenatal visit should include:

- a careful family medical history, individual medical history, and reproductive health history
- a comprehensive physical examination designed to evaluate potential risk factors
- routine prenatal laboratory screening
- individualized, risk-appropriate laboratory evaluation
- fetal assessment after the first trimester [fetal heart rate (FHR), fetal activity, kick counts] and individualized fetal surveillance as indicated [nonstress test (NST), ultrasonography (US), biophysical profile (BPP)].

Medical and Obstetrical History

Assessment of health factors that may influence pregnancy outcome includes careful evaluation of the woman's individual medical, gynecologic, and obstetric history. In addition, pertinent family history of both the woman and her partner is necessary for complete evaluation. Maternal family reproductive health history (e.g., preeclampsia, hypertension, and preterm birth) may be particularly significant. Chronic conditions (e.g., diabetes, hypertension, or cardiac disease) are known to be affected by the additional physiologic stress of pregnancy. Likewise, factors such as a history of frequent sexually transmitted diseases (STD) or chemical dependency may be indicative of lifestyle behaviors that threaten maternal-fetal wellbeing.

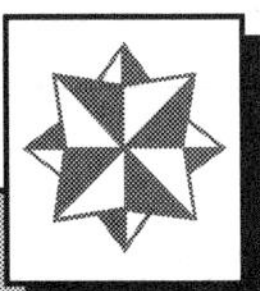

Display 6-2

Risk Assessment

OB History

- History of infertility
- Grand multiparity
- Incompetent cervix
- Uterine/cervical anomaly
- Previous preterm labor/preterm birth
- Previous cesarean birth
- Previous macrosomic infant
- Previous ectopic/SAB
- Previous stillborn/neonatal death
- Previous multiple gestation
- Previous prolonged labor
- Previous LBW infant
- Previous midforceps delivery
- DES exposure in utero
- Two or more spontaneous or elective abortions
- Last pregnancy < 1 year before present conception
- Previous hydatidiform mole/choriocarcinoma
- Previous infant with neurological deficit/birth injury/congenital anomaly

Medical History

- Cardiac disease
- Metabolic disease
- Gastrointestinal disorders
- Chronic hypertension
- Seizure disorders
- Malignancy
- Pulmonary disease
- Renal disease/repeat urinary tract infections/bacteriuria
- Endocrine disorders
- Hemoglobinopathies
- Sexually transmitted diseases
- Surgery during pregnancy
- Reproductive tract anomalies
- Emotional disorders/mental retardation
- Family history of severe inherited disorders
- Previous surgeries, particularly involving the reproductive organs
- History of abnormal Pap smear

Current OB Status

- Inadequate prenatal care
- Intrauterine growth restricted fetus
- Large for gestational age fetus
- Pregnancy-induced hypertension/preeclampsia
- Polyhydramnios
- Placenta previa
- Abnormal presentation
- Maternal anemia
- Weight gain < 10 lb
- Weight loss ≥ 5 lb
- Over/under weight
- Immunization status
- Fetal/placental malformations
- Abnormal fetal surveillance tests
- Rh sensitization
- Preterm labor
- Multiple gestation
- Premature rupture of membranes
- Abruptio placentae
- Postdatism
- Fibroids
- Fetal manipulation
- Cervical cerclage
- Sexually transmitted diseases
- Maternal infection

DISPLAY 6-2 (cont.)

Psychosocial Factors

Inadequate finances	Poor housing
Social problems	Unwed/Father of baby uninvolved
Adolescent	Minority status
Poor nutrition	Parental occupation
More than 2 children at home/no help	Inadequate support systems
Unacceptance of pregnancy	Dysfunctional grieving
Attempt/ideation of suicide	Psychiatric history

Demographic Factors

Maternal age <16 or >35	Education <11 years

Lifestyle

Smokes >10 cigarettes/day	Alcohol intake
Substance abuse	Heavy lifting/long periods of standing
Long commute	Unusual stress
Non-use of seat belts	No in-home smoke detectors

Obstetrical history, such as length of previous labors, birth weight, gestational age, history of preterm labor/preterm birth, operative birth, grand multiparity, elective or spontaneous abortion, previous stillbirth, or uterine or cervical anomaly may indicate potential risks for the current pregnancy (Fogel & Lewallen, 1995). Familial history, including cardiac disease, diabetes, bleeding disorders, etc., should be noted. The woman may also be affected by her mothers obstetrical history. Daughters born to mothers who maintained their pregnancy through use of diethylstilbestrol (DES) may have uterine anomalies that increase their risk for preterm labor. There is a familial predispostion to develop preeclampsia. Finally, both the pregnant woman's and the father's family medical and genetic history serves to guide counseling and testing for predisposed genetic complications.

Socioeconomic Factors

Demographic factors, such as maternal age and education, have been linked to pregnancy outcomes. Optimal childbearing age is considered to be between 20 and 30 years of age, with an increased risk of perinatal morbidity after age 35. Children born to mothers less than 19 or more than 35 years of age have an increased risk of prematurity, congenital anomalies, and risks from other complications of pregnancy (Fogel & Lewallen, 1995). The incidence of genetic anomalies such as Down syndrome increases with advanced maternal age (Hook, 1981). Number of years of completed maternal education has been correlated to birth weight, perinatal mortality and morbidity, and neonatal neurological sequelae (Auman & Baird, 1993). In general, as years of maternal education increase, incidence of perinatal mortality and morbidity decrease. This association may be a reflection of education as an indicator of socioeconomic status. A disproportionate number of women of childbearing age are uninsured or underinsured. Women in lower socioeconomic groups tend to initiate prenatal care later than their middle socioeconomic group counterparts (York & Brooten, 1992).

Both maternal and paternal occupation and employment status has been linked to perinatal outcome. Overall, the highest incidence of perinatal loss occurs in families where the father is not present. In families where the father is present, the incidence of perinatal loss is higher when the father is a semiskilled or manual laborer, and lower in families where the father is a professional or a farmer (Auman & Baird, 1993). Multiple studies suggest marital status is associated with incidence of low birth weight. In a recent study evaluating perinatal outcomes of nearly 15,000 singleton pregnancies, women who were separated, divorced, or widowed had 43% more low-birth-weight infants than women who were married (McIntosh, Roumayah, & Bottoms, 1995).

Women in low-income positions or employed as unskilled laborers are at increased risk for preterm labor. The woman's occupation may require long commutes, heavy work, or long periods of standing or sitting, all of which contribute to the risk of preterm labor. However, decreasing or eliminating work during pregnancy may place the woman at greater socioeconomic risk by threatening her livelihood. Socioeconomic factors influence gestational age at entry to prenatal care, nutritional status, and availability of support systems.

Lifestyle Factors

Lifestyle/behavior factors have significant effects on women's health in general, and perinatal health specifically. Approximately 8–10% of birth defects occur due to environmental factors such as maternal infection, disease, or exposure to chemicals, drugs, and/or alcohol (Beckman & Brent, 1986; Robins & Mills, 1993). All of these factors can be linked to lifestyle issues and can be affected by positive healthcare decisions (Pletsch, 1990). Careful assessment of the woman's daily routine provides valuable information about potential lifestyle risk factors.

Nutritional care during the antepartum period should include nutritional assessment, nutritional counseling, and nutrient supplements as appropriate. The nutrition assessment includes diet information (1–3 day recall), monitoring weight gain, and hematologic assessment. Assessment of usual dietary patterns provides a basis for understanding nutritional health. Variations from the normal dietary routine, such as eating disorders, food shortages, and metabolic disorders such as diabetes, warrant additional interventions. Both the Institute of Medicine (1990) and ACOG (1993a) recommend a weight gain for women, based on their prepregnant weights and single births (Table 6-1). A weight gain of 35–45 lb is recommended for women with twins (ACOG, & Institute of Medicine). Weight gain should be carefully monitored during each prenatal visit (Muerer & Taren, 1993). Weight gain or loss may be indicative of maternal nutritional status or development of complications. Excessive weight gain, weight loss, or inadequate weight gain indicates a need for consultation with a nutritionist. Weight gain of more than 5–10 lbs in 1 week after 20 weeks' gestation requires evaluation for preeclampsia.

TABLE 6-1. Recommendations for Weight Gain During Pregnancy

Prepregnant Status	Pounds	
Underweight	28–40 lb	(12.7–18.2 kg)
Average Weight	25–35 lb	(11.4–15.9 kg)
Overweight	15–25 lb	(6.8–11.4 kg)
Obese	15 lb	(6.8 kg)

From Nutrition During Pregnacy, by Institute of Medicine, 1990, Washington, DC: National Academy Press; Nutrition During Pregnancy, ACOG Technical Bulletin, 179, by American College of Obstetricians and Gynecologists, 1993, Washington, DC: Author.

Cigarette smoking has been linked to an increased incidence of low birth weight and prematurity. Yet, in one study, less than 20% of pregnant women who smoked quit when pregnancy was confirmed (Hebel, Fox, & Sexton, 1988). The incidence of perinatal substance abuse increased during the early 1980s (Hoyme et al., 1990). Data from the 1991 National Household Survey on Drug Abuse indicate that over 4.5 million women of childbearing age had used some type of illicit drug in the month prior to the survey (U.S. Department of Health and Human Services, 1991).

Substance abuse or chemical dependency affects all body systems, and can cause cardiac, pulmonary, gastrointestinal, and psychiatric complications. Use of unsterile drug paraphernalia contributes to infection and disease transmission. When substance abuse occurs during pregnancy, maternal risk of abruptio placenta, preterm labor, sudden cardiac death, and stroke is increased (Chasnoff, 1989). It is important to note that substance abusers rarely abuse a single substance (ACOG, 1994c). The woman's lifestyle when using drugs (which may include alcohol abuse, cigarette smoking, inadequate prenatal care, poor nutrition, and sexual promiscuity) further complicates the pregnancy (Brown, & Zuckerman, 1991). Robins and Mills' (1993) comprehensive review of research on the effects of substance exposure in utero found that, overall, there is enough data to suggest substance exposure adversely affects some pregnancies. However, individual research studies have found the effects of substance exposure in utero to be transitory. It is difficult to determine to what extent complications of pregnancy may be attributed to actual drug use or to lifestyle factors associated with drug use (Robins & Mills). Because substance abuse or chemical dependency can adversely affect the health of both the woman and the fetus, it is essential to include drug use assessment and education strategies in prenatal and women's health care encounters (Chapter Appendix).

A moderate level of physical activity, in the absence of medical or obstetrical complications, maintains cardiorespiratory and muscular fitness throughout pregnancy (ACOG, 1994b). However, activities which cause excessive fatigue such as heavy work, strenuous activities, job-related stress, climbing more than three flights of stairs on a routine basis, or daily commutes of 1.5 to 2 hours per day may stimulate uterine contractions. Research suggests that exhaustive occupations increase risk of perinatal complications (Papiernik, Keith, Bouyer, Dreyfus, & Lazar, 1989; Papiernik, 1993). However, one study found that unemployed women had higher preterm labor rates than their employed counterparts (Mamelle, Laumon, Munoz, & Collin, 1989). Household tasks may be a source of fatigue equal to or greater than job-related fatigue. Household stress is further influenced by home ownership (private or government housing); quality of comfort (heat, water); housekeeping burden; and number and age of children (Mamelle et al.). Unusual stressful events, such as death of a significant family member or friend, job loss, or a problematic relationship with the baby's father may increase risk of poor pregnancy outcome.

Current pregnancy status

Assessment of current pregnancy status includes the following: (1) examination of current pregnancy history, psychosocial factors, nutritional status, and laboratory data; (2) a review of symptoms that may reflect medical or pregnancy complications; and (3) a complete physical examination. Symptom review includes questions about nausea and vomiting, headache, abdominal or epigastric pain, visual changes, fever, viral illness, vaginal bleeding, dysuria, cramping, and other concerns. This screening process incorporates assessment of historical and social factors with current health status. Evaluation of current pregnancy status provides baseline data that guides planning for future evaluation and health promotion activities.

The physical examination is comprehensive and covers a review of the cardiovascular, respiratory, neurologic, endocrine, gastrointestinal, reproductive, and genitourinary systems. Particular attention should be directed to the anthropometric assessment including the woman's height, weight, and pelvimetry data because these physical characteristics can potentially influence the pregnancy course and birth (Witter, Caulfield, & Stoltzfus, 1995). Pelvic examination includes measurement of cervical length, a pap smear, and assessment for sexually transmitted diseases. The abdominal examination compares data from the woman's report of her last menstrual period with physical findings. Depending on weeks of gestation, the fetal heart rate may be auscultated.

Nutritional assessment is an integral component of the first visit since maternal weight may affect pregnancy outcome. Underweight women, or women who fail to gain the recommended 25–40 lbs (25–45 lbs with twins) during pregnancy (ACOG, 1993a), are at greater risk for delivering low-birth-weight infants. Women who are overweight, or who exceed the recommended prenatal weight gain, are at greater risk for developing preeclampsia or for delivering a large-for-gestational-age infant, increasing the risk for perinatal mortality and morbidity (Auman & Baird, 1993). There may be a relationship between the pattern and timing of maternal weight gain and infant birth weight. A recent study of healthy nonobese women suggests that the amount of weight gained during the second trimester is more predictive of infant birth weight than total maternal weight gain (Abrams & Selvin, 1995).

Selected laboratory data are valuable to the assessment process. Biochemical information provides information about current prenatal health, as well as general wellness status from a women's health perspective. Evaluation of specific laboratory data is discussed later in this chapter.

Psychological risk factors cannot be overlooked. Pregnancy affects the entire family, and therefore, assessment and intervention must be considered in a family-centered perspective. Stress has been suggested as a potential contributor to physical complications during pregnancy and birth, including prolonged labor, increased use of intrapartum analgesics and barbiturates, and other complications. Maternal anxiety has also been associated with interference in fetal and newborn development (Lederman, 1990). Other symptoms of dysfunctional family relationships, such as violence toward the pregnant woman, child abuse, or psychosomatic illnesses, are also indicative of risk and warrant investigation.

Ongoing Prenatal Care

Subsequent prenatal visits should be structured to promote continuous, rather than episodic, risk assessment.

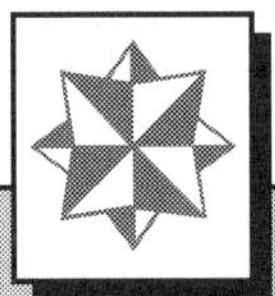

DISPLAY 6-3

Schedule of Prenatal Care

Initial Prenatal Visit

INTAKE ASSESSMENT

- Comprehensive medical and reproductive health history
- Comprehensive family history
- History of current pregnancy
- Psychosocial assessment (by social worker if possible)
- Nutrition assessment (by nutritionist if possible)
- Comprehensive physical examination

BIOCHEMICAL EVALUATION

- Complete blood count (CBC)
- Blood type and Rh; antibody screen
- PAP Smear
- Gonorrhea culture
- Chlamydia test
- Serology (RPR, VDRL)
- Rubella (unless previously noted to be immune)
- Hepatitis B Surface Antigen (HB_SAg)
- Urinalysis
- Urine culture and sensitivity
- Sickle cell screen (for women of African, Asian, or Middle Eastern descent)
- Tay Sachs screening (for women of Jewish or French-Canadian ancestry)
- Glucose Challenge Test (GCT) if woman is at risk, as indicated by:
  - History of fetal demise
  - Recurrent spontaneous abortion
  - History of prior macrosomic infant (birthweight > 4,000 g)
  - History of gestational diabetes
  - Maternal family history of diabetes (1st degree relatives)
  - Obesity
- Offer HIV testing (provide pretest counselling)
- PPD (tuberculin screen)
- Obtain if indicated:
  - TORCH titres
  - Group B Streptococcus culture
  - Ultrasound examination

DISPLAY 6-3 (cont.)

Subsequent Visits

ASSESSMENT (each visit)

Vital signs

Urine dipstick for glucose, albumin, and ketones

Weight

Fundal height

Fetal heart rate (FHR)

Fetal movement

Leopold's maneuvers to evaluate fetal lie/presentation

Assess presence/absence of edema

15–20 weeks

Maternal serum α-fetoprotein (MSAFP)

Begin preterm birth prevention education

20–24 weeks

Preterm birth prevention education

24–28 weeks

Cervical exam at 28 weeks as indicated by risk status

One hour GCT

Ongoing education about preterm birth prevention and warning signs of pregnancy complications

Initiate education regarding contraceptive options

28–36 weeks

CBC at 28 weeks for selected at–risk women

Blood group antibody screen at 28 weeks if Rh negative; RhoGAM if indirect Coombs negative

Cervical examination at 32 weeks as indicated by risk status

Follow up visit with dietitian/nutritionist

Breast assessment/educational preparation for breastfeeding

Ongoing education about preterm birth prevention and warning signs of pregnancy complications

Initiate parenting education

36–40 weeks

CBC if Hbg <11g/dl or Hct <33% at 28 weeks

Repeat GC, chlamydia, RPR, HIV, HB_SAg if indicated

Initiate education about signs of labor, preparation for birth (after 37 weeks' gestation)

Adapted from American Academy of Pediatrics & American College of Obstetricians and Gynecologists. (1992). Guidelines for perinatal care (3rd ed.). Elk Grove Village IL: Author and Shannon, M.T. (1990b) Initial prenatal visit. In W.L. Star, M.T. Shannon, L.N. Sammons, L. Lommel, & Y. Gutierrez (Eds.). Ambulatory Obstetrics: Protocols for nurse practitioners/nurse midwives (2nd ed.). San Francisco: School of Nursing, University of California.

Each prenatal visit should include a maternal-fetal physical assessment: vital signs, weight, fundal height, fetal heart rate, and fetal movement (Display 6-3).

Particular attention should be given to evaluation of blood pressure trends. During pregnancy, blood pressure values decrease slightly during the second trimester, but return to early pregnancy values by the third trimester. Ideally, during preconception care or early prenatal care, a baseline blood pressure is noted. It is important to evaluate and document blood pressure measurements in the same arm with the woman in the same position (e.g., sitting or semi-Fowlers) with the blood pressure cuff at the level of the heart. Use of the same device for assessing blood pressure is also critical to accuracy. Values obtained via automatic blood pressure devices do not compare to values obtained using the mercury cuff. Korotkoff sounds phase V are detected by automatic blood pressure devices during pregnancy, while Korotkoff sounds phase IV are more likely heard during auscultation when using a mercury cuff and a stethescope (Brown et al., 1994). Automatic blood pressure devices underestimate diastolic blood pressure by approximately 10 mmHg and slightly overestimate systolic blood pressure during pregnancy, when compared with values obtained using a mercury cuff (Franx et al., 1994). Thus a blood pressure of 140/80 obtained via an automatic blood pressure device can provide false reassurance that the woman is normotensive, when the value obtained via a mercury cuff would have been closer to 136/90.

TABLE 6-3. Common Prenatal Laboratory Tests

Test	Timing	Significant Values
CBC		
Hct	initial visit, 28, 36 weeks	< 32%
Hb	initial visit, 28, 36 weeks	<11g/dl
WBC	initial visit, 28, 36 weeks	>15,000/mm^3
Type & Rh	initial visit	mother Rh–, father Rh+
Antibody Screen	initial visit, 36 weeks	positive
Serology	initial visit, 36 weeks	positive
Rubella	initial visit	≤ 1:8; significant rise 50 g
1hr GCT	24–28 weeks	>140 g/dl
HB$_S$Ag	initial visit, as indicated	positive
Urinalysis	initial visit	positive
Urine C&S	initial visit	positive
Urine		
Glucose/protein	each visit	greater than 2+
PAP Smear	initial visit	abnormal cervical cytology
GC Culture	initial visit, 36 weeks	positive
Rh antibody	initial visit, 28 weeks	negative
HIV	initial visit (offer)	positive
MSAFP	15–20 weeks	≥ 2.0 (Multiples of the median)
Sickle Cell Screen	initial visit	positive for trait/anemia
Tay Sachs Screen	initial visit	carrier
PPD	initial visit	positive

From Auman, G.E., Baird, M.M. (1993). Risk assessment for pregnant women. In R.A. Knuppel & J.E. Drukker, High risk pregnancy: A team approach (p.p. 18-19). Philadelphia: W.B. Saunders.

Consistency in blood pressure monitoring, including the same arm, position, and equipment, allows for more accurate assessment and comparison across prenatal visits. Traditionally an elevation of systolic blood pressure of 30 mmHg and/or an elevation 15 mmHg diastolic blood pressure over prepregnancy or first trimester measurements was thought to be predictive of the development of preeclampsia, however recent data suggest this criteria may be of questionable value for diagnosis (Villar & Sibai, 1989). The predictive validity of elevated mean arterial pressure (MAP) during the second trimester is also low. There is a high incidence of false positives (MAP value >90 mmHg) in women who remain normotensive during pregnancy (Roberts, 1994; Villar & Sibai, 1989). The most important clinical data to assess are trends in blood pressure values and the concurrent development of proteinuria, headaches, dizziness, visual disturbances, epigastric pain, and/or edema.

Basic fetal surveillance includes assessment of fundal height, fetal heart rate (FHR), and fetal activity. Fundal height is the measurement of the uterus from the symphysis pubis to the top of the fundus. The measurement of the fundal height in centimeters (±2 cm) should correlate with gestational age between 22 and 34 weeks. Fundal height less than gestational age may be indicative of intrauterine growth restriction (IUGR). Fundal height greater than gestational age may be indicative of multiple gestation, polyhydramnios, fibroids, or other conditions which cause uterine distension. Fetal activity is an indirect measure of central nervous system function and is predictive of fetal well-being.

Selected biochemical screens may be repeated at specific intervals during pregnancy (see Table 6-3.) Subsequent prenatal visits usually include urinalysis via dipstick for evidence of proteinuria, glucosuria, and ketonuria. Although it is common practice, there are little data to suggest routine urinalysis via dipstick provides useful clinical information or is predictive of women who will develop complications of pregnancy (Gribble, Fee, & Berg, 1995). After a baseline complete blood count (CBC) is obtained, periodic assessment of hematocrit and hemoglobin values may be indicated for certain at-risk populations.

Based on medical and obstetrical history, clinical symptoms, and assessment information, more extensive laboratory data may be indicated, including screening for sexually transmitted diseases (AAP & ACOG, 1992). Recent data indicate risk of maternal-fetal transmission of the human immunodeficiency virus (HIV) can be reduced by prophylactic administration of zidovudine during the antepartum and intrapartum periods to pregnant women who are HIV seropositive and to their infants (Connor et al., 1994). Thus all pregnant women should be offered screening for HIV in order to initiate timely treatment. Appropriate counseling and referral services should be available for women with positive test results.

Serum glucose evaluation prior to 28 weeks' gestation may be indicated based on family history, or maternal factors, such as previous macrosomic infant, previous unexplained fetal loss, maternal obesity, or previous gestational diabetes mellitus (GDM) (Plovie, 1991). Pregnant women who have not been identified as glucose intolerant should have a Glucose Screening Test (GST) between 24 and 28 weeks' gestation (ACOG, 1994b). A level of ≥ 140 mg/dl 1 hour after consuming a 50 g glucose load warrants further evaluation with an Oral Glucose Tolerance Test (OGTT) (Avery & Rossi, 1994). Diagnosis of GDM is based on two or more abnormally elevated venous plasma glucose values (Metzger, 1991) (Table 6-2).

Women diagnosed with GDM require education about appropriate nutrition, self-management, and self-glucose monitoring and referral for appropriate medical care and counseling.

Risk status in pregnancy is a dynamic process that affects both clinical and nonclinical parameters (Muerer & Taren, 1993). Psychosocial factors, socioeconomic factors, and lifestyle patterns also require ongoing evaluation. Employment status, family economic status, and relationship status could change from visit to visit. These changes affect the woman's psychosocial stress level, potentiating existing risk factors. In general, factors with potential to affect the pregnancy are in a constant state of fluctuation and require continued surveillance.

TABLE 6-2. Normal Oral Glucose Tolerance Test Values

Fasting Blood Sugar (FBS)	105mg/dl
1 hour	190 mg/dl
2 hour	165 mg/dl
3 hour	145 mg/dl

From Metzger, B. (1991). Summary and recommendations of the third international workshop-conference on gestational diabetes melitus. Diabetes, 40(2 Suppl), 197-201.

Laboratory assessment

Laboratory data such as complete blood count (CBC), urinalysis, blood type & Rh, antibody screen, rubella titre, rapid plasma reagin test (RPR), hepatitis B surface antigen (HB_SAg), gonorrhea culture (GC), chlamydia culture, and cervical cytology should be evaluated in all pregnant women. Additional laboratory tests (e.g., STD screens, Group B Streptococci, TORCH titres, tuberculin testing, toxicology screens, and genetic screens) should be performed as indicated, based on historical indicators and/or clinical findings (AAP & ACOG, 1992; ACOG, 1992a; ACOG, 1992b).

Maternal serum alpha-fetoprotein (MSAFP) screening should be offered to all pregnant women between 15 and 20 weeks' gestation (Baumann & McFarlin, 1994). Alpha-fetoprotein is a protein which is produced in the fetal yolk sac during the first trimester and in the fetal liver during later gestation (Shannon, 1990a). Abnormally elevated MSAFP levels have been associated with birth defects and chromosomal anomalies, such as open neural tube defects, open abdominal defects, and congenital nephrosis (Main & Menutti, 1986). High MSAFP levels may also be due to multiple gestations. Low MSAFP levels have been associated with Down syndrome and other chromosomal anomalies (Drugan et al., 1989; Knight, Palomaki, & Haddow, 1988). Triple marker screening (TMS) is also available to screen for trisomy 21 and neural-tube defects although it is costly and not offered as frequently as the MSAFP. In addition to the MSAFP, the TMS evaluates two other maternal serum

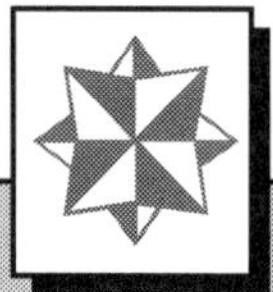

Display 6-5

Patient Teaching Tool for Genetic Transfer of Sickle Cell Disease/Trait

1. Two parents affected with sickle cell trait:
   SA + SA = 25% of children will have sickle cell disease
   50% of children will have sickle cell trait
   25% of children will not be affected by the trait or disease
2. One parent affected with sickle cell trait, one parent affected with sickle cell disease:
   SA + SS = 50% of children will have sickle cell disease
   50% of children will have sickle cell trait
   0% of children will not be affected by the trait or disease
3. Two parents are affected by sickle cell disease:
   SS + SS = 100% of children will have sickle cell disease
   0% of children will have sickle cell trait
   0% of children will not be affected by the disease
4. One parent affected by sickle cell disease, one parent unaffected:
   SS + AA = 100% of children will have sickle cell trait
   0% of children will have sickle cell disease
   0% of children will not be affected by trait
5. One parent affected by sickle cell trait, one parent unaffected:
   SA + AA = 50% of children will have sickle cell trait
   50% of children will not be affected by the trait
   0% of children will not be affected by sickle cell disease

SA=sickle cell trait; SS=sickle cell disease; AA=unaffected.

From Larrabee, K. & Cowan, M. (1995) Clinical nursing management of sickle cell disease and trait during pregnancy. Journal of Perinatal and Neonatal Nursing, 9 (2) 29–41.

markers; unconjugated estriol and human chorionic gonadotropin (hCG). Average hCG levels are higher and unconjugated estriol levels are lower in Down syndrome pregnancies. Both hCG and estriol levels are lower in trisomy 18 pregnancies (Heyl, Miller, & Canick, 1990; Palomaki et al., 1992). The TMS combines the data from all three tests along with maternal age, race, weight, diabetes, and smoking habits, to calculate individual risks. Benefits include increased accuracy in diagnosis because more parameters are evaluated; for women under age 35, TMS detects approximately 60% of pregnancies with trisomy 21, with a false-positive rate of approximately 5% (Hendricks, Von Eschen, & Grady, 1995). The woman should be made aware of the tests available, including benefits and risks of each procedure.

Hemoglobin electrophoresis is used to detect genetic hemoglobin disorders, including sickle cell anemia, sickle cell-C disease, and thalassemia. These recessive inherited conditions occur in the United States primarily in families of African descent, but can also be found in families of Asian, Middle Eastern, or Mediterranean area descent (Larrabee & Cowan, 1995). Women of African descent are routinely screened for these disorders. Although prevalence of sickle cell trait is common among African Americans (8–12%), information related to inheritance patterns is not well known to those at risk. Display 6-5 provides a teaching tool that may be helpful in explaining the genetic transfer of sickle cell trait and sickle cell disease to women and their partners (Larrabee & Cowan, 1995). Tay-Sachs disease is another recessive disorder common in families of Jewish ancestry. This disease causes poorly metabolized lipid substances to accumulate with resultant fatty deposits causing neural tissue degeneration within 6 months of birth and death by five years of age (Paritsky, 1985). Approximately 1 in 30 Ashkenazi Jews are carriers and should be screened prenatally (Baumann & McFarlin, 1994) (Table 6-2).

Prenatal Diagnosis

Prenatal diagnostic evaluation should be considered for families with any of the following: maternal age of 35 years or more; a family history of chromosomal anomalies; parental balanced translocation carrier; the mother a known or at-risk carrier for X-linked disorder; parents who are carriers of an autosomal recessive disorder detectable in utero; a parent affected with an autosomal dominant disorder detectable in utero; a family history of neural tube defects (Bauman & McFarlin, 1994; Matthews & Smith, 1993; Pletch, 1994). See Display 6-6.

Amniocentesis. Amniocentesis is the collection of a sample of amniotic fluid from the amniotic sac for (1) identification of genetic diseases, selected birth defects, and fetal lung maturity; (2) therapy for polyhydramnios; and (3) progressive evaluation of isoimmunized pregnancies. Amniocentesis for genetic evaluation may be performed between 15 and 20 weeks' gestation. Genetic amniocentesis allows for detection of chromosomal anomalies, biochemical disorders, neural tube defects, some ventral wall defects, and DNA analysis for a number of single gene disorders. Early amniocentesis between 12 and 14 weeks' gestation is offered at some centers, but data regarding fetal loss following early amniocentesis remain under investigation (Matthews & Smith, 1993). Prior to testing, families should be given information about indications for amniocentesis, how the procedure is done, risks involved, and ramifications of findings.

Chorionic Villus Sampling. Chorionic villus sampling (CVS) involves the removal of a small sample of chorionic (placental) tissue via a catheter inserted through the cervix. The villi are harvested and cultured for chromosomal analysis and processed for DNA and enzymatic analysis as indicated. CVS can be done at 9–12 weeks' gestation and karyotype results can be available within 4 days (Matthews & Smith, 1993). As with amniocentesis, information about benefits and risks must be provided prior to the procedure.

Ultrasonography. Ultrasonography (fetal imaging via intermittent high-frequency sound waves) is the most commonly used prenatal diagnostic procedure. Approximately 70% of pregnant women in the United States have at least one ultrasound examination during pregnancy (ACOG, 1993b). Indications vary widely and are dependent on gestational age and on type of diagnostic information sought. During early pregnancy, ultrasound is frequently used to determine presence of an intrauterine gestational sac, fetal number, cardiac activity, and to measure crown-rump length. Ultrasound during the second and third trimesters can be useful when there is a discrepancy between the woman's last menstrual period and uterine size, to detect fetal anatomical defects, and for placental localization and amniotic fluid volume estimates (ACOG, 1993b). When maternal or fetal complications are suspected or identified, ultrasonography serves as a valuable tool to confirm the diagnosis and follow-up on

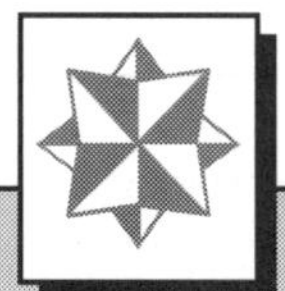

Display 6-6

Conditions with Incidences and Carrier Frequencies Calling for Prenatal Diagnosis and Counseling

Conditions	*Carrier Frequencies*	*Prenatal Diagnostic Methods*
Couples at an increased risk		
Maternal age >35 years		
Balanced chromosome rearrangement		
Previous child with chromosome abnormality		
Low maternal serum α-fetoprotein		
Family history of birth defects and/or mental retardation		
Congenital heart disease	8/1,000	Echocardiography
Neural tube defect	1.5/1,000	US, AC
Cleft lip and/or palate	1/700	US
Multiple congenital anomalies		US
Mental retardation		
Family history of known or suspected Mendelian genetic disorder		
Cystic fibrosis	1/2,500 (whites)-1/17,000 (blacks)	CVS
Hemophilia A	1/10,000 males	
B	1/1,500-1/2,000 males	FBS
Duchenne muscular dystrophy	1/4,000 males	CVS, AC
Becker muscular dystrophy		CVS, AC
Ethnicity		
African population		
Sickle cell disease	1/600 US blacks	
Trait carriers	1/12	CVS, AC
Mediterranean/Indian: β-thalassemia		CVS, AC
Jewish: Tay-Sachs disease		
Ashkenazic Jews	1/3,600	
Trait carriers	1/30	
General population	1/360,000	
Trait carriers	1/300	CVS
Exposure to possible teratogens		
Alcohol		US
Radiation		US
Occupational chemical exposures		US
Toxoplasmosis		US, FBS
Rubella		US, FBS
Cytomegalovirus		US, FBS
Syphilis		US
Insulin-dependent diabetes mellitus		US
Epileptic disorder: drugs		US, AC
Patients with low or high levels of maternal serum α-fetoprotein		US, AC
Fetal abnormalities diagnosed by ultrasonogram		CVS, AC, FBS
Consanguinity		US
Multiple pregnancy losses, stillbirth, infertility		US
Anxiety		US

US=ultrasound; AC=amniocentesis; FBS=fetal blood sampling; CVS=chorionic villus sampling

From Baumann, P., & McFarlin, B. (1994). Prenatal diagnosis, Journal of Nurse-Midwifery, Vol 39, No. 2 (Suppl).

fetal status. Ultrasonography is also used to guide the obstetrician during other diagnostic procedures such as CVS, amniocentesis, and fetal blood sampling.

Controversy exists related to the benefits of routine ultrasound examination for all pregnant women. Advocates suggest routine screening can decrease incidence of labor induction for suspected postdates pregnancies and avoid undiagnosed fetal anomalies and twin gestations. Based on a cost-benefit analysis, ACOG (1993b) does not support routine ultrasonography for women with no identified maternal or fetal risk factors.

Doppler flow studies allow assessment of flow patterns and velocities in a number of fetal arteries (ACOG, 1994a). The umbilical artery is most commonly evaluated. Data continue to emerge related to the predictive value of Doppler velocimetry; however, based on what is known at present, abnormal umbilical arterial flow patterns such as absent or reversed umbilical flow during fetal cardiac diastole are probably an indication of fetal compromise when other fetal diagnostic test findings are abnormal (ACOG, 1994a).

Fetal Blood Sampling. Fetal blood sampling also known as percutaneous umbilical blood sampling (PUBS) or cordocentesis, allows direct evaluation of fetal blood obtained from the umbilical cord. Using ultrasonography to guide placement, a needle is inserted into one of the umbilical vessels (usually the vein) and a small amount of blood is withdrawn. Valuable information can be gained from analysis of fetal blood including prenatal diagnosis of fetal blood disorders, isoimmunization, metabolic disorders, infections, and karyotyping (Cunningham, MacDonald, Gant, Leveno, & Gilstrap, 1993). Cordocentesis can also be used for fetal therapies such as red blood cell and platelet transfusions.

FETAL DEVELOPMENT

It is helpful to relate education about positive pregnancy outcome to fetal development. Throughout the pregnancy, the fetus is nourished and protected by placental functioning. This dependence on the placenta leaves the fetus vulnerable to insult from lifestyle factors such as substance abuse, smoking, and poor nutrition. However, education focusing first on the woman's own health needs is essential in establishing an environment of respect for her as an individual separate from a "maternal-fetal unit."

A number of factors contribute to risks for the woman and fetus throughout the pregnancy. Environmental agents may cross the placenta and affect the development of the embryo/fetus. Three critical periods of development exist: (1) fertilization and implantation; (2) the embryonic period, from day 18 through day 55; and (3) the fetal stage, from day 56 through birth. Factors influencing development in the first period include the quality of the sperm and ovum, the adequacy of the intrauterine environment, and maternal stores and nutrition. A critical window exists in which cells undergoing the most rapid growth are most vulnerable to teratogenic agents. Additionally, long-term exposure to noxious agents may impair development.

Approximately 10% of all human malformations are caused by environmental factors, 10% by genetic factors, and the remaining 80% are presumably the result of a combination of environmental and genetic factors (Sadler, 1995).

Teratogens are agents that cause congenital anomalies in the fetus. Major teratogenic influences include smoking during pregnancy, alcohol and drug use and abuse, occupational hazards, injuries, viruses, and nutritional deficiencies (Baumann & McFarlin, 1994). Exposure to teratogenic influences during the embryonic period can cause structural and functional defects. During the fetal period, when there is organ differentiation, structural defects as well as fetal growth retardation can occur (see Table 6-4).

Nurses interacting with the childbearing family in the prenatal period assess the well-being of the woman and the growth and well-being of the fetus. Nursing intervention is directed by the data obtained from ongoing comprehensive maternal-fetal assessments. Knowledge of beneficial and detrimental behaviors to pregnancy outcome is necessary if the nurse is to provide guidance to the childbearing family. Evaluation of the growth and development of the fetus can be shared with the parents to promote prenatal parent-infant attachment. Table 6-5 identifies normal fetal developmental events.

FETAL SURVEILLANCE

Fetal assessment is an integral component of prenatal care. Careful assessment of fetal well-being enhances perinatal outcome through early identification and intervention for fetal compromise. Ultrasonography may be used as indicated throughout the pregnancy

TABLE 6-4. Known and Potential Teratogens

Known Teratogenic Chemicals		Potential Teratogenic Maternal Conditions and Infections Agents	
Agent	**Related Effects**	**Agent**	**Related Effects**
Alcohol	Intrauterine growth restriction; mental retardation; maxillary hypoplasia; reduction in width of palpebral tissues; microcephaly	Cytomegalovirus	Central nervous system damage; intrauterine growth restriction
Anticancer drugs	Drug-specific effects, with wide variation from drug to drug	Diabetes mellitus	Affects various systems; caudal dysplasia or caudal regression syndrome; insulin therapy protects fetus
Anticonvulsants, hydantoins, diones	Orofacial clefts; cardiac and skeletal defects; hydantoin syndrome; trimethadione syndrome; central nervous system anomalies; developmental delay	Endocrinopathies	Effects similar to those of administering the hormone; masculinization of female fetus
Androgenic hormones, progestogenic hormones	Genital malformations; masculinization of female fetus with high doses	Herpes simplex	Central nervous system anomalies; microcephaly; intracranial calcification; eye defects
Aspirin	Heavy use related to low birth weight microcephaly;	Phenylketonuria	Fetal death; mental retardation; intrauterine growth restriction
Coumadin anticoagulants	Skeletal defects; nasal hypoplasia; stippling of secondary epiphysis; intrauterine growth restriction; anomalies of eyes, hands, neck, and central nervous system	Rubella virus	Cardiovascular malformation; deafness; mental retardation; cataracts; glaucoma; microphthalmia
Diethylstilbestrol	Masculinization of female fetus; vaginal carcinoma; cervical and uterine anomalies; possible male effects	Syphilis	Maculopapular rash; hepatosplenomegaly; deformed nails; osteochondritis at joints of extremities; congenital neurosyphilis; abnormal epiphyses; chorioetinitis
Lithium carbonate	Cardiovascular malformation; neural tube defects	Toxoplasmosis	Hydrocephaly; microphthalmia; chorioretinitis

Methylmercury	Cental nervous system anomalies; Minamata disease; microcephaly; mental retardation; blindness	Varicella-zoster (chickenpox)	Skin and muscle defects; intrauterine growth restriction; limb and eye defects
Radiation	Microcephaly; mental retardation; intrauterine growth restriction;	Venezuelan equine encephalitis	Hydroanencephaly; microphthalmia; luxation of hip
Smoking/nicotine	Intrauterine growth restriction; placental lesions		
Thyroid and antithyroid drugs	Hypothyroidism or goiter		
Tetracycline	Hypoplastic tooth enamel; bone and tooth anomalies		
Vitamin A isoretinoin	Urogenital anomalies (large doses); ear, palate, facial, and neural tube defects		
Thalidomide	Limb reduction defects; facial, esophageal, duodenal, and external ear defects; heart or kidney defects		

From Beckman & Brent. (1986). Mechanism of known environmental teratogens: Drugs and chemicals. Clinical Perinatology, 13(3), 649-687.

to assess fetal growth and development (Gegor & Paine, 1992). Doppler ultrasound may be used during the second half of pregnancy to assess blood flow changes in the fetal heart, aorta, or cerebrum, and the uterine and umbilical arteries (Lommel, 1990). This allows for evaluation of the fetus at risk for intrauterine compromise or death. Recent data indicate cervical ultrasonography may be useful in identifying women at risk for preterm birth. In one study, a cervical length of at least 30 mm, when evaluated between 24 and 35 weeks' gestation, predicted a low likelihood of preterm birth (Iams, Paraskos, Landon, Teteris, & Johnson, 1994).

Assessment of Fetal Activity

Fetal movement counting ("kick counts") has been proposed as a primary method of fetal surveillance for all pregnancies. Cessation of fetal movement is correlated with fetal death. The mother's observations of fetal movement has been validated through an 80–90% correlation of maternal perception of movement with movement detected on real-time ultrasonography (Moore & Piacquadio, 1989).

Several methods of fetal movement counting have been proposed; however, neither the ideal number of kicks nor the ideal interval for movement counting has been defined (ACOG, 1994a). The Cardiff Count-to-Ten method involves beginning fetal movement counting at the same time each day. Less than 10 fetal movements in a 10-hour period for two consecutive days, or no fetal movements in a 10-hour period, are reported to the healthcare provider (Gegor & Paine, 1992). The count-to-ten method is based on the assumption that less than 10 movements in a 12-hour

TABLE 6-5. Major Events of Fetal Period (9th to 40th week)

Normal Events

Weeks 9 to 12
CRL doubles between 9 and 12 weeks
Upper limbs develop to normal proportions, while lower limbs remain less developed
Male and female genitalia are recognizable by 12 weeks
Production of RBCs transfers from the liver to the spleen at 12 weeks

Weeks 13 to 16
Rapid fetal growth occurs
Fetus doubles in size
Lanugo begins to grow
Fingernails are formed
Kidneys begin to secrete urine
Fetus begins to swallow amniotic fluid
Fetus appears human
Placenta fully formed

Weeks 17 to 23
Fetal growth slows
Lower limbs fully formed
Fetal body is covered with lanugo
Vernix caseosa covers the body to protect skin from amniotic fluid
Brown fat forms

Weeks 24 to 27
Skin growth is rapid and skin appears red and wrinkled
The eyes open and eyelashes and eyebrows are formed
The fetus becomes viable at 26 to 27 weeks

Weeks 28 to 31
Subcutaneous fat is deposited
If the fetus is born at this time with immature lungs, RDS may occur.

Weeks 32 to 36
Lanugo has disappeared from the body but remains on the head
Weight gain is steady
Fingernails are growing
The fetus has a good chance of surviving if born

Weeks 37 to 40
Subcutaneous fat builds and fetal contours appear round
Both testes have descended in the male
The skull is fully developed

From May, K.A, & Mahlmeister, L.R. (1994). Maternal and neonatal nursing (3rd ed., p. 265). Philadelphia: J.B. Lippincott.

period is cause for concern (Moore & Piacquadio, 1989) and should be reported to the healthcare provider. The Sadovsky method of monitoring fetal movement involves the mother setting aside a consistent time to do "kick counts" three times each day. This method defines fetal activity as four or more movements in 1 hour. Less than four movements in 2 hours should be reported to the healthcare provider (Freda et al., 1993). Freda et al. found no evidence that women prefer or are more compliant with either method. Regardless of technique, monitoring of fetal movement is recommended for pregnant women at increased risk for antepartum fetal death beginning at 28 weeks' gestation (ACOG, 1994a). Although only one randomized controlled study of maternal fetal movement assessment demonstrated a reduction in the rate of antepartum fetal death (Neldam, 1980), because of the simplicity and relative effectiveness, all women could benefit from instruction on fetal activity assessment.

While fetal activity is a reassuring sign, decreased fetal movement is not necessarily ominous. A healthy fetus usually has ten perceivable movements within 10 to 60 minutes (Lommel, 1990). However, fetal movement can be influenced by many factors, including time of day, gestational age, glucose loading, maternal smoking, maternal medications, and decreased uterine space as gestation increases. Decreased fetal movement may also be due to a fetal sleep state. Early identification of conditions which can affect pregnancy outcome can minimize perinatal morbidity by allowing for the establishment of an appropriate treatment plan and referrals (AAP & ACOG, 1992). Report of decreased fetal movement is an indication for further assessment. The woman should be instructed to have something to eat and drink, rest, and focus on fetal movement for 1 hour. Four movements in 1 hour are considered reassuring. If less than four movements are perceived in 2 hours, the woman should call her primary healthcare provider immediately.

Non Stress Test (NST)

The NST is one of the most common methods of antenatal screening and involves electronic fetal heart rate monitoring for approximately 20 minutes. The NST is based on the premise that the normal fetus moves at various intervals and that the central nervous system and myocardium responds to movement with acceleration of the fetal heart rate. Acceleration of the FHR during fetal activity is a sign of fetal well-being (Lommel, 1990). Consensus does not exist in the literature or in clinical practice related to criteria for a reactive NST; however, most commonly, an NST is considered to be reactive when a minimum of two fetal heart rate accelerations of 15 bpm above baseline and lasting at least 15 seconds occur within a 20-minute time frame (ACOG, 1994a). NSTs that do not meet this criteria are nonreactive. A reactive NST is reassuring, indicating less than a 1% chance of fetal death within 1 week of a reactive NST (Field, 1989). Most deaths within 1 week of a reactive NST fall into nonpreventable categories such as abruptio placentae, sepsis, and cord accidents. However, a nonreactive NST is not necessarily an ominous sign. Rather, the nonreactive NST indicates a need for further testing and should be followed by a Oxytocin Challenge Test (OCT) or BPP(Gegor & Paine, 1992).

Oxytocin Challenge Test (OCT)

The OCT, or Contraction Stress Test (CST), evaluates FHR response to uterine contractions. FHR and uterine activity are assessed via an electronic fetal monitor. A baseline monitor tracing is obtained for 20 minutes. If spontaneous uterine contractions do not occur, uterine stimulation is produced via IV oxytocin infusion or breast self-stimulation, until three contractions of at least 40 seconds duration occur within a 10-minute time frame. CSTs are evaluated as follows (ACOG, 1994a):

- Negative CST (normal)–No late decelerations
- Positive CST (abnormal)–Late decelerations following ≥ 50% of contractions even if the contraction frequency is less than three in 10 minutes
- Suspicious (equivocal) CST –Intermittent late or significant variable decelerations
- Unsatisfactory CST–Fewer than three contractions per 10 minutes or quality of tracing inadequate for interpretation

The negative CST is reassuring and is associated with a low fetal death rate within 1 week of a negative test. A positive CST requires further evaluation or birth. The CST false-positive rate of 30–50% warrants evaluation of the OCT within the context of the total clinical picture (Lommel, 1990).

Biophysical Profile (BPP)

The BPP combines electronic fetal heart rate monitoring with ultrasonography to evaluate fetal well-being based on multiple biophysical variables. Five parameters are assessed: fetal muscle tone, fetal movement, fetal breathing movements, amniotic fluid volume, and fetal heart rate reactivity as demonstrated by NST. Each item has a maximum score of two, with a summative score of 8-10 indicating fetal well being. The BPP has a lower false-positive rate than single variable tests and is a more accurate predictor of fetal compromise (Gegor & Paine, 1992).

PLAN FOR NURSING CARE AND INTERVENTION

Nursing interventions are based on nursing diagnoses and a collaborative approach to the identification of strengths and problems. Together, the nurse and woman set goals and strategize ways to implement a plan of care to meet these goals. During the antepartum period, nursing care typically includes comfort promotion (e.g., measures to relieve discomforts caused by the physiologic changes of pregnancy), family adaptation in planning the addition of a new member, and encouraging behaviors to enhance maternal and fetal well-being. In addition, providing information, especially for the woman pregnant for the first time, is an important aspect of antepartum care. The nurse has the opportunity and the responsibility to teach the woman and her family about beneficial and detrimental lifestyle practices, potential risks, and care required to promote maternal and fetal well-being. The staff nurse in ambulatory care provides anticipatory planning, assesses all available data, and structures education and nursing interventions accordingly. Inherent in competent perinatal nursing practice is the ability to differentiate between normal pregnancy variations and high-risk complications, and the initiation of appropriate nursing interventions (NAACOG, 1991).

COLLABORATIVE MANAGEMENT AND FOLLOW UP

Total care management of the childbearing family requires cooperation, collaboration, and communication across disciplines. It is important to remember that risk factors must be evaluated in terms of individual risk versus benefit in order to be effective. Healthcare providers are charged with the task of finding the goodness of fit between the recommended healthcare regimen and the individual's reality in order to optimize outcome. Case management allows for a single healthcare professional to coordinate healthcare management in collaboration with the pregnant woman (NAACOG, 1991).

Case Management

The childbearing woman and her family are the core of the perinatal healthcare team. When families are included in healthcare decision-making, satisfaction with care received and adherence to the recommended regimen is increased (Giuliano & Poirer, 1991; NAACOG, 1991). The nurse's role as case manager, advocate, and educator is of primary importance in facilitating a family-friendly system that validates the woman's own knowledge and promotes empowered healthcare decision-making. (See Appendixes I and J for examples or care paths that begin in the prenatal period and follow through to the postpartum home visit.)

Nutrition

The nutritionist is a valuable asset to the prenatal healthcare team. Nutrition assessment and counseling is a vital component of prenatal care. The woman may benefit from regularly scheduled appointments with the nutritionist during an early prenatal visit and again at 28 weeks' gestation. Additional visits with the nutritionist should be scheduled as indicated (e.g., for inadequate or excessive weight gain, anemia, of metabolic disorders such as GDM). Weight-gain charts, 24-hour diet recall, or simple, self-report dietary assessment tools are valuable education resources.

Nutritional status may change due to availability of appropriate foods and financial resources for groceries. The most significant food shortages for low-income women occur at the end of the month when federal and local resources are depleted (Taren, Clark, Chernesky, & Quirk, 1990). Likewise, religious practices may dictate fasting during specific times of the year (i.e., Lent or Ramadan), thus limiting the woman's food intake. Awareness and ongoing assessment of these factors allows for timely interventions and appropriate referral to nutrition counseling, social work, and community support services. Referrals to food and nutrition supplement programs may be warranted. Women in the United States should be referred to the Special Supplemental Feeding Program for Women, Infants, and Children (WIC). Other supplemental food and nutrition programs are available to childbearing families on a regional or local basis (Muerer & Taren, 1993). The prenatal healthcare team must be knowledgeable about such resources in their area.

Confidence-building strategies that promote breastfeeding are an important component of prenatal nutrition education. Providing information about breastfeeding convenience, infant benefits, and potential formula cost savings can enhance maternal motivation. Acknowledging that some women may feel embarrassed or uncomfortable about breastfeeding and providing tips for discreet breastfeeding techniques are also helpful approaches. Anticipated length of breastfeeding is an important prenatal factor associated with breastfeeding duration (O'Campo, Faden, Geilen, & Wang, 1992). There is a positive correlation between increased breastfeeding duration and increased maternal confidence (O'Campo et al.). A session with the nutritionist, focusing on nutrition during lactation, may be helpful in encouraging initiation of breastfeeding and in a successful breastfeeding experience. (See Chapter 15 for a more indepth discussion of breastfeeding.)

Social Services

The emphasis on an individualized, holistic approach to prenatal care, encompassing physiologic and psychosocial needs, promotes a move toward a prevention oriented model of care (Young, 1990). The World Health Organization (WHO)(1985) advocates the need to unite the medical approach and the social approach in the further development of services during pregnancy and birth and following birth. Today's families face multiple factors, such as unemployment, homelessness, chemical dependency, increased family and neighborhood violence, and lack of support systems that may precipitate crises and affect perinatal outcome. It is possible to identify women prenatally who are at risk for experiencing parenting difficulties. More than two address changes in the year prior to birth, history of psychiatric or emotional problems, unrealistic expectations of the baby, or dropping out of prenatal classes are examples of criteria for determining parenting risk (Egan et al., 1990). Risk factors such as previous psychological disorders, disintegration of significant relationships, or difficulty during the prenatal and/or intrapartum period are indicative of risk for postpartum depression (Boyer, 1990). Assessment for psychosocial risk factors should be incorporated into prenatal assessment. Early recognition of potential risk allows for prompt intervention and referral. The role of the perinatal social worker is critical in providing interventions that relieve stress, provide for woman's basic needs, follow crisis situations, and facilitate healthcare decision making (Walther, 1990). Social work referrals are appropriate for pregnant women experiencing medical, psychological, or socioeconomic crises. Psychosocial and socioeconomic factors are evaluated on a continuing basis, with referral to social services as needed. (See Chapter 5 for a more indepth discussion of psychological factors related to pregnancy.)

Education and Counseling

Educational and health promotional activities that include the father must be integrated into prenatal care. Prenatal education should focus not only on a positive labor and birth experience but, more importantly, on laying the groundwork for a successful pregnancy outcome and family experience (NAACOG, 1991). Therefore, education regarding nutrition, sexuality, stress reduction, lifestyle behaviors, and hazards in the work place are appropriate to include in prenatal education (Display 6-4). (See Chapter 17 for a more comprehensive review of prenatal education.)

Early identification of conditions that can affect pregnancy outcome can minimize perinatal morbidity by allowing for the establishment of an appropriate treatment plan and referrals (AAP & ACOG, 1992). Therefore, it is important that women receive information regarding risk factors, warning signs, and criteria for provider notification. One study of the effect of prenatal education on birth outcome in a high-risk population found that lack of advice to call the healthcare provider if preterm labor was suspected, emerged as a more important predictor of preterm labor/low-birth-weight risk than lack of education in recognition of preterm labor (Libbus & Sable, 1991). In this population of high-risk, potentially disenfranchised women, the permission to act on their own instinct and self-knowledge was found to be of equal or greater value than specific educational content (Libbus & Sable). Routine prenatal care should include education to enhance recognition of warning signs of preterm labor, specifically identification of contractions. It is sometimes helpful to describe contractions as feeling "hard like your forehead" and a relaxed uterus as feeling "soft like the tip of your nose", or having the woman palpate her upper arm as she flexes and relaxes the muscle to simulate a contraction. Education regarding warning signs of pregnancy must also include information concerning recognition of signs of preeclampsia, such as headaches, visual disturbances, edema, and epigastric pain.

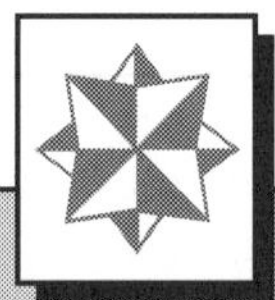

DISPLAY 6-4

Prenatal Education Topics

First Trimester

Smoking cessation
Alcohol avoidance
Illicit drug avoidance
Work/rest patterns
Physiologic changes of pregnancy
Emotional changes of pregnancy
Healthy lifestyle
Screening/diagnostic tests
Nipple assessment/breastfeeding promotion
Teratogen avoidance
Nutrition
Seat belt use
Safe sex
Sexuality
Discomforts of pregnancy
Importance of early prenatal care
What to expect during prenatal care

Warning signs of pregnancy complications
Criteria and mechanism for notification of health care provider
(Information may be given at individual prenatal care visit or early pregnancy class)

Second Trimester

Smoking cessation
Alcohol avoidance
Illicit drug avoidance
Physiologic changes of pregnancy
Emotional changes of pregnancy
Discomforts of pregnancy
Fetal growth/development
Breastfeeding promotion
Perineal exercises
Teratogen avoidance
Nutrition
Prenatal laboratory tests
Sexuality
Healthy lifestyle
Family roles
Infant car seat use
Childbirth education

Preterm Birth Prevention
Preeclampsia precautions

Third Trimester

Smoking cessation
Alcohol avoidance
Illicit drug avoidance
Physiologic changes of pregnancy
Emotional changes of pregnancy
Discomforts of pregnancy
Fetal growth/development
Breastfeeding promotion
Postpartum self-care choices
Postpartum emotional changes
Teratogen avoidance
Nutrition
Prenatal laboratory tests
Sexuality
Reproductive health
Healthy lifestyle
Newborn care
Childbirth education

Preparation for childbirth
Where to go - Who to call

Adapted from Expert Panel on the Content of Prenatal Care. (1989) Caring for our Future:The content of prenatal care. Washington DC: Public Health Service and Murer, J., & Taren, D.L., (1993). Prevention and public health in Obstetrics. In RA. Knuppel & J.E. Drukker. High risk pregnancy:A team approach. Philadelphia:W.B. Saunders.

With current postpartum length of stay, it is increasingly difficult to teach the woman and family all they need to know about maternal-newborn care during hospitalization. The last trimester of pregnancy may be a potentially effective time to introduce maternal-newborn care content, including parenting issues and contraceptive choices. Education programs with the goal of modifying behaviors during pregnancy are most effective when they are targeted to all women, rather than a select population. Currently, there is no accurate way to predict which women will develop postpartum emotional disorders (Boyer, 1990). Therefore, it is important that every childbearing woman and family are provided information about postpartum depression and where to seek help (Boyer). Although risk-assessment tools for postpartum emotional illness with adequate validity and reliability are not yet available, a self-administered risk assessment is one way to heighten women's awareness about postpartum depression. A psychological illness in the mother will interfere with healthy adaptation and affect all family members.

The childbearing continuum is a transition involving each family member. Childbirth education provides the opportunity for enhancement of family systems and facilitation of empowered behaviors that will last a lifetime (Starn, 1993). Thirty years ago, the first childbirth education classes began as a means to provide information for women wishing to be awake, active participants in the birth of their child. Since then, childbirth education focusing on coping strategies for labor has been shown to decrease use of anesthesia in labor and enhance maternal confidence and satisfaction. Today, childbirth education goes well beyond basics to include information about birth as a natural process; environments that enhance the woman's ability to give birth; care options; and, most importantly, the tools necessary to make informed healthcare decisions that are appropriate for individual families. Childbirth education must expand to meet consumers' need for information concerning preconception wellness, care provider and birthing options, and maternal-newborn care during the postpartum period (Lothian, 1994). Current, accurate information, effective coping skills, and intact support systems fostered by childbirth education provide families with the skills to explore alternatives and make informed decisions that are congruent with their personal goals (Lothian, 1993). It is important that childbirth education is available to all women. Perinatal nurses are challenged to move childbirth education from traditional series to time frames and locations that meet consumer needs.

Health Promotion

Preconception health promotion is increasingly recognized as an important factor influencing perinatal outcome. Anticipatory guidance and health promotion information are most useful when provided prior to conception (Barron, Brown, & Ganong, 1987). Health promotion and health education, beginning with children in school, is essential to improving pregnancy outcome for the next generation (March of Dimes, 1993). Programs should emphasize healthy lifestyle behaviors, self-esteem, and decision-making skills. If women have not been exposed to this information prior to pregnancy, healthcare professionals should seize the opportunity to provide information and experiences that promote these activities during prenatal care. Awareness of reproductive risk, healthy lifestyle behaviors, and reproductive options is essential in improving pregnancy outcome. Reproductive awareness dialogue should be incorporated into general medical care for both men and women (March of Dimes).

Prenatal care provides numerous opportunities for increasing reproductive awareness from a woman's health perspective. Aside from providing valuable information regarding the current pregnancy, laboratory evaluation also provides indicators of general health status and opportunities for health promotion. Screening tests that allow for health promotion are also offered during pregnancy. HIV testing and counseling is available and should be offered to all women. Barbacci, Repke, and Chaisson (1991) found that screening only women with known risk factors for HIV accounted for only 57% of detected cases; however, when HIV counseling and testing was offered to all pregnant women, the detection rate rose to 87%. HIV pretest counseling should include assessment of individual risk, benefits of testing, test procedure and meaning of results, and confidentiality of procedure. Posttest counseling should include discussion of results, limitations of results, review of potential modes of transmission, and discussion regarding risk-reduction behaviors and safe-sex practice. For example, the woman with a negative HB_SAg may be offered the hepatitis B immunization series during her pregnancy, and the woman with a negative rubella titre may plan to receive a rubella vaccine after birth at discharge from the postpartum unit (ACOG, 1992b).

SUMMARY

Nursing care during the prenatal period is multifaceted, requiring knowledge of the psychosocial tasks and issues surrounding the childbearing continuum, as well as knowledge of normal physiologic processes and potential risks. Anticipatory guidance during the prenatal period has the potential to have a significant impact on perinatal outcome. Education, based on individual assessment, empowers women and underscores their partnership in healthcare decision-making. The goal of prenatal care must go a step farther than targeting a positive physical outcome. Rather, we must work toward providing care and education that facilitates holistic family wellness.

REFERENCES

Abrams, B., & Selvin, S. (1995). Maternal weight gain pattern and birth weight. Obstetrics and Gynecology, 86(2), 163-169.

American Academy of Pediatrics & American College of Obstetricians and Gynecologists. (1992). Guidelines for perinatal care (3rd ed.). Elk Grove Village, IL: Author.

American College of Obstetricians and Gynecologists. (1992a). Group B streptococcal infections in pregnancy (Technical Bulletin), No. 170. Washington, DC: Author.

American College of Obstetricians and Gynecologists. (1992b). Guidelines for hepatitis B virus screening and vaccination during pregnancy (Committee Opinion No. 111. Washington, DC: Author).

American College of Obstetricians and Gynecologists. (1993a). Nutrition during pregnancy (Technical Bulletin No. 179). Washington, DC: Author.

American College of Obstetricians and Gynecologists. (1993b). Ultrasonography in pregnancy (Technical Bulletin No. 200). Washington, DC: Author.

American College of Obstetricians and Gynecologists. (1994a). Antepartum fetal surveillance (Technical Bulletin, No. 188). Washington, DC: Author.

American College of Obstetricians and Gynecologists. (1994b). Diabetes and pregnancy (Technical Bulletin No. 200). Washington, DC: Author.

American College of Obstetricians and Gynecologists. (1994c). Exercise during pregnancy and the postpartum period (Technical Bulletin, No. 189). Washington, DC: Author.

American College of Obstetricians and Gynecologists. (1994d). Substance abuse in pregnancy (Technical Bulletin No. 195). Washington, DC: Author.

American College of Obstetricians and Gynecologists (1995a). Preconceptional care (Technical Bulletin No. 205). Washington, DC: Author.

American College of Obstetricians and Gynecologists (1995b). Preterm labor (Technical Bulletin No. 206). Washington, DC: Author.

Arnold, L.S., & Grad, R.K. (1992). Low birth weight and infant mortality: A health policy perspective. NAACOG's Clinical Issues in Perinatal and Women's Health Nursing, 3(1), 1-12.

Atrash, H.K., Rowley, D., & Hogue, C.J. (1992). Maternal and perinatal mortality. Current Opinion in Obstetrics and Gynecology, 4(1), 61-71.

Auman, G.E., & Baird, M.M. (1993). Risk Assessment for Pregnant Women. In R.A. Knuppel & J.E. Drukker (Eds.), High risk pregnancy: A team approach (pp. 8-35). Philadelphia: W.B. Saunders.

Avery, M.D., & Rossi, M.A. (1994). Gestational diabetes. Journal of Nurse-Midwifery, 39 (Suppl. 2), 9-19.

Baldwin, L.M., Raine, T., Jenkins, L.D., Hart, G., & Rosenblatt, R. (1994). Do providers adhere to ACOG standards? The case of prenatal care. Obstetrics and Gynecology, 84 (4, Pt. 1), 549-556.

Barbacci, M., Repke, J.T., & Chaisson, R.E. (1991). Routine prenatal screening for HIV infection. Lancet, 337 (8743), 709-711.

Barron, M.L., Brown, M.C., & Ganong, L.H. (1987). PREPARED for pregnancy: A counseling guide . . . preconception counseling model. Clinical Nurse Specialist, 1(3), 111-115.

Baumann, P., & McFarlin, B. (1994). Prenatal diagnosis. Journal of Nurse-Midwifery, 39 (Suppl. 2), 35-51.

Beckman, D.A., & Brent, R.L. (1986). Mechanisms of known environmental teratogens: Drugs and chemicals. Clinics in Perinatology, 13(3), 649-687.

Boyer, D. (1990). Prediction of post partum depression. NAACOG's Clinical Issues in Perinatal and Women's Health Nursing, 1(3), 359-368.

Brown, E.R., & Zuckerman, B. (1991). The infant of the drug abusing mother. Pediatric Annals, 20(10), 555-563.

Brown, M.A., Reiter, L., Smith, B., Buddle, M.L., Morries, R., & Whitworth, J.A. (1994). Measuring blood pressure in pregnant women: A comparison of direct and indirect methods. American Journal of Obstetrics and Gynecology, 171(3), 661-667.

Brown, S.A., & Grimes, D.E. (1993). A meta-analysis of process of care, clinical outcomes, and cost-effectiveness of nurses in primary care roles: Nurse practitioners, and certified nurse midwives. Washington, DC: American Nurses' Association.

Burks, J.A. (1992). Factors in the utilization of prenatal services by low-income black women. Nurse Practitioner: American Journal of Primary Health Care, 17 (4), 34, 46, 49.

Carpenter, M.B. (1995). The impact of legislation designed to reduce infant mortality. Journal of Perinatal and Neonatal Nursing, 9(1), 19-30.

Centers for Disease Control and Prevention. (1995a). Differences in maternal mortality among black and white women—United States, 1990. Morbidity and Mortality Weekly Report, 44(1), 6-7, 13-14.

Centers for Disease Control and Prevention. (1995b). Rates of cesarean delivery—United States, 1993. Morbidity and Mortality Weekly Report, 44(15), 303-306.

Chasnoff, I.J. (1989). Drug use and women: Establishing a standard of care. Annals of the New York Academy of Sciences, 562, 208-210.

Children's Defense Fund. (1994). The state of America's children yearbook 1994. Washington, DC: Author.

Connor, E., Sperling, R., Gelber, R., Kiselev, P., Scott, G., O'Sullivan, M., VanDyke, R., Bev, M., Shearer, W., Jacobson, R., Jimenez, E., O'Neill, E., Bazin, B., Delfraissy, J., Culnane, M., Coombs, R., Elkins, M., Moye, J., Stratton, P., Balsey, J., & the Pediatric AIDS Clinical Trials Group. (1994). Reduction of maternal-infant transmission of human immunodeficiency virus type I with zidovudine treatment. New England Journal of Medicine, 331(18), 1173-1180.

Cunningham, F.G., MacDonald, P.C., Gant, N.F., Leveno, K.J., & Gilstrap, L.C. (1993). Williams obstetrics, Norwalk, CT: Appleton & Lange.

Drugan, A., Dvorin, E., Koppitch, F.C., Greb, A., Krivchenia, E.L., & Evans, M.I. (1989). Counseling for low maternal serum alpha feto-protein should emphasize all chromasomal anomalies, not just Down's Syndrome. Obstetrics & Gynecology, 73(2), 271-274.

Edenfield, S.M., Thomas, S.D., Thompson, W.O., & Marcotte, J.J. (1995). Validity of the Creasy risk appraisal instrument for prediction of preterm labor. Nursing Research, 44(2), 76-81.

Egan, T.G., Monaghan, S.M., Muir, R.C., Gilmore, R.J., Clarkson, J.E., & Crooks, T.J. (1990). Prenatal screening of pregnant mothers for parenting difficulties: Final results from the Queen Mary Child Care Unit. Social Science & Medicine, 30(3), 289-295.

Ellerbrock, T., Atrash, H.K., Hogue, C.J., & Smith, J. (1988). Pregnancy mortality surveillance: A new initiative. Contemporary Obstetrics and Gynecology, 31(6), 23-34.

Enkins, M.W. (1994). Risk in pregnancy: The reality, the perception, and the concept. Birth: Issues in Perinatal Care and Education, 21(3), 131-134.

Expert Panel on the Content of Prenatal Care. (1989). Caring for our future: The content of prenatal care. Washington, DC: Public Health Service.

Field, D.R. (1989). Changing patterns in antepartum surveillance. In J.T. Parer (Ed.), Antepartum and intrapartum management. Philadelphia: Lea & Febinger.

Finnegan, L. (1990). Maternal addiction. Special currents: Maternal addiction (pp. 1-3). Columbus, OH: Ross Laboratories.

Fogel, C.I., & Lewallen, L.P. (1995). High-risk childbearing. In C.I. Fogel & N.F. Woods (Eds.), Women's health care: A comprehensive handbook (pp. 427-453). Thousand Oaks, CA: Sage.

Franx, A., van der Post, J.A.M., Elfering, I.M., Veerman, D.P., Merkus, H.M.W.M., Boer, K., & van Montfrans, G.A. (1994). Validation of automatic blood pressure recording in pregnancy. British Journal of Obstetrics and Gynaecology 101(1), 66-69.

Freda, M.C., Mikhail, M., Mazloom, E., Polizzotto, R., Damus, K., & Merkatz, I. (1993). Fetal movement counting: Which method? American Journal of Maternal Child Nursing, 18(6), 314-321.

Gegor, C.L., & Paine, L.L. (1992). Antepartal fetal assessment techniques: An update for today's perinatal nurse. Journal of Perinatal & Neonatal Nursing, 5(4), 1-15.

Giuliano, K.K., & Poirier, C.E. (1991). Nursing care management: Critical pathways to desirable outcomes. Nurse Management, 22(3), 52-55.

Givens, S.R., & Moore, M.L. (1995). Status report on maternal and child health indicators. Journal of Perinatal and Neonatal Nursing, 9(1), 8-18.

Goldenberg, R.L., Patterson, E.T., & Freese, M.P. (1992). Maternal demographics, situational, and psychosocial factors and their relationship to enrollment in prenatal care: A review of the literature. Women & Health, 19(2-3), 133-151.

Gribble, R.K., Fee, S.C., Berg, R.L. (1995). The value of routine urine dipstick screening for protein at each prenatal visit. American Journal of Obstetrics and Gynecology, 173(1), 214-217.

Haller, K.B. (1992). Primary care in rural America and your own backyard. Journal of Obstetric, Gynecologic, and Neonatal Nursing, 21(4), 269.

Handler, A., & Rosenberg, D. (1992) Improving pregnancy outcomes: Public versus private care for urban, low-income women. Birth: Issues in Perinatal Care and Education, (19)3, 123-130.

Harvey, S.M., & Faber, K.S. (1992). Obstacles to prenatal care following implementation of a community-based program to reduce financial barriers. Family Planning Perspectives, 25(1), 32-36.

Hebel, J.R., Fox, N.L., & Sexton, M. (1988). Dose response of birth weight to various measures of maternal smoking during pregnancy. Journal of Clinical Epidemiology, 41(5), 483-489.

Hendricks, S.K., Von Eschen, M., & Grady, M.C. (1995). Preconception counseling and care of common medical disorders. In D.P. Lemcke, J. Pattison, L.A. Marshall & D.S. Crowley (Eds.), Primary care of women (pp. 518-530). Norwalk, CT: Appleton & Lange.

Heyl, P.S., Miller, W., & Canick, J.A. (1990). Maternal serum screening for aneuploid pregnancy by alpha-fetoprotein, HCG, and unconjugated estriol. Obstetrics & Gynecology, 76(6), 1025-1031.

Hook, E.B. (1981). Rates of chromosome abnormalities at different maternal ages. Obstetrics and Gynecology, 58(3), 282-285.

Horton, J. (Ed.). (1995). The Women's Health Data Book: A Profile of Women's Health in the United States (2nd ed.). Washington, DC: Elsevier.

Hoyme, H. E., Jones, K.L., Dixon, S.D., Jewett, T., Hanson, J.W., Robinson, L.K., Msall, M.E., & Allanson, J.E. (1990). Prenatal cocaine exposure and fetal vascular disruption. Pediatrics, 85(5), 743-747.

Iams, J.D., Paraskos, J., Landon, M.B., Teteris, J.M., & Johnson, F.F. (1994). Cervical sonography in preterm labor. Obstetrics and Gynecology, 84(1), 40-45.

Institute of Medicine. (1985). Preventing low birthweight. Washington, DC: National Academy of Sciences.

Institute of Medicine. (1990). Nutrition during pregnancy. Washington, DC: National Academy.

Jamieson, D.J., & Buescher, P.A. (1992). The effect of family planning participation on prenatal care use and low birth weight. Family Planning Perspectives, 24(5), 214-218.

Kiely, M. (Ed.), (1991). Reproductive and perinatal epidemiology. Boca Raton, FL: CRC.

Knight, G.J., Palomaki, G.E., & Haddow, J.E. (1988). Use of maternal serum alpha fetoprotein measurements to screen for Down's Syndrome. Clinical Obstetrics & Gynecology, 31(2), 306-327.

Larrabee, K., & Cowan, M. (1995). Clinical nursing management of sickle cell disease and trait during pregnancy. Journal of Perinatal and Neonatal Nursing, 9(2), 29-41.

Lederman, R.P. (1990). Anxiety and stress in pregnancy: Significance and nursing assessment. NAACOG's Clinical Issues in Perinatal and Women's Health Nursing, 1(3), 279-288.

Libbus, M.K., & Sable, M.R. (1991). Prenatal education in a high-risk population: The effect on birth outcomes. Birth: Issues in Perinatal Care and Education, 18(2), 78-82.

Lommel, L. (1990). Antepartal fetal surveillance. In W.L. Star, M.T. Shannon, L.N. Sammons, L. Lommel, & Y. Gutierrez (Eds.), Ambulatory obstetrics: Protocols for nurse practitioners/nurse midwives (2nd ed.). San Francisco: School of Nursing, University of California.

Lothian, J.A. (1993). Critical dimensions in perinatal education. AWHONN's Clinical Issues in Perinatal and Women's Health Nursing, 4(1), 20-27.

Lothian, J.A. (1994). Is childbirth education obsolete? The Journal of Perinatal Education, 3(2), 5-6.

Main, D.M., & Menutti, M.T. (1986). Neural tube defects: Issues in prenatal diagnosis and counseling. Obstetrics & Gynecology, 67(1), 1-16.

Mamelle, N., Laumon, B., Munoz, F., & Collin, D. (1989). Life Style. In E. Papiernik, L.G. Keith, J. Bouyer, J. Dreyfus & P. Lazar (Eds.). Effective prevention of preterm birth: The French experience at Hagenau (pp. 73-86). White Plains, NY: Author.

March of Dimes Birth Defects Foundation. (1993). Toward improving the outcome of pregnancy: The 90's and beyond. White Plains, NY: March of Dimes Birth Defects Foundation.

Matthews, A.L., & Smith, A.C.M. (1993). Genetic counselling. In R.A. Knuppel & J.E. Drukker (Eds.), High-risk pregnancy: A team approach, (pp. 664-703). Philadelphia: W.B. Saunders.

May, K.A., & Mahlmeister, L.R. (1994). (Eds.), (1994) Comprehensive maternity nursing (3rd ed., pp. 55-58, 390-421). Philadelphia: J.B. Lippincott.

McAnarney, E.R., & Hendee, W.R. (1989). Adolescent pregnancy and its consequences. Journal of American Medical Association, 262(1), 74-77.

McClanahan, P. (1992). Improving access to and use of prenatal care. Journal of Obstetric, Gynecologic, and Neonatal Nursing, 21(4), 280-284.

McIntosh, L.J., Roumayah, N.E., & Bottoms, S.F. (1995). Perinatal outcome of broken marriages in the inner city. Obstetrics and Gynecology, 85(2), 233-236.

Metzger, B. (1991). Summary and recommendations of the third international workshop-conference on gestational diabetes melitus. Diabetes, 40 (Suppl. 2), 197-201.

Moore, T.R., & Piacquadio, K. (1989). A prospective evaluation of fetal movement screening to reduce the incidence of antepartum fetal death. American Journal of Obstetrics and Gynecology, 160 (5, Pt. 1), 1075-1080.

Morrison, J.C. (1990). Preterm birth: A puzzle worth solving. Obstetrics & Gynecology, 76,(1) (Suppl), 5S-12S.

Muerer, J., & Taren, D.L. (1993). Prevention and public health in obstetrics. In R.A. Knuppel & J.E. Drukker. High risk pregnancy: A team approach. Philadelphia: W.B. Saunders.

National Center for Health Statistics. (1993a). Advance report of final mortality statistics, 1991. Monthly Vital Statistics Report, 42 (Suppl 2), 1-64.

National Center for Health Statistics. (1993b). Advance report of final natality statistics, 1991. Monthly Vital Statistics Report, 42(3), 1-2.

National Center for Health Statistics. (1994). Advance report of final natality statistics, 1992. Monthly Vital Statistics Report, 43(5), 6-7.

Neldam, S. (1980). Fetal movements as an indicator of fetal well-being. Lancet, 1(8180), 1222-1224.

Nurses' Association of the American College of Obstetricians and Gynecologists. (1991). NAACOG Standards for the Nursing Care of Women and Newborns. Washington, DC: Author.

O'Campo, P., Faden, R.R., Geilen, A.C., & Wang, M.C. (1992). Prenatal factors associated with breastfeeding duration: Recommendations for prenatal interventions. Birth: Issues in Perinatal Care and Education, 19(4), 195-201.

Palomaki, G.E., Knight, G.J., Haddow, J.E., Canick, J.C., Saller, D.N., & Nanzza, D.S. (1992). Prospective intervention trial of a screening protocol to identify fetal trisomy 18 using maternal serum alpha-fetoprotein unconjugated estriol, and human chorionic gonadotropin. Prenatal Diagnosis, 12(11), 925-930.

Papiernik, E., Keith, L.G., Bouyer, J., Dreyfus, J., & Lazar, P. (Eds). (1989). Effective prevention of preterm birth: The French experience at Hagenau. White Plains, NY: March of Dimes.

Papiernik, E. (1993). Prevention of preterm labor and delivery. Balliere's Clinical Obstetrics and Gynecology, 7(3), 499-521.

Paritsky, J.F. (1985). Tay Sachs: The dreaded inheritance. American Journal of Nursing, 8(3), 260-264.

Pearson, L. (1994). Annual update of how each state stands on legislative issues affecting advanced nursing practice. Nurse Practitioner, 19(1), 11-53.

Pletsch, P. (1990). Birth defect prevention: Nursing interventions. Journal of Obstetric, Gynecologic, and Neonatal Nursing, 19(6), 482-488.

Pletsch, P. (1994). The genetic code and fetal development. In K.A. May & L.R. Mahlmeister (Eds.), Maternal and neonatal nursing: Family centered care (pp. 251-274). Philadelphia: J.B. Lippincott.

Plovie, B. (1991). Diabetes in pregnancy. White Plains, NY: March of Dimes Birth Defects Foundation.

Raine, T., Powell, S., & Krohn, M.A. (1994). The risk of repeating low birth weight and the role of prenatal care. Obstetrics and Gynecology, 84 (4, Pt. 1), 485-489.

Roberts, J. (1994). Current perspectives on preeclampsia. Journal of Nurse-Midwifery, 39(2), 70-90.

Robins, L.N., & Mills, J.L. (Eds.). (1993). Effects of in utero exposure to street drugs. American Journal of Public Health, 83 (Suppl.), 9-32.

Sadler, T.W. (1995). Medical embryology. Baltimore: Williams & Wilkins.

Shannon, M.T. (1990a). Alpha-fetoprotein screening. In W.L. Star, M.T. Shannon, L.N. Sammons, L. Lommel, & Y. Gutierrez (Eds.), Ambulatory obstetrics: Protocols for nurse practitioners/nurse midwives. San Francisco: School of Nursing, University of California.

Shannon, M.T. (1990b). Initial prenatal visit. In W.L. Star, M.T. Shannon, L.N. Sammons, L. Lommel, & Y. Gutierrez (Eds.), Ambulatory obstetrics: Protocols for nurse practitioners/nurse midwives (2nd ed.), San Francisco: School of Nursing, University of California.

Starn, J. (1993). Strengthening family systems. AWHONN's Clinical Issues in Perinatal and Women's Health Nursing, 4(1), 35-43.

Taren, D.L., Clark, W., Chernesky, M., & Quirk, E. (1990). Weekly food servings and participation in social programs among & low income families. American Journal of Public Health, 80(11), 1376-1378.

Tyson, J., Guzick, D., & Rosenfeld, C.R., (1990). Prenatal care evaluation and cohort analyses. Pediatrics, 85(2), 195-204.

United States Department of Health and Human Services. (1991). Drug abuse and drug treatment. The third triennial report to Congress from the Secretary, Department of Health and Human Services (Publication No. (ADM) 91-1704). Rockville, MD: National Institute on Drug Abuse.

Villar, M.A., & Sibai, B.M. (1989). Clinical significance of elevated mean arterial blood pressure in second trimester and threshold increase in systolic or diastolic blood pressure during third trimester. American Journal of Obstetrics and Gynecology, 160(2) 419-423.

Walther, V.N. (1990). Emerging roles of social work in perinatal services. Social Work in Health Care, 15(2), 35-48.

Wilson, B.L. (1989). Delivery outcomes of low-risk births: Comparison of certified nurse midwives and obstetricians. Journal of the American Academy of Nurse Practitioners, 1(1), 9-13.

Witter, F.R., Caulfield, L.E., & Stoltzfus, R.J. (1995). Influence of maternal anthropometric status and birth weight on the risk of cesarean delivery. Obstetrics and Gynecology, 86(6), 947-951.

World Health Organization. (1985). Having a baby in Europe: Report on a study. Public Health in Europe 26. Copenhagen, Denmark: Author.

Young, D. (1990). How can we "enrich" prenatal care? Birth: Issues in Perinatal Care and Education, (17)1, 12-14.

York, R., & Brooten, D. (1992). Prevention of low birth weight. NAACOG's Clinical Issues in Perinatal and Women's Health. 3(1), 13-24.

CHAPTER 6 APPENDIX

PERINATAL SUBSTANCE ABUSE ASSESSMENT GUIDE

Drug and alcohol use among women of childbearing age presents many challenges to health care professionals. Maternal chemical dependence has been associated with numerous medical, obstetrical, and neonatal complications. Comprehensive assessment strategies are necessary to identify women at risk for or currently using drugs and alcohol in pregnancy. Thorough assessment includes observation of the woman's physical appearance and behavioral characteristics, as well as a complete medical, obstetrical, psychosocial, and substance abuse history. The following information provides recommendations and suggested approaches to assessment which may lead to early identification of substance abuse.

Medical History

Factors associated with chemical dependence may include a history of:

Cellulitis	Septicemia	Undocumented seizure disorder or blackouts
Cirrhosis	Pneumonia	Victim of physical or sexual abuse
Depression	Acute hypertension	Recent sexually-transmitted disease
Endocarditis	Suicide attempt	Multiple drug allergies
Hepatitis	HIV Infection	Use of mood-altering prescription drugs
Pancreatitis	AIDS	

Obstetrical History

Factors associated with chemical dependence may include a history of:

Abruptio placentae	Low birth weight	Meconium staining
Unexplained fetal death	Spontaneous abortion	Premature rupture of membranes
Preeclampsia/eclampsia	Placental insufficiency	Unexplained preterm labor/preterm delivery
Gestational diabetes	Amnionitis	Sudden Infant Death Syndrome

Present Pregnancy

Factors associated with chemical dependence may include:

Preterm labor	Inactive/hyperactive fetus	Late, no, or sporadic prenatal care
Poor weight gain	Spotting or bleeding	Sexually-transmitted diseases

Psychosocial History

Family personal factors associated with chemical dependence may include:

Dysfunctional family	Psychiatric history	History of marked emotional deprivation
Drunk driving record	Lack of religiosity	Minimal coping and communication skills
Arrest record	Self-destructive behaviors	Self-induced social isolation
Low self-esteem	Previous child in foster care	Family history of substance abuse
Unstable lifestyle	Major depressive episodes	Poor relationship with family members

Partner has history of/current substance abuse problem

Physical Appearance and Demeanor

Aspects of the physical appearance associated with chemical dependency include:

Untidy appearance	Pupil changes	Looks physically exhausted
Track marks	Abscesses	Inflamed/indurated nasal mucosa
Rhinitis	Cardiac arrhythmias	Thrombophlebitis/sclerosed veins
Alcohol on breath	Weight loss	Liver/abdominal tenderness
Edema of extremities	Fundal size less than dates	Lung congestion/diminished breath sounds

Behavioral Characteristics

Behavioral characteristics associated with chemical dependency include the following:

<u>Behavioral Cues</u>

Slurred speech	Inappropriate behavior	Agitation/restlessness
Emotional lability	Ataxia	Nystagmus
Mistrust of authority figures or other professionals		

<u>Coping Mechanisms</u>

Denial	Rationalization	Minimizing
Blaming		

<u>Withdrawal/Crash Symptoms</u>

Increased respiratory rate	Lacrimation	Diaphoresis
Yawning	Diarrhea	Rhinorrhea
Tremors/muscle spasms	Piloerection	Irritability
Anxiety	Dilated pupils	Insomnia
Nausea/vomiting	Tachycardia	Abdominal cramps
Anorexia	Chills/flushing	Hypertension
Weakness		

Substance Abuse History

The substance abuse history is an effective means for assessment of risk status of **all** pregnant women. It is important that the substance abuse history is conducted in a nonthreatening, nonjudgmental manner. The following questions provide an outline for substance abuse assessment, which may be helpful in guiding the assessment process.

1. TOBACCO

_____ Have you ever smoked cigarettes?

_____ Before you found out you were pregnant, how many cigarettes did you smoke per day?

_____ How many cigarettes do you smoke in one day?

_____ Are there times when you seem to smoke more?

II. ALCOHOL

_____ Have you ever drank alcohol (beer, wine, wine coolers, mixed drinks, or hard liquor)?

_____ Before you found out you were pregnant, how many drinks did you have per day? Per week?

_____ How many beers/glasses of wine/glasses of hard liquor do you drink per week now?

_____ How many beers/glasses of wine/glasses of hard liquor do you drink per day?

_____ What other types of beverages containing alcohol, such as wine coolers, champagne, champalle, mixed drinks (such as margaritas, wine spritzers, etc.) do you like to drink?

_____ Are there times that you seem to drink more often?

III. OVER-THE-COUNTER MEDICATIONS

_____ How often do you use over-the-counter medications (such as aspirin, Tylenol, etc.)?

_____ How often have you taken over-the-counter medications during this pregnancy?

_____ What have you taken these medications for?

_____ How often do you take sleeping pills, diet pills, laxatives, water pills, cough medicine, antihistamines, etc.?

_____ When was the last time you used any of these medications? Reason?

IV. PRESCRIPTION MEDICATIONS

_____ How often have you taken prescription medications during this pregnancy?

_____ Are you currently taking medicines requiring a prescription? What are they?

_____ Why are you taking them? How often?

_____ Were the medications prescribed for you?

_____ Who prescribed them?

_____ Does your obstetrician know that you are taking them?

_____ Does the prescribing physician know that you are pregnant?

_____ Are there times when you tend to use more of this medication?

V. ILLICIT DRUGS

_____ Have you ever used marijuana, cocaine, etc. ?

_____ How often did you use drug (name specifics) before you found out you were pregnant?

_____ How often have you used this drug during this pregnancy?

_____ Are there times when you use more?

_____ How do you take the drug (IV, smoke, snort, etc.)?

_____ When was the last time you used this drug?

It is important to be familiar with drugs available in your area and interview regarding list of specific drugs (i.e., crack, cocaine, marijuana, speed, primos, etc.).

VI. OTHER HELPFUL QUESTIONS

Significant other or family members' past or current substance abuse history is also a recognition cue. The following questions may be helpful:

_____ Does your significant other/family member use drugs/alcohol?

_____ What are you doing while they are using/partying?

_____ Where are you when they are using?

If answers to the previous questions indicate the need for further exploration of drinking and drugging patterns, asking the following questions may be helpful:

_____ Have you ever tried to cut down your use of __________? What was that like for you?

_____ Do you feel annoyed by criticism of your drinking/drug use?

_____ Do you feel guilty about your drinking/drug use?

_____ Do you ever experience memory lapses (blackouts)?

_____ Do you get sick from drinking or drug use afterwards?

_____ Do you ever regret what you have done while drinking or using drugs?

_____ Do you ever use _____________ first thing in the morning to steady your nerves or get rid of a hangover?

_____ Do you ever get shaky or edgy if you don't use _____________ ?

References

Chappel, J.N. (1987). Alcohol and drug dependencies: How to spot; what steps to take. Consultant, 27(4), 60-75.

Chasnoff, I.J. (1987). Perinatal effects of cocaine. Contemporary OB/GYN, 26(5), 163-179.

Chisum, G.M. (1990). Nursing interventions with the antepartum substance abuser. Journal of Perinatal and Neonatal Nursing, 3(4), 26-33.

Finkellstein, N., Duncan, S.A., Derman, L., & Smeltze, J. (1990). Getting sober, getting well. Cambridge, MA: The Women's Alcoholism Program of C.A.S.P.A.R.

Glans, J.C., & Woods, J.R. (1991). Obstetrical issues in substance abuse. Pediatric Annals, 20(10), 531-539.

Hoegerman, G., & Schnoll, S. (1991). Narcotic use in pregnancy. Clinics in Perinatology, 18(1), 51-73.

Ryall, J. (1989). Eliciting a history of pathological drinking from women. A & D News, 1-4.

Starr, K.L., & Chisum, G.M. (1992). The chemically dependent pregnant woman. In L. K. Mandeville, & N.H. Troiano (Eds.), High risk intrapartum nursing (pp. 115-145). New York: J.B. Lippincott.

Common Perinatal Complications

Mary Ellen Burke
Judy Poole

Pregnancy and childbirth are natural processes. The majority of women during pregnancy do well with periodic assessments, supportive measures, and encouragement, requiring minimal intervention. However, complications in pregnancy can frequently occur with little or no warning. Life-threatening events such as hemorrhage from a placenta previa or accreta, preterm labor at 26 weeks gestation, or an eclamptic seizure place the woman and fetus at risk for significant morbidity and mortality.

Providing safe and effective care for the woman during pregnancy requires a joint effort from all members of the healthcare team, with each member contributing unique skills and talents to provide maximum outcome for mother and infant. The nurse in the perinatal setting must quickly assess and identify changes in maternal-fetal condition and adjust care accordingly. Comprehensive nursing assessments are essential in recognizing alterations from the normal process during the antepartum, intrapartum, and postpartum periods. Anticipatory nursing care is invaluable in preventing a complication from becoming a crisis. Notifying the primary healthcare provider immediately of signs or symptoms of alterations from expected clinical progression during pregnancy can facilitate early intervention and determine the proper course and placement of treatment.

This chapter discusses the nursing management of three of the more common perinatal complications: hypertension, bleeding, and preterm labor. Suggestions for homecare management of women in stable condition and guidelines for maternal transfer to a tertiary center are also included.

HYPERTENSION IN PREGNANCY

Significance and Incidence

Hypertensive disorders of pregnancy are the most common medical complication of pregnancy. Hypertension is a significant contributor to maternal and perinatal morbidity and mortality and is estimated to complicate approximately 7–10% of all pregnancies

(Working Group on High Blood Pressure in Pregnancy, 1990). In the United States, preeclampsia ranks second only to embolic events as a cause of maternal mortality and is directly responsible for 15% of maternal deaths (Rochat, Koonin, Atrash, & Jewett, 1988). Of the women with hypertension during pregnancy, between one half to two thirds are diagnosed with preeclampsia or eclampsia (Brown, 1991).

Morbidity and Mortality

Hypertension in pregnancy predisposes the woman to potentially lethal complications such as abruptio placentae, disseminated intravascular coagulation (DIC), cerebral hemorrhage, cerebral vascular accident, hepatic failure, and acute renal failure (Poole, 1993; Roberts, 1994; Working Group on High Blood Pressure in Pregnancy, 1990). Cerebral hemorrhage and cerebral vascular accident (CVA), resulting from severe preeclampsia and eclampsia, are the major maternal hazards.

Maternal hypertension contributes to intrauterine fetal death and perinatal mortality (Repke & Villar, 1991; Wen, Goldenberg, Cutter, Hoffman, & Cliver, 1990; World Health Organization [WHO], 1980; York & Brooten, 1992). The main causes of neonatal death are placental insufficiency and abruptio placentae. In addition, intrauterine growth restriction (IUGR) is common in infants of women with preeclampsia (Roberts, Taylor, Friedman, & Goldfien, 1990; Sibai, 1990a).

Risk Factors

Preeclampsia is a subtle and insidious disease process. The signs and symptoms of preeclampsia become apparent relatively late in the course of the disease, usually during the third trimester of pregnancy. However, the underlying pathophysiology may be present as early as 8 weeks' gestation (Friedman, Taylor, & Roberts, 1991).

Historically, several well-defined risk factors have been identified for the development of preeclampsia. These risk factors can be found in Display 7-1. Although risk factors are identified, the individual predictive value of the risk factors for screening and risk identification purposes have not been verified.

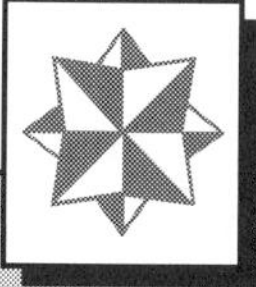

Display 7-1

Risk Factors For The Development of Preeclampsia

- First pregnancy or a pregnancy of new genetic makeup (Chesley & Cooper, 1986; Cunningham & Leveno, 1988)
- Multifetal gestation (Thompson, Lyons, & Makowski, 1987)
- Presence of preexisting diabetes, collagen vascular disease, hypertension, or renal disease (Mabie, Pernoll, & Biswas, 1986; Cunningham, Cox, Harstad, Mason, & Pritchard, 1990; Siddiqi, Rosenn, Mimouni, Khoury, & Miodovink, 1991)
- Hydatidiform mole (Page, 1939)
- Fetal hydrops (Barron, 1991)
- Maternal age (Spellacy, Miller, & Winegar, 1986)
- African American race (Cunningham & Leveno, 1988)
- Family history of pregnancy-induced hypertension (Chesley & Cooper, 1986)
- Antiphospholipid syndrome (Branch, Silver, Blackwell, Reading, & Scott, 1992)
- Angiotensinogen gene T235 (Ward, Hata, & Jeunemaitre, 1993)
- Socioeconomic status (Guzick et al., 1987)
- Failure to demonstrate hemodilution (Hays, Cruikshank, & Dunn, 1985)
- Failure to demonstrate a decrease in systemic vascular resistance and second trimester mean arterial pressures (MAP) (Ales, Norton, & Druzin, 1989; Gavette & Roberts, 1987).

Definitions

Terminology used to describe the hypertensive disorders of pregnancy is associated with imprecise usage, causing confusion for healthcare providers caring for women with hypertensive complications during pregnancy and childbirth.

The American College of Obstetricians and Gynecologists' (ACOG, 1986) Technical Bulletin, *Management of Preeclampsia,* outlines current accepted terminology. It should be noted that this technical bulletin is presently in revision and for an update, readers should refer to new version, *Hypertension in Pregnancy,* to be published in December 1995.

Clinically, there are two basic types of hypertension during pregnancy—chronic hypertension and pregnancy-induced hypertension (PIH)—with the distinction based on the onset of hypertension in relation to the pregnancy.

Chronic Hypertension

Chronic hypertension is hypertension that predates the pregnancy or hypertension continuing beyond 42 days postpartum (Sibai, 1991b; Working Group on High Blood Pressure in Pregnancy, 1990).

Pregnancy-Induced Hypertension

Pregnancy-induced hypertension is the onset of hypertension, generally after the twentieth week of pregnancy, appearing as a marker of a pregnancy-specific vasospastic condition (Roberts, 1994). These two types of hypertension may occur independently or simultaneously.

Once PIH is present, it is further classified according to the maternal organ systems affected.

Preeclampsia. Preeclampsia is characterized by renal involvement as evidenced by the onset of proteinuria. The disease process is said to be either mild or severe, based on maternal or fetal findings.

HELLP Syndrome. HELLP Syndrome is characterized by hepatic involvement as evidenced by hemolysis, elevated liver enzymes, and low platelets.

Eclampsia. Eclampsia is characterized by the onset of seizure activity or coma in the woman diagnosed with PIH, with no history of preexisting neurologic pathology.

Pathophysiology of Preeclampsia

Preeclampsia has been called the "disease of theories." There is not one agreed upon etiology; however, research is ongoing to identify the pathophysiology of this process. Although the exact mechanism is unknown, preeclampsia is thought to occur secondary to changes within the maternal cardiovascular, hematologic, and renal systems.

Normal physiologic adaptations to pregnancy include an increase in plasma volume, vasodilation of the vascular bed, decreased systemic vascular resistance, elevation of cardiac output, and increased prostacyclin production. Physical assessment findings consistent with these changes are dilutional anemia, lower systemic blood pressures and mean arterial pressure, a slight increase in heart rate, and peripheral edema (Harvey, 1991).

With preeclampsia these normal adaptations are altered. Instead of plasma volume expansion and hemodilution, there is a decrease in circulating plasma volume resulting in hemoconcentration. This is evidenced by increased hemoglobin and hematocrit concentrations and increased blood viscosity leading to a decrease in maternal organ perfusion, including the uteroplacental unit. The vascular bed demonstrates increased sensitivity to vasoactive substances, resulting in vasoconstriction and an increased vascular tone. Vasoconstriction results in increased systemic vascular resistance and hypertension. This hypertension is further aggravated by arterial vasospasms; the underlying mechanism for observed signs and symptoms of the disease process.

Vasoconstriction and a further increase in cardiac output above the normal pregnancy elevation (Easterling, Benedetti, Schmucker, & Millard, 1990), results in arterial vasospasms, endothelial damage, and an imbalance in endothelial prostacyclin and thromboxane ratios (Sibai, 1991a; Zeeman & Dekker, 1992). See Display 7-2 for highlights of the pathophysiology of disease progression and multiple organ system improvement.

Clinical Manifestations of PIH

Historically, the classic triad for preeclampsia has included hypertension, proteinuria, and edema. However, not all of these parameters have to be present for the diagnosis of PIH. Hypertension and proteinuria are the most significant indicators. Edema is significant only if hypertension, proteinuria, or signs of multisystem organ involvement are present.

The clinical manifestations of PIH are directly related to the presence of vascular vasospasms. These vasospasms result in endothelial injury, red blood cell destruction, platelet aggregation, increased capillary

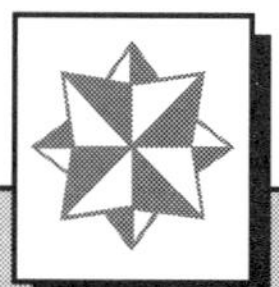

DISPLAY 7-2

Physiologic and Pathophysiologic Changes Associated With Preeclampsia

Feature	Normal Pregnancy Change	Preeclampsia Alteration
Blood volume	50% increase	A lesser increase
Plasma volume	50% increase	small or no increase
Red cell mass	20% increase (physiologic anemia)	increase (hemoconcentration)
Cardiac output	40–50% increase	Variable
Blood pressure	Decline Nadir—midtrimester with return to prepregnancy level by third trimester	Hypertension
Peripheral vascular resistance	Decline	Increases Increased vascular reactivity Vasospasm
Renal function	Enhanced secondary to increased perfusion	Decreased
RPF	75% increase	Decrease
GFR	50% increase	Decrease
by 2nd trimester	Urea nitrogen—decreases Creatinine clearance—increases	BUN increases Creatinine increases (clearance decreases)
	Uric acid—decreases	Uric acid increases
Renin–angiotensin–aldosterone system	Markedly activated and responds appropriately to posture and salt intake	Plasma renin concentration and activity suppressed along with loss of antagonists (vasodilators) to AII
Coagulation system		
Fibrinogen	Increased	Remains normal initially (decreased in severe preeclampsia)
Factors VII, VIII, IX, X	All increased	Increase in ratio of von Willebrand factor to factor VII, coagulant activity increased—leading to consumption of factor VIII
Fibrinolytic activity	Decreased	Increased
Platelet count	Normal or slight increase	Decreased
Bleeding time	Normal	Prolonged

RPF=renal plasma flow; GFR=glomerular filtration rate; BUN=blood urea nitrogen; AII=angiotensin II.

Adapted from Roberts, J. (1994). Current perspectives on preeclampsia. Journal of Nurse–Midwifery, 39 (2), 76.

permeability, increased systemic vascular resistance, and renal and hepatic dysfunction.

Hypertension

Although controversy exists as to the most appropriate definition of hypertension, one of the following criteria may be used: (1) a sustained blood pressure elevation of 140/90 mmHg after the twentieth week of gestation, as recorded on two or more measurements, or (2) elevation of 30 mmHg systolic or 15 mmHg diastolic over the first trimester or prepregnancy baseline values. Current research is ongoing; however, this criteria is of questionable value for diagnosis. MacGillivray, Rose, & Rowe (1969) reported that 73% of nulliparous women with normal pregnancies demonstrated an increase in diastolic blood pressure of more than 15 mmHg during pregnancy, while 57% of these women demonstrated an increase in diastolic pressure of more than 20 mmHg. Later studies have confirmed these findings (Moutquin, Rainville, & Giroux, 1985; Villiar & Sibai, 1989), suggesting that further study is required to determine the degree of elevation that is significant for the prediction of preeclampsia.

Earlier research suggests that an increase in mean arterial pressure in the second trimester (MAP-2) of greater than 85 mmHg is diagnostic in predicting the women at risk for developing hypertension during pregnancy (Page & Christianson, 1976). Several authors have correlated an elevation of MAP-2 with an increased risk for maternal hypertension, and fetal and neonatal risks (Ales, Norton, & Druzin, 1989; Chesley & Sibai, 1987; Gavette & Roberts, 1987; O'Brien, 1990). However, more definitive research is needed.

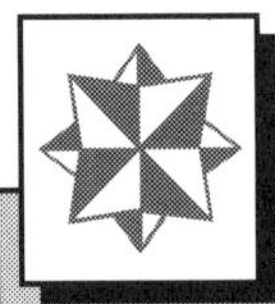

DISPLAY 7-3

Criteria for Severe Preeclampsia

- Systolic blood pressure of 160 mmHg or diastolic blood pressure of 110 mmHg on two occasions at least 6 hours apart with the patient on bedrest. However, if this degree of hypertension is sustained, blood pressure measurements should be taken more frequently.
- Proteinuria of 5 g or greater in 24 hours, or 3–4+ on dipstick
- Oliguria: less than 400–500 ml of urine output over 24 hours or altered renal function tests. Look for trends of decreasing urinary output. A kidney that is adequately perfused and oxygenated should produce a minimum of 30 ml/hr or 100 ml/4 hr of urine.
- Elevated serum creatinine >1.2
- Intrauterine growth restriction
- Cerebral or visual disturbances including (but not limited to) altered level of consciousness, headache, scotomata, or blurred vision (magnesium sulfate may cause headache or blurred vision if serum concentration is in the high therapeutic range)
- Impaired liver function demonstrated by right upper quadrant or epigastric pain and/or altered liver function tests (increased aspartate transaminase [AST or SGOT] or alanine transaminase [ALT or SGPT] liver enzymes). With significant hepatic involvement there is increased risk for coagulation defects and hypoglycemia.
- Thrombocytopenia: platelet count <150,000; coagulopathies generally not present until platelet counts drop below 100,000
- Pulmonary or cardiac involvement: may present as pulmonary edema, cyanosis, chest pain, cardiac dysrhythmias
- Development of eclampsia
- Development of HELLP Syndrome

Proteinuria

Proteinuria is defined as the excretion of 0.1 g/L (100 mg/L) in a random specimen, or 0.3 g/L in a 24-hour specimen (300 mg/L), or 1–2+ on dipstick. The presence of proteinuria indicates a worsening of the disease process, increasing the risk to the woman and fetus. There is a positive correlation between the degree of proteinuria and perinatal mortality and fetal growth restriction (Tervila, Goecke, & Timonen, 1973).

Edema

Edema is a common finding of pregnancy and is not necessary for the diagnosis of PIH. Intracellular and extracellular edema is present, representing a generalized and excessive accumulation of fluid in tissue. As vasospasms worsen, there will be capillary endothelial damage resulting in increased systemic capillary permeability (leakage), which facilitates hemoconcentration and increases the risk of pulmonary edema.

Mild Versus Severe Preeclampsia

In order to identify the progression of PIH from mild to severe disease, nursing management will require accurate and thorough observation and assessments. See Display 7-3 for criteria for severe preeclampsia and Display 7-4 for the potential maternal and fetal complications of severe preeclampsia.

In caring for the woman with a hypertensive disorder of pregnancy, nursing assessments focus on identification of the disease progression. PIH is a systemic disease in which one or more organ systems are involved. The wide range of symptoms and multiple organ system involvement can sometimes result in misdiagnosis and delay in treatment. Cocaine intoxication, lupus nephritis, chronic renal failure, and acute fatty liver of pregnancy are examples of conditions which may mimic preeclampsia and eclampsia (O'Brien, Mercer, Friedman, & Sibai, 1993; Simpson, 1993). The care of the woman with severe preeclampsia or HELLP syndrome is best referred to a tertiary perinatal center.

Nursing Assessment and Interventions for Preeclampsia

The only definitive therapy for preeclampsia is birth. The decision of delivery versus expectant management must be individualized.

Homecare Management. Mild preeclampsia may be managed at home with frequent follow-up care including daily telephone contact between the woman and a high-risk perinatal nurse, and periodic nurse home visits. Criteria for home management varies with primary perinatal healthcare provider and homecare agency. The woman must be in stable condition with no evidence of worsening maternal or fetal status (Grohar, 1994).

Diagnostic criteria and considerations suggested for homecare referral for management of woman with mild PIH can be found in Chapter Appendix 7-1 (Grohar, 1994; Simpson, 1992).

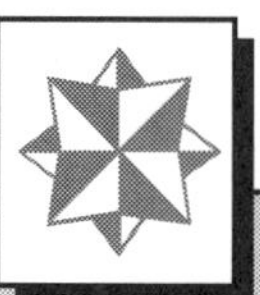

DISPLAY 7-4

Maternal and Fetal Complications From Severe Preeclampsia

- Cardiovascular: severe hypertension, hypertensive crisis, pulmonary edema
- Renal: oliguria, acute renal failure
- Hematologic: hemolysis, decreased oxygen-carrying capacity, thrombocytopenia, coagulation defects including DIC
- Neurologic: eclampsia, cerebral edema, cerebral hemorrhage, cerebral vascular accidents, amaurosis (blindness)
- Hepatic: hepatocellular dysfunction, hepatic rupture, hypoglycemia
- Uteroplacental: abruptio placentae, fetal growth restriction, fetal death, fetal intolerance to labor

Inpatient Management

Women with mild preeclampsia may also be evaluated in the inpatient setting and remain hospitalized. Women with severe preeclampsia and eclampsia are managed in the hospital. Those patients at an early gestational age, usually less than 34 weeks, are generally managed in a tertiary center because of the ability to provide advanced neonatal care if delivery is indicated.

Nursing care involves accurate and astute observations and assessments. A comprehensive knowledge base regarding pharmacologic therapies, management regimens, and possible complications is also required.

The most important aspect of care for women with hypertension in pregnancy is recognition of the abilities of the facility and the obstetric staff to handle potential emergencies. It is best to not attempt to expectantly manage patients with severe preeclampsia (antepartum or postpartum) unless in a tertiary care center. However, providers of obstetric care must be able to stabilize the woman prior to transport.

Controversial Management Protocols

Some management protocols are considered to be inappropriate in the care of women with preeclampsia. Diuretics and/or the administration of high concentrations of colloid solutions (albumin, Hespan) should not be used to decrease peripheral edema due to further depletion of intravascular volume and an increased risk of pulmonary edema and uteroplacental insufficiency (Repke, 1993; Dildy, Phelan, & Cotton, 1992). Valium is no longer the first-line agent to stop seizure activity due to the depressant effect on the fetus and depression of the maternal gag reflex. Seizure precautions should be followed according to institution protocol. It is important to avoid insertion of a padded tongue blade to the back of the throat; a nasopharyngeal airway may be appropriate, if available. Finally, heparin should not be administered as prophylaxis against coagulopathies; it will increase the risk for intracranial bleeding.

Activity Restriction

Activity restriction, varying from frequent rest periods with legs elevated to bedrest therapy in the full lateral position, is frequently prescribed for women with PIH. While on bedrest, blood pressure (BP) decreases and interstitial fluid is mobilized into the intravascular space, thus enhancing flow to the uterus and kidneys

Controversy exists as to whether the reduction of systolic BP associated with bedrest actually improves maternal or fetal outcomes. For pregnancies complicated with nonproteinuric hypertension, bedrest does not appear to significantly improve outcome; however, in women with proteinuric preeclampsia, bedrest does seem to be of some benefit. It is unclear at this point whether bedrest in a hospital setting improves outcomes because of concurrent intensive inpatient maternal/fetal assessments and appropriate medical intervention, or bedrest is beneficial when considered as an independent factor (Goldenberg et al., 1994).

Ongoing Assessments

Preeclampsia can occur without warning or with the gradual development of symptoms. A key goal is early identification of women at risk for development of preeclampsia.

A review of the major organ systems adds to the database for detecting changes from baseline in BP, weight gain, pattern of weight gain, increasing edema, and presence of proteinuria. It is also important to note whether the woman complains of unusual, frequent, or severe headaches; visual disturbances; and/or epigastric pain. Lack of specific reliable diagnostic tests currently hinder early detection and treatment of preeclampsia.

Accurate and consistent BP assessment is important for establishing a baseline and monitoring subtle changes throughout the pregnancy. BP readings are affected by maternal position and measurement techniques. Consistency must be ensured in that proper equipment and cuff size are used, the woman is correctly positioned, there is a rest period before recording the pressure, and that Korotkoff phase IV are used (Sibai, 1988). Ideally, BP measurements should be recorded with the woman in a semi-Fowler's position with the arm at heart level (Sibai, 1991b). If the initial measurement indicates an elevation, the woman should be allowed to relax and have a repeat measurement performed, again in a semi-Fowler's position (Sibai, 1988). When using electronic BP devices, there is a widening of pulse pressure compared to manual readings; however, mean arterial pressure (MAP) is unchanged (Marx, Schwalbe, Cho, & Whitty, 1993). The main point to remember is that BP measurements should be taken in a consistent manner. Assessment focuses on BP trends, not on a single reading.

Presence of edema, in addition to hypertension, warrants additional investigation. Edema, assessed by distribution and degree, is described as dependent or pitting. If periorbital or facial edema is not obvious, the pregnant woman is asked if it was present when she awoke.

Deep tendon reflexes (DTRs) are evaluated if preeclampsia is suspected. The biceps and patellar reflexes and ankle clonus are assessed and the findings recorded. The evaluation of DTR is especially important if the woman is being treated with magnesium sulfate; absence of DTR is an early indication of impending magnesium toxicity.

Proteinuria is determined from dipstick testing of a clean-catch or catheter urine specimen. A reading greater than +1 on two or more occasions, at least 4 hours apart, should be followed by a 24-hour urine collection (Gilbert & Harmon, 1992). A 24-hour collection for protein and creatinine clearance is more reflective of true renal status. Proteinuria is usually a late sign in the course of preeclampsia (Working Group on High Blood Pressure in Pregnancy, 1990). Urine output is assessed for volume of at least 25–30 ml/hr or 100 ml/4 hr. Placement of an indwelling Foley catheter with urometer will facilitate accurate assessment of fluid balance and early signs of renal compromise.

An important ongoing assessment will be determination of fetal status. Uteroplacental perfusion is decreased in women with preeclampsia, thereby placing the fetus in jeopardy. The spiral arteries of the placental bed are subject to vasospasm. When this occurs, perfusion between maternal circulation and the intervillous space is compromised, decreasing blood flow and oxygenation to the fetus. Oligohydramnios, intrauterine growth restriction, fetal compromise, and intrauterine fetal death all are associated with preeclampsia. The fetal heart rate (FHR) should be assessed for baseline rate, variability, and reassuring versus nonreassuring patterns. The presence of abnormal baseline rate, decreased or absent variability, or late decelerations are indications of fetal intolerance to the intrauterine environment. The presence of variable decelerations, antepartum or intrapartum, are suggestive of decreased amniotic fluid volumes (oligohydramnios), increasing the risk of umbilical cord compression and fetal compromise. Biophysical or biochemical monitoring for fetal well-being may be ordered: fetal movement counts (FMC), nonstress test (NST), contraction stress test (CST), biophysical profile (BPP), and serial ultrasonography (Phelan, 1991). As long as the fetus continues to grow in an appropriate manner, it can be inferred that the placenta and uterine blood flow are appropriate (Working Group on High Blood Pressure in Pregnacy, 1990). Until birth, the woman with preeclampsia should be encouraged to rest in a lateral recumbent position to increase uterine perfusion.

Uterine tonicity is evaluated for signs of labor and abruptio placentae. If labor is suspected, a vaginal examination for cervical changes is indicated.

Assessments target signs of deterioration from mild preeclampsia to severe preeclampsia or eclampsia. Signs of liver involvement (e.g., epigastric pain, elevated liver function test, and thrombocytopenia), renal failure, worsening hypertension, cerebral involvement, and developing coagulopathies must be assessed and documented. Respirations are assessed for rales (crackles) or diminished breath sounds, which may indicate pulmonary edema. Noninvasive assessment parameters include level of consciousness (LOC), blood pressure, hemoglobin oxygen saturation (pulse oximetry), electrocardiogram (ECG) findings, and urine output. Invasive hemodynamic monitoring with a flow-directed pulmonary artery catheter (Swan-Ganz) may be indicated in selected patients (Clark, Cotton, Hankins, & Phelan, 1994).

Laboratory Tests

The nurse assists in obtaining a number of blood and urine specimens to aid in diagnosis of preeclampsia, HELLP syndrome, or chronic hypertension. At present no known laboratory tests predict the development of preeclampsia (Gavette & Roberts, 1987). Baseline laboratory test information is useful in the early diagnosis of preeclampsia and for comparison with results obtained to evaluate progression and severity of disease. See Display 7-5 for common laboratory values assessed in the woman with hypertension during pregnancy.

Pharmacologic Therapies

Pharmacologic therapies are instituted for two purposes: seizure prophylaxis and antihypertensive management.

Magnesium Sulfate. Magnesium Sulfate ($MgSO_4$) is the drug of choice in the management of preeclampsia to prevent seizure activity. $MgSO_4$ is administered as a secondary infusion via an infusion controlled device, to achieve serum levels of approximately 5–8 mg/dl (4–7 mEq/dl). The loading dose is a 4–6 g bolus IV over 15 to 30 minutes followed by a maintenance infusion of 2–3 g/hr.

The action of $MgSO_4$ as an anticonvolusant is controversial, but it is thought to decrease neuromuscular irritability and block the release of acetylcholine at neuromuscular junctions, depressing the vasomotor center, thereby depressing central nervous system irritability.

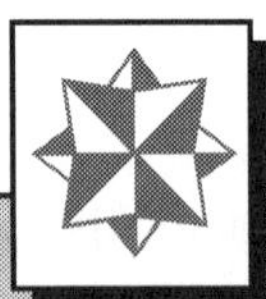

DISPLAY 7-5

Laboratory Values Assessed in the Patient with Hypertension in Pregnancy

Complete Blood Count
- Hemoglobin
- Hematocrit
- Platelet count

Chemistry
- Electrolytes
- Blood urea nitrogen (BUN)
- Serum creatinine
- Serum albumin
- Uric acid
- Serum calcium
- Serum sodium
- Serum magnesium
- Liver function tests: LDH, AST (SGOT), ALT (SGPT)

Urine
- Urinalysis for protein
- 24-hour creatinine clearance may be measured in patients with chronic hypertension or renal disease
- 24-hour urine for sodium excretion
- Specific gravity

Coagulation Profile
- Platelet count
- PT/PTT
- Fibrinogen
- FSP/FDP
- Bleeding time
- D-Dimer

Side effects of magnesium sulfate are dose dependent and include flushing, nausea, vomiting, headache, lower maternal temperature, blurred vision, respiratory depression, and cardiac arrest. The effect of $MgSO_4$ on fetal heart baseline variability is controversial.

Nursing responsibilities and assessments for women receiving $MgSO_4$ include (1) assessing maternal baseline vital signs (VS), DTR, and urinary output prior to initiation of therapy and reassessing per institution protocol; (2) preparing $MgSO_4$ according to protocol; (3) establishing primary IV and administering $MgSO_4$ IV piggyback via control infusion device; (4) documenting $MgSO_4$ infusion in g/hr; (5) continuous fetal assessment; (6) keeping calcium gluconate at bedside; (7) being cautious with concurrent administration of narcotics, central nervous system (CNS) depressants, calcium channel blockers, and β-blockers; and (8) discontinuing $MgSO_4$ and notifying the physician if signs of toxicity (including loss of knee-jerk reflexes, respiratory depression, oliguria, respiratory arrest, and cardiac arrest) or if the woman complains of shortness of breath or chest pain.

Phenytoin (Dilantin). Phenytoin has also been proposed for eclampsia prophylaxis; however, it is not a first-line therapy in the United States. Clinical studies have not demonstrated better results with phenytoin when compared with $MgSO_4$. Due to a lack of experience with phenytoin and significant maternal side effects, $MgSO_4$ remains the first-line drug in the United States.

Antihypertensive Therapy. Pharmacologic therapies directed at the control of significant hypertension include a variety of agents. There are several general precautions to be considered when antihypertensive agents are ordered: (1) antihypertensive therapy is initiated when BP is sustained or greater than 110 diastolic to prevent maternal cerebral vascular accident; (2) effect of the agent may be dependent upon intravascular volume status, and hypovolemia secondary to increased capillary permeability and hemoconcentration may need correction prior to the initiation of therapy; and (3) maintain diastolic BP between 90–100 mmHg to maintain uteroplacental perfusion.

Hydralazine Hydrochloride (Apresoline). Hydralazine hydrochloride is considered by many to be the first-line agent to decrease hypertension. Dosage regimens vary, but intermittent IV boluses generally work equal to continuous infusions; there is also less chance of rebound hypotension with intermittent boluses. Side effects of hydralazine include flushing, headache, maternal and fetal tachycardia, palpitations, uteroplacental insufficiency with subsequent fetal tachycardia, and late decelerations. Because hydralazine increases maternal cardiac output and heart rate, hypertension may worsen.

Labetalol. Labetalol has recently been used in place of hydralazine for the management of hypertension. Dosage regimens vary, based on physician experience and preference. Labetalol is contraindicated in women with asthma and those with greater than first-degree heart block (Chez & Sibai, 1994). Due to labetalol's alpha- and beta- adrenergic blockage, transient fetal and neonatal hypotention, bradycardia, and hypoglycemia are possible.

Nifedipine (Procardia). Nifedipine may be used as a third-line agent in the treatment of hypertension. As with other pharmacologic agents, protocols vary. With the administration of nifedipine, a calcium channel blocker, care must be taken with concomitant administration with $MgSO_4$ and β-blockers.

Postpartum Management

Immediate postpartum curettage has been associated with a more rapid recovery for women with severe preeclampsia, though more research is needed in this area (Magann et al., 1993). Most women will be clinically stable within 48 hours after birth. However, because of the risk of eclampsia during the first 24 to 48 hours postpartum, careful monitoring is essential and should include frequent assessments of vital signs, LOC, DTRs, urinary output, and laboratory data. Intravenous $MgSO_4$ is usually continued for 24 hours postpartum. It is important to be alert for early signs and symptoms of complications of preeclampsia such as postpartum hemorrhage, DIC, pulmonary edema, HELLP syndrome, increased intracranial pressure, and intracranial hemorrhage. Intensity of monitoring and progression of activity are based on patient condition. After vital signs and mental status are stable, laboratory data indicate condition is improving, urinary output is reassuring, and IV $MgSO_4$ is discontinued, frequency of maternal assessments are decreased from 1 to 2 hours to 4 to 8 hours, the Foley catheter is removed, and the patient is encouraged to ambulate. It is important to provide assistance and assess stability during initial ambulation, after bedrest and IV administration of $MgSO_4$ during the intrapartum and postpartum period. Efforts should be made to initiate maternal-newborn attachment by bringing the newborn, if stable, to visit the mother. Photographs of the newborn can be taken and provided to the woman if maternal or newborn condition prevents visitation.

HELLP Syndrome

HELLP Syndrome, a multisystem disease, is a form of severe preeclampsia in which the woman presents with a variety of complaints and exhibits common laboratory markers for a syndrome of hemolysis (H), elevated liver enzymes (EL), and low platelets (LP). This subset of women progresses from preeclampsia to the development of multiple organ involvement and damage. The complaints range from malaise, epigastric pain, nausea and vomiting, to nonspecific viral-syndrome-like symptoms. On presentation, these patients are generally in the second or early third trimester and initially may show few signs of preeclampsia. Because of the presenting symptomatology, these patients often receive a nonobstetric diagnosis delaying treatment and increasing maternal and perinatal morbidity and mortality (Sibai, 1990b; Weinstein, 1985).

Assessments and management of the woman diagnosed with HELLP Syndrome are the same as for the woman with severe preeclampsia.

Eclampsia

Eclampsia is the development of seizures or coma or both, in a woman with signs and symptoms of preeclampsia. Other causes of seizures must be excluded. Eclampsia can occur antepartum, intrapartum, or postpartum; approximately 50% of cases occur antepartum (Fairlie & Sibai, 1993).

The immediate care during a seizure is to ensure a patent airway. Once this has been attained, adequate oxygenation must be maintained by use of supplemental oxygen. $MgSO_4$ (and amobarbital sodium for recurrent convulsions) is given per institution protocol (Sibai, 1990c).

Aspiration is a leading cause of maternal morbidity following an eclamptic seizure. After initial stabilization and airway management, the nurse should anticipate orders for a chest x-ray and possibly arterial blood gases (ABG) to rule out the possibility of aspiration.

A rapid assessment of uterine activity, cervical status, and fetal status are performed. During the seizure, membranes may rupture and the cervix may dilate because the uterus becomes hypercontractile and hypertonic. If birth is not imminent, the timing and route of delivery and the induction of labor versus cesarean birth is dependent upon maternal and fetal status. All medications and therapy are merely temporary measures.

Summary

Hypertensive disorders of pregnancy are the most common medical complication of pregnancy. Nurses caring for women diagnosed with one of the hypertensive disorders must be fully aware of risk factors, diagnostic criteria, appropriate management regimens, and potential complications for both the woman and fetus.

BLEEDING IN PREGNANCY

Significance and Incidence

Hemorrhagic disorders in pregnancy are medical emergencies. Maternal mortality has decreased significantly in recent years; however, hemorrhage remains a major cause of maternal death. From 1979 to 1986, hemorrhage accounted for 30.2% of all maternal deaths in the United States (Atrash, Rowley, & Hogue, 1992). Most maternal deaths from hemorrhage occur due to complications of ectopic pregnancy rupture; however, approximately 18–20% of maternal hemorrhagic deaths occur during the second or third trimester (Atrash et al., 1992). Current research estimates that approximately 15% of maternal cardiac output (1 L/min) flows through the placental bed at term; unchecked bleeding can result in complete exsanguination in 8–10 minutes (O'Brien, 1993, Thorp, 1993).

It is estimated that one in five pregnancies are complicated by bleeding; the incidence and type of bleeding varies by trimester (Thorp, 1993). Most bleeding occurring in the first trimester of pregnancy is related to spontaneous abortion and is generally not life threatening. Placenta previa, one of the most common causes of bleeding during the second and third trimester, occurs in approximately 1 in 200 pregnancies (Cunningham, MacDonald, Gant, Leveno, & Gilstrap, 1993). The incidence of abruptio placentae varies in the literature, from 0.5–1.5% of pregnancies, and is dependent on the risk status of populations studied (Saftlas, Olson, Atrash, Rochat, & Rowley, 1991).

Abnormalities of placental implantation and development may lead to hemorrhage. Abnormal implantation of the placenta is a rare occurrence with the most common abnormality being placenta accreta. Vasa previa, related to velamentous umbilical cord insertion, is a rare but life-threatening complication for the fetus (Cunningham et al., 1993), which may exsanguinate before a cesarean birth can be accomplished.

Bleeding is possible due to uterine trauma or rupture. Rupture of a low transverse uterine scar occurs in less than 1% of women with a previous cesarean birth (Cunningham et al., 1993). Incidence of rupture of a vertical scar from a prior cesarean birth is not well documented. The incidence of spontaneous uterus inversion is approximately 1 in 2,500 births (Zahn & Yeomans, 1990). Improper management of the third stage of labor increases the likelihood of iatrogenic uterine inversion.

The actual incidence of postpartum hemorrhage is unknown but is thought to occur in 5–10% all births (Arias, 1992). Hemorrhage occurring immediately after birth is most commonly caused by uterine atony or cervical or vaginal wall lacerations.

Any bleeding in pregnancy is associated with increased risk of maternal or fetal morbidity and mortality. Maternal blood loss decreases oxygen-carrying capacity, which predisposes the woman to increased risk for hypovolemia, anemia, infection, preterm labor and preterm birth and adversely effects oxygen delivery to the fetus. Fetal risks from maternal hemorrhage include blood loss/anemia, hypoxemia, hypoxia, anoxia, and preterm birth. Bleeding that is fetal in origin is always significant because of the small fetal blood volume.

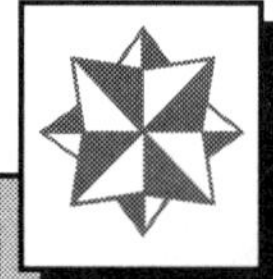

DISPLAY 7-6

Risk Factors for Placenta Previa

- History of a prior placenta previa
- Increased parity
- Advanced materal age
- Multiple cesarean births
- Three or more induced abortions
- Repeated curettage or uterine surgeries
- Multiple gestation
- Fetus with erythroblastosis fetalis
- Large placenta
- Endometritis

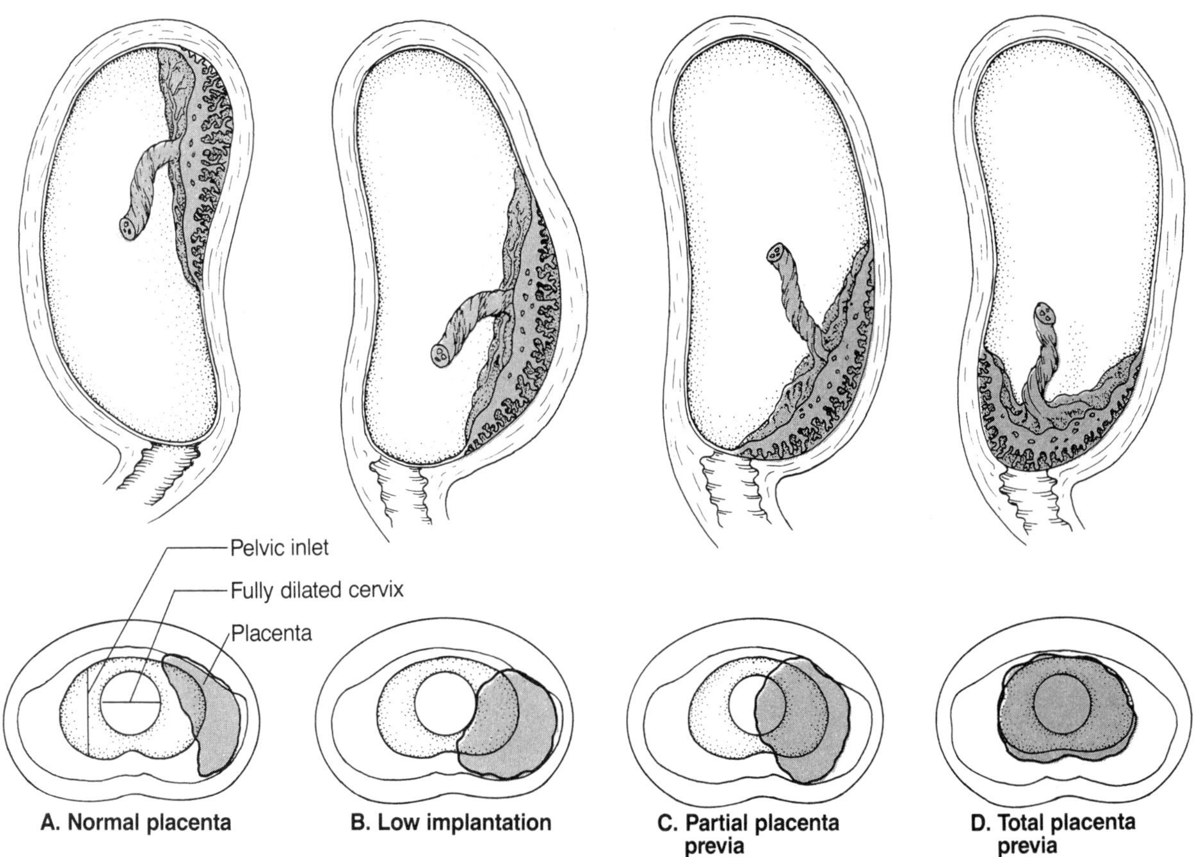

Figure 7-1. A. Placenta previa. **B.** Low implantation. **C.** Partial placenta previa. **D.** Total placenta previa.

From: Reeder et al. (1992). Maternity nursing (17th ed.). Philadelphia: JB Lippincott.

The nurse must be alert to the symptoms of hemorrhage and shock and be prepared to act quickly to minimize blood loss and hasten maternal stabilization. Placenta previa, abruptio placentae, abnormal placenta adherence, postpartum hemorrhage, and uterine rupture are critical events for the woman and fetus.

Definitions and Clinical Manifestations

The definitions, etiology, pathophysiology, and clinical manifestations of the most frequently occurring causes of bleeding in pregnancy are described as follows. Also, a diagnosis-specific summary of expected management is included. A more detailed summary of nursing interventions for bleeding in pregnancy concludes this section.

Placenta Previa

Placenta previa is the abnormal implantation of the placenta in the lower uterine segment. The degree to which the internal cervical os is covered by the placenta determines how the placenta previa is classified. See Figure 7-1 for classification of placental previa. By term, the incidence of placenta previa is 0.5–1% (Lavery, 1990). It is theorized that uterine scarring plays a role in the development of placenta previa. Late development and implantation of the ovum may also play a role; this may be seen more frequently in older women (Poziac, 1991). See Display 7-6 for risk factors for placenta previa.

Clinical Manifestations. Painless uterine bleeding, especially during the third trimester, characterizes placenta previa. The first significant bleeding episode usually occurs between 29 and 30 weeks' gestation. Rarely is the first episode life threatening or a cause of hypovolemic shock. The bright-red bleeding may be intermittent, or continuous.

Diagnosis. Currently, the standard for the diagnosis of placenta previa is a transabdominal ultrasound. If ultrasound reveals a normally implanted placenta, a speculum examination is performed to rule out local causes of bleeding (e.g., cervicitis, polyps, or carcinoma of the cervix) and a coagulation profile is obtained to rule out other causes of bleeding.

Diagnosis of placenta previa has increased dramatically with the advent of obstetrical ultrasound, especially with a vaginal transducer. Placenta previa is suspected when a woman presents with painless vaginal bleeding and is diagnosed by ultrasound. It may also be diagnosed prior to the onset of bleeding by ultrasound examination for other indications. The majority of placenta previas are noted in the second trimester as the uterus continues to develop, except for complete placenta previa. Women will have questions concerning position of the placenta and how it is possible for this condition to resolve as pregnancy progresses. A demonstration by drawing a "placenta" on the neck of a white balloon, and then blowing the balloon up can provide reassurance to the woman and her support person.

Management. Conservative management (see Homecare Management) is usually possible when the fetus is not mature and maternal status is stable. When fetal lung maturity is achieved and survival is likely, the delivery is accomplished.

After the diagnosis of placenta previa has been made, the woman may remain in the hospital under close supervision. The gestational age of the pregnancy should be confirmed and, except in an emergency, birth postponed until after the thirty-sixth week. If the woman has greater than a 30% placenta previa or if bleeding is excessive, cesarean birth is indicated.

Abruptio Placentae

Abruptio placentae, or premature separation of the placenta, is the detachment of part or all of the placenta from its implantation site, typically occurring after the twentieth week of pregnancy (Figure 7-2). Premature separation of the placenta is a serious event and accounts for about 15% of all perinatal deaths (Abdella, Sibai, Hays, & Anderson, 1984). More than 50% of these deaths are the result of preterm delivery; others die from intrauterine hypoxia.

Identified risk factors that increase a woman's risk for experiencing a placental abruption can be found in Display 7-7. Despite these risk factors, the exact etiology is unknown. Of the known risk factors, a previous abruption is a significant risk for the woman. The risk of recurrence ranges from 10–30%, which yields a relative risk of 30–40 times over that of the general pregnant population (Thorp, 1993).

Clinical Manifestations. Abruptio placentae is suspected in the woman presenting with sudden onset, intense, usually localized, uterine pain or uterine tenderness with or without vaginal bleeding. Visible blood loss from a abruptio placentae may not be proportional to the area of placental detachment, because blood becomes trapped behind the placenta. Marginal separations and large abruptions are associated with bright-red bleeding and are almost always accompanied

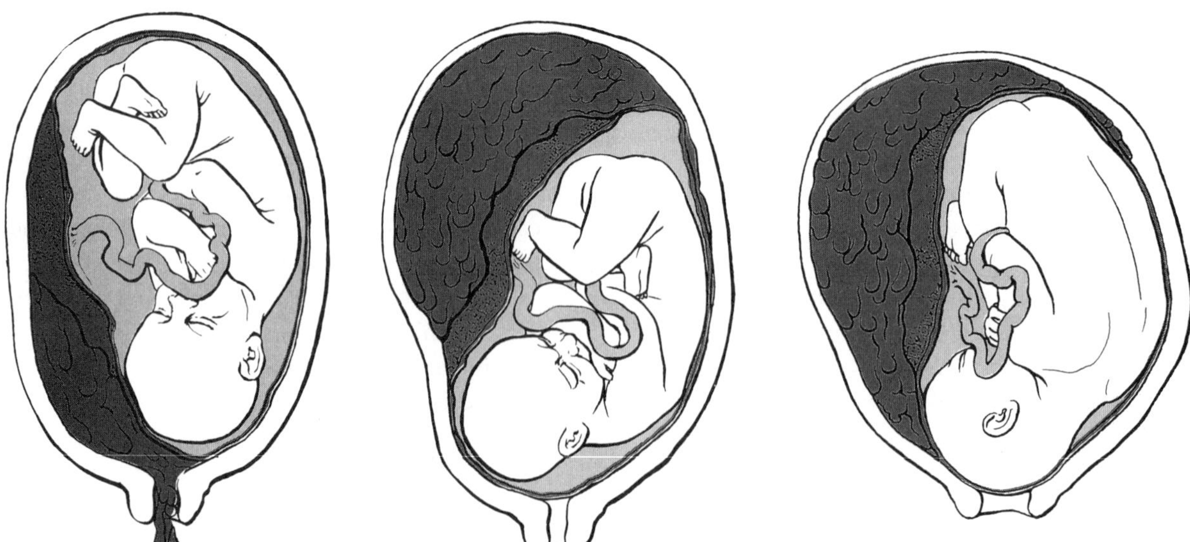

Figure 7-2. Abruptio placentae at various separation sites. (Left) External hemorrhage. (Center) Internal or concealed hemorrhage. (Right) Complete separation.

From Reeder, S.J., Martin, L.L., & Koniak, D. (1992). Maternity Nursing (17th ed.). Philadelphia: JB Lippincott.

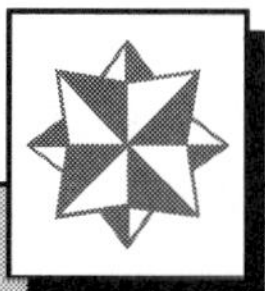

DISPLAY 7-7

Risk Factors for Abruptio Placentae

Prior abruptio placentae
(recurrence risk of 10–30%, which increases relative risk by 30–40 times that of a woman with no history)
Hypertension
Rapid decompression of the uterus
Delivery of first-order, multiple fetuses
Amniotic fluid reduction therapy in polyhydramnios
Preterm premature rupture of membranes at <34 weeks of gestation
Blunt abdominal trauma
Increased parity
Multiple gestation
Cocaine use
Cigarette smoking
Uterine fibroids
Short umbilical cord
Supine hypotensive syndrome

by contractions that are usually of low amplitude and high frequency (Green, 1994). Contractions may be difficult to palpate or record if there is an increase in uterine resting tone. The woman may present with preterm contractions/labor with an occult abruption; ultrasound may reveal an echogenic area consistent with a retroplacental clot. Fetal response to a abruptio placentae is dependent on the volume of blood loss and the extent of uteroplacental insufficiency. Be suspicious of an abruption if there is fetal tachycardia, bradycardia, loss of variability, presence of late decelerations, or a sinusoidal fetal heart rate pattern.

The mother's serum and/or vaginal blood may be tested for the presence of fetal cells. Fetal to maternal transfer of blood is documented by the presence of fetal cells in maternal serum. Depending on fetal age and size, the number of fetal cells present in maternal blood can be calculated to estimate the fetal blood loss. Formulas for this calculation can be found in the maternal-fetal medicine literature and in laboratory manuals.

Women with an abruption may demonstrate very rapid labor progress (Mahon, Chazotte, & Cohen, 1994). However, in women who are not at term or not in labor, the pregnancy may be continued if the abruption is small and the fetus is stable. Chronic abruptio placentae may develop, with the woman experiencing episodic bleeding, subjecting the fetus to prolonged stress. Risk of developing DIC exists during abruption due to release of thromboplastin from the site into the maternal bloodstream.

Diagnosis. The diagnosis of abruptio placentae is based on the woman's history, physical examination, and laboratory studies. Ultrasonography is used to rule out placenta previa; however, it is not diagnostic (Lowe & Cunningham, 1990). Abruptions are classified as partial or complete, or only the margin of the placenta may be involved (Green, 1994). The abruption may be occult, or there may be evidence of vaginal bleeding.

Management. Treatment is dependent on maternal and fetal status. In the presence of fetal compromise, severe hemorrhage, coagulopathy, poor labor progress, or increasing uterine resting tone, a cesarean birth is performed. If the mother is hemodynamically stable, a vaginal birth may be attempted when the fetus is alive (with no signs of compromise) or if the fetus is dead. If the mother is hemodynamically stable and the fetus is showing sign of compromise, an emergency cesarean birth should be performed. If the mother is hemodynamically unstable, attempts should first be directed at maternal stabilization prior to birth, if possible.

Fluid resuscitation may be aggressive in the presence of hemorrhage. Blood replacement products and Ringer's lactate are infused in quantities necessary to maintain a urine output of 30–60 ml/hr and a hematocrit of approximately 30% (Lowe & Cunningham, 1990).

Abnormal Placental Implantation

Abnormal adherence of the placenta occurs for unknown reasons but is thought to be the result of zygote implantation in a zone of defective endometrium. Abnormal adherence of the placenta is diagnosed in only about 1 out of every 12,000 births. At least 15% of cases of abnormally adherent placenta (all types) are associated with placenta previa (Zahn & Yeomans, 1990).

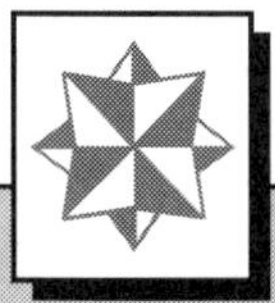

DISPLAY 7-8

Factors Associated with Abnormal Placental Implantation

Previous cesarean birth

Placenta previa, especially anterior

Placental implantation in the lower uterine segment

Multiparity

Uterine malformations

Infection

Fibroid tumors

The mother with an abnormally attached placenta is at increased risk for postpartum hemorrhage leading to hypovolemic shock. See Display 7-8 for factors associated with abnormal placental implantation.

Unusual placental adherence may be partial or complete. See Figure 7-3 for abnormal adherence of a placenta. The following degrees of attachment are recognized:

Placenta Accreta. Placenta accreta occurs when there is a lack of decidua basalis, so that the placenta is implanted directly into the myometrium. Complete accreta occurs when the entire placenta is adherent; partial accreta occurs with one or more cotyledons adherent; and focal accreta occurs with one piece of a cotyledon adherent.

Placenta Increta. Placenta increta is the abnormal invasion of the trophoblastic cells into the uterine myometrium.

Placenta Percreta. Placenta percreta occurs when the trophoblast cells actually penetrate the uterine musculature and the placenta develops on abnormal organs in the vicinity of the percreta.

Placenta accreta, increta, and percreta tend to occur if there is lack of decidua basalis in the area of uterus where the placenta would normally implant. Elevated maternal serum α-fetoprotein (MSAFP) in the second trimester has been associated with placenta accreta, increta, and percreta in women whose pregnancies ended in a cesarean hysterectomy (Kupferminc, Tamura, Wigton, Glassenberg, & Socol, 1993).

The diagnosis of an abnormally adherent placenta generally is made when manual separation of a retained placenta is attempted. If the placenta will not separate readily (even a portion), immediate surgical intervention may be indicated.

Vasa Previa. Vasa previa is the result of a velamentous insertion of the umbilical cord. With a vasa previa, the umbilical vein and arteries are not surrounded by Wharton's jelly and have no supportive tissue. Thus the umbilical blood vessels are at risk for laceration at any time, but this occurs most frequently during rupture of the membranes (ROM) (Green, 1994). The sudden appearance of bright-red blood at the time of ROM, spontaneous or artificial, coupled with a sudden increase in the fetal heart rate when there are no other known risk factors, should immediately alert the nurse to the possibility of vasa previa.

Although it rarely occurs (less than 1 in 3,000 pregnancies), vasa previa is associated with high incidence of fetal morbidity and mortality because of the potential for fetal exsanguination (Thorp, 1993). Diagnosis prior to delivery is unusual, though there are reports of examiners palpating a pulsing vessel. The vasa previa may also be noted on ultrasound examination, or by direct visualization (Cunningham et al., 1993).

Uterine Rupture

Uterine rupture is usually a catastrophic event for both the woman and fetus, whether related to rupture of a uterine scar from prior uterine surgery, such as a cesarean birth or myomectomy, or spontaneous rupture of the uterus. The terms uterine rupture and uterine dehiscence are sometimes used interchangeably in the literature. Uterine rupture refers to the actual separation of the uterine myometrium or previous uterine scar, with rupture of the membranes and extrusion of the fetus or fetal parts into the peritoneal cavity. Dehiscence refers to a separation of the old scar, but

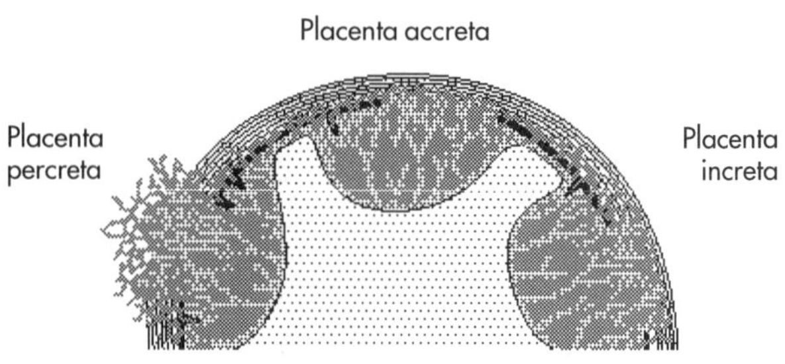

Figure 7-3. Abnormal adherence of the placenta.

the fetus generally remains inside the uterus. Hemorrhage usually occurs with uterine rupture, whereas bleeding is generally minimal with dehiscence.

Uterine rupture occurs most frequently in women with a previous uterine incision through the myometrium. Hyperstimulation of the uterus with oxytocin or prostaglandin can cause uterine rupture. Uterine rupture may also occur spontaneously where there is no history of uterine surgery or terminations of pregnancy. The pathophysiology related to spontaneous rupture is not fully understood. Invasive or blunt trauma, seen in women with knife or gunshot wounds or following a motor vehicle accident or fall, are additional causes of uterine rupture. See Display 7-9 for risk factors for uterine rupture.

Clinical Manifestations. The clinical presentation of the woman experiencing a uterine rupture is dependent upon the specific type of rupture. The clinical picture may develop over several hours with the woman complaining of abdominal pain and tenderness, vomiting, syncope, vaginal bleeding, tachycardia, pallor, and possibly absent fetal heart rate. Uterine contractions may not be present or may become less effective in progressing labor. If unrecognized, the bleeding can quickly progress to hypotension and shock.

A violent or traumatic rupture is apparent almost immediately in that the woman complains of sharp, tearing pain, "like something has given way." Uterine contractions are absent, and the fetus is easily palpated through the abdominal wall. Bleeding may be visible or may be into the abdominal cavity. Intraabdominal bleeding should be suspected if there is a tense, acute abdomen with shoulder pain. Signs of shock appear soon after the rupture, and complete cardiovascular collapse will follow.

A dehiscence of a prior low segment cesarean scar initially is asymptomatic. The woman will continue to contract without further dilation of the cervix; if an intrauterine pressure catheter is in place for labor assessments, there may be little if any change in intrauterine pressure or uterine resting tone pressures. If the dehiscence, extends past the scar tissue, the woman may begin to complain of pain in the lower abdomen that is unrelieved with analgesia or epidural anesthesia. Prolapse of the umbilical cord can occur through the dehiscence resulting in fetal bradycardia or repetitive variable decelerations following each contraction.

Diagnosis. The key for diagnosis is suspicion that uterine rupture has occurred. The nurse should immediately inform the primary healthcare provider at the first suspicion of a uterine rupture.

Management. Treatment includes maternal stabilization and immediate cesarean birth. If possible, the uterine defect is repaired.

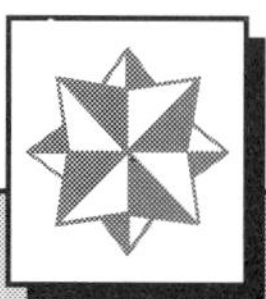

DISPLAY 7-9

Causes of Uterine Rupture

- Previous surgery, where the uterine cavity was entered
- Hyperstimulation of the uterine musculature
- Grand multiparity
- Abdominal trauma
- Obstructed labor
- Maneuvers within the uterus
- Midforceps rotation of the fetus

From Cunningham, F.G., MacDonald, P., Gant, N., Leveno, K., & Gilstrap, L. (1993). William's Obstetrics (19th ed., p. 545). Norwalk, CT: Appleton & Lange. Copyright 1993 by Appleton & Lange. Reprinted with permission.

Inversion of the Uterus

Inversion of the uterus (turning inside out) after birth is a potentially life-threatening complication. The incidence of uterine inversion is approximately 1 out of 2,500 births (Zahn & Yeomans, 1990).

Fundal pressure and traction applied to the cord may result in inversion. Other factors associated with inversion of the uterus include uterine atony, leiomyomas, and abnormally adherent placental tissue. Uterine inversion occurs most frequently in multiparous women and with placenta accreta and increta. Partial inversion occurs when the fundus inverts; a complete inversion occurs when the fundus passes through the opening of the cervix. Although proper management of the third stage of labor prevents the majority of uterine inversions, some are unavoidable. Regardless of the precipitating factor, once an inversion occurs, prompt recognition and correction is necessary to reduce maternal morbidity and mortality.

Clinical Manifestations. The primary presenting sign of uterine inversion is hemorrhage, and the woman experiences sudden agonizing pelvic pain. Attempts to massage the fundus are unsuccessful because the fundus has inverted into the uterus, vaginal vault, or completely through the introitus.

Management. Uterine inversion is an emergent situation requiring immediate attempts to replace the uterus within the pelvic cavity. Significant blood loss can occur. If attempts to replace the uterus are not quickly successful, administration of tocolytics or general anesthesia may be necessary.

Prevention—always the easiest, cheapest, and most effective therapy—is especially appropriate in the avoidance of uterine inversion. *One must not pull on the umbilical cord unless the placenta has definitely separated.* Uterine inversion may occasionally recur during a subsequent birth.

Management of this condition involves all of the following interventions (Kochenour, 1991, Zahn & Yeomans, 1990): (1) Combat shock, which invariably is out of proportion to the blood loss. Oxytocin is withheld until the uterus has been repositioned; (2) Replace the uterus after the woman has received tocolysis or is under deep anesthesia. Give the oxytocic as ordered;(3) Abdominal or vaginal surgery may be necessary to reposition the uterus if successful manual replacement fails; (4) Give the woman blood replacement therapy as indicated. Also initiated are broad-spectrum antibiotic therapy and a nasogastric tube to minimize paralytic ileus.

Postpartum Hemorrhage

Approximately 8% of all births are complicated by postpartum hemorrhage (Murahata, 1991). Postpartum hemorrhage, traditionally the loss of 500 ml of blood or more after birth, is the most common and most serious type of excessive obstetric blood loss. A more meaningful definition of postpartum hemorrhage is based not only on estimated blood loss (which is traditionally underestimated) but also on clinical signs and symptoms (Veronikis & O'Grady, 1994).

Postpartum hemorrhage is a leading cause of maternal morbidity and mortality accounting for approximately 13% of maternal deaths ([ACOG, 1990; Varner, 1991).

Complications of postpartum hemorrhage are either immediate or delayed. Hemorrhagic (hypovolemic) shock and death may occur from sudden, exsanguinating hemorrhage. Delayed complications provoked by postpartum hemorrhage include anemia, puerperal infection, and thromboembolism.

Risk Factors. Postpartum hemorrhage can occur secondary to uterine atony; abnormal implantation of the placenta; lacerations of the cervix, vagina, or perineum; uterine inversion; and DIC. Postpartum hemorrhage is further described as primary or secondary. Primary postpartum hemorrhage occurs within the time period immediately after the delivery of the placenta, up to 24 hours after birth; secondary postpartum hemorrhage occurs after 24 hours postbirth. Secondary postpartum hemorrhage is associated with subinvolution of the uterus and with retained placental tissue that may be the result of abnormal placental implantation (Khong & Khong, 1993). See Display 7-10 for causes of postpartum hemorrhage. A thorough discussion of postpartum hemorrhage is found in Chapter 12.

Uterine Atony. Uterine atony is marked hypotonia of the uterus. Because of the increased blood flow to the placenta in late pregnancy (approximately 500 ml/min), failure of the uterus to contract following placental separation can result in significant blood loss very rapidly.

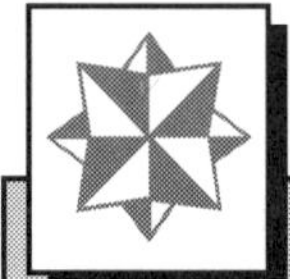

DISPLAY 7-10

Causes of Postpartum Hemorrhage

Uterine atony	Genital tract lacerations
Precipitous labor	Genital tract hematoma
Intraamniotic infection	Compound presentation
Macrosomia	Precipitous delivery
Multifetal gestation	Forceps delivery
History of uterine atony	Vacuum extraction
Retained products of conception	Episiotomy extension
Clotted blood in uterus	Coagulation defects
Polyhydramnios	High parity
Prolonged labor	
Oxytocin induction or augmentation	Prostaglandin ripening
Anesthesia effects	Sepsis

Trauma to genital tract: large episiotomy, including extensions; lacerations of the perineum, vagina, or cervix; ruptured uterus

Poorly perfused myometrium secondary to hypotension, hemorrhage, conduction anesthesia

Uterine atony occurs in at least 5% of births, particularly when the woman is a grand multipara; with hydramnios; when the fetus is large; or after the delivery of a multifetal gestation. In such conditions, the uterus is "overstretched" and contracts poorly. Other causes of atony include traumatic birth, use of halogenated anesthesia, magnesium sulfate, rapid or prolonged labor, chorioamnionitis, and use of oxytocin for induction or augmentation.

Lacerations of the Birth Canal. Lacerations of the birth canal are the second major cause of postpartum hemorrhage. Birth canal lacerations may include injuries to the labia, perineum, vagina, and cervix. Therefore, prevention, recognition, and prompt, effective treatment of birth canal lacerations are vitally important. Vaginal hematoma formation may develop slowly, with blood seeping into a small pocket that gradually expands and becomes more painful.

Continued bleeding despite efficient postpartum uterine contractions demands inspection or reinspection of the birth passage. Continuous bleeding from so-called minor sources may be just as dangerous as a sudden loss of a large amount of blood, although often it is ignored until shock develops.

Management. The first step in the treatment of uterine bleeding is to evaluate the uterus to determine if it is firmly contracted. The healthcare provider generally orders oxytocin 20–40 units to 1 liter of crystalloid to infuse at 10–15 ml/min (Veronikis & O'Grady, 1994; Zahn & Yeomans, 1990); this infusion should be continued at least 3 or 4 hours. If the uterus fails to respond to oxytocin, methylergonovine 0.2 mg intramuscularly produces tetanic uterine contractions and is effective in treating hemorrhage from uterine atony. However, its use is contraindicated in the presence of hypertension. If methylergonovine fails or is contraindicated, prostaglandin 15-methyl $f_{2\alpha}$ becomes the oxytocic of choice in the absence of maternal asthma or systemic lupus. Most hemorrhage can be controlled after one or two injections of 0.25 mg prostaglandin 15-methyl $f_{2\alpha}$ intramuscularly; the majority of failures occurred in women with chorioamnionitis (Zahn & Yeomans, 1990). Blood transfusion for the treatment of shock and blood replacement may be urgently needed.

The healthcare provider should hasten to palpate the interior of the uterus so that retained products of conception can be removed and possible rupture of the uterus diagnosed. If the blood being lost fails to clot, a coagulopathy (e.g., DIC) may have developed and prompt appropriate treatment may be life saving.

Nursing Assessment of Bleeding During Pregnancy

Assessment of the woman who is bleeding begins with careful evaluation of amount and color of blood loss, character of uterine activity, presence of abdominal pain, and stability of maternal-fetal vital signs. Bright-red vaginal bleeding is suggestive of current active bleeding, while dark or brown blood with clots may indicate past blood loss or pooling of blood in the vaginal vault.

Vital signs are important in assessing amount of blood loss. Maternal or fetal tachycardia and maternal hypotension are suggestive of hypovolemia; however, hypotension is a late sign. Frequency of vital signs depends on patient stability. Vital signs are repeated every 15 minutes until the bleeding is controlled and the vital signs remain or return to normal. Vital signs are performed more frequently (every 1–5 minutes) when there is evidence of instability, including systolic blood pressure less than 90 mmHg, maternal tachycardia above 100 bpm, and decreasing level of consciousness.

When using an automatic BP cuff, assess that the Doppler is directly over the brachial artery for an accurate recording. However, in severe hypotensive states the automatic BP device is less accurate. Many automatic BP monitors calculate MAP (MAP = Systolic BP + 2 × diastolic BP ÷ by 3), which provides a quick number for reference and is a more stable parameter of hemodynamic function. The normal value for MAP in the second trimester of pregnancy is approximately 80 mmHg (Page & Christianson, 1976).

When the BP can not be assessed with a BP cuff, systolic BP may be estimated by the presence of a radial, femoral, or brachial pulse. The presence of a radial pulse is associated with a systolic BP of approximately 80 mmHg, a femoral pulse with a BP of 70 mmHg, and a carotid pulse with a BP of 60 mmHg (Daddario & Johnson, 1992). Placement of an arterial line in the woman who is hemorrhaging allows for continuous, accurate, BP monitoring and provides a means for drawing blood for arterial blood gas analysis and other laboratory values. Invasive hemodynamic monitoring with a flow-directed pulmonary artery catheter (Swan-Ganz) may be indicated in selected patients (Clark et al., 1994).

Color of skin and mucous membranes are noted. Inspection also includes looking for oozing at the sites of incisions or injections and assessing for the presence of petechiae or ecchymosis in areas not associated with surgery or trauma.

A medical history should be obtained if possible, with attention focused on previous bleeding or bleeding disorders.

FHR is always continuously assessed. Auscultation of FHR (Nurses' Association of the American College of Obstetricians and Gynecologists [NAACOG], 1990) and palpation of uterine contractions may be used; however, in an emergent situation, application of electronic FHR monitoring provides continuous data about the fetus and allows the nurse time to simultaneously initiate other needed treatment.

The pregnant woman should be positioned in the lateral or modified Trendelenburg position, if possible. If the patient is in Trendelenburg or supine position, a wedge is placed under one hip to alleviate compression of the vena cava and aorta by the gravid uterus. Caution must be used in placing a woman still pregnant in Trendelenburg because the pressure of the gravid uterus may interfere with optimal cardiopulmonary functioning. Oxygen is administered preferably by nonrebreathing face mask at 10–12 L/min, to maintain maternal-fetal oxygen saturation. LOC is assessed frequently and provides additional indications of maternal blood volume and oxygen saturation.

Blood is drawn to assess the maternal hemoglobin, hematocrit, platelet count, and coagulation profile. See Display 7-11 for blood tests commonly ordered for the woman who is bleeding. In an emergent situation, blood may be drawn into a plain red top (clot) tube and then visually evaluated for clot formation. If no signs of clotting are evident within 7–10 minutes, coagulopathy should be suspected.

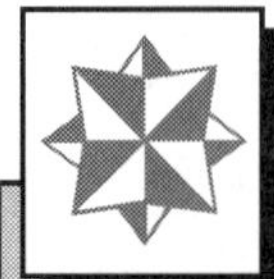

Display 7-11

Laboratory Values Assessed in Pregnant Women Who Are Bleeding

- Complete blood count
- Fibrinogen concentration
- Prothrombin time
- Activated partial thromboplastin time
- Fibrin degradation products/fibrin split products
- Platelet count
- Blood type, Rh, and antibody screen
- Clot retraction

Possibly indicated:

- Kleihauer-Betke test
- APT test
- Ivy bleeding time
- D-dimer
- Serum BUN
- Serum creatinine
- Urine creatinine clearance
- Urine sodium excretion
- Liver function test, including serum glucose
- Antithrombin III
- Arterial blood gases
- Urine/serum drug screen

Circulating volume is usually restored with IV crystalloid solution administration. Blood and blood products are administered as soon as they are available or as needed. Breath sounds should be auscultated prior to fluid volume replacement, if possible, to provide a baseline for future assessment. Massive fluid replacement in a pregnant or newly delivered woman who is hemorrhaging increases the potential for development of pulmonary edema. However, fluid replacement is necessary to restore circulatory volume, and the nurse should anticipate and assess for the development of peripheral and pulmonary edema.

Oxygen saturation should be monitored with a pulse oximeter. Pulse oximeters are an adjunct to assessment; however, they are not always accurate, especially in a patient in hypovolemic shock. In the hemorrhagic patient, blood flow to the extremities will be decreased, so the oxygen saturation displayed may not accurately reflect tissue oxygenation status. Blood gas analysis may therefore be necessary to determine oxygenation status in the woman who is hemorrhaging. A maternal oxygen saturation of at least 95% and a PaO_2 of at least 65 mmHg as determined by blood gas analysis are necessary for the fetus to maintain adequate oxygenation (Barth & Hankins, 1992).

Continuous electrocardiographic monitoring may be indicated for the woman who is hypotensive or tachycardiac, continuing to bleed profusely, or in shock. Maternal hypovolemia leading to hypoxia and acidosis may result in maternal heart rate dysrhythmias, including premature ventricular contractions, tachycardia, and atrial or ventricular fibrillation.

A Foley catheter with a urometer is inserted to allow for hourly assessment of urine output. The most objective and least invasive assessment of adequate organ perfusion and oxygenation is urinary output of at least 30 ml/hr (Veronikis & O'Grady, 1994). In addition to assessment of volume, urine also is assessed for the presence of blood and/or protein and specific gravity.

Nursing Interventions for Bleeding During Pregnancy

Evaluation and management of acute episodes of bleeding during pregnancy usually occur in the inpatient setting. An exception is spotting during early gestation. After stabilization and a period of hospitalization, selected women may be managed at home.

Homecare Management

Controversy exists concerning homecare management of women with placenta previa and marginal separation of the placenta; however, increasingly women in stable condition are being cared for in the home, with frequent visits by perinatal nurses and daily provider-initiated phone contact. Criteria for homecare management varies with primary perinatal provider and homecare agency. The woman must be in stable condition with no evidence of active bleeding and have resources to be able to return to the hospital immediately if active bleeding resumes.

See Chapter Appendix 7-1 for diagnostic criteria and considerations for homecare referral for management of women with antepartum bleeding (Grohar, 1994; Simpson, 1992).

Inpatient Management

With the woman's admission to the hospital, the nurse begins with an assessment of the bleeding. The woman with acute bleeding requires continuous, ongoing nursing assessments and interventions.

Maternal vital signs are assessed frequently according to individual clinical situations. Careful assessments are mandatory. Vital signs and noninvasive assessments of cardiac output (e.g., skin color, skin temperature, pulse oxymetry, LOC, and urinary output) are obtained frequently to observe for signs of declining hemodynamic status.

Electronic FHR and uterine activity monitoring should be continuous. Fetal status is continuously monitored if the fetus has survived the initial insult.

It is important to appreciate how rapidly maternal-fetal status can deteriorate as a result of maternal hemorrhage. Because of the potential for maternal-fetal mortality, it is essential to be prepared for an emergent birth at all times when caring for a pregnant woman who is bleeding. Supportive staff necessary for an emergency cesarean birth (e.g., anesthesia personnel, operating room [OR] team, and neonatal resuscitation team) should be notified and be on standby (if possible, in the hospital). Current guidelines suggest perinatal units should be able to initiate a cesarean birth within 30 minutes of the decision to deliver via that route, recognizing that hemorrhage from placenta previa, abruptio placentae, and uterine rupture require more expeditious delivery (American Academy of Pediatrics [AAP] & American College of Obstetricians and Gynecologists [ACOG], 1992).

To provide immediate venous access, at least one, preferably two, 18-gauge intracatheters are inserted into the woman who is bleeding. If consistent with institution policy, a 14- to 16-gauge intracatheter should be considered. The need to replace fluids and blood is determined by a number of parameters, including vital signs, actual amount of blood loss, mental status, and laboratory values.

Fluid replacement consists of administering lactated Ringer's or normal saline solution, packed red blood cells, fresh frozen plasma, and possibly platelets. Blood product replacement therapy is still indicated in life-threatening situations. Significant hemorrhage resulting in syncope or hypovolemic shock generally necessitates transfusion (see section on hemorrhagic shock).

Blood type, Rh, and antibody screen should be drawn on admission; crossmatching is no longer necessary because antibodies will be identified from a type and screen. Also, current ACOG guidelines provided in *Blood Component Therapy* (1994) suggest that the use of blood components, rather than whole blood, is usually a better treatment option because it provides only the specific components needed. By using only the specific products required for the emergency, blood resources are conserved and there is a decreased risk of blood replacement complications. Signs of a transfusion reaction demonstrated by chills, fever, tachycardia, hypotention, shortness of breath, muscle cramps, itching, convulsions, and ultimately cardiac arrest must be assessed throughout the procedure. In the event of a reaction, the transfusion must be immediately discontinued and the IV line flushed with normal saline. Treatment is then based on clinical symptoms. Risk for the development of anaphylaxis should be considered.

Careful fetal surveillance is critical to ensure fetal well-being during transfusion of multiple blood products. It is important to be aware of an increased incidence of uteroplacental insufficiency related to complications of coagulation factor replacement therapy (Simpson, 1993). Administration of multiple replacement blood products leads to increased intravascular fibrin formation. Deposition of fibrin in the decidual vasculature of the chorionic villi may cause fetal compromise.

Pregnant women may lose up to one third of their fluid volume prior to displaying signs of shock (Dorman, 1989). Women who are bleeding should be monitored carefully for the actual amount of blood loss although this is sometimes difficult in an emergent situation. All sheets, pads, etc., should be inspected and weighed, if possible. Accurate intake and output measurement and documentation is critical. Ideally, one nurse is assigned to monitor intake and output during a period of massive fluid and blood replacement. In an emergent situation where the obstetrician and anesthesiologist both may be ordering or actually adding replacement fluid to multiple IV lines, it becomes essential that one nurse records and maintains a running total of intake and output, in addition to signing for blood products and overseeing administration.

The possibility that the patient will develop a coagulopathy (See Display 7-12 for risk factors for DIC), pulmonary edema, and renal failure as evidenced by oliguria proceeding to anuria must be anticipated. Systolic blood pressures of less than 60 mmHg are associated with acute renal failure. The woman is at risk for development of acute tubular necrosis from lack of perfusion to the kidneys (prerenal failure). Prolonged periods of severe hypotention may result in renal cortical necrosis. Therefore urine output of less than 30 cc/hr should be reported immediately.

In the case of severe hemorrhage, control of abdominal bleeding may be achieved by the placement of medical antishock trousers (MAST suit), which are used in emergency/trauma units to control bleeding. Consensus does not exist related to the benefits of MAST suit use; however, they are used in many institutions.

Hemorrhagic shock. Hemorrhagic shock is an emergent situation in which the perfusion of body organs may become severely compromised and death may ensue. Aggressive treatment is necessary to prevent adverse sequelae (e.g., cellular death, fluid overload, shock lung, and oxygen toxicity).

Blood replacement therapy is not uncommon in the management of hemorrhage. Common clinical symptomatology of inadequate intravascular volume (hypovolemia) that necessitates blood replacement includes the following: (1) evidence of hemorrhage (loss of a large amount of blood externally or internally in a short period of time); (2) evidence of hypovolemic shock (increasing pulse, cool clammy skin, rapid breathing, restlessness, reduced urine output); or (3) decrease in hemoglobin and hematocrit below acceptable level for trimester of pregnancy or the nonpregnant state.

Aggressive fluid and blood replacement is not without risk. The 24 hours after the shock period are critical. Observe for fluid overload, adult respiratory distress syndrome (ARDS), and oxygen toxicity. Transfusion reactions may follow administration of blood or blood components. Even in an emergency, each unit should be checked per hospital protocol. Rapid transfusion with cold blood can chill the heart and cause arrhythmia or arrest. Banked blood may be calcium deficient, increasing the risk for arrhythmias and further bleeding.

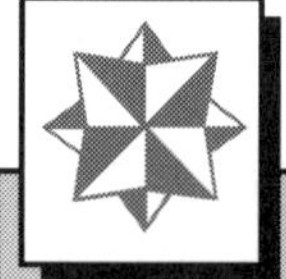

DISPLAY 7-12

Obstetrical Factors Associated with the Development of DIC

Abruptio placentae
Hemorrhage
Preeclampsia/eclampsia
Amniotic fluid embolism
Saline termination of pregnancy
Sepsis
Dead fetus syndrome
Cardiopulmonary arrest
Massive transfusion therapy

Infection is another complication of hemorrhage. Causes may include surgical procedures, multiple pelvic examinations, anemia, and loss of the white blood cell component of the blood.

Summary

Hemorrhagic disorders in pregnancy are medical emergencies requiring rapid and efficient teamwork from all members of the healthcare team. Perinatal nurses play an important role in the initial assessments, early interventions, and stabilization of the woman. Recognition that blood loss may reach 35% (Dorman, 1989) before hypovolemic shock occurs is important because initial vital signs may remain within normal range in the presence of a significant hemorrhage.

PRETERM LABOR

Significance and Incidence

Low-birth-weight and prematurity prevention are major concerns confronting obstetrical healthcare providers today as both are major contributors to perinatal morbidity and mortality in the United States (Garbaciak, 1992). Approximately 10% of all pregnancies in the United States end prior to 37 weeks' gestation (ACOG, 1995). The 1989 White House Task Force Report on Infant Mortality stated that of the 40,000 infants who died in 1989, nearly one quarter of those deaths could have been prevented in large part through reduction of low birth weight (Arnold & Grad, 1992). Worldwide, 21 million low-birth-weight infants were born in 1979, which accounted for 17% of all births and 75% or more of the neonatal and infant deaths in that year (WHO, 1980). Fuchs (1976) and Rush, Keirse, and Howat (1976) reported that when anomalies incompatible with life are excluded as a cause of perinatal death, preterm births are responsible for 75% of perinatal deaths.

Preterm births continue despite availability of new tocolytic agents, comprehensive birth prevention programs (Freda et al., 1990), prenatal risk assessment scoring systems, and various methods of detecting preterm contractions, such as self-uterine palpation and home uterine-activity monitoring (HUAM) (ACOG, 1995; Leveno, Little, & Cunningham,1990). It must also be remembered that despite the best medical efforts and technology, neonates will continue to be born at a preterm gestation. Of the preterm births today, approximately 20–25% are induced secondary to either maternal or fetal indications; these infants generally do well (Creasy, 1993).

Survival rates for the preterm infant are variable. Gestational age has a stronger correlation with survival prior to 29 weeks, while birthweight is a better predictor of outcome after 29 weeks (Copper, Goldenberg, & Creasy, 1993). Incidence and severity of neonatal complications decline sharply after 32 weeks of completed gestation and decrease to almost zero after 34 completed weeks (Higby, Xenakis, & Pauerstein, 1993).

The most common complications related to preterm birth are intraventricular hemorrhage (IVH), respiratory distress syndrome (RDS), patent ductus arteriosus (PDA), and necrotizing enterocolitis (NEC). Care of infants born prematurely is extremely costly emotionally as well as financially, and continued care for some infants may be a lifelong issue.

Definitions

Defining the concept "preterm" infant is difficult in that the terms low birth weight, prematurity, and immature are used interchangeably in the literature to describe the neonate that is either too small or born too early. Low-birth-weight infants comprise a mixed group of infants born at an early gestational age or infants who are born growth restricted, or both (Whitter, 1993). Preterm labor and preterm birth occur after 20 weeks' gestation and prior to 37 completed weeks' gestation (Creasy, 1994).

The definition of the concept of preterm has evolved since the 1935 American Academy of Pediatrics' definition of prematurity, which was based on birth weight. Any liveborn infant weighing 2,500 g or less was termed premature. The World Health Organization (WHO) expanded the concept of prematurity in 1961 by using gestational age as well as birth weight to determine prematurity. WHO defined premature infants as those delivering prior to 36 completed weeks' pregnancy and also introduced the separate concept of low birth weight, defined as 2,500 g or less at birth. Very-low-birth-weight infants (1,500 g or less) and extremely low-birth-weight infants (1,000 g or less) are terms that have evolved as the number of preterm survivors has increased, and improved outcomes have occurred even among the extremely low-birth-weight group (Cunningham et al., 1993; McCormick, 1991; WHO, 1980). Current practice focuses on gestational age, birth weight, and neonatal adaptation to the extrauterine environment.

Risk Factors

In recent years, preterm labor and preterm birth have been identified as a leading cause of infant morbidity and mortality. As a result, numerous epidemiologic studies have identified risk factors associated with this abnormal outcome of pregnancy. A detailed report from the Institute of Medicine (1985) describes these factors, with the most important identified as genetics, ethnic group, medical illness, malnutrition, and chronic deprivation. See Display 7-13 for risk factors associated with preterm labor and preterm birth and Display 7-14 for the predictive value of risk factors for preterm labor. It is important to note that many risk factors listed have no firm cause-and-effect relationship to preterm birth but instead are frequently identified in women who experience a preterm birth.

Pathophysiology

The precise identification of women at risk for developing preterm labor, as well as diagnosing preterm labor, is difficult at best. Differences in the etiology and incidence of preterm and low-birth-weight neonates are population dependent (Meis, Ernest, & Moore, 1987; United States Department of Health & Human Services, 1984; York & Brooten, 1992).

Prenatal care is available throughout the United States, but it is often difficult for women to access the system. Transportation and child-care issues are the two most frequent reasons that women cite for not attending prenatal visits (Dutton, 1981; O'Connell, 1987).

Demographically, women at either end of the childbearing-age continuum are at increased risk for preterm labor. Age, however, as an independent factor is difficult to assess in that lifestyle, use of prenatal care, and socioeconomic status also contribute to the incidence of preterm labor. Race of the woman also is significant to the risk of delivering a preterm infant. Virji and Cottington (1991) found a twofold increased rate of preterm delivery among Black women as compared to non-Black populations.

In comparing insured verses medicaid births, Meis, Ernest, & Moore (1987) demonstrated significant differences based on populations studied. Idiopathic premature labor was related to 47.1% of insured low-birth-weight infants as compared to 24.8% of medicaid births. With respect to low birth weight, term (26.7%) and premature rupture of the fetal membranes (33.7%) medicaid were more prevalent in medicaid

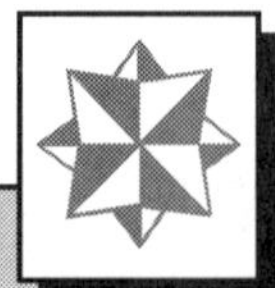

Display 7-13

Risk Factors Associated with Preterm Labor and Birth

Medical or obstetric risks antedating pregnancy:

- Prior preterm birth
- Previous second-trimester abortion
- Cervical incompetence
- Uterine or cervical anomalies
- Hypertension
- Diethylstilbestrol (DES) exposure

Current pregnancy-associated risks:

- Anemia
- Multiple gestation
- Placenta previa
- Abruptio placentae
- Fetal abnormality
- Hydramnios
- Abdominal surgery
- Maternal infection
- Maternal bleeding
- Cervical effacement of dilatation (more than 50% or 1 cm)
- Previous preterm labor
- Uterine distention
- Cervical incompetence

Demographic and behavioral risk factors:

- Age (less than 20 or more than 35 years)
- Non-White
- Low socioeconomic status
- Single parent
- Smoking
- Chemical use or dependence
- Prepregnancy weight of less than 100 lb
- Poor weight gain
- Inadequate prenatal care
- Psychological stress

From Mandeville, L.K., & Troiano, N.H. (1992). NAACOG: High risk intrapartum nursing (p. 61). Philadelphia: JB Lippincott. Copyright 1992 by JB Lippincott. Reprinted with permission.

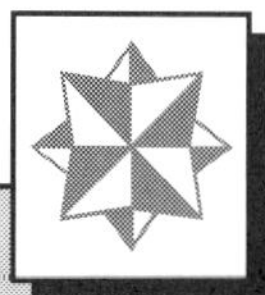

DISPLAY 7-14

Predictive Value of Risk Factors for Preterm Labor

RISK FACTOR	PRETERM LABOR RATE
Multiple gestations	51%
Dilated cervix at 32 weeks	43%
Abdominal surgery during pregnancy	41%
Effaced cervix at 32 weeks	33%
Uterine anomaly	33%
Exposure to DES	33%
Prior preterm birth	31%
Irritable uterus	29%
Hydramnios	26%
Prior preterm labor	25%
History of cone biopsy	22%
Bleeding after 12 weeks	21%
Two or more midtrimester abortions	20%
Febrile illness	17%
One second-trimester abortion	14%
Three or more first-trimester abortions	12%
Pyelonephritis	12%

From Iams, J.D., Johnson, F.F., & Creasy, R.K. (1988). Prevention of preterm birth. Clinical Obstetrics and Gynecology, 31(3), pp. 599-606.

low-birth-weight births than in insured births (13.8% and 23.0% respectively). Medical complications related to low-birth-weight births were present in 16.1% of insured births compared to 14.9% of the medicaid low-birth-weight births.

Lifestyle and work environment may contribute to preterm labor and birth. Cigarette smoking and the use of chemically addictive substances are reported as risk factors for preterm labor and birth; however, a direct cause and effect relationship is difficult to establish (Iams, Johnson, & Creasy, 1988; Zuckerman, Frank & Hingson, 1989).

In relation to normal physical activity and work environment, the woman with no other risk factors for preterm labor or birth does not appear to have an increased risk of delivering a preterm infant. A tentative association has been established between prolonged periods of standing and fatigue with preterm delivery (Klebanoff, Shiono & Selby, 1991; Mamelle, Laumon, & Lazar, 1984).

A woman's reproductive history is a major factor in determining the outcome of the current pregnancy. Women with a history of delivering prior to 37 completed weeks' gestation are at increased risk for a subsequent preterm birth (Owen, Goldenberg, & Davis, 1990). Care must be individualized for the woman with a history of preterm birth that presents with uterine activity, with or without cervical change (Copper, Goldenberg, & Davis, 1990; Katz, Goodyear, & Creasy, 1990).

The role of endogenous bacteria in the pathophysiology of preterm labor and birth has received considerable attention. Research by Romero and Mazor (1988), and Romero, et al. (1989) suggest a strong association between asymptomatic bacteriuria, genital tract infections, Group B streptococcus, and preterm labor and birth.

Clinical Manifestations of Preterm Labor

Preterm labor is subtle in presentation and may be misdiagnosed. The primary healthcare provider must establish a therapeutic relationship in which the woman feels comfortable reporting vague, nonspecific complaints. The woman must be encouraged to call her primary healthcare provider if she experiences any of the following signs or symptoms of preterm contractions and/or labor:

- Uterine cramping (menstrual-like cramps)
- Uterine contractions every 10–15 minutes or more frequently
- Low abdominal pressure
- Low backache (below curve of spine, intermittent, change in character of back pain)
- Any vaginal bleeding
- Increased vaginal discharge of clear or tan fluid
- Feeling that "something" is in the vagina
- Abdominal cramping with or without nausea, vomiting, or diarrhea
- Thigh pain which is intermittent or persistent

The diagnosis of preterm labor includes preterm, regular uterine activity and cervical change. However, diagnosis is difficult, and therapy may be initiated based on clinical presentation, not on cervical change. Appropriate medical management of preterm labor ranges from no intervention, or expectant management, to aggressive tocolytic therapy (Leonardi & Hankins, 1992). Additional therapies such as antibiotic therapy, corticosteroid therapy, subcutaneous terbutaline pump, and HUAM, may also be initiated.

Current medical regimens recognize that no single therapy is the panacea for preterm labor. Benefits of therapy, as well as risks, must be evaluated on an individual basis.

Nursing Assessment of Preterm Labor

Early identification by risk-assessment scoring, patient education related to preterm labor signs and symptoms, and contact between high-risk pregnant women and the primary healthcare provider appear to be an effective strategy in decreasing the incidence of preterm birth in women with risk factors other than a history of preterm birth. Report of the 12-year study of preterm birth prevention in a small region of eastern France is the basis of most preterm birth prevention programs in the United States today (Papiernik et al., 1985). Using a risk-assessment scoring system, women who were identified as high risk for preterm birth were provided early education about preterm labor signs and symptoms, encouraged to make life-style modifications, and seen more often during their pregnancy. During the course of the study interventions, the preterm birth rate and number of low-birth-weight infants decreased. Other researchers have reported similar results with comprehensive preterm birth prevention programs (Creasy, 1993; Hobel et al., 1994).

Early in the prenatal period, education about warning signs of preterm labor should be provided to all women. Reinforcement of this information should occur at each subsequent prenatal visit with review of any symptoms that may have been noted since the last visit.

Education of healthcare providers is an equally important component of preterm birth prevention. Attitudes of healthcare professionals can influence the woman's response to education about preterm labor. Women need encouragement to call with questions about signs and symptoms of preterm labor and need to be told that they should not feel silly or embarrassed if they call repeatedly. Women who do not get this reassurance may be less likely to call or to seek care and therefore increase their risk for active preterm labor.

Risk-assessment scoring systems have been used to screen pregnant women who may be at increased risk for preterm labor and birth. (See Chapter 6 for a more in-depth discussion of risk assessment during pregnancy). Women who have identified risk factors for preterm birth may have more prenatal visits, be encouraged to restrict activity, and be enrolled in preterm birth prevention programs that include frequent phone contact, home visits, and a method of monitoring uterine activity.

Women who have a shortened cervix are known to be at increased risk for preterm birth; therefore, use of vaginal ultrasound to measure cervical length may have potential for identifying women at risk and may improve accuracy of diagnosis in women treated for preterm labor. Research is in progress to determine if a specific length or change in length of the cervix could be used as indicators to predict preterm labor and birth. One group of researchers found that cervical length of at least 30 mm predicted a low likelihood of preterm birth (Iams, Paraskos, Landon, Teteris, & Johnson, 1994).

There has also been investigative research into using oncofetal fibronectin, a substance that is produced by the fetus and measured in the amniotic fluid. It is hypothesized that the finding of fetal fibronectin in cervicovaginal secretions may be a marker for the development of future preterm labor (Jackson, Edwin, Varner, Cassal, & Mitchell, 1993). Investigations are ongoing to determine if testing for oncofetal fibronectin, and thus allowing early interventions, will demonstrate a significant reduction in preterm delivery.

Women who are admitted to the hospital with symptoms of preterm labor are assisted to bed and encouraged to maintain a lateral position. The woman may be anxious and concerned about fetal well-being and the labor process. High levels of circulating catecholamines are present during anxiety and may induce further uterine activity (Neal & Bockman, 1992). Explaining nursing interventions and providing reassurance can decrease maternal stress (Myers & Nathanielsz, 1993). Baseline maternal vital signs are assessed and may provide clues as to etiology of preterm contractions. Uterine tenderness, maternal tachycardia, fetal tachycardia, or elevated maternal temperature may be early signs of intraamniotic infection, which is thought to be a frequent cause of preterm labor.

Accurate assessment of uterine activity begins with direct palpation, which provides information about contraction frequency, duration, intensity, and uterine resting tone. A visual inspection of the abdomen to note bruising or trauma, and Leopold's maneuver to determine fetal position are done concurrently with palpation. After initial assessment by palpation, external electronic fetal monitoring is used to assess frequency and duration of contractions. It is important to remember that because the standard external tocodynamometer detects abdominal wall changes during contractions and uterine relaxation, it is designed to be used in pregnant women near term when the position of the uterus is proximal to the abdominal wall. Reduced sensitivity of the standard tocodynamometer should be considered when using electronic fetal monitoring for women who are obese or less than 26 weeks pregnant (Eaganhouse & Burnside, 1992). Some fetal monitors are equipped with an additional tocodynamometer especially designed to detect preterm contractions.

Initial assessment also includes discussion of cramping or contraction onset and frequency and level of discomfort. Uterine tenderness may indicate intraamniotic infection. Some women do not have palpable contractions but instead report intermittent lower back or thigh pain and/or pelvic pressure. The woman should be asked if she has noticed any change in the character of vaginal discharge including watery mucous, bleeding, or amniotic fluid leakage. Sterile speculum examination assists in determining cervical and amniotic membrane status. Any fluid noted in the vaginal vault can be evaluated to rule out amniotic membrane rupture. Nitrazine paper is used to determine if fluid is alkaline, possibly indicating amniotic fluid; however, false positives can be obtained when blood is mixed with the fluid or mucous. A fluid specimen can be evaluated under the microscope for presence of a ferning pattern, as a more accurate indication of amniotic fluid. Following speculum examination, a digital examination to assess cervical softening, effacement, and dilation is usually done.

During assessment of clinical signs and symptoms of preterm labor, a maternal history is obtained including review of potential risk factors for preterm birth and obstetrical and medical history. Significant obstetric or medical history may preclude tocolytic therapy.

Fetal surveillance is usually accomplished via electronic fetal monitoring. Parameters to evaluate fetal well-being are slightly different in the preterm fetus. An FHR baseline of 150 to 160 bpm may be normal due to immaturity of the fetal parasympathetic nervous system. However, fetal tachycardia above 160 bpm may be an early sign of intraamniotic infection. Fetal movement may result in slight FHR decelerations instead of accelerations during the second trimester. In addition, instead of the usual 15-bpm acceleration of the FHR for 15 seconds, a 10-bpm acceleration lasting 10 seconds is reassuring for the fetus under 30 weeks' gestation (Eganhouse & Burnside, 1992). Biophysical profile assessment, with the knowledge that the nonstress test (NST) component may be zero so that the overall score is 8/10, is an effective measurement of fetal well-being in the fetus 24–30/32 weeks' gestational age in uncomplicated preterm labor.

Nursing Interventions for Preterm Labor

Evaluation and management of acute episodes of preterm labor usually occur in the inpatient setting; however, many women who have been successfully treated in the hospital and women with risk factors for preterm birth are managed in the home.

Homecare Management

Criteria for homecare management of women with preterm contractions or women at high risk for preterm birth vary with primary healthcare provider and homecare agency. See Chapter Appendix 7-1 for diagnostic criteria and considerations for homecare management of the woman at high risk for preterm birth (Grohar, 1994; Simpson, 1992).

HUAM has been introduced in an attempt to prevent preterm births; however, numerous prospective studies do not support the efficacy of this approach. There may be some evidence that HUAM is effective in decreasing preterm birth rates for women with a multiple gestation, but more confirmatory data is needed.

Research by Katz, Newman, and Gill (1986) suggested a 24- to 48-hour window of opportunity to prevent preterm births. In their study with a small sample of women, an increase in contraction frequency was noted 1 to 2 days prior to preterm birth. Thus, they felt HUAM could be effective in detecting this increase in uterine activity, allowing for treatment before cervical changes occurred leading to preterm birth. New data suggest that the time period during which contractions are detected either by HUAM or self-palpation is limited to 12 to 24 hours before overt preterm labor (Iams, Johnson, & Parker, 1994).

Daily provider-initiated telephone contact usually included with HUAM services may be effective in reducing the incidence of prematurity in a select group of women prospectively identified as at risk for preterm birth (ACOG, 1992). Prospective, randomized, blinded, clinical trials with sufficient sample size and statistical power to detect significant differences in outcomes in women at risk for preterm labor, using HUAM and self-palpation as methods for assessing uterine activity are needed. The role of daily healthcare provider contact (usually a perinatal nurse) as a separate factor also should be investigated. The question of whether reported reductions in preterm birth rates in studies of HUAM are related to the monitor, or frequent provider contact and patients' heightened awareness of signs and symptoms of preterm labor remain to be answered. Based on current published research data on efficacy, ACOG (1992) considers HUAM an investigational device and does not recommend it for clinical use.

According to ACOG (1995, p. 2), it has not been clearly demonstrated that HUAM can be used to actually affect the rate of preterm birth; however, the use of "this expensive and burden-some system" and "subsequent treatment has the potential for substantially increasing costs."

Inpatient Management

Many women experience preterm contractions. Currently there is no way to predict which preterm contractions cause cervical changes. It is known that all preterm contractions do not result in preterm labor, although preterm contractions are often treated empirically to prevent preterm labor and birth. Most healthcare providers in the United States and Canada treat preterm contractions even when cervical change has not occurred, in the hopes of preventing a preterm birth.

Bedrest. Bedrest is the oldest and most common treatment for preterm contractions. Bedrest in a lateral position increases blood flow to the uterus and is thought to decrease uterine activity. Although widely recommended as a clinical prevention strategy, there is no evidence to support the efficacy of bedrest therapy in preterm birth prevention (Goldenberg et al., 1994). Multiple, randomized, controlled, clinical trials have not shown an increase in length of gestation or improvement in neonatal outcomes in women prescribed bedrest therapy, compared with women who remained ambulatory during a pregnancy at high risk for preterm birth. Changes in practice have not occurred; most likely because no alternative effective treatment method has been identified.

Prolonged bedrest is associated with a variety of physical and psychosocial side effects (Maloni, 1993). These include muscle atrophy, muscle weakness, changes in cardiac output, bone loss, decreased gastric motility, and increased gastric reflux. Pregnant women prescribed complete bedrest may demonstrate decreased weight gain, weight loss, depression, anxiety, cardiovascular deconditioning, and changes in sleep cycles (Maloni). Bedrest in a semi-Fowlers position rather than lateral position may decrease some of the above complications.

Hydration. Patients who progress from preterm contractions to preterm labor, as evidenced by cervical change, may require other therapies such as hydration and pharmacologic agents to prevent preterm birth. Intravenous fluids are usually administered to increase vascular volume and possibly decrease oxytocin secretion (Lipshitz, Pierce, & Arntz, 1993). Definitive data related to efficacy of IV fluids, as a specific treatment for preterm contractions in women who are not dehydrated, do not exist. Similar to bedrest, IV fluid therapy is a traditional treatment for preterm contractions.

Tocolytic Agents. Since the administration of tocolytic agents may be the next therapy, an accurate intake and output record should be initiated including intake prior to admission. Many women, especially those in a HUAM program, will increase fluid intake at home in an effort to decrease uterine contractions. A baseline and then serial complete blood counts (CBCs) allow evaluation of a decrease in the hemoglobin and hematocrit, with the infusion of fluid and/or betamimetic therapy. A decrease of greater than 1–2 g in the hemoglobin is indicative of hemodilution from therapy, in the absence of maternal bleeding.

If bedrest and IV fluids are unsuccessful in inhibiting preterm labor, a tocolytic agent may be added to the treatment plan. Regional and institutional differences related to the decision to treat preterm contractions exist, ranging from a continuum of no treatment, bedrest, oral hydration, IV hydration, oral tocolytics, subcutaneous tocolytics, and IV tocolytics.

A comprehensive review of the literature on tocolytics, from 1930 to 1992, concluded that the only tocolytic agents which might be effective are prostaglandin inhibitors used between 24–32 weeks' gestation (Higby, Xenakis, & Pauerstein, 1993). All tocolytic agents carry some maternal risk, and this risk increases if dual tocolytic agent therapy is used. Recent cases of a maternal death and significant maternal morbidity related to IV terbutaline administration have been reported (Hudgens & Conradi, 1993; Levy, 1994).

BETAMIMETIC AGENTS. Ritodrine hydrochloride (Yutopar) is the only agent currently approved by the Food and Drug Administration (FDA) for use as a tocolytic in the United States.

Ritodrine and terbutaline (Brethine) are both β-agonists; they stimulate β-receptor cells located in smooth muscle. Theoretically, these agents work by relaxing the smooth muscle, which decreases or stops uterine contractions. β-receptors are also located in smooth muscle in the cardiovascular, pulmonary, and gastrointestinal systems. Effects of betamimetic agents are related directly to dosage and route of administration (Cunningham et al., 1993; Higby, Xenakis, & Pauerstein, 1993). (See Display 7-15 for summary of systemic effects of betamimetic therapy.) Fetal side effects are thought to be the same as those in the mother because they rapidly cross the placenta. Betamimetic agents are contraindicated in patients with known cardiac disease. They may be used in women with diabetes with concomitant intravenous insulin infusion; however, magnesium sulfate is the first agent of choice for these patients.

Betamimetic agents may be administered subcutaneously or intravenously as a secondary infusion, after baseline assessments (e.g., electrolytes, BUN, creatinine, serum glucose, and ECG) are obtained and a meticulous intake and output record is started. The infusion is titrated per institution protocol until uterine activity ceases, maximum dosages are reached, or the patient experiences severe side effects. Decreases in blood pressure, a widening pulse pressure, and maternal tachycardia will develop in most patients. Oral therapy is usually started 30 minutes before the intravenous solution is discontinued.

Use of oral betamimetic agents has not been associated with a significant increase in length of gestation. Oral doses have the same side effects as intravenous or subcutaneous dose, though the effects are usually milder. Oral agents sometimes cause an increase in blood glucose levels (Regenstein, Belluomini, & Katz, 1993).

Maternal pulse rate must be monitored for any patient who is administered a betamimetic agent. A pulse rate of 120 bpm or greater may warrant continuous ECG monitoring and discontinuation of tocolytic therapy. A heart rate of greater than 120 bpm is associated with a decreased ventricular filling time, and therefore, decreased cardiac output. Over the course of time, if the left ventricular filling time is decreased, less blood will be pumped to the myocardium, resulting in decreased myocardial perfusion. This will be reflected by patient complaints of chest heaviness, shortness of breath, or chest pain. Myocardial infarction may result if the agent is not discontinued.

MAGNESIUM SULFATE THERAPY. IV magnesium sulfate ($MgSO_4$) is frequently used to treat preterm contractions, though the exact mechanism of action is not known. Theoretically, magnesium interferes with calcium uptake in the cells of the myometrium. Since these myometrial cells are thought to need calcium in order to contract, decreasing the amount of calcium decreases or stops contractions. $MgSO_4$ relaxes smooth muscle throughout the body, so a decrease in BP may be noted with the administration of a loading dose or at high infusion doses.

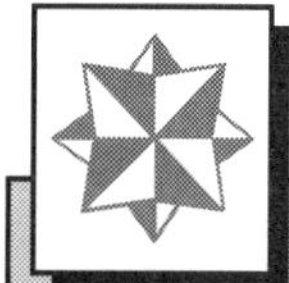

DISPLAY 7-15

Systemic Effects of Ritodrine and Terbutaline

Cardiovascular
- Increased heart rate
- Widened pulse pressure
- Decreased BP
- Increased cardiac output
- Cardiac dysrhythmia [preventricular contractions (PVC), paroxysmal atrial tachycardia (PAT)]
- Tachycardia
- Chest pain

Pulmonary
- Pulmonary edema

Metabolic
- Increased glucose
- Diabetic ketoacidosis
- Decreased serum potassium levels
- Increased antidiuretic hormone production

There are no prospective studies which demonstrate that intravenous $MgSO_4$ is an effective tocolytic agent. Many practitioners feel comfortable using this agent because they have widespread experience in the administration of $MgSO_4$ for the prevention of eclamptic seizures. Institution protocols should be followed. The therapeutic serum levels of $MgSO_4$ for the treatment of premature contractions/labor are not well documented; many practitioners use the 4–8 mEq/L (5–8 mg/dl) serum level that is known to be the therapeutic dosage for the prevention of seizures (Higby, Xenksis, & Pauerstein, 1993). Nursing care of the woman receiving $MgSO_4$ for tocolysis is the same as for the woman receiving $MgSO_4$ for seizure prophylaxis.

Few studies are available to assess the efficacy of long-term therapy with IV $MgSO_4$. However, long-term therapy is not contraindicated in women with normal renal function. One study that did follow the use of long-term IV $MgSO_4$ therapy suggested that maternal side effects were ileus, constipation, blurring of vision, and headache. Long-term $MgSO_4$ therapy has been associated with increased calcium excretion, which may affect bone mineralization (Cunningham et al., 1993; Maloni, 1993).

Oral administration of a variety of magnesium preparations, such as magnesium gluconate, has not been shown to have a significant role in increasing length of gestation, though it may decrease the frequency of recurrence of preterm contractions (Ricci, Hariharan, Helfgott, Reed, & O'Sullivan, 1991).

Calcium channel blockers. Calcium channel blockers may suppress contractions and cause the myometrial muscle to relax by interfering with the movement of extracellular calcium into the calcium channels of the cells. This prevents the electrical system from passing the current through the cells, thus preventing a contraction. These agents, especially nifedipine (Procardia) and nicardipine (Nicardipine) have been studied in Europe for use as tocolytic agents and have been demonstrated to be effective. Verapamil (Isoptin), a well-known calcium channel blocker, is not used as a tocolytic agent due to maternal cardiovascular side effects.

The use of calcium channel blockers in the United States remains limited due to animal research, suggesting that these agents may cause fetal acidosis and hypoxia when administered intravenously (Cunningham et al., 1993). Calcium channel blockers have also been associated with maternal hepatotoxicity when administered for preterm labor (Cunningham et al., 1993; Higby, Xenakis, & Pauerstein, 1993). Nifedipine causes neuromuscular blockade and when given in conjunction with $MgSO_4$, can increase $MgSO_4$, toxicity (Higby et al., 1993).

Prostaglandin inhibitors. Prostaglandin is a naturally produced agent that is thought to cause uterine contractions and cervical ripening in term pregnancies. There are absent or low amounts of prostaglandin secretions in the amniotic fluid of preterm pregnant women not in labor (Higby et al., 1993).

Several types of prostaglandins affect uterine contractions and cervical ripening. The most well-known and well-studied prostaglandin inhibitor for use as a tocolytic agent is indomethacin. Indomethacin competes with other factors in a long-term process, whereby prostacyclin is the end product blocking the production of prostaglandin. Indomethacin is not without fetal effects, however. After 34 weeks' gestation, indomethacin may cause premature closure of the ductus arteriosis and increase the risk of fetal pulmonary hypertension (Higby et al., 1993). Indomethacin also impairs fetal renal function which may result in oligohydramnios. This is a transient phenomenon, with fetal renal function returning to normal when the agent is discontinued. The renal effect makes indomethacin a therapeutic agent for use in preterm contractions/labor associated with polyhydramnios, since it may normalize fluid volume. Amniotic fluid status is monitored to observe for a decrease in volume. Indomethacin has been associated with a delay in the time from the onset of preterm labor contractions to delivery, potentially allowing for a course of antenatal steroids to enhance fetal lung maturity (Higby et al., 1993).

Oxytocin antagonists. Oxytocin antagonists compete with oxytocin at receptor sites in the myometrium in the prevention of uterine contractions. This is a new class of agents currently under investigation in multicenter, prospective, randomized trials in the United States. These studies are testing the oxytocin antagonists against the only current FDA-approved tocolytic agent, ritodrine. Initial studies indicated that uterine activity ceased in patients who received an oxytocin inhibitors, though some of the patients had further contractions and received betamimetic agents. Side effects reported to date have been minimal. The full reports of the multicenter study should be available by the mid-1990s.

Antibiotics. The use of antibiotics in the treatment of preterm labor remains controversial, though more evidence suggests that antibiotics may play a role in prolonging pregnancy and improving neonatal outcomes, especially in patients with preterm premature rupture of the membranes (PPROM) (Kirschbaum, 1993).

Acceleration of Fetal Lung Maturity. The second leading cause of neonatal mortality is RDS. Extending intrauterine life to enhance fetal lung maturity can dramatically reduce neonatal morbidity and mortality. Currently, several treatment modalities are being used in the United States to pharmacologically enhance fetal lung maturity.

Antenatal corticosteroid administration has been associated with approximately a 50% reduction in neonatal RDS (Crowley, Chalmers, & Keirse, 1990). A secondary benefit of antenatal corticosteroid administration is the reduction of neonatal mortality, IVH, and NEC (Crowley et al., 1990).

Thyrotropin-releasing hormone (TRH), when given in combination with glucocorticoid treatment, has shown early promise in reducing the number of ventilator days for neonates with RDS and decreasing the rates of bronchopulmonary dysplasia (Knight, Liggins, & Wealthall, 1994). However, further research is warranted.

A third therapy currently in use after birth is artificial surfactant therapy. In preterm infants treated prophylactically, artificial surfactant therapy appears to reduce neonatal mortality and morbidity, when compared with infants treated after the diagnosis of RDS (rescue therapy) (Kendig, Notter, & Cox, 1991). Further research is ongoing.

Nursing Issues Related to Pharmacologic Therapy

All tocolytic therapies carry maternal risks, so appropriate continuous assessment for the effects of the agents are indicated during administration. Intravenous tocolytics are given per institution protocol as a secondary infusion via a controlled infusion pump for accurate administration and monitoring of fluid intake. In addition to accurate intake and output, bilateral breath sounds, changes in vital signs, and mental status are continuously monitored to identify early signs of fluid overload and pulmonary edema. A maternal heart rate of 120 or greater, or a decrease in BP to less than 90 mmHg systolic or 40 mmHg diastolic indicates profound hemodynamic changes and should be reported immediately. The need for the tocolytic therapy with consideration of maternal side effects must be continuously reassessed by the perinatal team. The pregnant woman's wishes must be considered. Full disclosure of potential maternal-fetal benefits and risks of tocolytic therapy should be given to the woman and her family or support persons, by the primary healthcare provider.

Women who report chest heaviness, discomfort, or pain should have a repeat check of bilateral breath sounds and possibly a 12-lead ECG. If rales, crackles, or diminished breath sounds are noted, immediate notification of the physician is indicated. A chest x-ray may be obtained to rule out pulmonary edema. The woman is placed in Fowler's position and oxygen administration at 10–12 L/min may be initiated. A pulse oximeter or aterial blood gas results may be used to determine maternal oxygenation and acid-base balance. The repeat ECG is compared with the baseline ECG to determine if there are S-T segment changes correlating with myocardial ischemia or infarction. Tocolytic therapy is discontinued if the patient develops chest pain, heaviness, discomfort, or shortness of breath.

Women receiving oral agents are monitored for agent-specific side effects. Nifedipine may reduce maternal BP. Indomethacin is associated with a decrease in amniotic fluid volume; ultrasound measurements of amniotic fluid volume or amniotic fluid index are followed. If oligohydramnios does result, the fetus is monitored for variable decelerations of the FHR. Oral ritodrine and oral terbutaline may increase maternal blood glucose levels, requiring glucose monitoring. The use of corticosteroids to enhance fetal lung maturity will increase the risk of elevated maternal glucose levels in the presence of betamimetics.

Preterm premature rupture of the membranes with documented premature labor is most commonly followed by birth within 48 to 72 hours. In women who present with PPROM and no labor, where sterile speculum examination has documented a closed cervix, expectant management, usually in the hospital, is indicated. Ongoing assessment for maternal fever, fetal tachycardia, color and odor of amniotic fluid, uterine or abdominal tenderness and purulent discharge from the vagina is mandatory. Intraamniotic infection is treated with IV antibiotics and birth. Cervical cultures and amniocentesis may be performed on admission.

Controversy exists related to treatment for Group B-Streptococcus infection. Consideration should be given to the administration of IV antibiotics in the presence of preterm labor or PPROM. If preterm birth is imminent, IV antibiotics are usually administered in most settings.

The nurse works in collaboration with the physician to fully assess maternal-fetal status and to provide optimal care to both patients. The woman and any significant others need to be informed of the options, risks, and benefits of the treatment choices that may be available. The woman and significant others are then included in the decision-making process.

Summary

The ultimate goal of prevention and treatment of preterm labor or birth is the delivery of a healthy infant with optimal maternal outcome. Since neonatal adaptation to extrauterine life is enhanced by fetal lung maturity, extending intrauterine life by even a few days can dramatically reduce neonatal morbidity and mortality. Therefore, the perinatal nurse can be beneficial in the identification and education of the women at risk for a preterm birth.

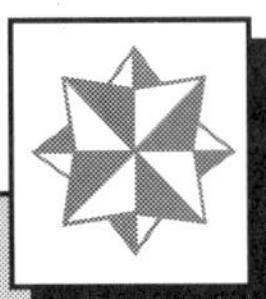

DISPLAY 7-16

Guidelines for Maternal Transfer

(All guidelines assume maternal and fetal stability)

From a Level I Institution:

Labor with cervical change less than 34–36 weeks' gestation

PPROM less than 34–36 weeks' gestation

Labor and/or PPROM where dating data is uncertain

Preterm labor with maternal or fetal complications

Bleeding less than 34–36 weeks' gestation

Twin or triplet gestation with contractions/labor less than 34–36 weeks

Severe preeclampsia

Eclampsia if maternal condition stabilized

Intrauterine growth restriction

Oligohydramnios

Polyhydramnios: Severe or uncertain origin

Fetal hydrops

Fetal anomalies, especially at gestational ages less than 34–36 weeks, which require specialized neonatal intervention (e.g., diaphragmatic hernia, oomphalocele, severe neural tube defects, etc.)

Fetal conditions requiring cordocentesis and/or transfusion

Maternal medical conditions outside of the scope of medical and nursing care available (e.g. liver transplant, renal dialysis, severe mitral stenosis, cancer, active lupus, pulmonary embolism, etc.)

Maternal (and possibly, fetal) trauma

Unusual fetal heart rate dysrhythmia: Complete fetal heart block, etc.

From a Level II Institution:

Any fetus requiring long-term ventilatory support as a newborn

Any fetus requiring neonatal care less than 30–34 weeks' gestation depending on the institution resources

Maternal complications listed above

MATERNAL TRANSFER

Maternal transfer from a Level I or Level II institution to a Level III institution is an option in the care of pregnant women. This is especially true of those patients less than 34–36 weeks' gestation in a Level II facility. Each case must be considered individually. (Suggested guidelines for transfer of care of the mother are listed in Display 7-16.) Before transfer, severity of the clinical situation and the time and distance to the receiving hospital is considered.

Maternal transport can be accomplished by either a one-way or two-way transfer of care. One-way transfer of care occurs when a referring hospital calls a receiving hospital to ask to transfer a pregnant patient. Once the patient is accepted verbally and initial physician report is given, the originating or referring hospital provides care throughout the transport process until the patient arrives at the receiving facility. Two-way transport occurs when the receiving facility accepts the patient verbally, then sends a team, including a registered nurse and possibly a physician, to transport the woman to the receiving facility. In this case, the transferring facility turns over the care and responsibility of the patient once the patient is under transport. Transport is accomplished by a variety of methods including private ambulance, public rescue vehicles, helicopters, and airplanes.

An accurate, thorough, nursing report is a critical element of transfer of care. A photocopy of the original record accompanies the patient. Any nursing or medical action performed enroute (e.g., vital signs, frequency of contractions, etc.) is documented, and a copy is left with the receiving hospital. Many institutions have specific forms for the transfer of obstetric patients. The decision as to the necessity of a nurse, physician, or both accompanying the patient in transfer is made in each individual case. If the nurse feels it inappropriate to transfer a specific patient without a physician present, and one has not been provided, institutional chain of command can provide a method for conflict resolution.

Based on an assessment of maternal-fetal status, appropriate equipment is required to ensure patient safety during the transfer process. For the patient with preeclampsia, a nasal airway, ambu bag, and anticonvulsant and antihypertensive agents should be included. Transport vehicles routinely are stocked with intravenous solutions and emergency equipment. Maternal transfer is less often initiated for women who are bleeding unless the patient is stable hemodynamically (i.e., the BP and pulse are within normal limits). When transferring women at risk for preterm labor, a delivery kit from the originating hospital should be included; the rescue kits on the ambulance are usually minimally stocked. A full delivery kit with DeLee catheters, suction bulb, blankets, fluid-absorbing pelches, and hat for the neonate is necessary. One-quart zip-lock plastic bags are useful to place the newborn in after birth, with the zip-lock closed on either side around the newborn's neck to prevent body heat loss. It is recommended that all patients have at least two infusion lines because attempting to start an IV line enroute is extremely difficult.

SUMMARY

Care of women with complications of pregnancy can be challenging for perinatal nurses, especially when they occur unexpectedly in the low-risk setting. A thorough knowledge of the nursing care for common perinatal complications including timely identification and appropriate interventions are requisite skills in order to ensure optimal maternal-fetal outcomes.

REFERENCES

Abdella, T.N., Sibai, B.M., Hays, J.M., & Anderson, G.M. (1984). Relationship of hypertensive disease to abruptio placentae. Obstetrics and Gynecology, 63(3), 365-370.

Ales, K.L., Norton, M.E., & Druzin, M.L. (1989). Early prediction of antepartum hypertension. Obstetrics and Gynecology, 73,(6) 928-933.

American Academy of Pediatrics & American College of Obstetricians and Gynecologists. (1992). Guidelines for perinatal care (2nd ed.). Elk Grove Village, IL: Author.

American College of Obstetricians and Gynecologists. (1986). Management of preeclampsia (Technical Bulletin No. 91). Washington, DC: Author.

American College of Obstetricians and Gynecologists. (1990). Diagnosis and management of postpartum hemorrhage (Technical Bulletin No. 143). Washington, DC: Author.

American College of Obstetricians and Gynecologists. (1992). Home uterine activity monitoring (Committee Opinion No. 115). Washington, DC: Author.

American College of Obstetricians and Gynecologists. (1994). Blood component therapy (Technical Bulletin No. 199). Washington, DC: Author.

American College of Obstetricians and Gynecologists. (1995). Preterm labor. (Technical Bulletin No. 206). Washington, DC: Author.

Arias, F. (1992). Practical guide to high-risk pregnancy and delivery. St. Louis: Mosby-Year Book.

Arnold, L.S., & Grad, R.K. (1992). Low birth weight and infant mortality: A health policy perspective. NAACOG's Clinical Issues in Perinatal and Women's Health Nursing, 3(1), 1-12.

Atrash, H.K., Rowley, D., & Hogue, C.J.R. (1992). Maternal and perinatal mortality. Current Opinion in Obstetrics and Gynecology, 4(1), 61-71.

Barron, W.M. (1991). Hypertension. In W.M. Barron & M.D. Lindheimer (Eds.), Medical disorders in pregnancy (pp. 1-42). Chicago: Mosby-Year Book.

Barth, W., & Hankins, G.D.V. (1992). Severe acute asthma in pregnancy. In S.L. Clark, D.B. Cotton, G.D.V. Hankins & J.P. Phelan (Eds.), Critical care obstetrics (2nd ed., pp. 371-392). Boston: Blackwell Scientific.

Branch, D.W., Silver, R.M., Blackwell, J.L., Reading, J.C., & Scott, J.R. (1992). Outcome of treated pregnancies in women with antiphospholipid syndrome: An update of the Utah experience. Obstetrics and Gynecology, 80(4), 614-620.

Brown, M.A. (1991). Pregnancy-induced hypertension: Pathogenesis and management. Australian and New Zealand Journal of Medicine, 21, 257-260, 262, 264-273.

Chesley, L.C., & Cooper, D.W. (1986). Genetics of hypertension in pregnancy: Possible single-gene control of pre-eclampsia and eclampsia in the descendants of eclamptic women. British Journal of Obstetrics and Gynaecology, 93(9), 898-908.

Chesley, L.C., & Sibai, B.M. (1987). Blood pressure in the midtrimester and future eclampsia. American Journal of Obstetrics and Gynecology, 157(5), 1258-1261.

Chez, R.A., & Sibai, B.M. (1994). Labetalol for intrapartum hypertension. Contemporary Obstetrics and Gynecology, (8), 37-38.

Clark, S.L., Cotton, D.B., Hankins, G.D.V., & Phelan, J.P. (1994). Handbook of critical care obstetrics. Boston: Blackwell Scientific.

Copper, R.L., Goldenberg, R.L., & Davis, R.O. (1990). Warning symptoms, uterine contractions, and cervical examination findings in women at risk of preterm delivery. American Journal of Obstetrics and Gynecology, 162(3), 748-754.

Copper, R.L., Goldenberg, R.L., & Creasy, R.K. (1993). A multicenter study of preterm birth weight and gestational age-specific neonatal mortality. American Journal of Obstetrics and Gynecology, 168(4), (1, Pt. 1), 78-84.

Creasy, R.K. (1993). Preterm birth prevention: Where are we? American Journal of Obstetrics and Gynecology, 168(4), 1223-1230.

Creasy, R.K. (1994). Preterm labor and delivery. In R.K. Creasy & R. Resnick (Eds.), Maternal-fetal medicine: Principles and practice (pp. 494-520). Philadelphia: W.B. Saunders.

Crowley P., Chalmers I., & Keirse M. (1992). The effects of corticosteroid administration before preterm delivery: An overview of the evidence from controlled trials. British Journal of Obstetrics and Gynaecology, 97(1), 11-25.

Cunningham, F.G., Cox, S.M., Harstad, T.W., Mason, R.A., & Pritchard, J.A. (1990). Chronic renal disease and pregnancy outcome. American Journal of Obstetrics and Gynecology, 163(2), 453-459.

Cunningham, F.G., & Leveno, K.J. (1988). Management of pregnancy-induced hypertension. In P.C. Rubin (Ed.), Handbook of hypertension: Vol. 10, Hypertension in pregnancy. Amsterdam: Elsevier Scientific.

Cunningham, F.G., MacDonald, P., Gant, N., Leveno, K., & Gilstrap, L. (1993). William's obstetrics (19th ed., pp. 819-852). Norwalk, CT: Appleton & Lange.

Daddario, J., & Johnson, G. (1992). Trauma in pregnancy. In L. Mandeville, & N. Troiano (Eds.), High-risk intrapartum nursing (pp. 256-279). Philadelphia: J.B. Lippincott.

Dildy, G.A., Phelan, J.P., & Cotton, D.B. (1992). Complications of pregnancy-induced hypertension. In S.L. Clark, D.B. Cotton, G.D.V. Hankins & J.P. Phelan (Eds.), Critical care obstetrics (2nd ed., pp. 251-288). Boston: Blackwell Scientific.

Dorman, K.F. (1989). Hemorrhagic emergencies in obstetrics, Journal of Perinatal and Neonatal Nursing 3(2), 23-32.

Dudley, D., Gagnon, D., & Varner, M. (1989). Long-term tocolysis with intravenous magnesium sulfate. Obstetrics and Gynecology, 73, (3, Pt. 1), 373-378.

Dutton, D. (1981). The select panel for the promotion of child health: Children's health care: The myth of equal access. Better health care for our children: A national strategy, 4 (DHHS Publication No. PHS 79-55071, pp. 357-440). Washington, DC: U.S. Government Printing Office.

Easterling, T.R., Benedetti, T.J., Schmucker, B.C., & Millard, S.P. (1992). Maternal hemodynamics in normal and preeclamptic pregnancies: A longitudinal study. Obstetrics and Gynecology, 76(6), 1061-1069.

Eganhouse, D.J., & Burnside, S.M. (1992). Nursing assessment and responsibilities in monitoring the preterm pregnancy. Journal of Obstetric, Gynecologic and Neonatal Nursing, 21(5), 355-363.

Fairlie, F.M., & Sibai, B.M. (1993). Hypertensive diseases in pregnancy. In E.A. Reece, J.C. Hobbins, M.J. Mahoney & R.H. Petrie (Eds.), Medicine of the fetus and mother. Philadelphia: J.B. Lippincott.

Freda, M., Anderson, H.F., Damus, K., Porest, D., Bruustman, L., & Merkatz, D. (1990). Lifestyle modification as an intervention for inner city women at high risk for preterm birth. Journal of Advanced Nursing, 15(3), 364-372.

Friedman, S.A., Taylor, R.N., & Roberts, J.M. (1991). Pathophysiology of preeclampsia. Clinics in Perinatology, 18(4), 661-682.

Fuchs, F. (1976). Prevention of prematurity. American Journal of Obstetrics and Gynecology, 126(7), 809-820.

Garbaciak, J.A. (1992). Prematurity prevention: Who is at risk? Clinics in Perinatology, 19(2), 275-289.

Gavette, L., & Roberts, J. (1987). Use of mean arterial pressure (MAP-2) to predict pregnancy-induced hypertension in adolescents. Journal of Nurse-Midwifery, 32(6), 357-364.

Gilbert, E.S., & Harmon, J.S. (1992). High-risk pregnancy and delivery (2nd ed.). St. Louis: Mosby-Year Book.

Goldenberg, R.L., Cliver, S.P., Bronstein, J., Cutter, G., Andrews, W., & Mennenmeyer, S. (1994). Bed rest in pregnancy. Obstetrics and Gynecology, 84(1), 131-136.

Green, J. (1994). Placenta previa and abrupio placenta. In R. Creasy, & R. Resnik (Eds.), Maternal-fetal medicine: Principles and practice (3rd ed., pp. 602-619). Philadelphia: W.B. Saunders.

Grohar, J. (1994). Nursing protocols for antepartum home care. Journal of Obstetric, Gynecologic, and Neonatal Nursing, 23(8), 687-694.

Guzick, D.S., Klein, V.R., Tyson, J.E., Lasky, R.E., Gant, N.F., & Rosenfeld, C.R. (1987). Risk factors for the occurrence of pregnancy-induced hypertension. Clinical Experiments in Hypertension of Pregnancy Part B: Hypertension in Pregnancy, 6, 281-297.

Harvey, M.G. (1991). Physiologic changes of pregnancy. In C. Harvey (Ed.), Critical care obstetrical nursing (pp. 1-33). Gaithersburg, MD: Aspen.

Hays, P.M., Cruikshank, D.P., & Dunn, L.J. (1985). Plasma volume determination in normal and preeclamptic pregnancies. American Journal of Obstetrics and Gynecology, 151(7), 958-966.

Higby, K., Xenakis, E.M., & Pauerstein, C.J. (1993). Do tocolytic agents stop preterm labor? A critical and comprehensive review of efficacy and safety. American Journal of Obstetrics and Gynecology, 168(4), 1247-1256.

Hobel, C.J., Ross, M.G., Bemin, R.L., Bragoier, J., Nessim, S., Sandhu, M., Bear, M., & Mori, B. (1994). The West Los Angeles Preterm Birth Preventions Project: Program impact on high-risk women. American Journal of Obstetrics and Gynecology, 170(1, Pt. 1), 54-62.

Hudgens, D.R., & Conradi, S.E. (1993). Sudden death associated with terbutaline sulfate administration. American Journal of Obstetrics and Gynecology, 169(1), 120-121.

Iams, J.D., Johnson, F.F., & Creasy, R.K. (1988). Prevention of preterm birth. Clinical Obstetrics and Gynecology, 31(3), 599-615.

Iams, J.D., Johnson, F.F., Parker, M. (1994). A prospective evaluation of the signs and symptoms of preterm labor. Obstetrics and Gynecology, 84(2), 227-230.

Iams, J.D., Paraskos, J., Landon, M.B., Teteris, J., & Johnson, F.F. (1994). Cervical sonography in preterm labor. Obstetrics and Gynecology, 84(1), 40-46.

Institute of Medicine. (1985). Preventing low birth weight. Washington, DC: National Academy.

Jackson, G.M., Edwin, S.S., Varner, M.W., Cassal, D., & Mitchell, M.D. (1993). Regulation of fetal fibronectin production in human chorion cells. American Journal of Obstetrics and Gynecology, 169(6), 1431-1435.

Katz, M., Goodyear, K., & Creasy, R.K. (1990). Early signs and symptoms of preterm labor. American Journal of Obstetrics and Gynecology, 162(5), 1150-1153.

Katz, M., Newman, R.B., & Gill, P.J. (1986). Assessment of uterine activity in ambulatory patients at high-risk of preterm labor and delivery. American Journal of Obstetrics and Gynecology, 154(1), 44-47.

Kendig, J.W., Notter, R.H., & Cox, C. (1991). A comparison of surfactant as immediate prophylaxis and as rescue therapy in newborns of less than 30 weeks gestation. New England Journal of Medicine, 324(13), 865-871.

Khong, T.Y., & Khong, T.K. (1993). Delayed postpartum hemorrhage: A morphologic study of causes and their relation to other pregnancy disorders. Obstetrics and Gynecology, 82(1), 17-22.

Kirschbaum, T. (1993). Antibiotics in the treatment of preterm labor. American Journal of Obstetrics and Gynecology, 168(4), 1239-1246.

Klebanoff, M.A., Shiono, P.H., & Carey, J.C. (1990). The effect of physical activity during pregnancy on preterm delivery and birth weight. American Journal of Obstetrics and Gynecology, 163, (1, Pt. 1) 1450-1460.

Klebanoff, M.A., Shiono, P.H., & Selby, J.V. (1991). Anemia and spontaneous preterm birth. American Journal of Obstetrics and Gynecology, 164, (1, Pt. 1), 59-63.

Kochenour, N.K. (1991). Intrapartum obstetric emergencies. Critical Care Clinics, 7(4), 851-864.

Kupferminc, M.J., Tamura, R.K., Wigton, T.R., Glassenberg, R., & Socol, M. (1993). Placenta Accreta is associated with elevated maternal serum alpha-fetoprotein. Obstetrics and Gynecology, 82(2), 266-269.

Lavery, J.P. (1990). Placenta previa. Clinical Obstetrics and Gynecology, 33(3),414-421.

Leonardi, M.R., & Hankins, G.D.V. (1992). What's new in tocolytics. Clinics in Perinatology, 19(2), 367-374.

Leveno, K.J., Little, B.B., & Cunningham, F.G. (1990). The national impact on Ritodrine Hydrochloride for inhibition of preterm labor. Obstetrics and Gynecology, 76(1), 12-15.

Levy, D.L. (1994). Morbidity caused by terbutaline infusion pump therapy. American Journal of Obstetrics and Gynecology, 170(6), 1835.

Lipshitz, J., Pierce, P., & Arntz, M. (1993). Preterm labor. In R.A. Knuppel & J.E. Drukker (Eds.), High-risk pregnancy: A team approach (pp. 396-421). Philadelphia: W.B.Saunders.

Lowe, T.W., & Cunningham, F.G. (1990). Placental abruption. Clinical Obstetrics and Gynecology, 33(3), 406-413.

Mabie, W.C., Pernoll, M.L., & Biswas, M.K. (1986). Chronic hypertension in pregnancy. Obstetrics and Gynecology, 67(2), 197-205.

MacGillivray, I., Rose, G.A., & Rowe, D. (1969). Blood pressure survey in pregnancy. Clinical Science, 37(2), 395-407.

Magann, E.F., Martin, J.N., Isaacs, J.D., Perry, K., Martin, R., & Meydrech, E. (1993). Immediate postpartum curettage: Accelerated recovery from severe preeclampsia. Obstetrics & Gynecology, 81(4), 502-506.

Mahon, T.R., Chazotte, C., & Cohen, W.R. (1994). Short labor: Characteristics and outcome. Obstetrics and Gynecology, 84(1), 47-51.

Mamelle, N., Laumon, B., & Lazar, P. (1984). Prematurity and occupational activity during pregnancy. American Journal of Epidemiology, 119(3), 309-322.

Maloni, J.A. (1993). Bed rest during pregnancy: Implications for nursing. Journal of Obstetrics, Gynecologic and Neonatal Nursing, 22, 422-426.

Marx, G.F., Schwalbe, S.S., Cho, E., & Whitty, J.E. (1993). Automated blood pressure measurements in laboring women: Are they reliable? American Journal of Obstetrics and Gynecology, 168, (3, Pt. 3), 796-798.

McCormick, M. (1991). Trends in rates of low birth weight in the United States. In H.L. Berendes, S. Kessel & S. Yaffee, Advances in the prevention of low birth weight: An international symposium (pp. 3-17). Washington, DC: National Center for Education in Maternal and Child Health.

Meis, P.J., Ernest, J.M., & Moore, M.L. (1987). Cause of low birthweight births in public and private patients. American Journal of Obstetrics and Gynecology, 156(5), 1165-1168.

Myers, D.A., & Nathanielsz, P.W. (1993). Biologic basis of term and preterm labor. Clinics in Perinatology, 20(1), 9-28.

Moutquin, J.M., Rainville, C., & Giroux, L. (1985). A prospective study of blood pressure in pregnancy: Prediction of preeclampsia. American Journal of Obstetrics and Gynecology, 151(2), 191-196.

Murahata, S.A. (1991). Third stage of labor and postpartum hemorrhage. In H. Frederickson & L. Wilkins-Haug (Eds.), OB/GYN secrets. St. Louis: Mosby-Yearbook.

Neal, A., & Bockman, V. (1992). Preterm labor and preterm premature rupture of the membranes. In L. Mandeville & N. Troiano (Eds.), High-risk intrapartum nursing (pp. 58-81). Philadelphia: J.B. Lippincott.

Nurses Association of the American College of Obstetricians and Gynecologists: The Organization for Obstetric, Gynecologic, and Neonatal Nurses. (1990). Fetal heart rate auscultation. OGN practice resource. Washington, DC: Author.

O'Brien, J.M., Mercer, B.M., Friedman, S.A., & Sibai, B.M. (1993). Amniotic fluid index in hospitalized hypertensive patients managed expectantly. Obstetrics and Gynecology, 82(2), 247-250.

O'Brien, W.F. (1990). Predicting preeclampsia. Obstetrics and Gynecology, 75(3, Pt. 1), 445-452.

O'Brien, W.F. (1993). Puerperal complications. In T.R. Moore, R.C. Reiter, R.W. Rebar & V.V. Baker (Eds.), Gynecology and Obstetrics: A longitudinal approach (pp. 637-654). New York: Churchill Livingstone.

O'Connell, J. (1987). Barriers to access to prenatal care in Rhode Island. Rhode Island Department of Health Internal Report.

Owen, J., Goldenberg, R.L., & Davis, R.O. (1990). Evaluation of a risk scoring system as a predictor of preterm birth in an indigent population. American Journal of Obstetrics and Gynecology, 163(3), 873-879.

Page, E.W., & Christianson, R. (1976). The impact of mean arterial pressure in the middle trimester upon the outcome of pregnancy. American Journal of Obstetrics and Gynecology, 125(6), 740-746.

Page, W.E. (1939). The relation between hydatid moles, relative ischemia of the gravid uterus, and the placental origin of eclampsia. American Journal of Obstetrics and Gynecology, 37, 291-293.

Papiernik, E., Bouyer, J., Drefus, J., Collin, D., Winisdorffer, G., Guegen, M., & Lazar, P. (1985). Prevention of preterm births: A perinatal study in Haguenaa, France. Pediatrics, 76(2), 154-158.

Phelan, J. (1991). Fetal considerations in the critically ill obstetric patient. In S. Clark, D. Cotton, G. Hankins & J. Phelan (Eds.), Critical Care Obstetrics (2nd ed., pp. 634-658). Boston: Blackwell Scientific.

Poole, J.H. (1993). HELLP syndrome and coagulopathies of pregnancy. Critical Care Nursing Clinics of North America, 5(3), 475-487.

Poziac, S. (1991). Hemorrhagic complications in pregnancy. In C. Harvey (Ed.), Critical care obstetrical nursing (pp. 115-146). Gaithersburg, MD: Aspen.

Regenstein, A., Belluomini, J., & Katz, M. (1993). Terbutaline tocolysis and glucose intolerance. Obstetrics and Gynecology, 81, (5, Pt. 1), 739-741.

Repke, J.T. (1993). Hypertension and preeclampsia. In T.R. Moore, R.C. Reiter, R.W. Rebar & V.V. Baker (Eds.), Gynecology and obstetrics: A longitudinal approach (pp. 463-477). New York: Churchill Livingstone.

Repke, J.T., & Villar, J. (1991). Pregnancy-induced hypertension and low birth weight: The role of calcium. American Journal of Clinical Nutrition, 54 (Suppl. 2), 237s-241s.

Ricci, J.M., Hariharan, S., Helfgott, A., Reed, K., & O'Sullivan, M.J. (1991). Oral tocolysis with magnesium chloride: A randomized controlled prospective clinical trial. American Journal of Obstetrics and Gynecology, 165(3), 603-610.

Roberts, J.M. (1994). Pregnancy-related hypertension. In R.K. Creasy & R. Resnick (Eds.), Maternal-fetal medicine: Principles and practice (3rd ed., pp. 804-843). Philadelphia: W.B. Saunders.

Roberts, J.M., Taylor, R.N., Friedman, S.A., & Goldfien, A. (1990). New developments in preeclampsia. Fetal Medicine Review, 2, 125-128.

Rochat, R.W., Koonin, L.M., Atrash, H.K., & Jewett, J.F. (1988). Maternal mortality in the United States: Report from the Maternal Mortality Collaborative. Obstetrics and Gynecology, 72(1), 91-97.

Romero R., & Mazor, M. (1988). Infection and preterm labor. Clinical Obstetrics and Gynecology, 31(3), 553-584.

Romero, R., Mazor, M., Oyarzun, E., Sirtori, M., Wu, Y.K., & Hobbins, J.C. (1989). Is there an association between colonization with group B Streptococcus and prematurity? Journal of Reproductive Medicine, 34(10), 797-801.

Rush, R.W., Keirse, M.J.N.C., & Howat, P. (1976). Contribution of preterm delivery to perinatal mortality. British Medical Journal, 2(6042), 965-968.

Saftlas, A.F., Olson, D.R., Atrash, H.K., Rochat, R.W., & Rowley, D. (1991). National trends in the incidence of abruptio placenta, 1979-1987. Obstetrics and Gynecology, 78(6), 1081-1086.

Sibai, B.M. (1988). Pitfalls in diagnosis and management of preeclampsia. American Journal of Obstetrics and Gynecology, 159, 1-5.

Sibai, B.M. (1990a). Eclampsia VI. Maternal-perinatal outcome in 254 consecutive cases. American Journal of Obstetrics and Gynecology, 163(3), 1049-1054.

Sibai, B.M. (1990b). The HELLP syndrome (hemolysis, elevated liver enzymes, and low platelets): Much ado about nothing? American Journal of Obstetrics and Gynecology, 162(2), 311-316.

Sibai, B.M. (1990c). Magnesium sulfate is the ideal anticonvulsant in preeclampsia-eclampsia. American Journal of Obstetrics and Gynecology, 162(5), 1141-1145.

Sibai, B.M. (1991a). Immunologic aspects of preeclampsia. Clinical Obstetrics and Gynecology, 34(1), 27-34.

Sibai, B.M. (1991b). Diagnosis and management of chronic hypertension in pregnancy. Obstetrics and Gynecology, 78 (3, Pt. 1), 451-461.

Siddiqi, T., Rosenn, B., Mimouni, F., Khoury, J.C., & Miodovink, M. (1991). Hypertension during pregnancy in insulin-dependent diabetic women. Obstetrics and Gynecology, 77(4), 514-519.

Simpson, K.R. (1992). Protocols for homecare management of high-risk pregnancies. St. Louis, MO: Healthy Homecomings.

Simpson, K.R. (1993). Acute fatty liver of pregnancy. Journal of Obstetric, Gynecologic, and Neonatal Nursing, 22(3), 213-219.

Spellacy, W.N., Miller, S.J., & Winegar, A. (1986). Pregnancy after 40 years of age. Obstetrics and Gynecology, 68(4), 452-454.

Tervila, L., Goecke, C., & Timonen, S. (1973). Estimation of gestosis of pregnancy (EPH-gestosis). Acta Obstetrics and Gynecology Scandanavia, 52(3), 235-243.

Thompson, S.A., Lyons, T.L., & Makowski, E.L. (1987). Outcomes of twin gestations at the University of Colorado Health Sciences Center, 1973-1983. Journal of Reproductive Medicine, 32(5), 328-339.

Thorp, J.M. (1993). Third-trimester bleeding. In T.R. Moore, R.C. Reiter, R.W. Rebar & V.V. Baker (Eds.), Gynecology and obstetrics: A longitudinal approach (pp. 479-485). New York: Churchill Livingstone.

United States Department of Health & Human Services. (1984). Public Health Service, National Center for Health Statistics: Vital statistics of the United States 1980: Vol. 1. Natality. Hyattsville, MD: Author.

Varner, M. (1991). Postpartum hemorrhage. Critical Care Clinics, 7(4), 883-897.

Veronikis, D.K., & O'Grady, J.P. (1994). What to do—or not to do—for postpartum hemorrhage. Contemporary Obstetrics and Gynecology, 39(8), 11.

Villiar, M.A., & Sibai, B.M. (1989). Clinical significance of elevated mean arterial blood pressure in second trimester and threshold increase in systolic or diastolic blood pressure during third trimester. American Journal of Obstetrics and Gynecology, 160(2), 419-423.

Virji, S.K., & Cottington, E. (1991). Risk factors associated with preterm deliveries among racial groups in a national sample of married mothers. American Journal of Perinatology, 8(5), 347-357.

Ward, K., Hata, A., & Jeunemaitre, X. (1993). A molecular variant of angiotensinogen associated with preeclampsia. Nature Genetics, 4(1), 59-61.

Weinstein, L. (1985). Preeclampsia/eclampsia with hemolysis, elevated liver enzymes, and thrombocytopenia. Obstetrics and Gynecology, 66(5), 657-660.

Wen, S.W., Goldenberg, R.L., Cutter, G.R., Hoffman, H.J., & Cliver, S.P. (1990). Intrauterine growth retardation and preterm delivery: Prenatal risk factors in an indigent population. American Journal of Obstetrics and Gynecology, 162(1), 213-218.

Whitter, F.R. (1993). Epidemiology of prematurity. In F.R. Whitter & L.G. Keith (Eds.), Textbook of prematurity (pp. 3-6). Boston: Little, Brown.

Working Group on High Blood Pressure in Pregnancy (Gifford, R.W., August, P., & Chesley, L.C.) (1990). National High Blood Pressure Education Program Working Group report on high blood pressure in pregnancy. American Journal of Obstetrics and Gynecology, 163, (5, Pt. 1), 1689-1712.

World Health Organization. The incidence of low birth weight: A critical review of available information. World Health Statistics Quarterly 33, 197-224, 1980.

York, R., & Brooten, D. (1992). Prevention of low birth weight. NAACOG's Clinical Issues in Perinatal and Women's Health Nursing 3(1), 13-24.

Zahn, C.M., & Yeomans, E.R. (1990). Postpartum hemorrhage: Placenta accreta, uterine inversion, and puerperal hematomas. Clinical Obstetrics and Gynecology, 33(3), 422-431.

Zeeman, G.G., & Dekker, G.A. (1992) Pathogenesis of preeclampsia: An hypothesis. Clinical Obstetrics and Gynecology, 35(2), 317-337.

Zuckerman, B., Frank, D.A., & Hingson, R.G. (1989). Effects of maternal marijuana and cocaine use on fetal growth. New England Journal of Medicine, 320(12), 762-768.

CHAPTER APPENDIX 7–1

GUIDELINES FOR HOMECARE MANAGEMENT OF COMMON PERINATAL COMPLICATIONS

General Guidelines for Homecare Management of Common Perinatal Complications

If homecare management is selected, patient education is a critical component of care. During the first visit, the woman and her family should be provided information about importance of adherence to the prescribed treatment plan and prompt notification to the primary healthcare provider of any signs or symptoms indicative of worsening disease. Education related to use of any technology or testing methods (e.g., daily weights, BP measurement, urinalysis using the dipstick method, fetal movement counting, uterine activity monitoring, and medications) and required documentation is also essential. Written materials provided to the woman and family members will reinforce teaching and serve as a resource for referral should questions arise at a later time.

Key points in homecare management include the following:

- Willingness of the woman and her family to adhere to prescribed treatment plan including activity restriction, fetal movement counting, blood pressure monitoring, daily weights, urinalysis, uterine activity monitoring, medications, and documentation
- Support systems in place to allow for activity restriction including childcare, if appropriate, and meal preparation
- Telephone service to allow daily phone contact between woman and perinatal nurse
- Knowledge of when to call the primary healthcare provider and/or come to the hospital
- Support persons should be identified to transport the woman to the hospital if necessary

Guidelines for Homecare Management of Preeclampsia

The following diagnostic criteria and considerations are suggested for homecare referral for management of women with mild preeclampsia:

- Gestational age >20 weeks
- BP <150/100 mmHg sitting or <140/90 mmHg in the lateral position
- Proteinuria <100 mg/L on urine dipstick or <1 g/24 hr
- No evidence of the following:
    1. headaches associated with visual disturbances
    2. epigastric pain judged to be related to preeclampsia
    3. marked edema or clonus
- Laboratory values: platelets >100,000 L; AST <50 U/L; ALT <200 U/L, serum creatine <1.32 mg/dl or within normal limits
- Ability to use electronic blood pressure (BP) equipment

The following parameters should be assessed based on the individual clinical situation. Standing protocols or physician orders are used to determine thresholds for each parameter:

- BP two to four times per day in the same arm in the same position
- Weight at the same time each day, usually in the morning, preferably on the same scale
- Urine dipstick for protein, using the first voided midstream specimen. A 24-hr urine collection may be ordered weekly
- Daily fetal movement counts
- Daily to twice weekly home visits for comprehensive maternal-fetal assessments including BP, fundal height, edema, reflexes, fetal well-being, and nonstress test (NST)
- Daily provider-initiated phone contact for assessment of signs and symptoms of PIH, review of BP, urinalysis, fetal movement, weight and activity level, and adherence to prescribed treatment plan

Indications of disease progression or fetal deterioration require admission to the hospital.

Guidelines for Homecare Management of Antepartum Bleeding

The following diagnostic criteria and considerations are suggested for homecare referral for management of women with antepartum bleeding:

- No evidence of active bleeding
- No evidence of signs and symptoms of preterm labor
- Home within reasonable distance to hospital (no more than 15 to 20 minutes from hospital)
- Emergency support systems in place for immediate transport to hospital

The following parameters should be assessed, based on the individual clinical situation. Standing protocols or physician orders are used to determine threshold for each parameter:

- Monitoring of vaginal discharge or bleeding after each urination or bowel movement, or more frequently as needed
- Daily fetal movement counts
- Daily uterine activity assessment either by self-palpation or electronic monitor or more frequently if needed
- Daily to twice weekly home visits for comprehensive maternal-fetal assessments including NST and fetal heart rate (FHR). Blood may be drawn for laboratory assessment of complete blood count (CBC) with differential
- Daily provider-initiated phone contact for assessment of uterine activity, bleeding, fetal well-being, activity level, and adherence to prescribed treatment plan

Guidelines for Homecare Management of Preterm Labor

The following diagnostic criteria and considerations are suggested for homecare referral for management of women with preterm labor:

- No evidence of active preterm labor
- No evidence of intraamniotic infection
- Cervical dilation less than 3 centimeters

The following parameters should be assessed, based on the individual clinical situation. Standing protocols or physician orders are used to determine thresholds for each parameter:

- Warning signs of preterm labor should be reviewed and a demonstration of uterine self-palpation provided. The nurse should observe the woman palpate for uterine activity
- At least twice daily uterine activity assessment either by self-palpation or electronic monitor
- Monitoring of vaginal discharge with heightened awareness of signs of SROM
- Assessment for urinary frequency, burning on urination or diarrhea, pelvic heaviness, pelvic pressure, maternal temperature, uterine tenderness, and cramping
- Frequent home visits for comprehensive maternal-fetal assessments including NST and FHR and possibly cervical examinations
- Daily provider-initiated phone contact for assessment of warning signs of preterm labor, fetal well-being, activity level, and adherence to prescribed treatment plan

Adapted from Simpson, K.R. (1992). Protocols for homecare management of high-risk pregnancies. St. Louis, MO: Healthy Homecomings, Inc. and Grohar, J. (1994). Nursing protocols for antepartum home care. Journal of Obstetric, Gynecologic, and Neonatal Nursing, 23(8), 687–694. Used with permission.

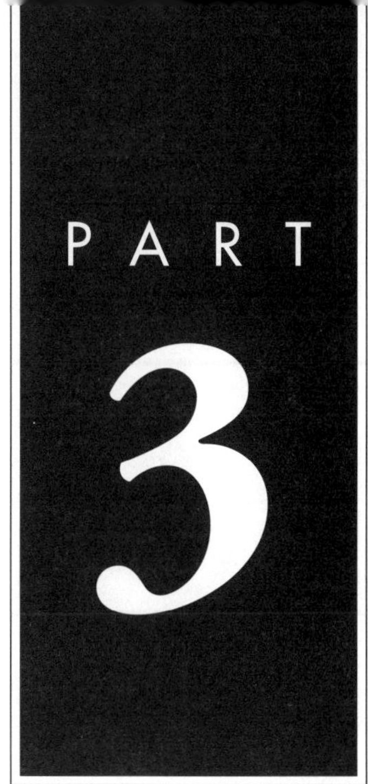

Intrapartum

Childbirth

Jean Bachman
Jo M. Kendrick

Childbirth is a natural process. During the intrapartum period, nurses use knowledge of physiologic and psychosocial aspects of birth to provide comprehensive care for women and families. The focus of this chapter is on researched-based nursing interventions that facilitate the birth process. A brief overview of the physiology of labor and birth is discussed. Maternal/fetal assessments, influence of maternal positioning on labor progression, and opportunities for supporting family attachment throughout the birth process are described. Clinical interventions including labor augmentation and induction, cervical ripening, and amnioinfusion are also presented. Strategies to ensure consistency with perioperative standards of care related to cesarean births are included, as well as controversial issues such as fundal pressure, suprapubic pressure, perineal massage, and open- versus closed-glottis pushing during the second stage.

OVERVIEW OF LABOR

Onset of Labor

Multiple theories have been proposed to explain the biophysiological factors that initiate labor; however, this process is not yet fully understood. It is likely that a combination of maternal-fetal factors influence labor onset (Display 8-1). Premonitory signs such as lightening, urinary frequency, pelvic pressure, changes in vaginal discharge, bloody show, loss of mucous plug, and irregular contractions are frequently reported several weeks before actual labor begins. Some women also describe changes in sleep patterns and increased energy levels in the final weeks of pregnancy. True labor is characterized by contractions which produce progressive effacement and dilation of the cervix with fetal descent into the maternal pelvis (Display 8-2).

Duration of Labor

Length of labor varies for each woman. The Friedman curve is most commonly used in the clinical setting to assess normal progression of labor; however, this guideline is used in the context of each woman's unique labor and birth experience. Generally, characteristics of most labors will be similar in length, progression, cervical changes, and fetal descent as outlined by Friedman, Niswander, and Bayonet-Rivera (1966). Parity influences the type of labor progression variances (Friedman, 1978). It is known that women in labor with their first child are more likely to experience

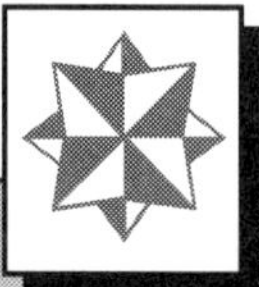

DISPLAY 8-1

Possible Causes of the Onset of Labor

Maternal Factor Theories

Uterine muscles stretched, causing release of prostaglandin.

Pressure on cervix stimulates nerve plexus, causing release of oxytocin by maternal posterior pituitary gland, the Ferguson reflex (Ferguson, 1941).

Oxytocin stimulation in circulating blood increases slowly during pregnancy, rises dramatically during labor, and peaks during second stage. Oxytocin and prostaglandin work together to inhibit calcium binding in muscle cells, raising intracellular calcium and thus activating contractions (Cunningham et al., 1993).

Estrogen/progesterone ratio change: estrogen excites uterine response; progesterone quiets uterine response. Decrease of progesterone allows estrogen to stimulate the contractile response of the uterus (Cunningham et al., 1993).

Fetal Factor Theories

Placental aging and deterioration triggers initiation of contractions.

Fetal cortisol, produced by the fetal adrenal glands, rises and acts on the placenta to reduce progesterone formation and increase prostaglandin. Anencephalic fetuses (no adrenal glands) tend to have prolonged gestation (Malpas, 1933; Anderson & Turnbull, 1973).

Prostaglandin, produced by fetal membranes (amnion and chorion) and the decidua, stimulates contractions. When arachidonic acid stored in fetal membranes is released at term, it is converted to prostaglandin (Wilson, 1989).

hypertonic uterine dysfunction, primary inertia, or a prolonged latent phase in early labor. During second and subsequent labors, deviations from the Friedman criteria during active labor, such as hypotonic uterine dysfunction, secondary inertia, and protraction or arrest of the active phase, are more common. Figure 8-1 provides graphic representations of an expected labor pattern and commonly seen deviations.

Stages of Labor and Birth

Labor and birth have traditionally been divided into four stages. The first stage is subdivided into the latent, active, and transition phases of labor. Cervical changes are used in assessing progression through each phase: latent phase, 0–3 centimeters; active phase, 4–7 centimeters; and transition 8–10 centimeters. Primigravid women usually experience complete cervical effacement prior to dilation. Increasing effacement usually occurs simultaneously with dilation in multiparas. Table 8-1 summarizes stages of labor, including average duration, cervical changes, uterine activity, maternal activity, and physical sensations.

Facilitating Labor and Birth

Nursing care during childbirth includes measures directed toward providing information so the woman knows what to expect, interpreting physical sensations, encouraging maternal position changes, reinforcing breathing and other relaxation efforts, coaching during second-stage pushing, and continued pain management. Attention is also given to the woman's partner/support person and family members in attendance. Areas in which there is a lack of consensus among practitioners in the literature as well as in practice include optimal maternal positions and strategies for second stage pushing. These issues are covered later in the chapter.

Nursing Assessments

Major roles of the perinatal nurse caring for laboring women include a thorough admission assessment and ongoing maternal/fetal assessments. This chapter's appendix contains a sample intrapartum admission assessment. Focus of this assessment is on prior obstetric history, current pregnancy, labor symptoms, and a history and physical examination emphasizing the respiratory, cardiovascular, gastrointestinal, urinary, and musculoskeletal systems. This initial interaction is also used to develop rapport with the woman and her family and to get a sense of their expectations for their birth experience. The amount of childbirth preparation and type of pain management anticipated during labor should be discussed at this time.

Guidelines for ongoing labor assessments are described in *Standards for the Nursing Care of Women and Newborns* (Nurses' Association of the American

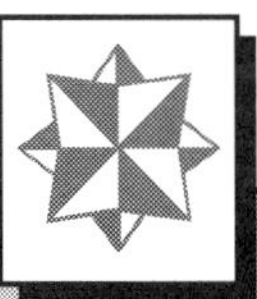

DISPLAY 8-2

Comparison of False and True Labor

False Labor	**True Labor**
Regular contractions	Regular contractions
Decrease in frequency and intensity; longer intervals	Progressive frequency and intensity; closer intervals
Discomfort in lower abdomen and groin	Discomfort begins in back, radiating to the abdomen
Activity has no effect or decreases contractions; disappear with sleep	Activity such as walking increases contractions; continue even when sleeping
No appreciable change in cervix	Progressive effacement and dilation of cervix
Sedation decreases or stops contractions	Sedation does not stop contractions
Show usually not present	Show usually present

TABLE 8-1. Stages of Labor

Stage	Duration	Contraction Frequency	Contraction Duration	Contraction Intensity	Physical Sensations	Maternal Behavior
FIRST STAGE						
Latent 0–3 cm	Primigravidas, 8.6 hr; Multigravidas, 5.3 hr	3–30 min; may be irregular	30–40 sec	Mild by palpation; 25 – 40 mm Hg by IUPC	Menstrual–like cramps, Low, dull backache; Light bloody show; Diarrhea; Possible rupture of membranes	Pain controlled fairly well; Able to ambulate and talk through most contractions; Range of emotions—excited, talkative, and confident versus anxious, withdrawn, and apprehensive
Active 4–7 cm	Primigravidas, 4.6 hr; Multigravidas, 2.4 hr	2–5 min	40–60 sec	Moderate to strong by palpation, 50–70 mm Hg by IUPC	Increasing discomfort; Trembling of thighs and legs; Pressure on bladder and rectum; Persistent backache with occipitoposterior fetal position	Begins to work at maintaining control during contractions; Accepts "coaching" efforts of perinatal staff and support persons; Quieter
Transition 8–10 cm	Primigravida 3.6 hr; Multigravida variable	1.5–2 min	60–90 sec	Strong by palpation, 70–90 mm Hg by IUPC	Increased bloody show; Urge to push; Increased rectal pressure; Membranes may rupture if they have not already	Ambulation difficult with uterine contractions; May be irritable and agitated; Self–absorbed, may appear to sleep between contractions;

						Need for support increases; Verbalizes feelings of discouragement and doubts her ability to cope
SECOND STAGE 10 cm to birth	Primigravida up to 3 hrs Multigravida 0–30 min	2–3 min	40–60 sec	Strong by palpation 70–100 mm Hg by IUPC	As presenting part descends, urge to push increases; Increased rectal and perineal pressure; Sensation of burning, tearing, and stretching of vagina and perineum	Excited and eager to push; Reluctant, ineffective at pushing
THIRD STAGE Birth of the infant to birth of the placenta	5–30 min				Mild uterine contractions; Feeling of fullness in vagina as placenta is expelled	Attention is focused on the newborn; Feelings of relief

Creehan, P.A. (1996)

A

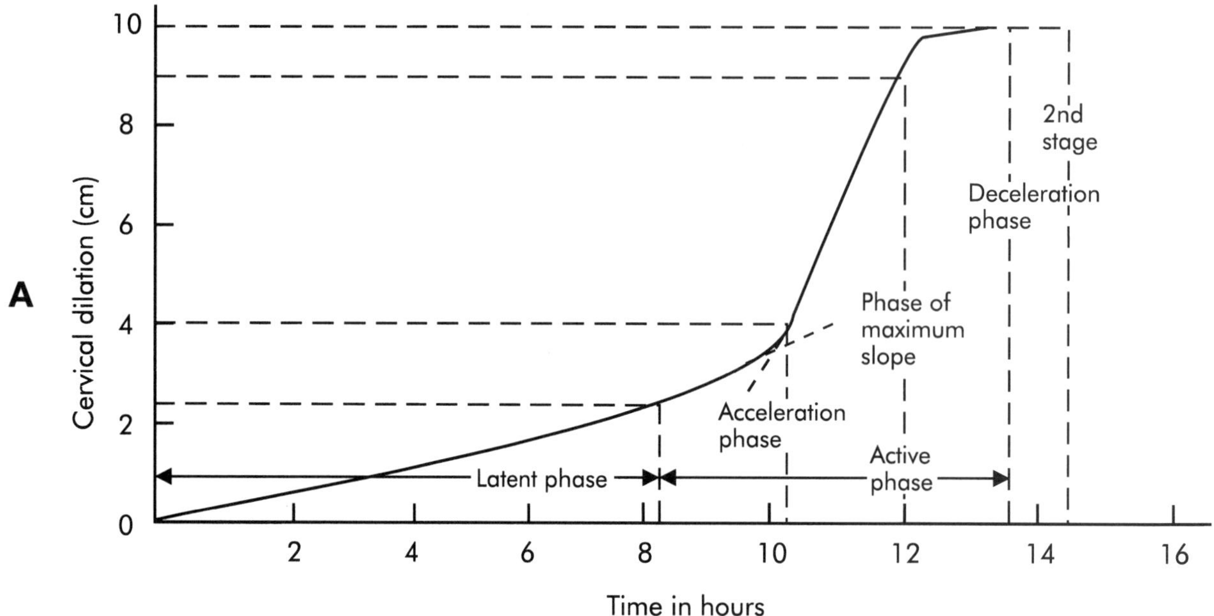

B

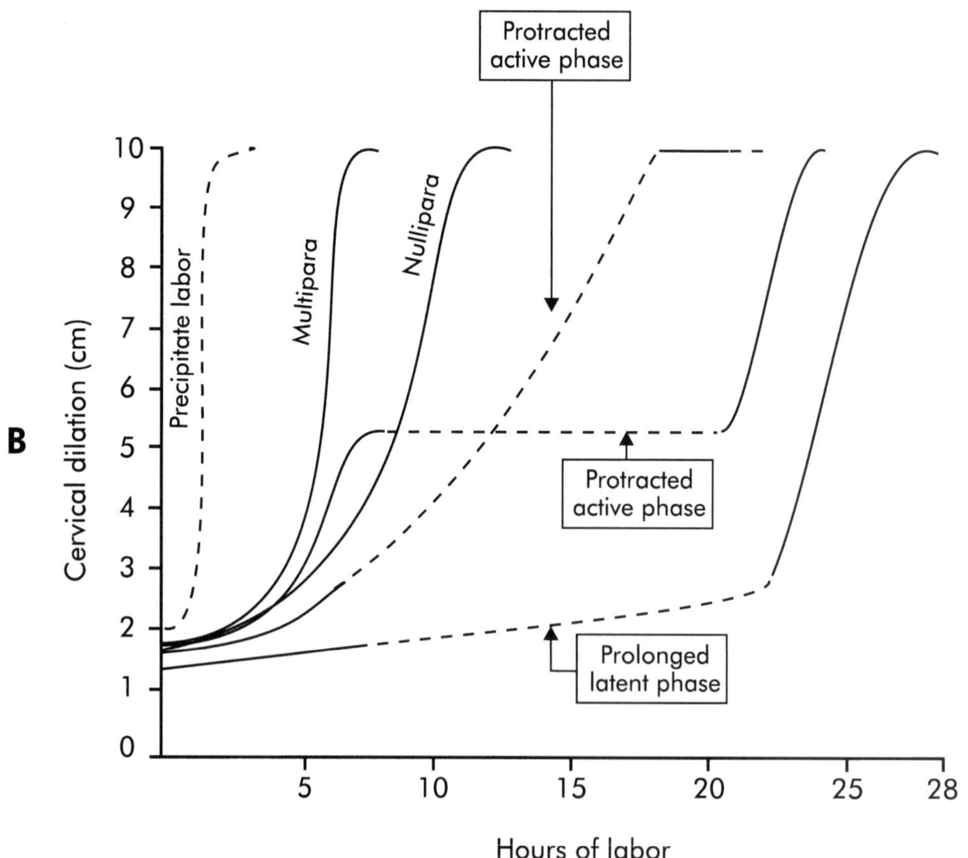

Figure 8-1. A. Partogram of a normal labor. **B.** Major types of deviation from normal progress of labor may be detected by noting dilation of cervix at various intervals after labor begins. If a woman exhibits an abnormal labor pattern, as depicted by broken lines, physician should be notified immediately.

From Bobak, I.M., & Jensen, M.D. (1991). Essentials of Maternity nursing (pp. 765). St. Louis, MO: Mosby-Year Book. Copyright 1991 by Mosby-Year Book. Reprinted with permission.

College of Obstetricians and Gynecologists [NAACOG], 1991), and *Didactic Content and Clinical Skills Verification for Professional Nurse Providers of Basic, High- Risk, and Critical-Care Intrapartum Nursing* (Association of Women's Health, Obstetric, and Neonatal Nurses [AWHONN], 1993). *Guidelines for Perinatal Care* (American Academy of Pediatrics & American College of Obstetricians and Gynecologists, [AAP & ACOG], 1992), Fetal Heart Rate Patterns: Monitoring, Interpretation, and Management (ACOG, 1995) maternity nursing textbooks, and some state board of health publications are other resources that provide guidelines for nursing assessments of women in labor. Based on these guidelines, each perinatal center develops standards of care related to maternal/fetal assessment. See Display 8-3 for suggested guidelines for maternal and fetal assessment during a normal, uncomplicated labor. While most providers choose continuous or intermittent EFM, institution policy should include guidelines for intermittent auscultation if electronic monitoring is unavailable or is not the preference of the patient, physician, or nurse-midwife.

Leopold maneuvers provide a systematic assessment of fetal position and presentation and thus should be performed prior to application of EFM, as part of the admission assessment. Information obtained while performing these maneuvers supports assessments made during vaginal examinations and assists in determining the best position to locate the fetal heart rate (Figure 8-2). Leopold maneuvers may be difficult with women who are obese, have tense or guarded abdominal muscles, or have polyhydramnios. In these situations an ultrasound may be necessary to determine fetal position and presentation.

Nurses should develop proficiency in performing vaginal examinations to assess labor progress. They must first be able to identify situations in which a vaginal examination is required and also recognize when a vaginal examination is contraindicated such as with unexplained vaginal bleeding or with premature rupture of the membranes. Developing clinical proficiency in performing vaginal examinations requires practice and assistance from a knowledgeable preceptor. Women undergoing a vaginal examination should be minimally exposed and advised of the necessity of the examination and the findings. The woman should also be positioned on her back with her head slightly elevated. The vaginal examination should be systematic, beginning with assessment of dilation and effacement, then fetal presentation, station, and position. The normal length of the pregravid cervix is 3.5–4 cm. The length of the cervix may vary in women who have had any cervical surgery such as conization or laser excision procedures. Assessment of station and position of the fetal head requires more skill. The ischial spines must be identified to assess station in relation to the biparietal diameter of the fetal head. The ischial spines may be identified by pressing in the sidewall of the vagina approximately one inch, with the examining fingers at approximately 3 and 9 o'clock, respectively. It is not necessary to identify both spines to assess station. The occiput of the fetal head should be at the level of the ischial spines, to be engaged or zero station. The examiner should not be confused by caput formation but instead identify the fetal skull for this assessment. The most difficult determination to make is that of fetal head position: occiput anterior or posterior. The examining nurse must be familiar with the location of the suture lines in the fetal skull more so than the shape of the anterior or posterior fontanelle since distortion or overlapping bones will alter fontanelle shape. The nurse should first identify the sagittal suture and then slide fingers to a fontanelle and count the number of suture lines extending from it exclusive of the sagittal suture. This can be accomplished by sweeping the examining finger 180° at a right angle to the sagittal suture. The anterior fontanelle has three suture lines extending from it and the posterior fontanelle has two suture lines. It is not necessary to palpate the posterior fontanelle to determine position of the fetal head. Determination of the position of the fetal head becomes necessary primarily during second stage when descent is slow. Repositioning the woman to a squatting or side-lying position to push may facilitate rotation of the fetal head.

Positioning

Culture often determines the position women assume during labor and childbirth, such as squatting, sitting, standing, kneeling, or on all fours (Engleman, 1884; Liu, 1989). Recumbency, a Western cultural tradition for the convenience of obstetricians, began when more women were hospitalized for childbirth. This practice gained favor with nurses with the advent of monitoring technology. Even today, maternal position during labor and birth remains controversial and is surrounded by myths. Myths such as, "she's not progressing so keep her in bed and monitor," "she's posterior, put her on her left side," "there's nothing you can do,

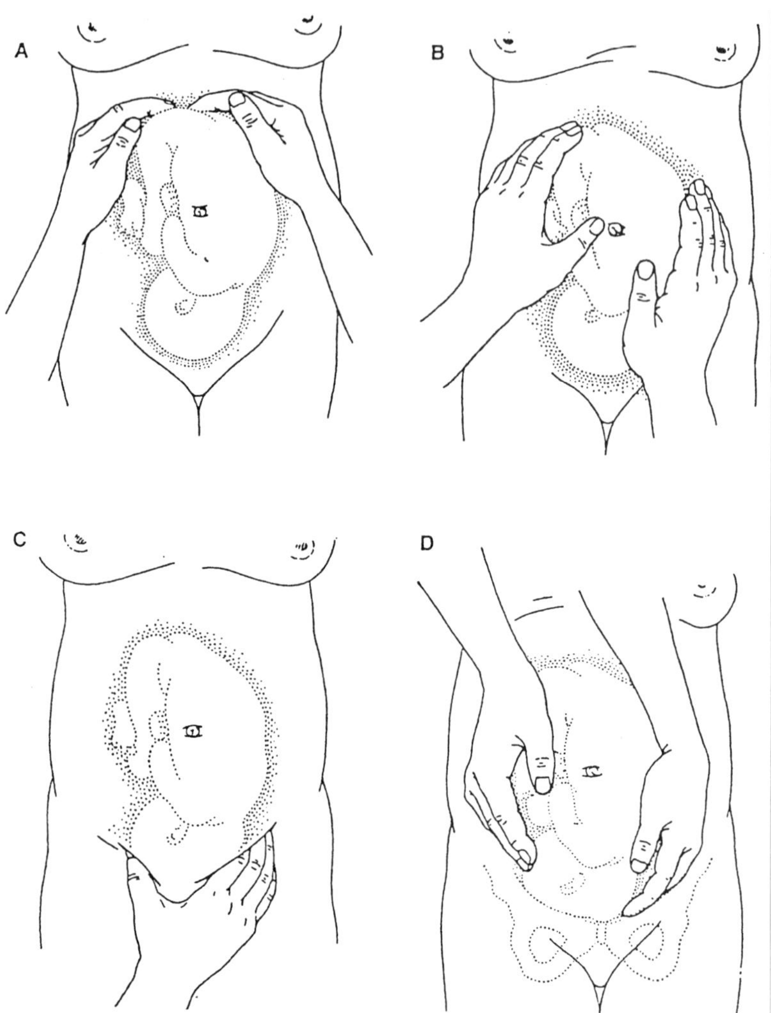

Figure 8-2. Leopold Maneuvers. **A**, First maneuver helps determine fetal presentation or the part of the fetus presenting at the inlet of the pelvis; usually presentations are head or breech. The examiner faces the woman's head and uses the tips of the fingers to palpate the fundus of the uterus. The fetal head feels smooth, globular, and firm and is mobile and ballotts. However, breech presentation feels irregular, rounded, and soft and is less mobile. **B**, Second maneuver helps to determine fetal position or identifies the relationship of the fetal back and small parts to the front, back, or sides of the maternal pelvis. The examiner continues to face the woman's head and places hands on either side of the uterus. While one hand stabilizes one side of the uterus, the other hand palpates the opposite side of the uterus to determine fetal back or small parts. Then the other side of the uterus is stabilized and palpated to locate the fetal back. The back is a long, smooth, hard plane. The small parts feel irregular and knobby and may be moving. **C**, Third maneuver helps to determine presenting part. While continuing to face the woman's head, the examiner uses the thumb and fingers of one hand to grasp the woman's lower abdomen just about the symphysis pubis and notes the contour, size, and consistency of the presenting part. The head feels firm and globular and is mobile if unengaged and immobile if engaged. A breech presentation feels smaller, softer, and irregular. **D**, Fourth maneuver helps to determine fetal attitude or the greatest prominence of the fetal head over the brim of the pelvis. The examiner faces the woman's feet and, using the tips of the first three fingers of each hand, presses deep in the direction of the pelvic inlet. The fingers of one hand will encounter a bony cephalic prominence. If the cephalic prominence is located on the opposite side from the back, it is the infant's brow, and the head is flexed. If the cephalic prominence is located on the same side as the back, it is the occiput, and the head is extended.

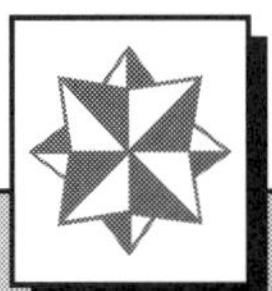

Display 8-3

Maternal-Fetal Assessments During Labor

Maternal Vital Signs

Assess temperature and pulse every 4 hours or more often if indicated (AAP & ACOG, 1992).

Assess blood pressure regularly (AAP & ACOG, 1992).

During oxytocin induction/augmentation, at a minimum, assess blood pressure before every dosage increase (AWHONN, 1993a).

Fetal Heart Rate

The intensity of FHR monitoring used during labor should be based on risk factors. When risk factors are present, the FHR should be assessed according to the following guidelines:

"During the active phase of the first stage of labor: If auscultation is used, the FHR should be evaluated and recorded at least every 15 minutes after a uterine contraction. If continuous electronic monitoring is used, the tracing should be evaluated every 15 minutes."

"During the second stage of labor: With auscultation, the FHR should be evaluated and recorded at least every 5 minutes. When electronic monitoring is used, the FHR should also be evaluated at least every 5 minutes."

"In the absence of risk factors, the standard practice is to evaluate and record the FHR at least every 30 minutes during the active phase of the first stage of labor and at least every 15 minutes during the second stage of labor."

(ACOG, 1995, pp. 2–3)

During oxytocin induction/augmentation, at a minimum, assess the FHR before every dosage increase (AWHONN, 1993a).

Uterine Activity/Labor Progress

Assess frequency, duration, and quality of uterine contractions regularly (AAP & ACOG, 1992).

During oxytocin induction/augmentation, at a minimum, assess uterine contractions before every dosage increase (AWHONN, 1993a).

Vaginal examinations should be kept to the minimum necessary to adequately monitor the progress of labor (AAP & ACOG, 1992) and should include assessment of dilation and effacement of the cervix, and station of the fetal presenting part (AWHONN, 1993b).

Additional Parameters

Assess maternal bladder status and encourage to void at least every 3 hours (AAP & ACOG, 1992).

Assess character and amount of amniotic fluid (AWHONN, 1993b).

Assess character and amount of bloody show/vaginal bleeding (AWHONN, 1993b).

Record intake and output (AAP & ACOG, 1992).

Assess maternal affect and response to labor (AWHONN, 1993b).

Assess level of maternal discomfort and effectiveness of pain management/pain relief measures (AWHONN, 1993b).

Assess labor support persons' abilities (AWHONN, 1993b).

When determining frequency of maternal-fetal assessments during labor, factors such as stage of labor, maternal-fetal risk status, and institutional policies, procedures, and protocols should be taken into consideration (AWHONN, 1993a). Collaboration between perinatal care providers and review of current published guidelines as outlined above can facilitate development of institutional guidelines for practice.

Simpson, K.R. (1996).

she'll be delivered by cesarean section for maternal distress," and "she doesn't know the best position," still prevail (Biancuzzo, 1993). Indeed, early medical research challenging the recumbent position was ignored (Mengert & Murphy, 1933; Vaughn, 1937). Recent research confirms that an upright position shortens labor. Duration of both first and second stage labor are shorter in women who labor 30° upright as compared to those in a flat recumbent position (Liu). Squatting births have shorter second stage labor (primiparas, 23 minutes; multiparas, 13 minutes), less oxytocin, fewer mechanically assisted births, and fewer and less-severe lacerations and episiotomies compared to semirecumbent births (Golay, Vedam, & Sorger, 1993). Women are often assisted to hands-and-knees position for certain nonreassuring fetal heart rate patterns but returned to a more standard position for birth. Last-minute change of maternal position for birth may be unwarranted because birth may be just as easily accomplished in hands-and-knees position (Gannon, 1992). Figure 8-3 and Figure 8-4 depict positions for labor and birth.

Pushing

Second stage of labor begins when the cervix is completely dilated. However, women often begin to have an involuntary urge to push prior to complete cervical dilation. This urge to push is triggered by the Ferguson reflex as the presenting fetal part stretches pelvic floor muscles. Stretch receptors are then activated releasing endogenous oxytocin, supporting the hypotheses that the urge to push is dependent more on station than dilation (Cosner & deJong, 1993; Noble, 1981). Women report well-defined urges to push which occur before, at, and after complete dilation (McKay, Barrows, & Roberts, 1990). These findings suggest that "when to push" should be individualized to maternal response rather than labor routines that dictate pushing at complete dilation.

There are generally two approaches to coaching women during second stage of labor. The traditional approach most prevalent in current nursing practice is to begin pushing and bearing-down instructions at complete dilation whether or not the woman feels the urge to push. In contrast, physiologic second-stage (PSS) management asserts that the second stage of labor is a normal physiological event that helps women push spontaneously and deliver with minimal intervention (Cosner & deJong, 1993). Women who deliver in an upright position without bearing-down instructions have a shorter labor, compared with women who receive routine bearing-down instructions in upright (26.4 minutes shorter) and recumbent (48.2 minutes shorter) positions (Liu, 1989). Women do, however, prefer assistance with breathing, relaxation, pushing techniques, and imagery (McKay & Smith, 1993). However, confusion can occur if several caregivers' pushing directions are different or at odds with body sensations (McKay & Smith, 1983). Individualized, consistent coaching (in coordination with the woman's expulsive efforts) that provides necessary instructions, support, and encouragement is important. Figure 8-5 provides an algorithm for PPS management.

Controversy exists between open–versus closed-glottis pushing. When the woman takes a deep breath and holds it (closed glottis), the Valsalva maneuver is instituted. This technique increases intrathoracic pressure, impairs blood return from lower extremities, and initially increases and then decreases blood pressure, resulting in a decrease in uteroplacental blood flow. In the newborn, hypoxemia, acidemia, and lower Apgar scores may result. Sustained pushing of 9–15 seconds can result in significant decelerations in the fetal heart rate (Caldeyro-Barcia et al., 1981). With involuntary pushing, women were observed to hold their breath for 6 seconds while bearing down, and took several breaths in between bearing-down efforts (Roberts, Goldstein, Gruener, Maggio, & Mendez-Bauer, 1985). This is in contrast to the traditional second-stage coaching instructions that encourage holding breath for 10 seconds while bearing down and allowing only one quick breath between pushes. Open-glottis or gentle pushing avoids fetal stress, has less impact on uteroplacental blood flow, allows for perineal relaxation, and is more natural physiologically (McKay & Roberts, 1985). The woman is more in control and responding to her body's own pushing cues, enhancing maternal confidence and satisfaction with the birth experience.

Fundal Pressure

Although fundal pressure is often used to decrease the second stage of labor in many institutions, intensity of the legal climate and the focus on published standards of care have caused nurses to scrutinize this clinical technique (Kline-Kaye & Miller-Slade, 1990). Correct procedure for applying fundal pressure is not taught; there are no legal or professional practice guidelines or standards; and the procedure is often not

Figure 8-3. Physiologic Positions for Labor

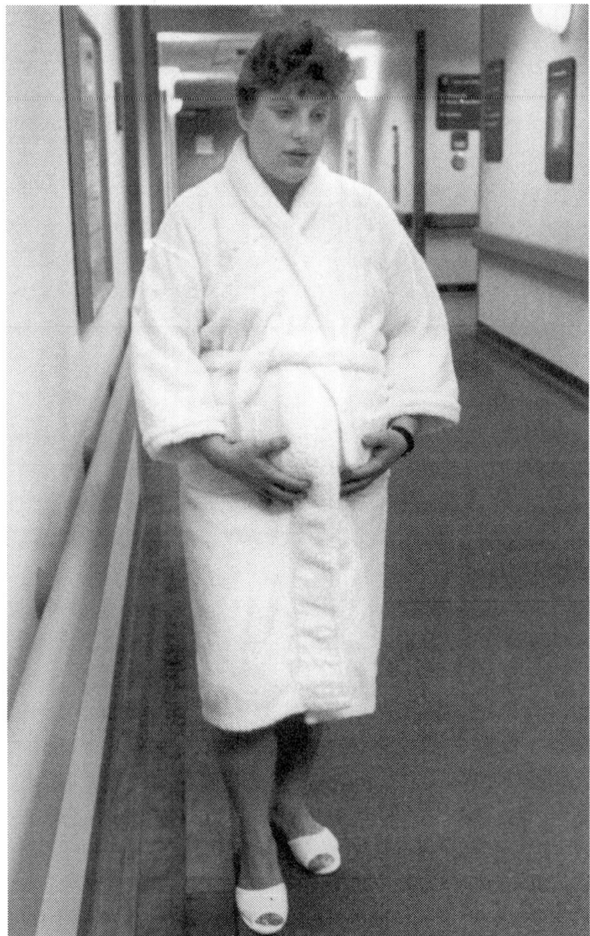

A. Walking

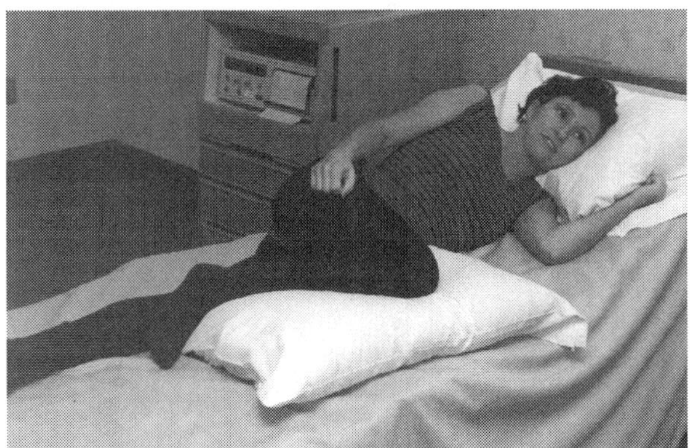

B. Sidelying with pillow support

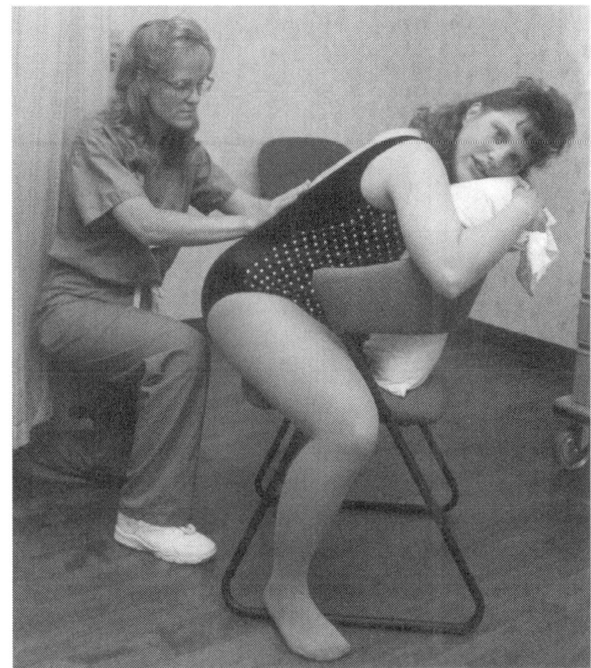

C. Sitting, leaning forward with pillow support

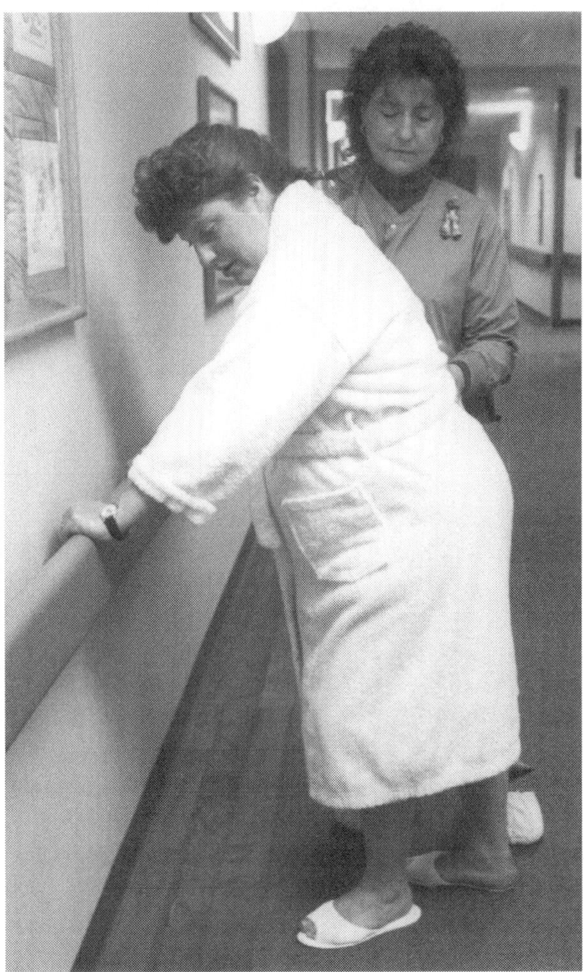

D. Standing, leaning forward

Figure 8-3 (cont.).

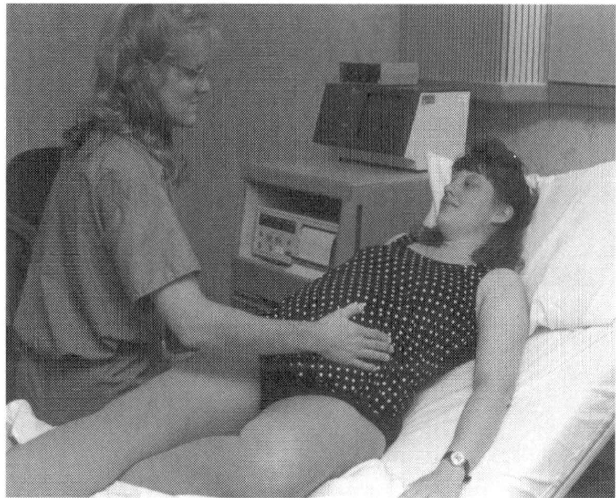

E. Reclining, head of bed elevated

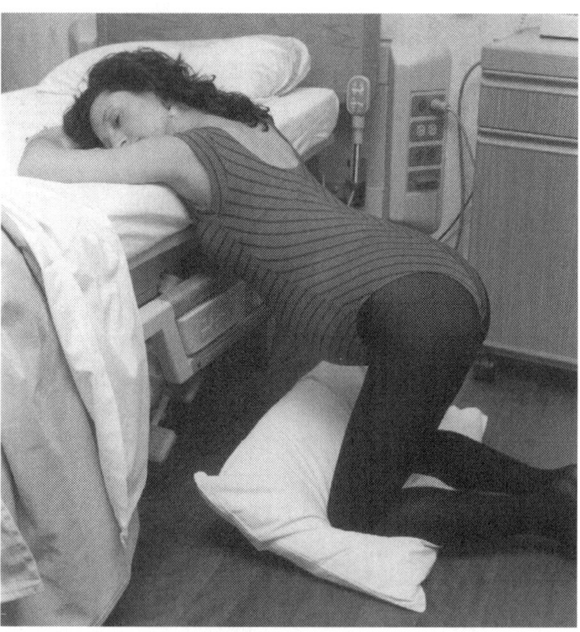

F. Kneeling, chest supported

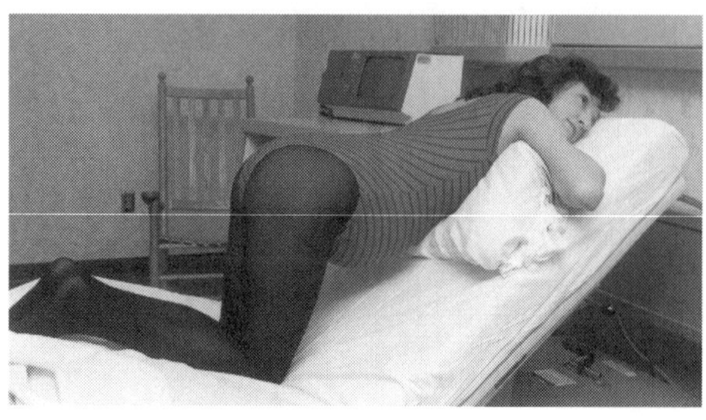

G. Kneeling, chest supported

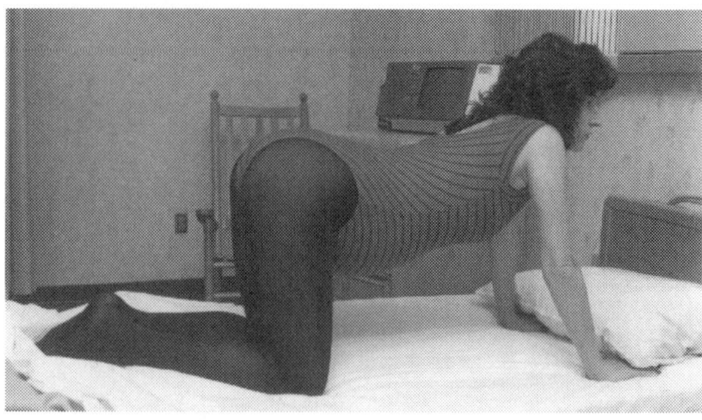

H. Hands and knees

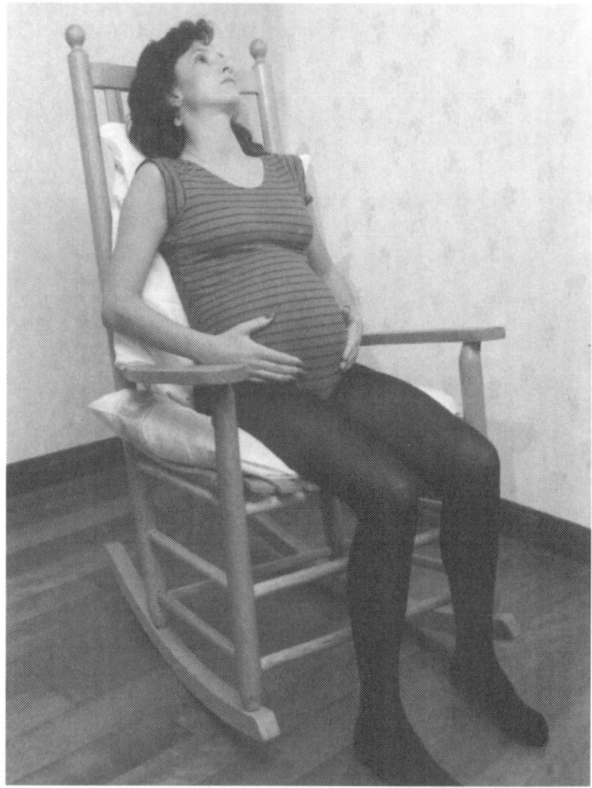

I. Rocking

Figure 8-4. Physiologic Positions for Birth

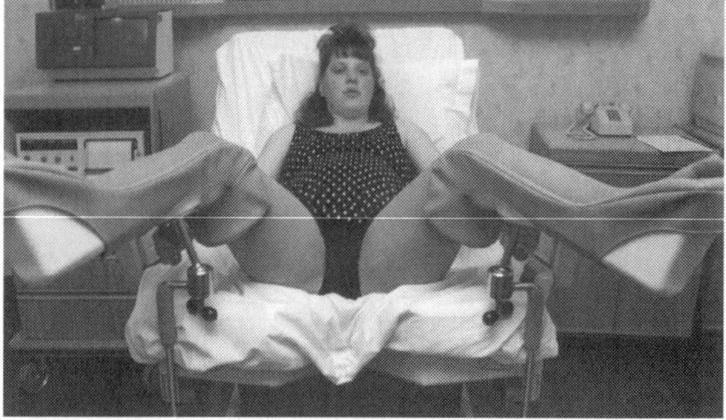

A. Semisitting, stirrup leg supports

Figure 8-4 (cont.)

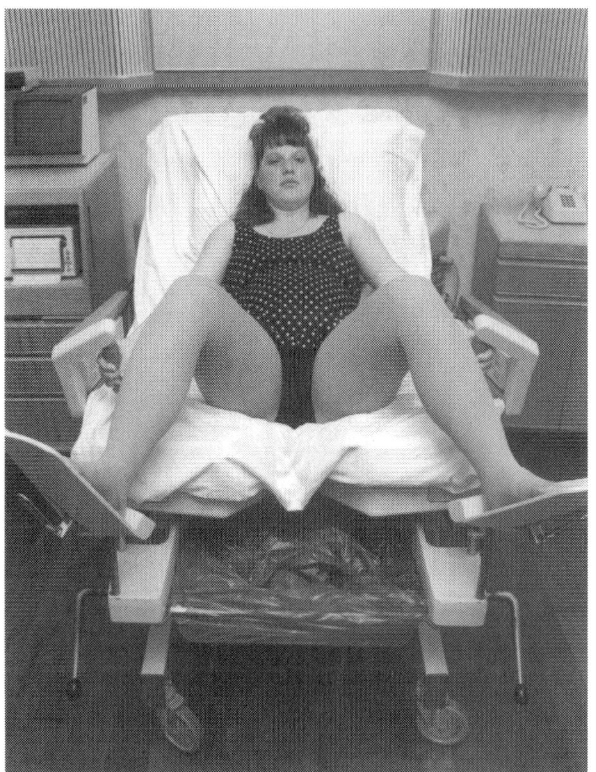

B. Semisitting, feet supported

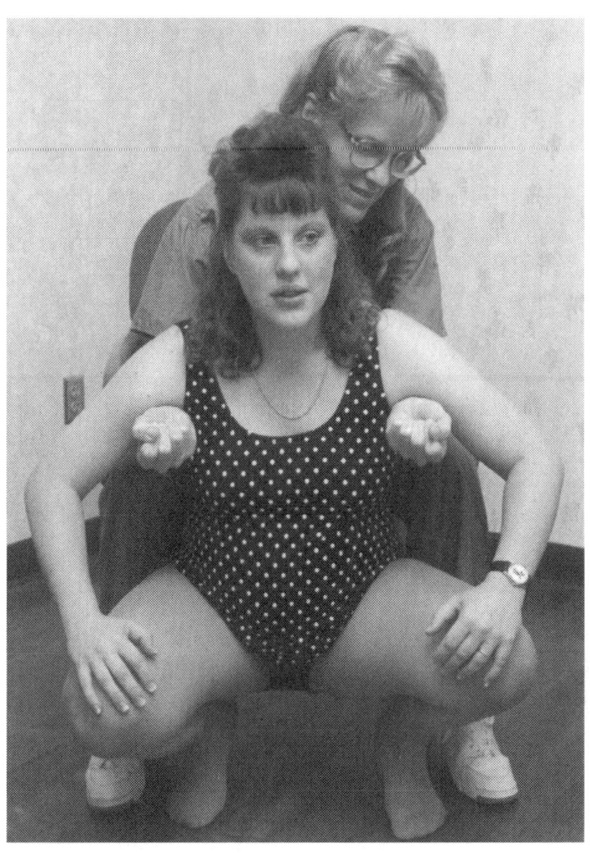

D. Squatting with support

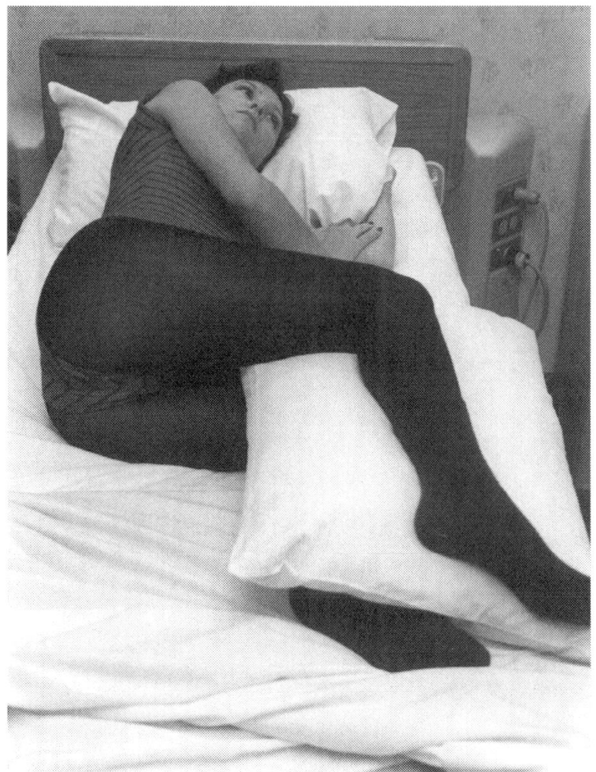

C. Side lying

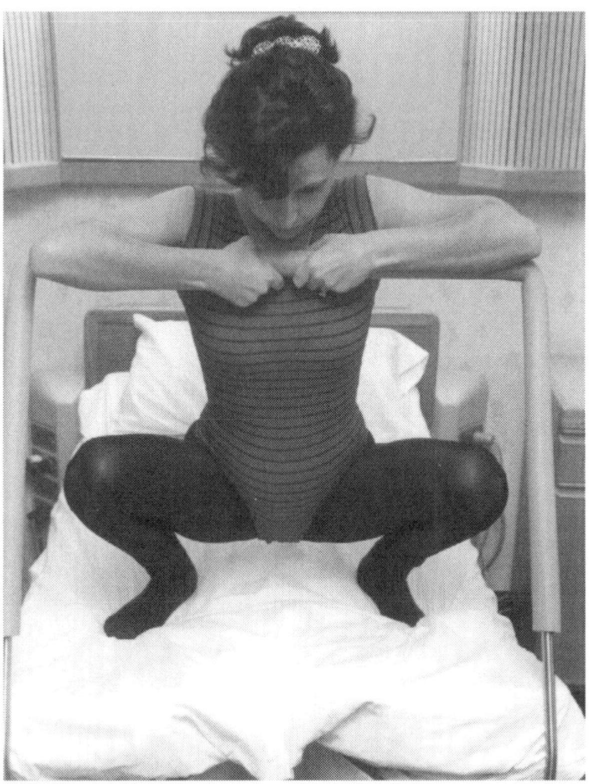

E. Squatting with support bar

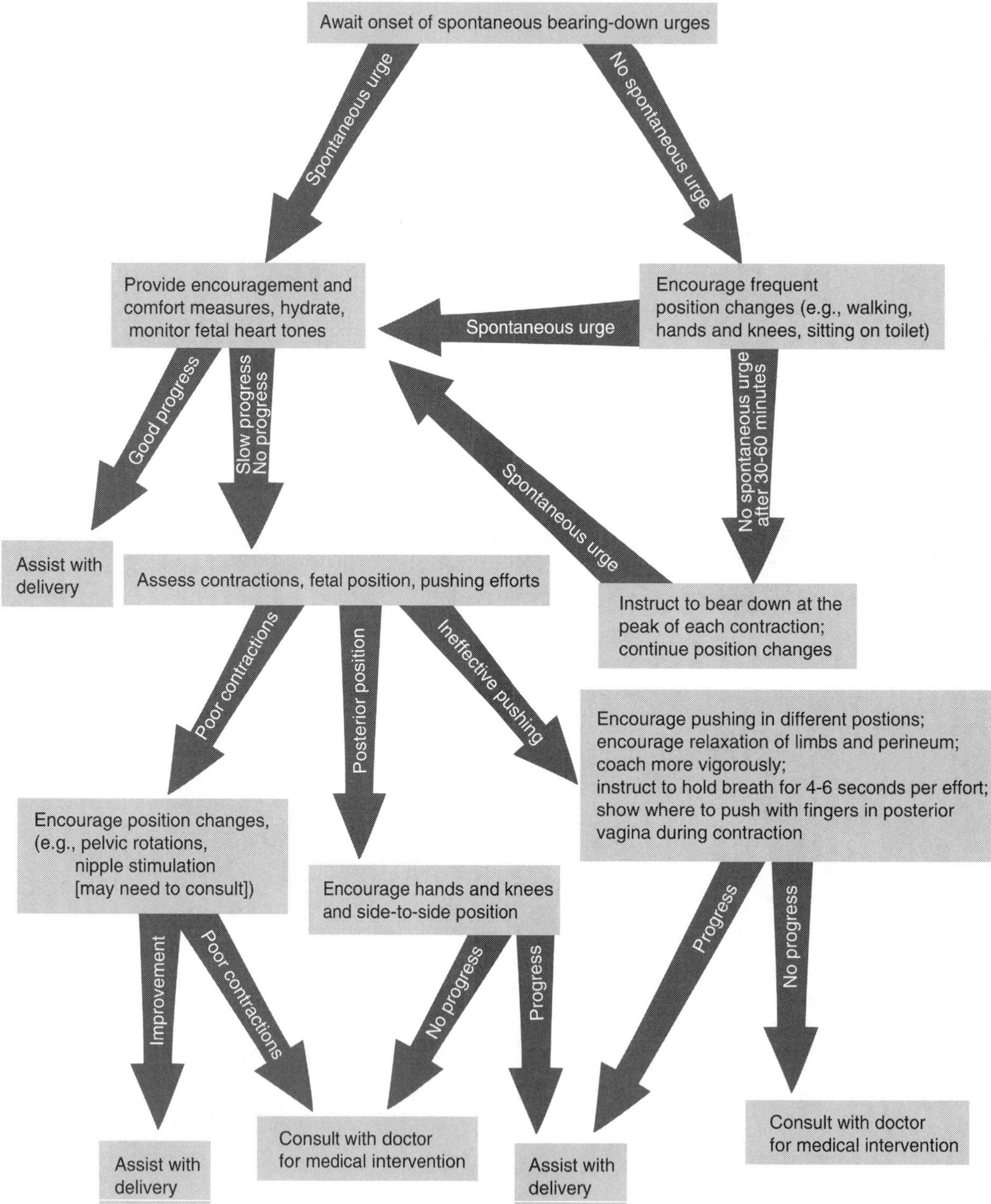

Figure 8-5.

From: Cosner, K.R., & deJong, E. (1993). Physiologic second-stage labor. Maternal Child Nursing, 18(1), 41.

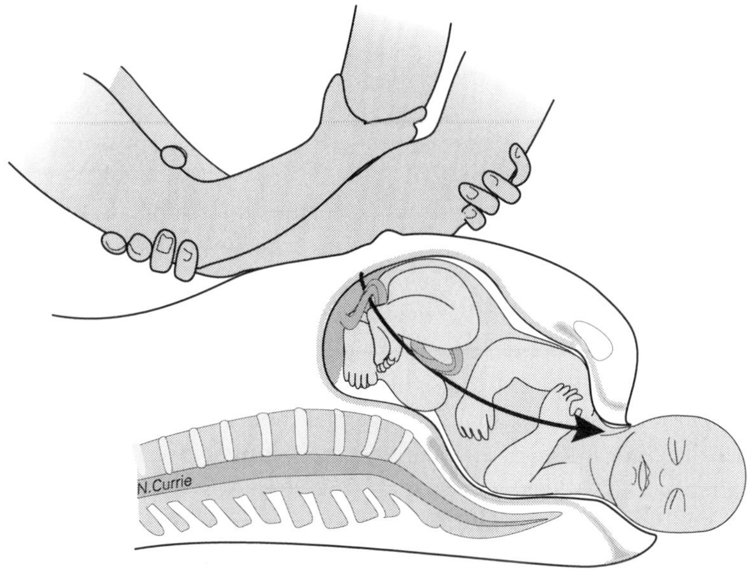

Figure 8-6. Nurse–assisted fundal pressure

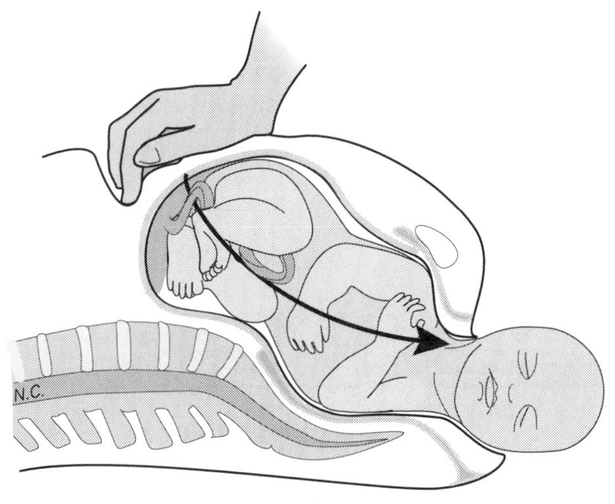

Figure 8-7. Fundal pressure

From Penney, D.S., & Perlis, D.W. (1992). When to use suprapubic or fundal pressure. American Journal of Maternal Child Nursing, 17, 34-36.

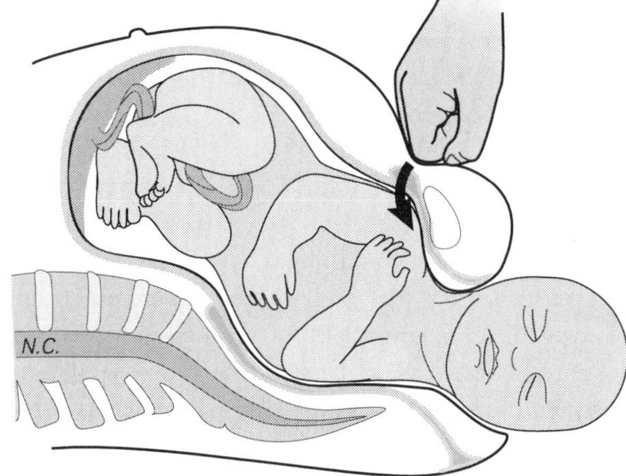

Figure 8-8. Suprapubic pressure

From Penney, D.S., & Perlis, D.W. (1992). When to use suprapubic or fundal pressure. American Journal of Maternal Child Nursing, 17, 34-36.

recorded, yet "the technique continues to be passed from generation to generation of healthcare professionals" (Kline-Kay & Miller-Slade, 1990). Examples of correct technique to apply fundal pressure in a longitudinal direction are shown in Figure 8-6 and Figure 8-7. When fundal pressure is applied, care should be taken to avoid perpendicular techniques, which result in direct vena caval compression. In the instance of shoulder dystocia, suprapubic pressure applied behind the pubic bone and under the symphysis (Figure 8-8) will relieve the impacted shoulder better than fundal pressure (Penney & Perlis, 1992). In fact, fundal pressure applied with a shoulder dystocia can further impact the fetal shoulder, resulting in an inability to deliver the fetal body. A knee-chest position while supine (McRoberts maneuver) has been found to reduce potential complications of shoulder dystocia, such as fetal clavicle fractures and brachial plexus stretching, without increasing maternal complications (Gonik, Stringer, & Held, 1983). The McRoberts maneuver may be accomplished by the mother, with assistance, and should be attempted prior to using any fundal pressure technique for the relief of shoulder dystocia (Figure 8-9). The supine knee-chest position may facilitate delivery without the use of invasive maneuvers that carry risks for the mother and fetus. Need for fundal pressure has not been well documented and efficacy of the procedure has not been proven. In some situations, use of fundal pressure may prove to be more detrimental to the fetus, limiting clinical usefulness of this technique. Excessive fundal pressure should be avoided. The perinatal nurse has the right to refuse to participate in fundal pressure application if uncomfortable with the clinical situation. In this case, institutional chain of command is the most appropriate process to resolve disputes among healthcare providers. Ideally, there is an understanding or written protocol related to the nurses' role in fundal-pressure application in each labor and delivery unit.

Episiotomy and Nursing Role

Episiotomy is an incision median or mediolateral into the perineum to permit easier passage of the baby. Advantages are that it (1) prevents perineal tearing; (2) is easier to repair, some believe; (3) reduces time and stress of second stage of labor; (4) relieves compression of fetal head, especially in premature birth; and (5) facilitates breech or forceps birth. Episiotomy is indicated when lacerations of the perineum, vagina, cervix, or (rarely) the body of the uterus may occur during birth (Cunningham, MacDonald, Leveno, Gant, Gilstrap, 1993). Lacerations of the vagina and perineum are classified according to degree as listed in Display 8-4. Episiotomy is not routinely required but should not be routinely avoided and is usually done when laceration is inevitable (Zlatnik, 1994).

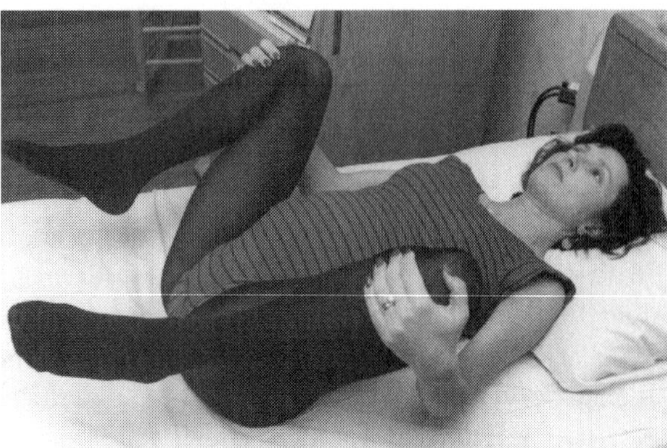

Figure 8-9. McRoberts maneuver to facilitate birth with shoulder dystocia.

However, episiotomy often results in more pain and potential for infection. Women without episiotomies have significantly better perineal healing than women with episiotomies (McGuinness, Norr, & Nacion, 1991). Upright position and open-glottis, gentle pushing with natural urges and sensations may aid perineal stretching, thus avoiding episiotomy. Women in lithotomy position are more likely to have an episiotomy than women in squatting, hands-and-knees, standing, or sitting positions (Rooks, Weatherby, & Ernst, 1992).

Other measures to enhance perineal stretching are the application of warm compresses, perineal massage, and warm oil perineal massage during the second stage of labor. Warm compresses and perineal massage are thought to soften and stretch perineal muscles. Perineal massage may reduce the rate of episiotomies (Avery & Burkett, 1986; Avery & Van Arsdale, 1987). However, in one study, women who were taught perineal massage reported pain, discomfort, irritation, fatigue, uneasiness with the concept, and negative physician comments (Mynaugh, 1991). More research is needed to determine whether perineal massage is effective in avoiding episiotomy or reducing the extent of lacerations. Intrapartum nurses are in a unique position to initiate and participate in this type of research.

DISPLAY 8-4

Perineal Lacerations

Type of Laceration	Involvement
First Degree	Perineal skin and vaginal mucous membrane
Second Degree	Skin and mucous membrane plus fascia and muscle of perineum
Third Degree	Skin, mucous membrane, muscle of perineum; extends into rectal sphincter
Fourth Degree	Extends into rectal mucosa to expose lumen of rectum

EMOTIONAL SUPPORT DURING LABOR AND BIRTH

Impact of the Psyche on Childbirth

The psyche plays a major role in the process of labor and birth. A high level of anxiety has been associated with decreased uterine activity and with longer and dysfunctional labor (Pernoll, 1991). Anxiety, uncertainty, loss of control, self-confidence, patterns of coping, support systems, fatigue, optimism, fatalism, and aloneness are some of the psychosocial factors to consider when caring for a women in labor. Previous birth experiences, present support systems, concerns/questions, anxiety or fear, and cultural considerations further contribute to attitudes and expectations for the current pregnancy experience.

Women with a history of sexual abuse have unique needs during the intrapartum period. Not all women report or remember sexual abuse. Sensations of labor and birth can mimic physical experiences of the abuse and sometimes cause flashbacks and extreme anxiety. Lack of control and lack of choice are the similarities between sexual trauma and gynecologic procedures (Chalfen, 1993). Pelvic examinations may evoke feelings of depersonalization and powerlessness (Kitzinger, 1990). Nurses caring for women with a history of sexual abuse should have a heightened awareness of potential behavior during labor. The woman may choose to discuss her history of sexual abuse with the nurse. This type of acknowledgement may be a sign of healing and indicate that the woman believes her feelings will be taken seriously (Chalfen). Not all women will be able to share the history of abuse with the nurse but may exhibit difficulty and anxiety during with pelvic examination. This behavior is a sign of possible previous sexual trauma requiring further exploration. Nurses should help the woman feel empowered to make choices about labor and birth by assuring the woman that she is in control and her wishes will be respected. Thorough explanations of all procedures and treatment should be provided and permission obtained before touching the woman. Minimal exposure and talking to the patient during a pelvic examination is vital. Examinations should not be forced. If the woman has not had counseling or is not presently in counseling, a referral would be appropriate; women who have been abused need ongoing support.

Fewer perinatal complications, fewer newborns admitted to the neonatal intensive care nursery, and shorter labors result when women have a support person as compared to women without support (Klaus, Kennel, Robertson, & Sosa, 1986; Norbeck & Anderson, 1989; Pascoe, 1993). Presence of a support person has also been found to reduce the rate of cesarean births (Klaus, Kennel, McGrath, Robertson, & Hinkley 1988, 1991). There is adequate research to validate significance of promoting support from family members/coach during the labor and birth experience.

Sibling presence during labor and birth also presents a unique opportunity for nurses to promote family attachment. Parents report that children present at labor and birth show a greater number of mothering and caretaking behaviors than did children not present (DelGiudice, 1986). Sibling classes to prepare children for the birth experience are imperative. These classes should be age related and include films on childbirth, discussion of maternal behavior and sounds in labor, and reassurance that pain experienced by the mother is temporary. Additionally, each child needs a support person to accompany the child and be familiar with the child's developmental level, so that both the child's curiosity and concerns for his/her mother and new brother/sister are answered.

Supporting Family Attachment

As the family is introduced to their newborn immediately at birth, explanation of umbilical cord clamping/cutting and inspection of the placenta help the family understand the final physiological separation of the newborn from the mother's life-support system. After stabilization, the nurse can unwrap the newborn and describe normal physical characteristics. Siblings can count fingers and toes. Encouraging interaction with the newborn sets the stage for successful attachment and integration into the family unit. All family members can hold the newborn after birth as desired, and opportunities for photographs should be provided.

Clinical Interventions for Laboring Women

The majority of labors are normal, requiring little or no intervention. However, some women require clinical interventions to optimize outcomes in pregnancies with identified maternal or fetal risk factors. It is important to remember that risk status for the woman and fetus may increase at any time during the pregnancy, labor and birth, or postpartum period. Nurses in perinatal settings must be able to quickly assess and identify changes in maternal-fetal status and adjust nursing care accordingly. For example, nursing management during labor may require intrauterine resuscitation techniques, when a nonreassuring fetal heart rate is noted, such as maternal position changes, intravenous fluids, oxygen administration, and discontinuation of oxytocin if infusing. Knowledge of appropriate nursing interventions for common maternal-fetal complications during labor is essential. The nurse must also be aware of changes in maternal-fetal status requiring physician or nurse midwife notification. The next section focuses on the clinical interventions of cervical ripening, induction and augmentation, assisted deliveries, and amnioinfusion. Implications for nursing care are presented with key points for assessment.

CERVICAL RIPENING

In some instances the cervix is not favorable when labor induction is indicated. In those cases the healthcare provider may improve the cervical readiness by using mechanical or pharmacologic methods of cervical ripening.

Mechanical Methods

Hygroscopic Dilator

Laminaria tents are stems of desiccated cold water seaweed that are sterile and are available in various sizes. When placed in the endocervix for 6–12 hours, laminaria increases in diameter by threefold to fourfold via water extraction (Trofatter, 1992). Cervical change is produced slowly. When cervical dilation is deemed adequate, the tents should be removed and induction by oxytocin infusion begun. The outpatient use of laminaria is currently under investigation and may prove to be successful, safe, and more cost effective.

Synthetic hygroscopic dilators have recently become available. Like laminaria, synthetic hygroscopic dilators come in a variety of sizes. The synthetic dilators enlarge much more rapidly (2–4 hours) and also work by water extraction. Serial applications within a 24-hour period to reach the desired cervical readiness may be required. Both synthetic dilators and laminaria have proven to be relatively inexpensive, safe to use, and effective in producing cervical dilation and softening. The Food and Drug Administration (FDA) has approved the use of hygroscopic dilators for pregnancy termination but not for preinduction cervical ripening. Both laminaria tents and synthetic hygroscopic dilators are nontoxic and can be used in pregnant women who have contraindications to the use of prostaglandins.

Stripping of the Amniotic Membranes

Separating the membranes from the lower uterine segment digitally has been used with some success to ripen the cervix and stimulate labor. Stripping of the membranes has been most successful in patients who are multiparous, with a well-applied vertex, some cervical effacement, and dilation of 1–2 centimeters (AWHONN, 1993). Risks involved with stripping of membranes are bleeding from a low-lying placenta, inadvertent rupture of the membranes with possible cord prolapse, and infectious morbidity (Trofatter, 1992). Many perinatal healthcare providers have abandoned use of membrane stripping, due to possible complications as well as patient discomfort.

Pharmacologic Methods

Prostaglandin Gel

Physicians and midwives have used prostaglandin E_2 gel preparations for preinduction cervical ripening with varying success for many years. These mixtures lacked consistent distribution, were possibly unstable, and lacked the bioavailability of the active agent (Trofatter, 1992). A commercially prepared gel became available in 1993 and has become the most widely reported pharmacologic method for cervical ripening (American College of Obstetricians and Gynecologists [ACOG], 1993). The gel is inserted intracervically using direct visualization by sterile speculum examination. Women are usually then monitored for a minimum of 1 hour via continuous EFM or by auscultation and palpation, to detect uterine hyperstimulation, hypertonus, or adverse fetal heart rate changes. Use of prostaglandin gel has not been recommended for outpatient use. Repeated applications at 6-hour intervals may be necessary to achieve the desired cervical ripeness. When cervical readiness is achieved, oxytocin can be administered 6–12 hours after the last gel application (ACOG, 1993). Specific protocols or nursing procedures for care of patients undergoing prostaglandin gel cervical ripening should include the following: (1) requiring the ready availability of a physician who is capable of performing a cesarean birth; (2) stipulating that administration only occur in a hospital setting; (3) exercising caution when administering gel to patients with a history of asthma, glaucoma, or pulmonary, hepatic, or renal disease; (4)

administering gel to patients who have a medical indication for induction and no contraindications; and (5) establishing intravenous access. Research is in progress to determine if prostaglandin gel can be safely used in the outpatient setting. If clinical studies demonstrate low risk of adverse outcomes after a specified period of observation following prostaglandin gel application has provided evidences of maternal–fetal wellbeing, women may be discharged home to wait for labor onset or scheduled to return the next day for oxytocin induction. Other pharmacologic agents for cervical ripening under investigation are estradiol cream and misoprostol.

Low-Dose Oxytocin Infusion

Low-dose oxytocin infusion has been used to produce cervical ripening without much success. A starting dose of 0.5 mU/min with hourly increases of 1 mU/min to a maximum of 4 mU/min is one such protocol (AWHONN, 1993). There is no published research to determine if complications associated with prolonged oxytocin use, such as water intoxication and fetal hyperbilirubinemia, are increased in patients who have had prolonged low-dose oxytocin infusions.

INDUCTION OF LABOR

Induction of labor refers to measures to initiate contractions prior to onset of spontaneous labor. Induction of labor may be indicated for fetal or maternal reasons. Display 8-5 lists maternal and fetal reasons for labor induction and absolute and relative contraindications. Because of potential risks involved, induction of labor without a medical indication is considered elective and should be avoided (ACOG, 1991).

Cervical status and fetal position should be evaluated immediately prior to induction (AAP & ACOG, 1992). Induction success may then be predicted using the Bishop scoring system for assessing readiness for induction. Table 8-2 lists the five parameters to assess prior to induction and the associated scores. A high probability of successful labor induction can be predicted with a total score of greater than six. Not all institutions require nurses to obtain and document a Bishop score prior to the initiation of induction nor is it a practice standard; however, this assessment is useful to provide anticipatory guidance to the woman experiencing induction.

Amniotomy

Amniotomy, or artificial rupture of the membranes, has been used effectively for labor induction in selected patients. Amniotomy, as a method of labor induction, usually initiates labor within 12 hours of rupture in near-term, parous patients with favorable cervices. If amniotomy does not result in labor within 12 hours, then an oxytocin infusion is started. Risks are involved with rupturing membranes prior to the onset of labor, so an amniotomy should be performed only in a labor and delivery area capable of emergency delivery. The presenting part should be low enough to avoid prolapse of the umbilical cord. Risk of developing chorioamnionitis or intraamniotic infection is increased with prolonged rupture of the membranes. After the membranes are ruptured, the woman should be observed for signs and symptoms of infection such as foul-smelling amniotic fluid, uterine tenderness, increasing white blood count (WBC), fever, and fetal tachycardia. Maternal temperature is usually assessed at least every 2 hours, or more frequently, depending on the clinical situation.

TABLE 8-2. Bishop Score for Assessing Readiness for Induction

	Assigned Value			
Factor	**0**	**1**	**2**	**3**
Cervical dilation	0	1–2 cm	3–4 cm	5 cm or more
Cervical effacement	0–30%	40–50%	60–70%	80% or more
Fetal station	−3	−2	−1,0	+1,+2
Cervical consistency	Firm	Moderate	Soft	
Cervical position	Posterior	Midposition	Anterior	

From Bishop, E.H. (1964). Pelvic scoring for elective induction. Obstetrics and Gyneclogy, 24, 266.

Fetal heart rate is assessed prior to rupture of membranes and immediately afterward via EFM or auscultation. Deceleration of the fetal heart rate may indicate umbilical cord prolapse and warrants an immediate vaginal examination to rule out the possibility. Color, consistency, odor, and amount of amniotic fluid should be noted. Women with polyhydramnios are at risk for placental abruption during amniotomy. Bloody amniotic fluid may be a sign of abruption. If placental abruption is suspected, the woman should be observed for vaginal bleeding, uterine tenderness, and hypertonus. Careful assessment of fetal status is also indicated. Nonreassuring fetal heart rate patterns, such as changes in baseline rate, decelerations, or loss of variability, require notification of the physician or nurse-midwife, intrauterine resuscitation measures, and continued close observation. Amniotic fluid will continue to leak until birth, requiring frequent underpad changes to keep the woman comfortable and dry. Women need to be reassured that continued leakage is expected.

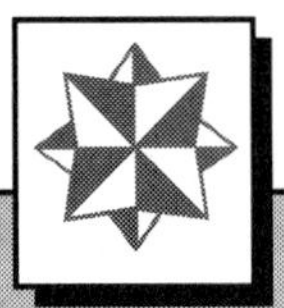

DISPLAY 8-5

Indications for Induction

Maternal	Fetal
Pregnancy induced hypertension/preeclampsia	Macrosomia
Medical illness (e.g., cardiac, pulmonary, diabetes)	Fetal demise
Premature rupture of membranes	Fetal anomaly
Chorioamnionitis/intraamniotic infection	Blood group sensitization
Abruptio placentae	Nonreassuring fetal testing
History of rapid labor	Fetal hydrops
Geographic distance from hospital	Intrauterine growth restriction
	Postdate pregnancy

Contraindications for Induction

Placenta previa or vasa previa
Classical uterine incision
Invasive cervical carcinoma
Nonreassuring fetal status
Abnormal fetal lie
Pelvic abnormalities
Active genital herpes
Absolute cephalopelvic disproportion
Fundal uterine scar

Relative Contraindications for Induction

Grand multiparity
Overdistended uterus
- polyhydramnios
- multiple gestations

Pharmacologic Induction: Oxytocin

Oxytocin is the only pharmacologic agent approved by the FDA for use for induction of labor. It is a synthetic hormone that stimulates uterine contractions by increasing myometrial cell membrane permeability to the sodium ion, thus increasing the number of contracting myofibrils. Uterine responsiveness to oxytocin increases with gestation but may also dramatically increase during labor. Oxytocin enhances cervical ripening indirectly, by stimulating the active syntheses of prostaglandin 15 methyl and $f_{2\alpha}$ in the decidua. It is cleared via the kidney and liver and thus should be given with caution in women with hepatic or renal disease. Oxytocin has an intrinsic antidiuretic effect and changes both maternal and fetal osmotic pressure to sodium ion concentration. It also increases water reabsorption at the glomerular filtrate. Maternal water intoxication and fetal hyperbilirubinemia have been associated with prolonged oxytocin infusions (≥ 24 hrs) at high dosages (≥ 25 mU/min) (Johnson, Aldrich, & Angelus, 1984; Loong, Lao, & Chin, 1988). Using intravenous solutions containing sodium or physiologic electrolyte solutions decreases risk of water intoxication, and fetal hyperbilirubinemia. The nurse should be alert for signs and symptoms of water intoxication, including headache, nausea and vomiting, mental confusion, decreased urinary output, hypotension, tachycardia, and cardiac arrhythmias (Davis, 1992; Pozaic, 1992). Oxytocinase released from the placenta destroys oxytocin, may contribute to its relatively short half-life, and may be an endogenous protective mechanism.

Physiological effects of oxytocin include an initial slight increase in maternal blood pressure, increased cardiac output and stroke volume, and decreased urinary output. Women with cardiac or hypertensive disease are monitored closely for signs and symptoms of decompensation during oxytocin-induced labor. Accurate assessment and documentation of intake and output is essential. The goal is to maintain urinary output of greater than 25 cc per hour. The most common adverse effects produced by oxytocin administration are uterine hyperstimulation and impaired fetal oxygenation. Uterine hyperstimulation is defined as a resting tone of 20 mmHg or greater, more than 5 contractions in 10 minutes, or contraction duration of greater than 90 seconds (Foster, Jacobson, & Valenzuela, 1988). Coupling of contractions is also a sign of hyperstimulation. Hyperstimulation may lead to uteroplacental insufficiency, fetal compromise, uterine rupture, or tumultuous labor with the potential for cervical and/or lower uterine lacerations. Oxytocin should be discontinued if uterine hyperstimulation or a nonreassuring fetal heart rate pattern is noted, and intrauterine resuscitation measures should be instituted.

Oxytocin should be administered intravenously by a controlled infusion device not affected by needle size. A secondary line containing the oxytocin admixture should be piggybacked at the lowest site on the primary line. Both the primary infusion and the oxytocin should be mixed in physiologic electrolyte solutions. Although *Guidelines for Perinatal Care* (AAP & ACOG, 1992) indicates that intermittent auscultation at frequencies prescribed for high-risk patients is equivalent to continuous EFM during oxytocin infusion, most perinatal centers use EFM as the method of fetal assessment for induction/augmentation procedures. During external EFM, manual palpation is necessary to access contraction intensity and uterine resting tone between contractions. Data from the tocodynamometer is limited to contraction frequency and duration. If unable to obtain an interpretable tracing with an external monitor, rupture of the membranes allows placement of a fetal scalp electrode and an intrauterine pressure monitor for more accurate assessment of fetal and uterine response to labor. A 1:1 nurse-patient ratio is recommended during oxytocin dosage adjustment. Maternal-fetal assessment during oxytocin infusion should occur at least before each dosage increase; however, other factors such as stage of labor and maternal-fetal risk status should be considered when determining frequency (AWHONN, 1993). Nursing and medical policies, procedures, and protocols for oxytocin administration should be developed and revised as necessary. Oxytocin should not be administered without a physician readily available who is capable of performing an emergency cesarean birth (AAP & ACOG).

There are a variety of oxytocin protocols that differ in the initial dose, the dosing increment, and the maximum dose. Most induction protocols differ from augmentation protocols. The dosing interval varies from 15 to 60 minutes. The exact half-life of oxytocin is unknown. The physiologic steady state of oxytocin is believed to be approximately 40 minutes. The American College of Obstetrics and Gynecologists (1991) recommends dosing increments of 1 mU/min (if the dosing interval is 15 minutes) or 1–2 mU/min increases (if the dosing interval is 40–60 minutes). The latter protocol has a starting dose of 0.5–1.0 mU/min (ACOG, 1991). Regardless of the protocol used, nursing responsibilities remain the same. The nursing goals should be individual management, assessing uterine activity, cervical dilation rate, and maternal-fetal response.

AUGMENTATION OF LABOR

Labor augmentation is necessary when contractions become ineffective or cease altogether after true labor has begun. Abnormal labor progress has been discussed previously. Refer to Figure 8-1B for a graphic display of abnormal labor progress that may indicate augmentation. Amniotomy, as a method of augmentation or stimulation of labor, has not been proven effective for labor enhancement but is frequently used. After amniotomy, many women report more painful contractions, possibly the result of decompression of the uterus or the lack of a buffer to the fetal head. Although contractions may be perceived as more painful, they do not result in higher intraamniotic pressures as measured by intrauterine pressure monitoring. Nipple and breast stimulation, which cause release of endogenous pitocin, have also been used to enhance labor.

Oxytocin infusion is the most common method for labor enhancement. Hyperstimulation and hypertonus may result if oxytocin infusion is not carefully titrated to uterine response. Most oxytocin-augmentation protocols recommend a lower starting dose and a longer dosing interval. Intrauterine pressure monitoring is helpful during labor induction/augmentation for direct assessment of quality of contractions as well as uterine resting tone.

ACTIVE MANAGEMENT OF LABOR

Active management of labor is an augmentation protocol directed toward reducing the cesarean birth rate due to dystocia in nulliparous women. This proposed management of augmentation was introduced in Dublin, Ireland and now is being used in the United States. The goal of active management of labor is birth of a healthy infant within 12 hours of admission to the labor unit. Inclusion criteria for active management of labor requires nulliparity, at least 37 weeks gestation, singleton pregnancy, and spontaneous labor. Spontaneous labor is defined differently in various protocols but usually refers to uterine contractions occurring at 5-minute intervals that have produced complete cervical effacement. Admission to the labor unit is restricted until complete cervical effacement has occurred or, in some protocols, 3–4 cm dilation. Artificial rupture of the membranes is performed within 2 hours of admission if rupture does not spontaneously occur. If cervical dilation does not progress at a rate of 1 centimeter per hour following amniotomy, then oxytocin infusion is begun. The initial dosage of oxytocin is 6 mU/min with 6 mU/min incremental increases every 15 minutes until a maximum dosage of 36–40 mU/min is reached. Labor is monitored closely for signs and symptoms of hyperstimulation and fetal compromise. Active management of labor in the United States is still under investigation. This oxytocin regimen should not be initiated in multiparous women or for women with pregnancies complicated by medical problems or any other disease process that might adversely affect uteroplacental perfusion.

ASSISTED DELIVERY

Forceps

Forceps are used to extract the fetal head when birth must be facilitated for the health of the mother or fetus. Maternal conditions that may necessitate use of forceps are medical complications such as cardiac or pulmonary disease, maternal exhaustion, or excessive analgesia/anesthesia. The fetus may exhibit signs of compromise via EFM during second-stage labor, requiring facilitated birth, such as bradycardia, marked tachycardia, prolonged and severe decelerations, or late decelerations. Forceps should not be considered unless the cervix is completely dilated, membranes are ruptured, head is engaged, and the woman has adequate anesthesia. Classification of forceps procedures is listed in Table 8-3. All perinatal nurses should be familiar with this classification so that documentation of the procedure is accurate. Forceps are associated with vaginal and cervical tears, extension of the episiotomy, uterine rupture, bladder trauma, fracture of the coccyx, and increased vaginal bleeding with uterine atony. Newborns delivered by forceps should be observed for lacerations, bruising, skull fractures, and intracranial hemorrhages.

Vacuum Extraction

Some physicians use vacuum extraction in lieu of forceps, usually dependent on their training and experience. A vacuum extractor consists of a Silastic cup that comes in various sizes that has a suction device attached.

TABLE 8-3. Criteria of Forceps Deliveries According to Station and Rotation

Types of Procedure	Criteria
Outlet forceps	1) Scalp is visible at the introitus without separating labia
	2) Fetal skull has reached pelvic floor
	3) Sagittal suture is in anteroposterior diameter or right or left occiput anterior or posterior position
	4) Fetal head is at or on perineum
	5) Rotation does not exceed 45°
Low forceps	Leading point of fetal skull is at station ≥ + 2 cm and not on the pelvic floor
	a. Rotation ≤ 45° (left or right occiput anterior to occiput anterior, or left or right occiput posterior to occiput posterior)
	b. Rotation>45°
Midforceps	Station above +2 cm but head engaged
High	Not included in classification

American College of Obstetricians and Gynecologists. (1994). Operative vaginal delivery. ACOG Technical Bulletin No. 196, Washington, DC: Author. Reprinted by permission.

The cup is placed on the fetal head and suction is increased gradually until a seal is formed. Gentle traction is then applied to deliver the fetal head. Indications and prerequisites for vacuum extraction or for the use of forceps are the same. Proponents of vacuum extraction feel that its use causes less tissue damage to both the woman and newborn. Actually, complications from both vacuum extraction and forceps use are similar, depending primarily on skill of the practitioner.

Nurses have a role in educating and reassuring the woman when an assisted birth is anticipated. Maternal comfort level should be assessed prior to the application of forceps or vacuum extraction. If a nonreassuring fetal heart rate pattern is the indication for the immediate birth, then the nurse must be prepared for newborn resuscitation assuring that appropriate equipment, supplies, and personnel are available. Nurses should also be aware of potential complications related to forceps and vacuum use and observe both the woman and newborn for associated signs and symptoms. Parents should be prepared and shown any forceps or vacuum extraction marks on the infant and be reassured that they should disappear in a few days.

AMNIOINFUSION

Amnioinfusion is a procedure during which saline or lactated Ringer's solution is introduced transcervically into the uterus to correct oligohydramnios or to dilute thickly stained amniotic fluid. The goal is to minimize or prevent fetal effects such as umbilical cord compression or meconium aspiration. Amniotic fluid serves to cushion the fetus from external pressure and trauma and also provides a stable thermal environment (Kulb, 1990). Pathologic decreases in amniotic fluid volume (AFV) can occur secondary to maternal or fetal conditions. The most common fetal conditions related to decreased AVF are renal or cardiac system abnormalities. Regardless of etiology of oligohydramnios, the condition is often associated with poor fetal outcome. Compression of the fetal body and/or umbilical cord, resulting from oligohydramnios, is often reflected by variable decelerations of the fetal heart rate.

Intrapartum amnioinfusion was first investigated as a treatment for variable and prolonged decelerations (Miyazaki & Taylor, 1983). Since then, amnioinfusion has been studied in the treatment of oligohydramnios as prophylactic prevention of cord compression with positive results (Nageotte, Bertucci, Towers, Lagrew, & Modanlou, 1991; Schrimmer, Macri, & Paul, 1991; Strong, Hetzler, Sarno, & Paul, 1990). However, not all investigators found prophylactic amnioinfusion for the prevention of cord compression to be beneficial (Ogundipe, Spong, & Ross, 1994). As investigation of intrapartum amnioinfusion continued, an interesting and unexpected finding consistently emerged; incidence of meconium aspiration was reduced. Research of intrapartum amnioinfusion

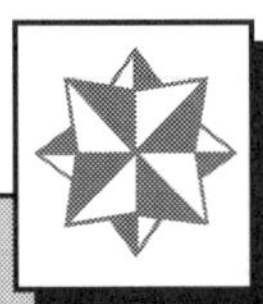

DISPLAY 8-6

Perioperative Cesarean Birth Care

Preoperative

- Admission assessment comparable to that for all women admitted for labor and birth.
- Obtain a 20 to 30 minute baseline FHR tracing via EFM. If the woman is not in active labor and the FHR is reassuring, EFM may be discontinued after this initial assessment.
- Provide a thorough explanation of what to expect in preparation for, during, and after, the surgery to the woman and her support person.
- Ensure that the woman has remained NPO as per institutional protocol.
- Initiate intravenous fluids.
- Witness informed consent signature for cesarean birth.
- Obtain surgical laboratory blood specimens if not done prior to admission.
- Shave abdomen.
- Insert Foley catheter; note amount and color of urine; delay until after epidural catheter is placed and dosed if possible.
- Administer preoperative medications as per physician order.
- If woman is in labor, periodic assessments of maternal-fetal status should continue as per institutional protocol.
- Transport the woman to the surgical suite/operating room.

Intraoperative

- Position the woman on the surgical table with a hip wedge in place.
- If EFM is used, continue monitoring until the abdominal prep is initiated.
- If a fetal scalp electrode is in place, EFM continues until the abdominal prep is completed. The electrode should be removed prior to birth.
- Prepare abdomen for surgery as per institutional protocol.
- Apply grounding device according to manufacturer's instructions.
- Note maternal vital signs, FHR, condition of the skin prior to incision, and the woman's emotional status.
- Assist the support person to a position at the head of the surgical table as per institutional protocol.
- Ensure that newborn resuscitation equipment is assembled and ready and personnel responsible are in attendance. Responsibility for resuscitation and stabilization of the healthy, full-term newborn differs by institution and could include the circulating nurse, an additional nurse, pediatrician, or neonatal nurse practitioner.
- Perform duties of circulating nurse as per institutional protocol
- Ensure that sponge, needle, and equipment counts are correct as per institutional protocol.
- Assist with application of abdominal dressing.
- Note maternal and newborn status prior to transport to the postanesthesia care unit (PACU).
- Assist with transport.

Postanesthesia Recovery Care

- Postoperative assessments are per PACU protocols and should be comparable to care provided in the main hospital PACU.

DISPLAY 8-6 (cont.)

- Initial and ongoing assessments include:

Review of intraoperative course, including medications and intravenous fluids received.

Respiratory assessment
- airway patency
- oxygen needs
- rate, quality, and depth of respirations
- auscultation of breath sounds
- arterial oxygen saturation via pulse oximetry

Circulation assessment
- blood pressure
- pulse
- ECG
- color

Level of consciousness
- orientation
- response to verbal, tactile, and painful stimulation

Obstetrical status
- uterine fundus position and contraction
- abdominal dressing
- maternal-newborn attachment
- lochia amount and color
- newborn condition
- breastfeeding desires

Intake and output
- intravenous fluids
- urinary output via Foley catheter

Pain/comfort level
- patient desires
- medications given

Discharge from PACU care occurs after the recovery period and when the woman is stable as determined by PACU discharge criteria.

A scoring system including the following parameters is useful to assess readiness for discharge:
- level of consciousness
- neuromuscular activity
- level of sensation
- circulation
- respiration
- color

(See Figure 8-9 for a sample PACU discharge scoring tool; using this sytem, the patient's score must be at least ten prior to discharge)

Additional assessment prior to PACU discharge include:
- vital signs
- urinary output via Foley catheter
- uterine fundus position and contraction
- abdominal dressing
- intravenous fluids/oral intake
- pain/comfort level
- lochia amount and color
- maternal-newborn attachment

The anesthesia provider is involved in the decision to discharge from PACU care.

If responsibility for care is transferred to another nurse after discharge, a complete report of intraoperative and postanesthesia course is vital.

Simson, K.R. and Creehan, P.A. (1996).

as a dilution technique for thick meconium fluid has shown reduction in fetal compromise, neonatal acidemia, meconium below the vocal cords, and cesarean births (Sadovsky, Amon, Bade, & Petrie, 1989; Eriksen, Hostetter, & Parisi, 1994).

Amnioinfusion is not without risks and should not be introduced on an intrapartum unit without first having policies, procedures, and protocols to ensure patient safety. The infusate should be lactated Ringer's solution or normal saline. Glucose solutions may increase the risk for infection and also have been associated with neonatal hyperglycemia, possibly due to fetal swallowing. An infusion pump should be used for amnioinfusion so that flow rate is accurate and an exact amount is infused, calculated, and documented. During bolus of the infusion and maintenance rate, amount of fluid returning should be calculated and recorded to avoid iatrogenic polyhydramnios. If 250 cc have infused with no return, the amnioinfusion should be discontinued until the fluid has returned. Lateral maternal position is indicated during infusion. A dual-lumen intrauterine catheter is preferred so that estimate of uterine resting tone can be assessed during the infusion; however, similar results can be achieved using two single-lumen, fluid-filled catheters. Turbulence at the end of the catheter does not allow for accurate recording of uterine resting tone (URT) during the procedure. If the URT exceeds 20 mmHg, discontinue the infusion and reassess resting tone; if it is below 20 mmHg, resume the infusion. Contraction intensity and frequency should be continually assessed during the procedure. If the flow rate for the bolus exceeds 600 cc per hr, then the infusate should be warmed to body temperature. The safest method to warm the infusate is by use of an electronic blood/fluid warmer. If variable decelerations are the indication for amnioinfusion, decelerations should improve very soon after initiating amnioinfusion. If decelerations do not improve, continuation is not necessary. Explain the procedure and indications to the woman and support persons prior to initiation. Continued reassurance during amnioinfusion helps to allay fears and concerns the woman and family may have.

CESAREAN BIRTH

Incidence of cesarean birth has risen in this country from about 5% to more than 20% in the past 15 to 20 years (Hale & Danforth, 1991). Perioperative perinatal nursing blends the specialties of obstetrics and surgery to deliver comprehensive care to women undergoing cesarean birth (NAACOG, 1991). While cesarean births have been performed in perinatal units for many years, only recently has attention been paid to ensuring that perinatal units maintain the same standards of care as the operating room/recovery room. The perinatal nurse should receive didactic orientation to preoperative, intraoperative, and postoperative care. Perioperative assessments and documentation forms used on the perinatal unit should be the same as those used in the main hospital operating room and postanesthesia recovery area. Ongoing quality assessment and improvement is conducted to ensure that all aspects of the program are maintained. Display 8-6 contains guidelines for the perioperative cesarean birth. During the critical first hour of postoperative recovery, nurse-patient ratio on the perinatal unit must be the same as the recovery room. If care during recovery occurs in an OB recovery room, the nurse is able to care for more than one patient. In settings where the postoperative patient returns to an LDRP immediately after surgery, the perinatal nurse remains at the bedside until cardiac monitoring is discontinued and the patient is stable. Postoperative patients may be discharged from postoperative status when the following criteria are met: (1) vital signs are stabilized for at least three consecutive readings with intervals of 15 minutes; (2) airway is clear and danger of vomiting and aspiration has passed; (3) patients recovering from general anesthesia must have regained consciousness and be oriented to time, place, person, or equivalent preoperative level of orientation; and (4) patients who have received spinal or epidural anesthesia must have progressive increase in movement of extremities. A PACU discharge scoring tool as shown in Figure 8-10 is helpful in conducting a systematic assessment and determining readiness for discharge. See Display 8-7 and Display 8-8 for critical components of obstetric postanesthesia nursing and necessary equipment.

Supporting Attachment in Women Experiencing Cesarean Birth

Whether anticipated or unexpected, the need for surgical births increases the families' anxiety, places additional strain on the maternal-newborn relationship, makes postpartum more difficult for the family, and creates a need for accepting the altered birth experience. Studies of women who had planned and unplanned cesarean births conclude that women who deliver via cesarean have special needs for information, presence of the partner throughout cesarean birth, and sustained contact with their newborn (Reichert, Baron, & Fawcett, 1993). Primigravid women who had an emergency cesarean birth reported that failure of communication was a major problem that occurred prior to, during, and after cesarean birth (Hillan, 1992). The father's presence in the delivery room and early contact with the infant were predicative of self-reported attachment behaviors in women experiencing either cesarean or vaginal births (Fortier, 1988). Thus, in order to facilitate a positive birth experience and attachment to the newborn, consideration should be given to ongoing attention of the families' understanding of cesarean birth, ways to maintain the father's presence throughout the birth experience, and early and sustained contact with the newborn.

Vaginal Birth After Cesarean

Until the last decade, women who had previous cesarean births were expected to have surgical deliveries for all subsequent pregnancies. It was believed that the prior uterine scar would rupture during labor. Research supports a trial of labor following a previous cesarean with minimal risks for uterine rupture. Most wound dehiscence from prior surgery occurs prior to onset of labor. Women who have had previous cesareans are now encouraged to attempt a vaginal birth. An obvious benefit is the shorter recovery period and inpatient stay following a vaginal birth. Overall morbidity and mortality is lower with vaginal births compared with surgical births, making a trial of labor a safer and less-expensive option. Not all women are candidates for trial of labor. Any contraindication for vaginal birth precludes the option for labor, such as malpresentation, a nonreassuring fetal heart rate pattern, placental previa, severe maternal disease, or cephalopelvic disproportion. Previous classical (horizontal) uterine incisions are also a contraindication to a trial of labor. Some women who labored prior to their cesarean birth may not want to attempt a vaginal birth, for fear that they will face a long uncomfortable labor and still require a cesarean. These concerns and fears must be

Figure 8-10. Sample PACU Discharge Scoring Tool

POST ANESTHESIA RECOVERY SCORE			
	CRITERIA	SCORE	DISCHARGE
CONSCIOUSNESS	Fully awake Arousable on calling Not responding	2 1 0	
NEUROMUSCULAR ACTIVITY	Move 4 extremities Move 2 extremities Move 0 extremites	2 1 0	
SENSATION	Normal None below pubis None below xiphoid	2 1 0	
CIRCULATION	B/P 10–20 mmHg ± admission B/P 10–50 mmHg ± admission B/P >51mmHg ± admission	2 1 0	
RESPIRATION	Deep breathing or cough Dyspnea Apnea	2 1 0	
COLOR	Pink Pale, blotchy, jaundiced, other Cyanotic	2 1 0	
Signature:	Date: Total Time		

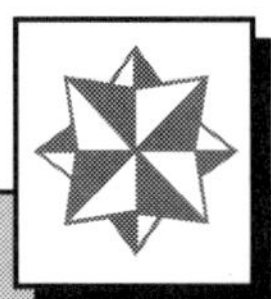

DISPLAY 8-7

Critical Components of Obstetric Postanesthesia Nursing

1. Women in the obstetric postanesthesia period after major regional or general anesthetic shall receive care equivalent to that available in the surgical PACU.
2. The anesthesiologist or nurse anesthetist is responsible for determining whether the condition of the woman warrants PACU or routine obstetric postpartum recovery care.
3. If the woman is admitted to obstetric PACU care, surgical PACU standards shall be followed until PACU discharge criteria are met and routine postpartum recovery care ensues.
4. Before patient arrival, the obstetric postanesthesia recovery area shall have required equipment in place. Otherwise, the woman should remain monitored by the anesthesiologist or nurse anesthetist until the recovery area is appropriately equipped to ensure patient safety.
5. A woman transported to the obstetric PACU shall be accompanied by a member of the anesthesia care team, who shall provide a verbal report to the responsible obstetric PACU nurse and remain in the obstetric PACU until the obstetric PACU nurse accepts responsibility for the nursing care of the patient.
6. Once the woman is admitted to obstetric PACU care, she shall be continually observed and monitored by methods appropriate to her medical condition. Particular attention should be given to monitoring oxygenation, ventilation, circulation, and temperature. Additional staff may be needed to interact with family members and the newborn infant. Once PACU discharge criteria are met, postpartum care should continue per obstetric standards.
7. Each hospital is responsible for developing guidelines, policies, and procedures collaboratively among the obstetric department, anesthesia department, and surgical PACU (e.g., assessment criteria, PACU discharge criteria, documentation, malignant hyperthermia, crisis management, medications and equipment, staff education and qualifications, and staffing requirements).
8. Each hospital shall ensure that advanced cardiac life support (ACLS) care is readily available at all times (e.g., code team). ACLS certification is not required for obstetric nurses providing postanesthesia care. This practice is supported by the Association of Women's Health, Obstetric, and Neonatal Nurses Position Statement on Postanesthesia Nursing for Obstetric Patients (1993).
9. For optimal skill development, obstetric postanesthesia education should include both didactic and practice components. A period of observation in the surgical PACU is strongly recommended to enhance the obstetric nurses perspective on recovery room practices.
10. Hospitals in which obstetric postanesthesia patients are consistently recovered in the surgical PACU (e.g., some level I obstetric services) may choose to omit this education for their obstetric staff.

From Obrien-Abel, N., Reinke, C., Warner, P., & Nelson, C. (1994). Critical components of obstetric postanesthesia nursing. Journal of Perinatal and Neonatal Nursing, 8 (3) pp. 4-16. Copyright 1994 by Aspen. Reprinted with permission.

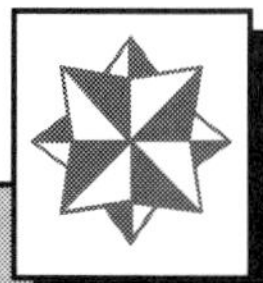

DISPLAY 8-8

Equipment for Obstetric Postanesthesia Care

A. Each postanesthesia recovery bed should have the following:
   1. oxygen delivery system
   2. constant and intermittent suction
   3. blood pressure monitoring equipment
   4. ECG monitoring equipment
   5. pulse oximeter
   6. adjustable lighting
   7. means to ensure patient privacy
B. The obstetric PACU should have the following:
   1. method to monitor patient temperature
   2. adult bag-valve-mask and emergency airway supplies
   3. portable oxygen, suction, and cardiac monitoring equipment for those patients requiring such equipment during transport
   4. method of calling for assistance in emergency situations
   5. emergency cart:
      a. supplies for insertion of arterial line, central venous lines, and pulmonary artery catheters
      b. emergency drugs and equipment
      c. airway/respiratory equipment
   6. blanket warmer
   7. supplies to treat malignant hyperthermic crisis:
      a. means to deliver 100% oxygen
      b. dantrolene (Dantrium), 1.0–2.5 mg/kg up to total of 10.0 mg/kg
      c. preservative-free, sterile water for reconstitution (60-ml vials)
      d. mannitol
      e. sodium bicarbonate
      f. regular insulin
      g. cool intravenous fluids and a cooling blanket

From Obrien-Abel, N., Reinke, C., Warner, P., & Nelson, C. (1994). Critical components of obstetric postanesthesia nursing. Journal of Perinatal and Neonatal Nursing, 8 (3) pp. 4-16. Copyright 1994 by Aspen. Reprinted with permission.

addressed, and then a joint decision made between the woman and primary healthcare provider. Increasingly, third-party-payors are mandating a trial of labor by refusing reimbursement or providing reduced reimbursement, for women with a history of prior cesarean birth who have no documented contraindications for vaginal birth after cesarean (VBAC).

Women undergoing a trial of labor require specialized and skilled nursing care. The patient and family need additional reassurance and support. Contraction pattern and fetal response should be observed closely. The nurse should note the rate of cervical dilation and fetal descent, being alert to abnormal progress. Close attention should be paid to any complaints of severe pain in the area of the prior incision. Impending rupture may be preceded by increasing uterine hypertonus, followed by an apparent lack of uterine activity postrupture. Rupture of the uterus is a perinatal emergency. Maternal-fetal survival depends on speed of identification and surgical intervention. Blood and blood products should be readily available. Policies, procedures, and protocols should be written and evaluated to ensure optimum care for women who are having a trial of labor.

SUMMARY

Nurses who care for women during the intrapartum period require knowledge of the labor process and a thorough understanding of techniques and interventions that enhance labor. Age-old nursing traditions surrounding birth are not always scientifically based and are now being questioned. Positioning for labor and birth is evolving from dorsal lithotomy to positions that are more patient and fetus oriented. Nurse-coached closed-glottis, second-stage pushing techniques should be carefully reexamined. Routine episiotomy should become a thing of the past. Nurses can influence changes related to routine childbirth practices by keeping abreast of current research in intrapartum nursing and using this knowledge in caring for laboring women. Labor induction/augmentation, cervical ripening procedures, amnioinfusion, and assisted births are interventions necessary for some women to promote optimal maternal and fetal outcome, but the least invasive approach should be the first considered. Nurses must also have expertise in perioperative standards for women experiencing cesarean births. This chapter has presented an overview of nursing considerations for clinical practice during childbirth. Perinatal care based on national standards and current research will enhance quality outcomes for women and newborns. The nurse has an important role in facilitating a positive childbirth experience. Attendance at the birth of a healthy newborn and sharing the joy with the new mother is one of the most rewarding experiences in perinatal nursing practice.

References

American Academy of Pediatrics, & American College of Obstetricians and Gynecologists. (1992). Guidelines for perinatal care (3rd ed.). Elkgrove, IL: Author.

American College of Obstetricians and Gynecologists. (1991). Induction and augmentation of labor (ACOG Technical Bulletin No. 157). Washington, DC: Author.

American College of Obstetricians and Gynecologists, (1993). Prostaglandin E2 gel for cervical ripening (ACOG Committee Opinion No. 123). Washington, DC: Author.

American College of Obstetrics and Gynecologists. (1995). Fetal heart rate patterns: Monitoring, interpretation, and management (ACOG Technical Bulletin No. 207). Washington, DC: Author

Anderson, A.B., & Turnbull, A.C. (1973). Comparative aspects of factors involved in the onset of labour in bovine and human pregnancy. In A. Kloopert & J. Gardner (Eds.), Endocrine factors in labour (p. 141). Cambridge University Press.

Association of Women's Health, Obstetric, and Neonatal Nurses. (1993a). Cervical ripening and induction and augmentation of labor. Washington, DC: Author

Association of Women's Health, Obstetric, and Neonatal Nurses (1993b). Didactic content and clinical skills verification for professional nurse providers of basic, high risk, and critical care intrapartum nursing. Washington, DC: Author.

Avery, M.D., & Burkett, B.A. (1986). Effect of perineal massage on the incidence of episiotomy and perineal laceration in a nurse-midwifery practice. Journal of Nurse-Midwifery, 31(3),128-134.

Avery, M.D., & Van Arsdale, L. (1987). Perineal massage: Effect on the incidence of episiotomy and laceration in a nulliparous population. Journal of Nurse-Midwifery, 32(3),181-184.

Biancuzzo, M. (1993). Six myths of maternal posture during labor. Maternal Child Nursing,18(5), 264-269.

Caldeyro-Barcia, R., Giussi, G., Storch, E., Poseiro, J.J., Kettenhuber, K., & Ballejo, G. (1981). The bearing down efforts and their effects on fetal heart rate, oxygenation, and acid-base valance. Journal of Perinatal Medicine, 9 (Suppl. 1), 63-67.

Chalfen, M.F. (1993). Obstetric-Gynecologic care and survivors of childhood sexual abuse. AWHONN'S Clinical Issues in Perinatal and Women's Health Nursing, 4(2), 191-195.

Cosner, K.R., & deJong, E. (1993). Physiologic second-stage labor. Maternal Child Nursing, 18(1), 38-43.

Cunningham, F.G., MacDonald, P.C., Leveno, K.J., Gant, N.F., & Gilstrap, L.C. (1993). Williams obstetrics (19th ed.). Norwalk, CT: Appleton Lange.

Davis, L.K. (1992). Nursing care protocols and procedures. In L.K. Mandeville & N.H. Troiano (Eds.), High-risk intrapartum nursing (p. 283-322). Philadelphia: J.B. Lippincott.

DelGiudice, G.T. (1986). The relationship between sibling jealousy and presence at a sibling's birth. Birth, 13(4), 250-254.

Engelman, G.J. (1884). Labor among primitive peoples (3rd ed.). St. Louis, MO: J.H Chambers.

Eriksen, N.L., Hostetter, M., & Parisi, V.M. (1994). Prophylactic amnioinfusion in pregnancies complicated by thick meconium. American Journal Obstetrics and Gynecology, 171, 1026-1030.

Ferguson, J.K.W. (1941). Study of motility of intact uterus at term. Surgery, Gynecology and Obstetrics, 73, 359-366.

Fortier, J.C. (1988). The relationship of vaginal and cesarean births to father-infant attachment. Journal of Obstetric, Gynecologic, and Neonatal Nursing 17(2), 128-134.

Foster, T.C., Jacobson, J.D., & Valenzuela, G.J. (1988). Oxytocin augmentation of labor: A comparison of 15 and 30 minute dose increment intervals. Obstetrics and Gynecology, 71(2), 147-149.

Friedman, E.A. (1978). Labor: Clinical evaluation of management (2nd ed.). New York: Appleton-Century-Crofts.

Friedman, E.A., Niswander, K.R., & Bayonet-Rivera, N.P. (1966). Relationship of prelabor evaluation to inducibility and the course of labor. Obstetrics and Gynecology, 28, 495-501.

Gannon, J.M. (1992). Delivery on the hands and knees: A case study approach. Journal of Nurse-Midwifery, 37(1), 48-52.

Golay, J., Vedam, S., & Sorger, L. (1993). The squatting position for the second stage of labor: Effects on labor and on maternal and fetal well being. Birth: Issues in Perinatal Care and Education 20(2), 73-78.

Gonik, B., Stringer, C.A., & Held, B. (1983). An alternate maneuver for management of shoulder dystocia. American Journal of Obstetrics and Gynecology, 145(7), 882-884.

Hale, R.W., & Danforth, D.N. (1991). Operative delivery. In M.L. Pernoll (Ed.), Current obstetric-gynecologic diagnosis & treatment (7th ed.). Norwalk, CT: Appleton & Lange.

Hillan, E.M. (1992). Issues in the delivery of midwifery care. Journal of Advanced Nursing 17(3), 274-278.

Johnson, J.D., Aldrich, M., & Angelus, P. (1984). Oxytocin and neonatal hyperbilirubinemia: Studies of bilirubin production. American Journal of Diseases in Children, 138(11),1047-1050.

Kitzinger, J. (1990). Recalling the pain: Medical procedures can bring back memories of sexual violence. Nursing Times, 86(3), 8-40.

Klaus, M.H., Kennel, J.H., McGrath, S., Robertson, S.S., & Hinkley, C. (1991). Continuous emotional support during labor in a U.S. hospital: A randomized control trial. Journal of the American Medical Association, 265(17), 2197-2201.

Klaus, M.H., Kennel, J.H., McGrath, S., Robertson S.S., & Hinkley, C. (1988). Medical intervention: The effect of social support during labor. Pediatric Research, 23(4), 211A. (Part 2 abstract).

Klaus, M.H., Kennel, J.H., Robertson, S.S, & Sosa, R. (1986). Effects of social support during parturition and maternal and infant morbidity. British Medical Journal, 293, (6547).

Kline-Kaye, V., & Miller-Slade, D. (1990). The use of fundal pressure during the second stage of labor. Journal of Obstetric, Gynecologic, and Neonatal Nursing, 196(6), 511-517.

Kulb, N. (1990). Abnormalities of the amniotic fluid. In K. Buckley & N. Kulb (Eds.), High-risk maternity nursing manual (pp. 335-347). Baltimore: Williams & Wilkins.

Loong E.P., Lao T.T., & Chin, R.K. (1988). Changes in neonatal transcutaneous bilirubinometer index following intravenous fluid and oxytocin infusion during labor. Asia Oceania Journal Obstetric Gynaecology, 14(4), 411-414.

Liu, Y.C. (1989). The effects of the upright position during childbirth. IMAGE, 21(1), 14-18.

Malpas, P. (1933). Postmaturity and malformations of the fetus. Journal of Obstetrics and Gynaecology British Empire, 40,1046-1053.

May, K.A., & Mahlmeister, L.R. (1994). Maternal & neonatal nursing family centered care, (3rd ed.). Philadelphia: J.B. Lippincott.

McGuinness, M., Norr, K., & Nacion, K. (1991). Comparison between different perineal outcomes on tissue healing. Journal of Nurse-Midwifery, 36(3), 192-198.

McKay, S., Barrows, T., & Roberts, J. (1990). Women's view of second-stage labor as assessed by interviews and videotapes. Birth: Issues in Perinatal Care and Education, 17(4), 192-198.

McKay, S., & Roberts, J. (1985). Second stage labor: What is normal? Journal of Obstetric, Gynecologic, and Neonatal Nursing 14(2), 101-106.

McKay, S., & Smith, S.Y. (1983). What are they talking about? Is something wrong? Information sharing during the second stage of labor. Birth: Issues in Perinatal Care and Education, 20(3),142-147.

Mengert, W., & Murphy, D. (1933). Intra-abdominal pressures created by voluntary muscular effort. Surgery and Gynecologic Obstetrics, 57, 745-751.

Miyazaki, F., & Taylor, N.A. (1983). Saline amnioinfusion for relief of variable or prolonged decelerations: A preliminary report. American Journal of Obstetrics and Gynecology, 146(6), 670-678.

Mynaugh, P.A. (1991). A randomized study of two methods of teaching perineal massage: Effects on practice rates, episiotomy rates, and lacerations. Birth: Issues in Perinatal Care and Education, 18(3), 153-159.

Nageotte, M.P., Bertucci, L., Towers, C.V., Lagrew, D., & Modanlou, H. (1991). Prophylactic amnioinfusion in pregnancies complicated by oligohydramnios: A prospective study. Obstetrics and Gynecology, 77(5), 677-680.

Noble, E. (1981). Controversies in maternal effort during labor and delivery. Journal of Nurse Midwifery, 26(2), 13-22.

Norbeck, J.S., & Anderson, N.J. (1989). Psychosocial predictors of pregnancy outcomes in low-income black, hispanic, and white women. Nursing Research, 38(4), 204-209.

Nurses' Association of the American College of Obstetricians and Gynecologists (NAACOG). (1991). Standards for the nursing care of women and newborns. Washington, DC: Author.

Ogundipe, O.A., Spong, C.V., & Ross, M.G. (1994). Prophylactic amnioinfusion for oligohydramnios: A reevaluation. Obstetrics and Gynecology, 84(4), 544-548.

Pascoe, J.M. (1993). Social support during labor and duration of labor: A community based study. Public Health Nursing, 10(2), 97-99.

Penney, D.S., & Perlis, D.W. (1992). Shoulder dystocia: When to use suprapubic or fundal pressure. Maternal Child Nursing, 17(1), 34-36.

Pernoll, M.L. (Ed.). (1991). Current obstetric and gynecologic diagnosis & treatment (7th ed.). Norwalk, CT: Appleton & Lange.

Pozaic, S. (1992). Induction and augmentation of labor. In L.K. Mandeville & N.H. Troiano (Eds.). High-risk intrapartum nursing (pp. 101-114). Philadelphia: J.B. Lippincott.

Reeder, S.J., Martin, L.L., & Koniak, D. (1992). Maternity nursing: Family, newborn and women's health care (17th ed.). Philadelphia: J.B. Lippincott.

Reichert, J.A., Baron, M., & Fawcett, J. (1993). Changes in attitudes toward cesarean birth. Journal of Obstetric, Gynecologic, and Neonatal Nursing, 22(2), 159-167.

Roberts, J.E., Goldstein, S.A., Gruener, J.S., Maggio, M., & Mendez-Bauer, C. (1987). A descriptive analysis of involuntary bearing-down efforts during the expulsive phase of labor. Journal of Obstetric, Gynecologic, and Neonatal Nursing, 16(1), 48-55.

Rooks, J.P., Weatherby, N.L., & Ernst, E.K.M. (1992). The national birth center study: Intrapartum and immediate postpartum and neonate care, part 2. Journal of Nurse-Midwifery, 37(5),301-330.

Sadovsky, Y., Amon, E., Bade, M.E., & Petrie, R. (1989). Prophylactic amnioinfusion during labor complicated by meconium: A preliminary report. American Journal of Obstetrics and Gynecology, 161(3), 613-617.

Schrimmer, D.B., Macri, C.J., & Paul, R.M. (1991). Prophylactic amnioinfusion as a treatment for oligohydramnios in laboring patients: A prospective, randomized trial. American Journal of Obstetrics and Gynecology, 165(4Pt.1), 972-975.

Strong, T.H.J., Hetzler, G., Sarno, A.P., & Paul, R.M. (1990). Prophylactic intrapartum amnioinfusion: A randomized clinical trial. American Journal of Obstetrics and Gynecology, 162(6), 1370-1374.

Trofatter, K.F. (1992). Cervical ripening. Clinical Obstetrics and Gynecology, 35(3), 476-486.

Vaughn, K.O. (1937). Safe childbirth: The three essentials. London: Ballière, Tindall, and Cox.

Wilson, T., Liggens, G.C., & Joe, L. (1989). Purification and characterization of a uterine phospholipase inhibitor that loses activity after labor onset in women. American Journal of Obstetrics and Gynecology, 160(3), 602-606.

Zlatnik, F.J. (1994). Normal labor and delivery and its conduct. In J.R. Scott, P.J. DiSaia, C.B. Hammond, & W.N. Spellacy (Eds.), Danforth's obstetrics and gynecology (6th ed., pp. 161-188). Philadelphia: J.B. Lippincott.

CHAPTER 8 APPENDIX

Name: ______ Age: ____ Admission date: ___ / ___ / _____ Time: _____ a.m. p.m.
Name patient wishes to be addressed by: ______ Support person/relationship: ______
Arrived by: ☐ Ambulatory ☐ Wheelchair ☐ Cart
Obstetrician ______ Pediatrician ______
Childbirth preparation: ☐ None ☐ Lamaze ☐ Refresher ☐ Cesarean ☐ PCH Instructor ______

Reason for admission:
☐ Labor ☐ R/O labor ☐ Induction ☐ Cesarean: ☐ Primary ☐ Repeat ☐ Delivered prior to admission
☐ ROM ☐ Vaginal bleeding ☐ Other ______

GRAV	TERM	PREM	ABORTION	LIVING	ECTOPIC	MULT. BIRTHS	STILLBORN	NEONATAL DEATHS:	LMP	EDC	GEST. IN WEEKS
			Spont. Induced:				Term: Prem:	Term: Prem:			

INITIAL EVALUATION: Vital Signs: Temp _____ Pulse _____ Resp _____ B/P _____
Weight: Present _____ Prepregnant _____ # Gain _____ Height: _____
FHT: _____ ☐ reg. ☐ irreg. Blood Type/Rh: _____
Allergies: ☐ None ☐ Iodine ☐ Adhesive tape ☐ Food _____ **Last Meal:** ___ / ___ / _____
☐ Drugs _____ ☐ Other _____ at _____ a.m. / p.m.
Describe reaction: _____ ☐ Fluids ☐ Solids

VAGINAL EXAM
☐ None
☐ Sterile Speculum
Dilation _____
Effacement _____
CERVIX
☐ Posterior
☐ Midposition
☐ Anterior
CONSISTENCY
☐ Firm
☐ Soft
Station _____
☐ Ballotable

MEMBRANES
☐ Intact
☐ Ruptured
_____ Date _____ Time
☐ Leaking
COLOR
☐ Clear
☐ Bloody
☐ Meconium
☐ Other _____
AMOUNT
☐ Small
☐ Medium
☐ Large
ODOR
☐ Normal
☐ Foul
NITRAZINE
☐ Negative
☐ Positive
☐ Inconclusive

PRESENTATION
☐ Vertex
☐ Brow
☐ Face
☐ Transverse
☐ Indeterminate
☐ Other
_____
BREECH
☐ Frank
☐ Complete
☐ Footling

CONTRACTIONS
☐ Absent
☐ Present
_____ Date & Time Began
☐ Regular
☐ Irregular
Frequency _____ mins.
Duration _____ secs.
Intensity
☐ Mild
☐ Moderate
☐ Strong
☐ Uterus relaxed between contractions

VAGINAL BLEEDING
☐ None
☐ Spotting
☐ Blood Show
☐ Frank Bleeding
☐ Associated w/ abdominal pain

SPECIAL PROCEDURES
☐ None
☐ NST
☐ OCT
☐ Ultrasound
☐ Amnio.
☐ Biophysical Profile
☐ Prenatal Rhogam: Date: _____
☐ Cervical Cultures: Result: _____

Fetal Activity: ☐ Present ☐ Diminished ☐ Absent
Prenatal Care: ☐ Yes ☐ No Date began: ___ / ___ / _____
OB complications/hospitalizations during this pregnancy: ______

Medications: (include prescription, over-the-counter, iron, prenatal vitamins)
Name Dose/Time Time Last Taken

Type of pain management discussed with M.D.: ______

PALOS COMMUNITY HOSPITAL
PALOS HEIGHTS, ILLINOIS

LABOR AND DELIVERY
ADMISSION ASSESSMENT

P-566
Rev. 7/93

RISK FACTORS

Past History/Family History (P = Patient & F = Family. Indicate specific family member)

KEY: M=Mother F=Father S=Siblings GP=Grandparents

	P	F		P	F
1. Diabetes			10. Infectious/communicable disease		
2. Headaches			11. Back/hip/knee problems		
3. Heart disease			12. Respiratory disease/asthma/TB		
4. Hypertension			13. Seizure disorder		
5. Phlebitis, varicosities			14. Blood transfusion		
6. Hepatitis			15. Anemia/clotting disorders		
7. Kidney disease/Pyelonephritis/UTI			16. Multiple births		
8. Birth defects/Genetic			17. Adverse reaction to anesthesia		
9. Sexually transmitted disease			18. Other		

Describe positive patient findings/previous hospitalizations/problems during previous pregancies/labor history: __________

Use Of:

Alcohol
☐ No
☐ Yes
What __________
How much __________
How often __________
How long __________

Cigarettes
☐ No
☐ Yes
day ______

Caffeinated Beverages
☐ No
☐ Yes
______ cups/day

Recreational/Street Drugs
☐ No
☐ Yes
What __________
How much __________
How often __________
How long __________

REVIEW OF SYSTEMS:

Skin

Temperature
☐ Warm
☐ Hot
☐ Cool

Humidity
☐ Dry ☐ Clammy
☐ Diaphoretic

Color
☐ Pink ☐ Flushed
☐ Pale ☐ Cyanotic
☐ Rash __________
☐ Other __________

Respiratory
☐ No distress ☐ Dyspnea
☐ Cough ☐ Orthopnea
☐ dry ☐ Shallow
☐ productive

Breath sounds
☐ Clear
☐ Diminshed
☐ Equal/bilateral
☐ Unequal
☐ Other __________

Cardiovascular
☐ Asymptomatic ☐ Chest pain
☐ Palpitations

Lower extremities
☐ Asymptomatic
☐ Other __________

☐ Pitting edema
☐ 1+2mm ☐ 3+6mm
☐ 2+4mm ☐ 4+8mm

Quantitative edema
☐ 1+Minimal edema of the pedal & pretibial areas
☐ 2+Marked edema of the lower extremities
☐ 3+Edema of the face and hands, lower abdominal wall & sacrum.
☐ 4+Anasarca (Generalized massive edema) & ascites

Homan's Sign
Right: ☐ Neg. ☐ Pos.
Left: ☐ Neg. ☐ Pos.

DTR's

Right	Left
___+1	___+1
___+2	___+2
___+3	___+3
___+4	___+4

Gastrointestinal
☐ Asymptomatic ☐ Diarrhea
☐ Nausea ☐ Constipation
☐ Vomiting ☐ Hemorrhoids
☐ Other __________

Urinary
☐ Asymptomatic Protein ______
☐ Urgency Glucose ______
☐ Burning Ketones ______

Musculoskeletal
☐ Asymptomatic
☐ Limitation in ROM ______
☐ Pain ☐ Weakness
☐ Stiffness ☐ Swelling

Neurologic
☐ Asymptomatic ☐ Syncope
☐ Headache ☐ Dizziness
☐ Visual disturbance

Present Behavior
☐ Appropriate/cooperative
☐ Apprehensive
☐ Demanding
☐ Lethargic
☐ Uncooperative
☐ Flat affect

Prostetics: ☐ None ☐ Glasses ☐ Contact lenses: ☐ hard ☐ soft ☐ extended wear ☐ Other __________

Dentures: ☐ None ☐ upper ☐ lower ☐ partial ☐ other __________

Orientation: ☐ Call system ☐ Bed controls ☐ Visiting ☐ Smoking ☐ TV ☐ Phone ☐ Single room maternity care ☐ Inpatient classes

Feeding Method: ☐ Breast ☐ Bottle

Signature: __________ **Date/Time Assessment Completed:** __________

FETAL HEART RATE

EFM ON = +
EFM OFF = Ø

SHORT TERM VARIABILITY
Present = +
Absent = Ø

PERIODIC PATTERN
L = Late
V = Variable
E = Early
A = Accelerations w/contractions
*Refer to Progress Notes

LONG TERM VARIABILITY
Ø = Absent 0-2 bpm
↓ = Minimal 3-5 bpm
+ = Average to Moderate 6-25 bpm
↑ = Marked greater than 25 bpm

MD
✓ = With patient
N = Notified
O = Orders received
T = Telephoned in

CONTRACTION

Frequency in Minutes
I = Irregular
Ø = Absent

INTENSITY
M = Mild
Mod = Moderate
S= Strong

RESTING TONE
R = Between contractions uterus relaxed when palpated
mmHG = When IUPC in place
* = If not relaxed refer to Progress Notes

SHOW / VAGINAL BLEEDING
SS = Small show
MS = Moderate show
HS = Heavy show
SFB = Small frank bleeding
MFB = Moderate Frank bleeding
HFB = Heavy Frank bleeding
Ø = None

AMNIOTIC FLUID

AMOUNT
S = Small
M = Moderate
L = Large
Ø = None

COLOR
Cl = Clear
D = Cloudy
B = Bloody
M = Meconium
TH = Thin
M = Moderate
TK = Thick

STATION
F = Floating
B = Ballotable
# of cms

SAFETY
1 or 2 = Side rails up
C = Call light within reach
F = Family member in room

***Indicates further documentation in Integrated Progress Notes**

Date/Time														
Temperature														
Pulse														
Respiration														
Blood Pressure														
FHR: EFM														
FHR: Baseline or FHR														
FHR: Short Term Variability														
FHR: Long Term Variability														
FHR: Periodic Pattern*														
Contractions: Frequency														
Contractions: Duration														
Contractions: Intensity														
Contractions: Resting Tone														
Vaginal Exam: Exam by														
Vaginal Exam: Dilatation														
Vaginal Exam: Effacement														
Vaginal Exam: Station														
Show/Vaginal Bleeding														
Amniotic Fluid: Amount														
Amniotic Fluid: Color														
Position														
Activity														
Response To Labor														
Affect														
Comfort Measures														
Oxygen														
MD														
Pitocin mu/min.														
IV Site														
Safety														
Initials														

Allergies:

Medication														
Date/ Time														

POSITION
L = Lithotomy
S = Supine
R = Right lateral
LL = Left lateral
T = Trendelenberg
SF = Semi fowlers
C = Chair
S = Squatting
S/LB = Squatting w/labor bar
L/S = Laboring in shower
HF = High fowlers
RC = Rocking chair
HK = Hands & knees
E = Recliner
X = Position change encouraged/patient reluctant

RESPONSE TO LABOR
O = Unaware of contractions
T = Talking through contractions
BW = Breathing well through contractions
MC = Minimal coaching by RN to maintain controlled breathing during contractions
IC = Intense coaching by RN to maintain controlled breathing during contrations
NC = Intense coaching by RN; unable to maintain controlled breathing
TH = Thrashing
R = Reassurance and encouragement given
UP = Urge to push
IP = Involuntary pushing
PC = Pushing w/contractions

AFFECT
R = Relaxed
A = Anxious
App = Apprehensive
C = Cooperative
UC = Uncooperative
G = Angry
F = Fatigued
U = Uncomfortable

ACTIVITY
D = Dozing between contractions
S = Sleeping
TV = Watching TV
T = Talking
R = Resting between contractions
BP = On bed pan
BR = Bathroom
A = Ambulating
E = Eating
P = Pushing

COMFORT MEASURES
MC = Mouth care
P = Pericare
HP = Hot pack
CP = Counter pressure
I = Ice packs
M = Massage
CC = Cool cloth
PP = Positioned w/pillows

OXYGEN
# of liters
FM = Face mask
C = Cannula
D/C = O2 removed

IV SITE
✓ = Patent, no signs of infection
* = Refer to Progress Notes

														Date/Time
														Temperature
														Pulse
														Respiration
/	/	/	/	/	/	/	/	/	/	/	/	/	/	Blood Pressure
														FHR: EFM
														FHR: Baseline or FHR
														FHR: Short Term Variability
														FHR: Long Term Variability
														FHR: Periodic Pattern*
														Contrac-tions: Frequency
														Contrac-tions: Duration
														Contrac-tions: Intensity
														Contrac-tions: Resting Tone
														Vaginal Exam: Exam by
														Vaginal Exam: Dilatation
														Vaginal Exam: Effacement
														Vaginal Exam: Station
														Show/Vaginal Bleeding
														Amni-otic Fluid: Amount
														Amni-otic Fluid: Color
														Position
														Activity
														Response To Labor
														Affect
														Comfort Measures
														Oxygen
														MD
														Pitocin mu/min.
														IV Site
														Safety
														Initials

Intrapartum Fetal Monitoring

Cydney Afriat Menihan

- **Historical Perspectives**
- **Intermittent FHR Auscultation**
- **Electronic Fetal Monitoring**
- **Nurse-Patient Collaboration**
- **Physiologic Basis for FHR Monitoring**
- **FHR Baseline**
  - Baseline Changes in Rate
    - Tachycardia
    - Bradycardia
    - Baseline Variability
- **Periodic FHR**
  - Decelerations
    - Early Decelerations
    - Late Decelerations
    - Variable Decelerations
    - Prolonged Decelerations
  - Periodic Accelerations
- **Nonperiodic Changes**
- **Uterine Activity Assessment**
- **Fetal Blood Flow**
- **FHR Pattern Interpretation**
  - Reassuring Patterns
  - Nonreassuring Patterns
- **Systematic Assessment and Management Strategies**
- **Fetal Blood Sampling**
  - Progression of Fetal Hypoxia
  - Acute Fetal Insults
- **Unusual FHR Patterns**
- **Dysrhythmia Detection**
- **EFM Education and Competency Validation**
- **Summary**
- **Acknowledgments**

The 1990s represent the third decade of electronic fetal monitoring (EFM), a technology that has had far-reaching impact on women's healthcare and the practices of both nursing and medicine. Debate continues about advantages and limitations, effects on perinatal mortality and morbidity, and its role in healthcare costs and medical malpractice litigation (Ocak et al., 1992; Phelan, 1991; Schifrin, 1982; Shy et al., 1990). Regardless of one's professional opinion or choice in method of fetal surveillance, development of EFM has improved fetal outcome simply by increasing the attention of perinatal healthcare providers and researchers to fetal heart rate (FHR) as an indicator of fetal status (Ellison, Foster, Sheridan-Pereira, & MacDonald, 1991). This chapter discusses the physiologic basis for FHR monitoring and defines and describes basic FHR patterns. Systematic maternal/fetal assessments and nursing management are also presented.

HISTORICAL PERSPECTIVES

Fetal heart tones were first heard and described in the 17th century. During the 1800s, researchers in France, Germany, Switzerland, and the United States reported findings in the medical literature. Kilian in 1848 (Goodlin, 1979) was perhaps the first physician to describe FHR patterns indicative of fetal distress. He developed criteria, based on FHR, warranting a rapid forceps delivery. Early data about fetal heart rate also concerned ability to predict fetal sex and weight based on average beats per minute (Munde, 1880). While listening to the FHR during labor, Munde discovered that a decrease in rate after a contraction was potentially ominous. He was possibly the first to describe this pattern, later known as a late deceleration. In 1893, Von Winckel (Goodlin) reported other signs of fetal distress including tachycardia, bradycardia, and irregularities in the FHR rhythm. It is interesting to note that although methods of assessing FHR have evolved over the years, this early research about nonreassuring FHR patterns is still considered valid.

After invention of the fetoscope in the early 1900s, fetal heart sounds were commonly assessed during the prenatal period. In later years, intermittent auscultation of the FHR became routine practice during labor. In 1958, Hon published the first report of continuous fetal electrocardiographic monitoring using a device placed on the maternal abdomen. Other researchers were attempting to perfect similar equipment, but not until 1968 was the first commercially available electronic fetal monitor introduced. Coinciding with the development of EFM technology was the emergence of data to suggest limitations of intermittent auscultation. The Benson, Shubeck, Deutschberger, Weiss, & Berendes (1968) study of over 24,000 births concluded that FHR auscultation during labor was unreliable in determining fetal distress except in extreme cases. Based on this report and rapid technologic advances, FHR auscultation began to fall into disfavor. Over the next two decades, EFM became the primary method of fetal surveillance during the intrapartum period in the United States and Canada.

INTERMITTENT FHR AUSCULTATION

Prior to electronic fetal monitoring, the FHR was assessed using a manual fetoscope for a period of 1 minute every hour during the early period of the first stage of labor, every half hour during the active phase of labor, and every five minutes during the second stage of labor. Contractions were manually palpated (Fitzpatrick, Reeder, & Mastroianni, 1971). Current recommendations for using auscultation during the intrapartum period are outlined by the Nurses' Association of the American College of Obstetricians and Gynecologists (NAACOG) (1990) Practice Resource, *Fetal Heart Rate Auscultation* and the 1995 American College of Obstetricians and Gynecologists (ACOG) Technical Bulletin, *Fetal Heart Rate Patterns: Monitoring, Interpretation, and Management.* In the absence of risk factors, auscultation of the FHR every 30 minutes in the first stage of labor and every 15 minutes in the second stage of labor is suggested. When risk factors have been identified, assessment frequency is increased to every 15 minutes in the active phase of the first stage of labor and every 5 minutes in the second stage. When auscultation is used as the primary method of fetal surveillance during labor, a 1 to 1 nurse-fetus ratio is required.

The decision to use intermittent auscultation or EFM rests with the healthcare provider but is made in collaboration with the laboring woman. The decision is based on many factors, including patient history, fetal condition, risk classification, hospital policies and procedures, and the standard of practice. The selected method of fetal assessment must be performed by educated, competent personnel who are well versed in that technique. Both intermittent auscultation and electronic monitoring are effective in fetal evaluation when used appropriately (American Academy of Pediatrics [AAP] & ACOG, 1992).

ELECTRONIC FETAL MONITORING

Complete consensus on EFM nomenclature has not been achieved within the United States and Canada and is dependent on the descriptive terminology of various researchers, authors, and equipment manufacturers. Since communication is the essence of quality and safety, common nomenclature should be established among the members of the same perinatal healthcare team. This assures that all members comprehend the meaning of pattern implications. Definitions and terms used in this chapter are commonly found in the literature (ACOG, 1995; Afriat, 1989; Association of Women's Health, Obstetric, and Neonatal Nurses [AWHONN], 1993a; Chez & Harvey, 1994; Freeman, Garite, & Nageotte, 1991; Parer, 1983; Schifrin, 1990; Tucker, 1996).

NURSE-PATIENT COLLABORATION

As with all nursing procedures, preparation for the application of the monitoring equipment requires an explanation of EFM and time for answering the woman and support person's questions. Most women know prior to labor that some form of fetal monitoring may be used. Ideally, objections or concerns regarding EFM will have been discussed between the woman and primary healthcare provider prior to admission. However, if the woman does refuse EFM, the nurse should follow institutional procedure for any patient refusing medical treatment. A positive attitude in discussing the rationale for EFM is most effective. One approach is to explain to the woman and support person that the fetal monitor can provide reassurance of fetal well-being.

PHYSIOLOGIC BASIS FOR FHR MONITORING

EFM is a technique of fetal assessment based on the premise that the FHR is reflective of fetal oxygen status. Maternal factors (e.g., cardiac output, position, and arterial oxygen concentration and hemoglobin level) have a direct influence on adequate maternal oxygen delivery to the placenta and, therefore, on fetal oxygenation. At term, approximately 10–15% of maternal cardiac output, or 500–750 cc of blood volume, perfuses the uterus each minute. Oxygenated blood from the mother is delivered to the placenta via the uterine arteries. Blood enters the intervillous space under positive arterial pressure from the uterine spiral arterioles, surrounds the villi, and then drains back to the uterine veins. Fetal deoxygenated blood is carried to the placental chorionic villi via the two umbilical arteries. Maternal/fetal exchange of oxygen and other nutrients occurs in the placental intervillous space. Oxygen is exchanged through passive diffusion from an area of high concentration (maternal side) to an area of low concentration (fetal side). Carbon dioxide and other fetal waste products are returned to the placenta and the maternal circulatory system to be excreted by the mother. In the absence of uterine activity, lower uterine pressure allows free blood flow across the intervillous space. Fetal and maternal blood do not mix directly. A thin membrane, comprised of a microscopic layer of fetal trophoblasts, permits exchange of respiratory gases, nutrients, and wastes. Oxygenated blood is then delivered to the fetus through the umbilical vein. The transport and transfer of oxygen and carbon dioxide are complex processes dependent on many physiologic and biochemical factors, including intervillous space blood flow, diffusing capacity of the placenta, placental area and vascularity, membrane permeability and thickness, oxygen tension of uterine and umbilical blood vessels, hemoglobin affinity and concentration of maternal and fetal blood, and fetal umbilical blood flow (Tucker, 1996). Mechanisms of exchange of other nutrients and wastes across the placental membrane include passive diffusion, facilitated diffusion, active transport, bulk flow, pinocytosis, and breaks or leaks in chorionic villi (Figure 9-1).

The regulatory control of the FHR is influenced by a number of factors. Display 9-1 summarizes the location, actions, and effects of factors regulating the FHR.

FHR BASELINE

Baseline FHR is assessed over a minimum of a 10-minute time frame, observing for a rise or fall in the FHR or changes in variability during this time period (Figure 9-2). Assessment occurs between contractions and between decelerations or accelerations in the heart rate; therefore, baseline FHR is the rate in the absence of contractions or periodic changes. The normal FHR ranges between 110 to 160 beats per minute (bpm). Rates between 110 and 120 bpm can be considered normal in the fetus over 40 weeks' gestation. In the preterm fetus the FHR may be in the upper range of normal, but the healthy preterm fetus does not usually exhibit a FHR above 160 bpm.

Baseline Changes in Rate

Changes in baseline rate that can occur are (1) tachycardia demonstrating a rate greater than 150–160 bpm, (2) bradycardia with a rate below 110 bpm, (3) a persistent rise in the baseline rate of 20 bpm or greater even within the normal range, (4) or a falling baseline rate when the baseline rate is 20 beats or more below the prior baseline rate (Display 9-2).

Tachycardia

A baseline tachycardia (FHR >150 to 160 bpm for 10 minutes or more) may be caused by fetal conditions such as hypoxemia, anemia, infection, prematurity, cardiac dysrhythmias, and congenital anomalies or by maternal conditions such as fever, dehydration, infection, anxiety, or medical problems as in thyroid

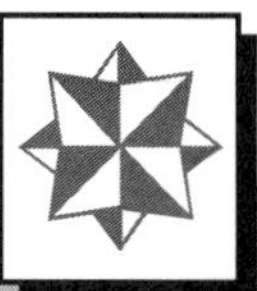

DISPLAY 9-1

Factors Regulating Fetal Heart Rate	Location
Parasympathetic division of autonomic nervous system	Vagus nerve fibers supply sinoatrial (SA) and atrioventricular (AV) node
Sympathetic division of autonomic nervous system	Nerves widely distributed in myocardium
Baroceptors	Stretch receptors in aortic arch and carotid sinus at the junction of the internal and external carotid arteries
Chemoceptors	Peripheral—in cartoid and aortic bodies
	Central—in medulla oblongata
Central nervous system	Cerebral cortex
	Hypothalamus
	Medulla oblongata
Hormonal regulation	Adrenal medulla
	Adrenal cortex
	Vasopressin (plasma catecholamine)
Blood volume/capillary fluid shift	Fluid shift between capillaries and interstitial spaces
Intraplacental pressures	Intervillous space
Frank-Starling mechanism	Based on stretching of myocardium by increased inflow of venous blood into right atrium

From Tucker, S.M. (1996) Fetal Monitoring, St. Louis, MO: Mosby-Year Book.

Action	Effect
Stimulation causes release of acetylcholine at myoneural synapse	Decreases heart rate Maintains beat-to-beat variability
Stimulation causes release of norepinephrine at synapse	Increases FHR Increases strength of myocardial contraction Increases cardiac output
Responds to increase in blood pressure by stimulating stretch receptors to send impulses via vagus or glossopharyngeal nerve to midbrain, producing vagal response and slowing heart activity	Decreases FHR Decreases blood pressure Decreases cardiac output
Responds to a marked peripheral decrease in O_2 and increase in CO_2	Produces bradycardia sometimes with increased variability
Central chemoceptors respond to decreases in O_2 tension and increases in CO_2 tension in blood and/or cerebrospinal fluid	Produces tachycardia and increase in blood pressure with decrease in variability
Responds to fetal movement	Increases variability
Responds to fetal sleep	Decreases variability
Regulates and coordinates autonomic activities (sympathetic and parasympathetic)	
Mediates cardiac and vasomotor reflex center by controlling heart action and blood vessel diameter	Maintains balance between cardioacceleration and cardiodeceleration
Releases epinephrine and norepinephrine with severe fetal hypoxia, producing sympathetic response	Increases FHR Increases strength of myocardial contraction and blood pressure Increases cardiac output
Low fetal blood pressure stimulates release of aldosterone, decreases sodium output, increases water retention, which increases circulating blood volume	Maintains homeostasis of blood volume
Produces vasoconstriction of nonvital vascular in the asphyxiated fetus	Distributes blood flow to maintain FHR and variability
Responds to elevated blood pressure by causing fluid to move out of capillaires and into interstitial spaces	Decreases blood volume and blood pressure
Responds to low blood pressure by causing fluid to move out of interstitial space into capillaires	Increases blood volume and blood pressure
Fluid shift between fetal and maternal blood is based on osmotic and blood pressure gradients; maternal blood pressure is about 100 mmHg and fetal blood pressure about 55 mmHg; therefore balance is probably maintained by some compensatory factor	Regulates blood volume and blood pressure
In the adult the myocardium is stretched by an increased inflow of blood, causing the heart to contract with greater force than before and pump out more blood; the adult then is able to increase cardiac output by increasing heart rate and stroke volume; this mechanism is not well developed in the fetus	Cardiac output is dependent on heart rate in the fetus: ↓ FHR = ↓ cardiac output ↑ FHR = ↑ cardiac output

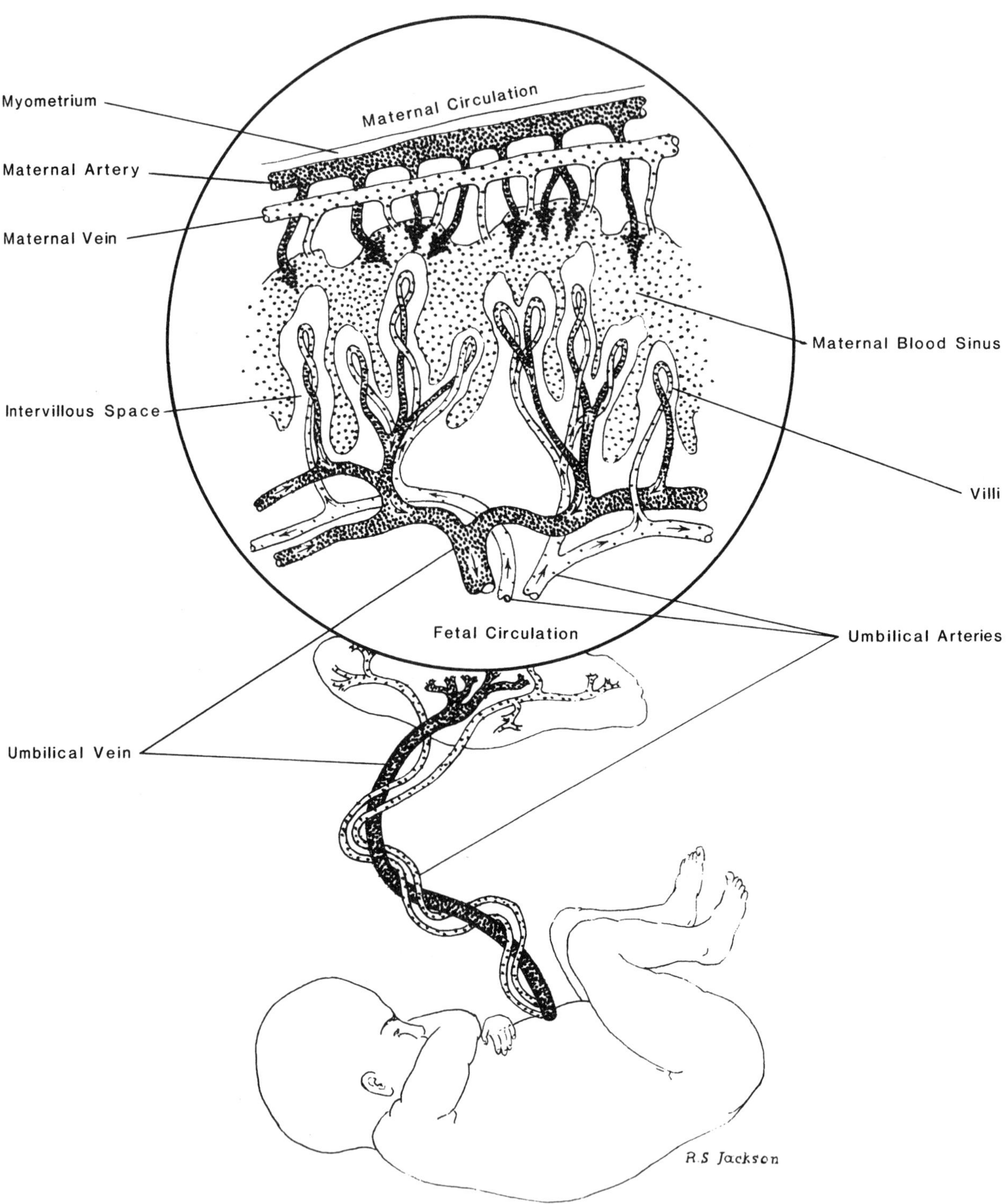

Figure 9-1. Maternal–Placental–Fetal Exchange.

From Afriat, C.I. (1989). Electronic fetal monitoring. Rockville, MD: Aspen.

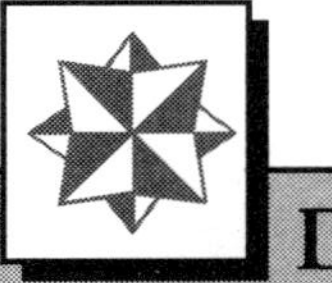

DISPLAY 9-2

Causes of Baseline Changes in Fetal Heart Rate

Tachycardia

Acute Hypoxemia/Hypoxia
- Decreased blood flow to fetus causing
  - –stimulation of baroreceptors
  - –decreased oxygen flow to fetus
  - –increased carbon dioxide level
  - –stimulation of chemoreceptors
  - –increase in FHR to eliminate excess carbon dioxide

Maternal Fever
- Increase in maternal temperature
- Increase in fetal temperature

Medications
- Fetal cardiac and central nervous system response to β-blockers such as atropine and scopolamine

Maternal Anxiety
- Increased maternal heart rate (may be reflected in FHR)

Persistent Tachycardia

Prematurity
- Inherently higher FHR (although rarely more than 160 bpm)

Dysrhythmia
- Supraventricular tachycardia
- Atrial tachycardia
- Ventricular tachycardia

Hypoxemia/Hypoxia (associated with decelerations)
- Maintenance of high FHR in attempt to eliminate excess carbon dioxide
- Return of FHR to normal with subsequent bradycardia and death due to asphyxia
- Decreased variability or variable decelerations with overshoot in chronic distress

Bradycardia

Hypoxemia/Hypoxia
- Terminal bradycardia preceding death
- Failure of compensatory mechanism to eliminate excess carbon dioxide from circulation

Medications
- Paracervical block causing
  - –uterine hyperstimulation with resultant decreased uteroplacental blood flow
  - –maternal supine position with resultant decreased uteroplacental blood flow
  - –direct fetal injection with resultant drug toxicity

Fetal Hypothermia
- Diving reflex (bradycardia) caused by cold water used to flush intrauterine pressure catheter

Vagal Response
- Stimulation of fetal parasympathetic nervous system

Congenital Defect
- Heart block
- Cardiac anomaly
- Central nervous system anomaly

Adapted from Afriat, CI, (1989) Electronic Fetal Monitoring, rockville, MD: Aspen

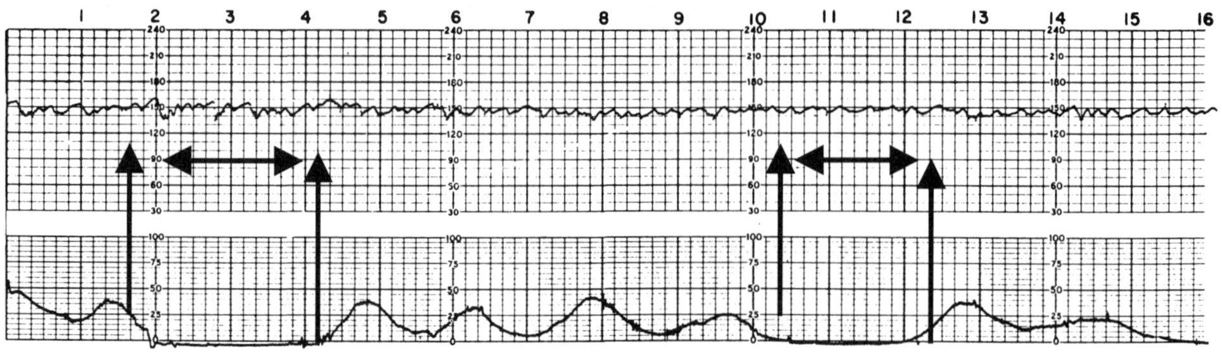

Figure 9-2. The baseline fetal heart rate is the rate between contractions, between decelerations, or when no contractions are present.

From Afriat, C.I. (1989). Electronic fetal monitoring. Rockville, MD: Aspen.

disease. Beta sympathomimetic drugs such as terbutaline and ritodrine may also cause both maternal and fetal tachycardia.

Management of tachycardia includes assessing maternal temperature and hydration, gestational age determination, and a review of maternal history for preexisting medical conditions and medication use. Tachycardia represents increased sympathetic and/or decreased parasympathetic autonomic tone and is therefore generally associated with a loss of variability (Freeman, Garite, & Nageotte 1991). Tachycardia with average short-term variability (STV) in the absence of FHR decelerations usually is not of particular concern. It should be closely observed, however, especially if there is not an obvious explanation, as listed above.

Conversely, a rising baseline rate following late or variable decelerations indicates the need for further evaluation to rule out hypoxemia. Evaluation includes fetal scalp stimulation to elicit an acceleration of the FHR, maternal position change, infusion of IV fluids, oxygen administration at 8–12 L/min by mask, and possibly fetal blood sampling.

Bradycardia

A baseline bradycardia (FHR <110–120 bpm for 10 minutes or more) may be caused by fetal conditions such as hypoxemia or asphyxia from a chronic or acute situation causing decreased oxygen flow to the fetus, vagal stimulation, cardiac or other anomalies, or hypothermia. FHR bradycardia in the presence of average variability is frequently associated with an occiput-posterior position or transverse position and is probably the result of increased vagal tone (Freeman, Garite, Nageotte, 1991).

Sustained fetal bradycardia with normal fetal movement is usually caused by complete atrioventricular (AV) heart block associated with clinical or serologic evidence of maternal collagen vascular disease, especially systemic lupus erythematosus (Hohn & Stanton, 1992). In a fetus with complete AV heart block, a FHR between 60 and 70 bpm without variability may be present (Tucker, 1996). Interventions during the intrapartum period are usually not warranted; however, the neonatal team should be notified. The newborn may require cardioversion after birth or pacemaker insertion. Other causes of fetal bradycardia and complete heart block are severe structural congenital cardiac disease (Hohn & Stanton, 1992) and cytomegalovirus (Freeman, Garite, Nagotte, 1991). An ultrasound examination to rule out structural cardiac disease and verify that the heart rate recording is not maternal in origin is the best approach in the presence of fetal bradycardia.

Variations in bradycardias exist. Bradycardia occurs occasionally during the second stage of labor, following a previously normal FHR pattern. It may be due to increased vagal tone as with forcep application or cord compression. If the short-term variability remains average and the FHR does not fall below 80 to 90 bpm, expediting birth is not generally warranted. However, methods to improve blood flow should be instituted (Figure 9-3).

The woman should be encouraged to push in either lateral position, avoiding the supine position. If possible, she should push with alternating contractions

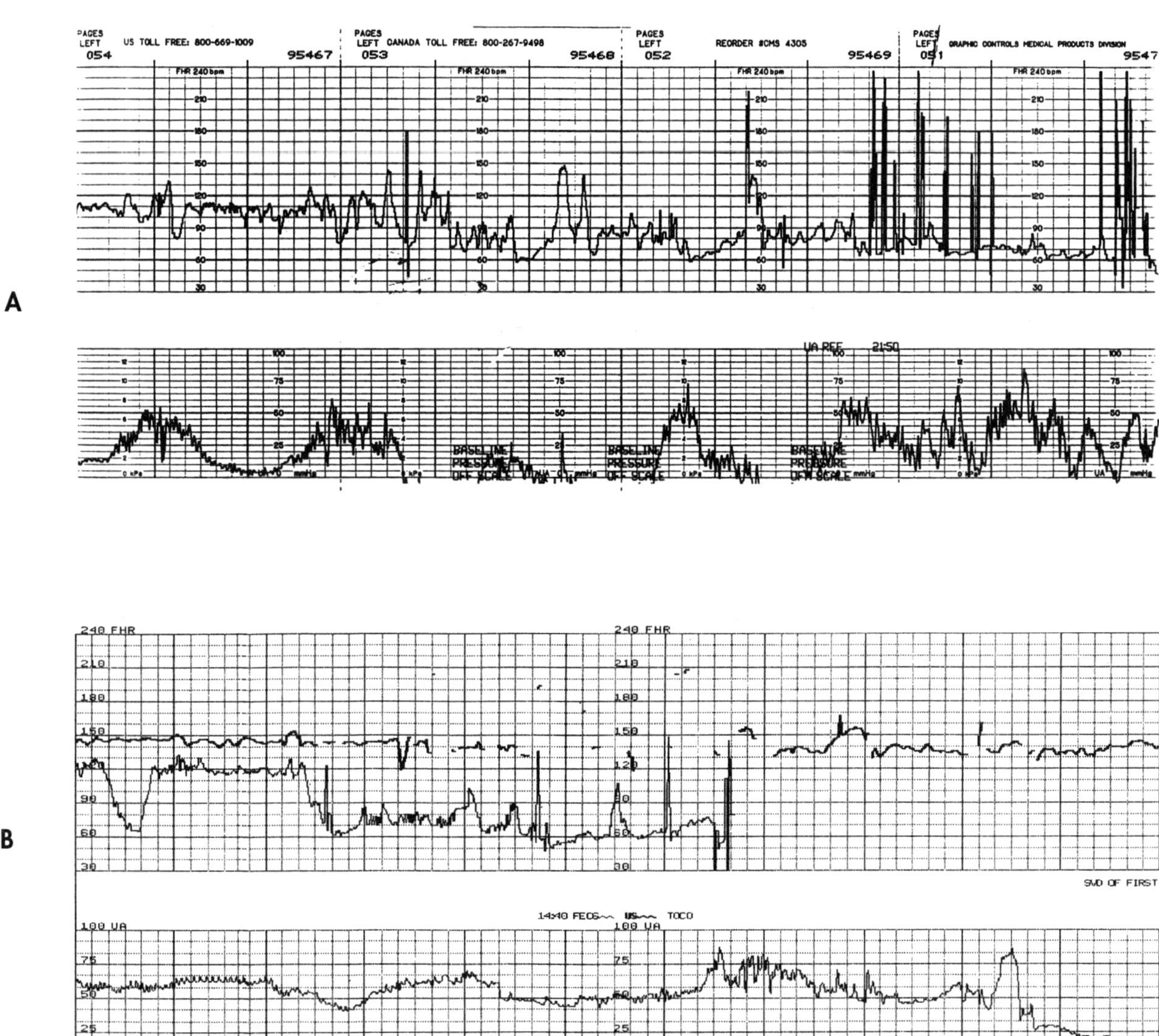

Figure 9-3. A. Second stage bradycardia secondary to forceps application. **B.** Second stage Bradycardia during birth of first twin. Other twin's FHR is reassuring.

to allow the fetus to gain a few added minutes of improved blood flow. Coaching a laboring woman to push with every other contraction may be difficult if she has no anesthesia, so this strategy may only be possible with regional anesthesia in place.

A terminal bradycardia is preceded by a nonreassuring tracing evidenced by either decelerations, absent or decreased variability, and possibly a tachycardia. This type of bradycardia warrants concern and may require cesarean birth since it generally precedes death in utero if it is a result of hypoxia. All methods to improve blood flow as described above should be instituted, as well as scalp stimulation and possibly fetal blood gas sampling (Figure 9-4).

Baseline Variability

In predicting fetal status, the most important aspect of the FHR is variability. Variability is the term used to characterize the baseline FHR variations from beat to beat (short-term variability) and fluctuations over 1-minute time intervals (long-term variability) (AWHONN, 1993a) (Figure 9-5). It is the normal irregularity of cardiac rhythm, resulting in a continuous balance between the sympathetic (cardioacceleration)

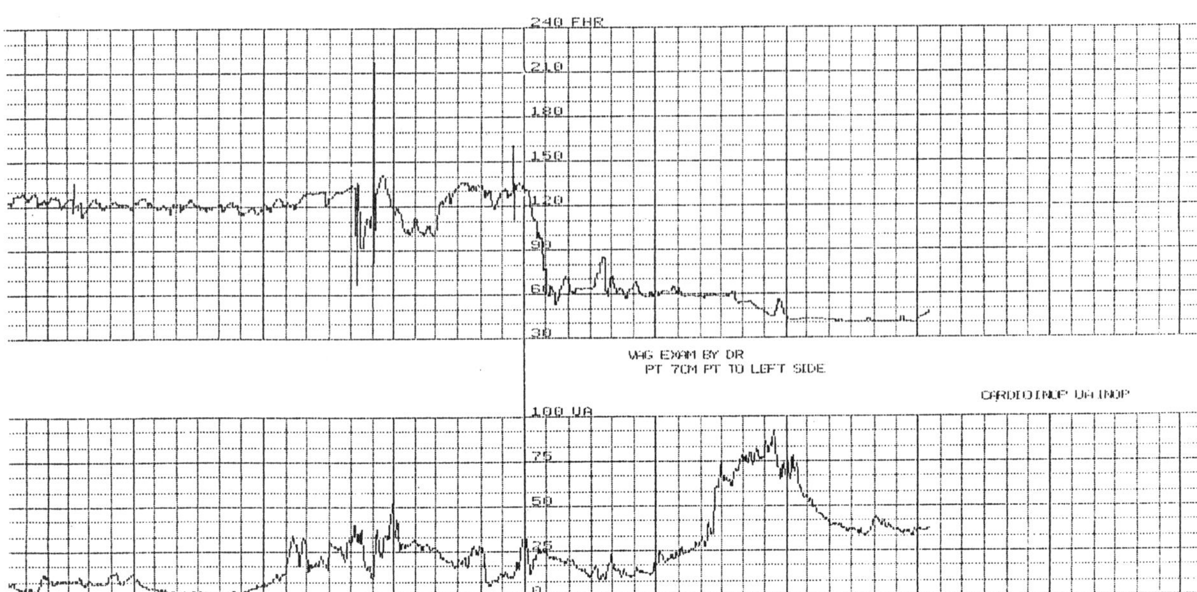

Figure 9-4. Terminal bradycardia as the result of a abruptio placentae. A cesarean birth was performed with good neonatal outcome and evidence of a 75% abruption.

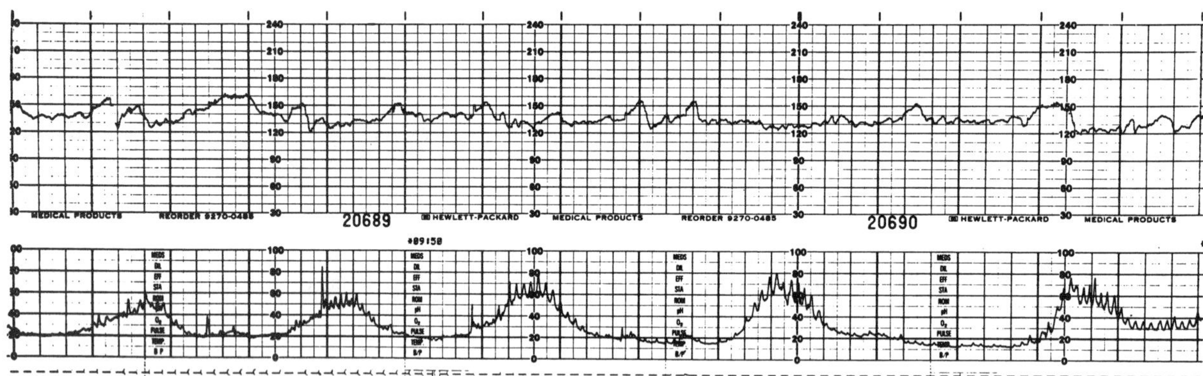

Figure 9-5. The tracing was obtained with a direct fetal electrode. Note the presence of both average short-term variability (beat to beat) and average long-term variability (fluctuations throughout the entire segment of tracing). This is a reassuring tracing.

and parasympathetic (cardiodeceleration) divisions of the autonomic nervous system (ANS) (Tucker, 1996). Normal variability of the FHR is a reflection of intact neurological modulation of the FHR and normal cardiac responsiveness (Freeman, Garite, Nagoette, 1991).

Long-term variability (LTV) appears as rhythmic fluctuations or waves, generally at a frequency of 3–6 cycles per minute, and is best assessed over time or a period of heart rate cycles. Changes in LTV are most evident in the fetus during "sleep-wake" cycles. In the presence of decreased LTV after a previously reassuring FHR pattern, attempts to stimulate the fetus, such as manual manipulation or noise, will result in a return of normal LTV if the pattern was due to fetal sleep.

STV in the FHR is a fluctuation from one heart beat to the next heart beat. It is an inaudible change in rate that occurs in milliseconds, representing the interval differences between R waves of the QRS complex of the fetal cardiac cycle. These fluctuations in rate appear on the fetal tracing as tiny ups and downs in rate that are visible due to slow paper speed. STV is an indication of fetal central nervous system (CNS) function. The interplay between the parasympathetic and sympathetic causes a "tug of war" effect. The parasympathetic pulls the heart rate down and the sympathetic pulls the heart rate up, with the balance achieved constituting the presence of STV. When there is an oxygen deficit in the CNS, the interplay malfunctions, resulting in a loss of variability. Therefore, STV is an indication of fetal oxygen reserve. However, most changes in variability are nonpathologic. Many other factors can affect the fetal CNS and cause a decrease in STV. The most common causes are narcotics, tranquilizers, and other analgesics administered to women during labor, including narcotics that are added to epidural and spinal anesthetics. These agents will suppress both STV and LTV. Other causes of decreased STV include fetal tachycardia, prematurity, cardiac and CNS anomalies, and fetal sleep.

Both STV and LTV are assessed during the baseline of the fetal heart rate, not during a deceleration. STV is most accurately recorded with a direct spiral electrode or maternal abdominal wall fetal ECG monitoring. The ultrasound devices on the most current generation of fetal monitors produce a recording that closely correlates with a direct electrode. However, when in doubt about the accuracy of the STV or if it appears decreased with the external transducer, an electrode should be applied, if possible.

Application of a fetal electrode is invasive and increases risk of maternal-fetal infection. As a result, there is a trend to reduce frequency in the use of direct fetal electrodes. Further, there is evidence to suggest that application of a direct electrode could enhance maternal-fetal transmission of the human immunodeficiency virus (HIV) when used in women who are HIV seropositive (Craven, Steger, & Jarek, 1994), however data are inconclusive. Therefore, until more information is known about risks of HIV transmission to the fetus via scalp electrodes, external monitoring or auscultation should be used for these women (ACOG, 1992). External EFM provides information about FHR reactivity. It has been widely established that if the FHR pattern is reactive, it is as reassuring as having average STV. A fetus must have a well-oxygenated ANS in order to have a reactive heart rate.

A reactive FHR pattern has variable accelerations of the heart rate that are greater than 15 beats above the baseline and last longer than 15 seconds (Figure 9-6A). In the absence of decelerations, this is a reassuring pattern and consistent with good fetal outcome. A nonreactive tracing indicates the absence of reactivity of the heart rate, an absence of accelerations that meets the above-mentioned criteria (Figure 9-6B). Nonreactivity, however, is not an indication of fetal compromise. In most cases it indicates a fetal sleep cycle and requires no intervention other than stimulation of the fetus to elicit an acceleration.

Several factors may account for loss of STV (Display 9-3). Anything that has an impact on the CNS will influence STV. It is not unusual to see a loss of STV following narcotic, tranquilizer, or anesthetic administration if a normal FHR preceded the administration. If the loss of STV can be traced to the administration of analgesia or anesthesia, no intervention is warranted nor is it necessary to withhold medication. Obtaining a reactive tracing prior to the administration of any medication is recommended; if a loss of STV results the etiology will be evident.

Other causes of decreased or absent STV include fetal tachycardia, prematurity due to an immature CNS, fetal sleep, and dysrhythmias. Persistent loss of STV of unknown etiology is suggestive of fetal hypoxemia or cardiac or CNS anomalies. Nursing intervention includes repositioning the woman to a lateral position, administration of IV fluids and oxygen, and notification of the physician or nurse-midwife. Fetal stimulation and/or fetal blood sampling may be initiated.

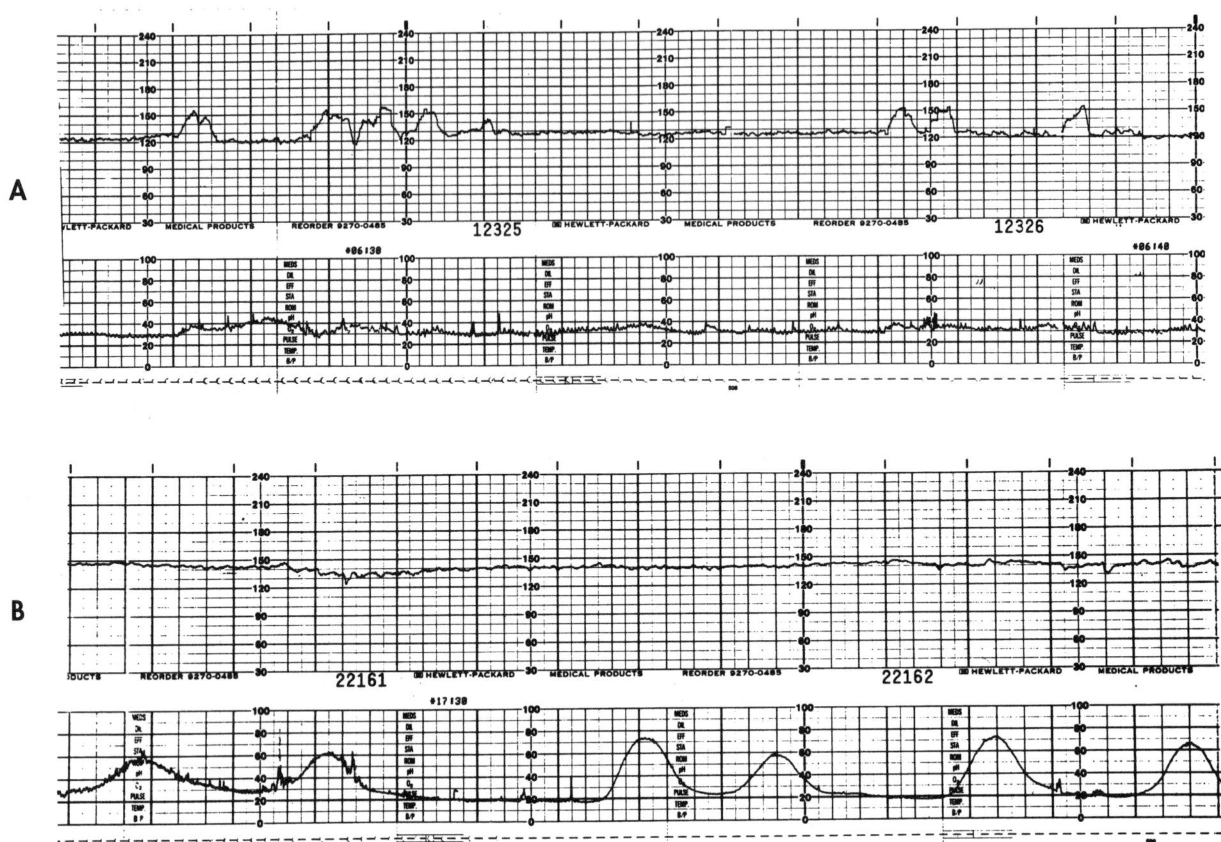

Figure 9-6. A. Reactive fetal heart rate pattern, with accelerations in response to fetal stimulation. **B.** Nonreactive fetal heart rate pattern, with no accelerations.

Causes of increased STV include fetal stimulation following the application of the direct fetal electrode or during maternal expulsive efforts. It is usually a normal response; however, some researchers believe that increased STV may be an early sign of fetal hypoxia (Freeman, Garite, Nageotte, 1991). Systematic evaluation of other aspects of the FHR tracing with identification of potential reasons for increased STV and continued fetal surveillance are indicated.

Since consensus in the literature and among perinatal healthcare providers does not exist, the most commonly used nomenclature related to STV and LTV are presented in Display 9-4. Quantifying changes in FHR variability, based on the beats-per-minute parameters outlined in Display 9-5, is useful for the novice learning to evaluate variability. However, FHR variability in clinical practice is most often described as absent, minimal or decreased, average, or increased. A visual inspection of variability displayed assists in selecting the appropriate description. No one nomenclature is superior. To ensure consistency in medical record documentation and to facilitate collaboration and communication, members of the perinatal healthcare team at each institution should decide on terminology to be used.

PERIODIC FHR

Periodic changes in heart rate are short-term changes in rate rather than baseline changes, lasting anywhere from a few seconds to 1 or 2 minutes. They are referred to as accelerations and decelerations. They are termed periodic because they occur repetitively or at periodic intervals. The four types of FHR decelerations are early, late, variable, and prolonged decelerations (Figure 9-7). The accelerations are referred to as uniform, shoulders (or variable accelerations), and rebound overshoots (Figure 9-8). Each is described.

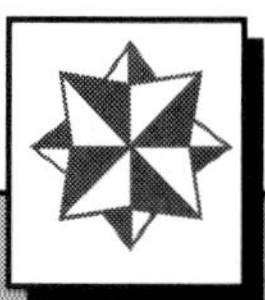

DISPLAY 9-3

Causes of Decreased Short-Term Variability

Cause	Rationale
Medications	Drugs that cross the placenta have the same effect on the fetal CNS as on an adult
Prematurity	Immature central nervous system
Fetal sleep	Central nervous system at rest
Fetal dysrhythmia	Central nervous system or cardiac anomaly
Anesthetic agents	Anesthetics cross the placenta and affect the fetal central nervous system
Central nervous system damage, anomaly, or ischemic injury	Loss of cardiac function secondary to central nervous system dysfunction
Hypoxemia/Hypoxia	Decreased oxygen flow to the fetal central nervous system

Adapted from Afriat, C.I. (1989). Electronic fetal monitoring. Rockville, MD: Aspen.

Decelerations

Early Decelerations

Early decelerations are believed to be caused by fetal head compression. Altered cerebral blood flow causes the decrease in heart rate through a vagal reflex (Display 9-6). When the contraction occurs, the fetal head is pressed into the maternal pelvis, stimulating the vagus nerve. The heart rate begins to drop at the onset of the contraction when the head compression begins and returns to the baseline rate at the end of the contraction when the head is no longer compressed. Generally, early decelerations mirror the contraction causing it; this means that the longer the contraction lasts and the stronger it is, the longer the deceleration lasts, and the deeper it is. Therefore, early decelerations reflect the intensity and duration of the contraction. They are benign decelerations, requiring no intervention or treatment and are not associated with fetal hypoxia or low Apgar scores.

Late Decelerations

Late decelerations may be precipitated by the following physiologic events: altered maternal blood flow to the placenta, reduced maternal arterial oxygen saturation, or placental changes altering maternal-fetal gas exchange (AWHONN, 1993a). Decreased uterine blood flow is a much more common cause of late decelerations than poor maternal-fetal exchange from other causes (Freeman, Garite, Nageotte, 1991). Alteration in blood flow may be either chronic (due to deterioration of the placenta as sometimes seen in women with diabetes, pregnancy-induced hypertension, or collagen disease), or an acute change in physiologic function (such as that resulting from uterine hyperstimulation, placental abruption, or maternal hypotension).

With all uterine activity, a physiologic decrease in blood flow occurs as the contraction builds, with minimal or absent exchange by the peak of a contraction. Normal, healthy fetuses have a reserve of oxygen that is used during this time with every contraction. Some fetuses, however, have less reserve and will demonstrate late decelerations. Generally, the beginning of the late deceleration occurs with the peak of the contraction, when the blood flow and exchange of gases is minimal or absent. Recovery to the baseline rate does not occur until the contraction has ended, blood flow has resumed, and reoxygenation of the fetus has occurred. Therefore, FHR recovery occurs well after the contraction ends.

Late decelerations mirror the contraction in terms of shape: the stronger and longer the contraction is, the deeper and longer the deceleration usually lasts. If hypertonus occurs and the contraction lasts 3 minutes, late deceleration will mirror the contraction. Late decelerations are also repetitive with contractions that are of equal duration and amplitude (Display 9-6). After prolonged periods of fetal hypoxemia, late decelerations may become more subtle, reflecting the inability of the chronically compromised fetus to respond to the stress of uterine activity.

Late decelerations should be evaluated in the context of other FHR characteristics. For example, late decelerations with average baseline rate and variability,

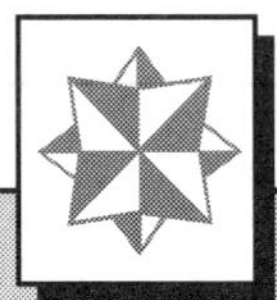

DISPLAY 9-4

Variability Nomenclature

Author	Short Term Variability (STV)	Long Term Variability (LTV)
Afriat (1989)	Absent Decreased Average Increased	Decreased Present
AWHONN Fetal Heart Monitoring Principles and Practices (1993)	Absent Present	Decreased/Minimal (0–5 bpm) Average/Within Normal Limits (6–25 bpm) Marked/Saltatory (>25 bpm)
Parer (1983)	Absent Present	Absent (0–2 bpm) Decreased (<6 bpm) Normal (6–25 bpm) Saltatory (>25 bpm)
Murray (1996)	Absent Present	Absent (0–2 bpm) Decreased/Minimal (3–5 bpm) Average/Within Normal Limits (6–25 bpm) Marked/Saltatory (>25 bpm)
Schifrin (1990)	Absent Decreased Average Increased	Absent (<2 bpm) Decreased (<5 bpm) Average (5–15 bpm) Increased (>15 bpm)
Tucker (1992)	STV and LTV tend to decrease and increase together; they are described as a unit None (0–2 bpm) Minimal (3–5 bpm) Average (6–10 bpm) Moderate (11–25 bpm) Marked (>25 bpm)	
Freeman, Garite, & Nageotte (1991)	STV and LTV tend to decrease and increase together; they are described as a unit Absent Decreased Good Increased	

Simpson, K.R. (1996)

DISPLAY 9-5

<table>
<tr><th colspan="5">Examples of Variability Nomenclature</th></tr>
<tr><td>0–2 bpm</td><td>Absent</td><td>Absent</td><td rowspan="2">Decreased</td><td rowspan="2">Absent</td></tr>
<tr><td>3–5 bpm</td><td>Minimal</td><td>Minimal</td></tr>
<tr><td>6–15 bpm</td><td>Average</td><td rowspan="2">Average</td><td rowspan="2">Average</td><td rowspan="3">Present</td></tr>
<tr><td>15–25 bpm</td><td>Moderate</td></tr>
<tr><td><25 bpm</td><td>Marked</td><td>Marked</td><td>Increased</td></tr>
</table>

Chez, B.F., & Harvey, C. (1994) Essentials of electronic fetal monitoring (Videotape Series, 2nd ed.). Baltimore, MD: Williams & Wilkins.

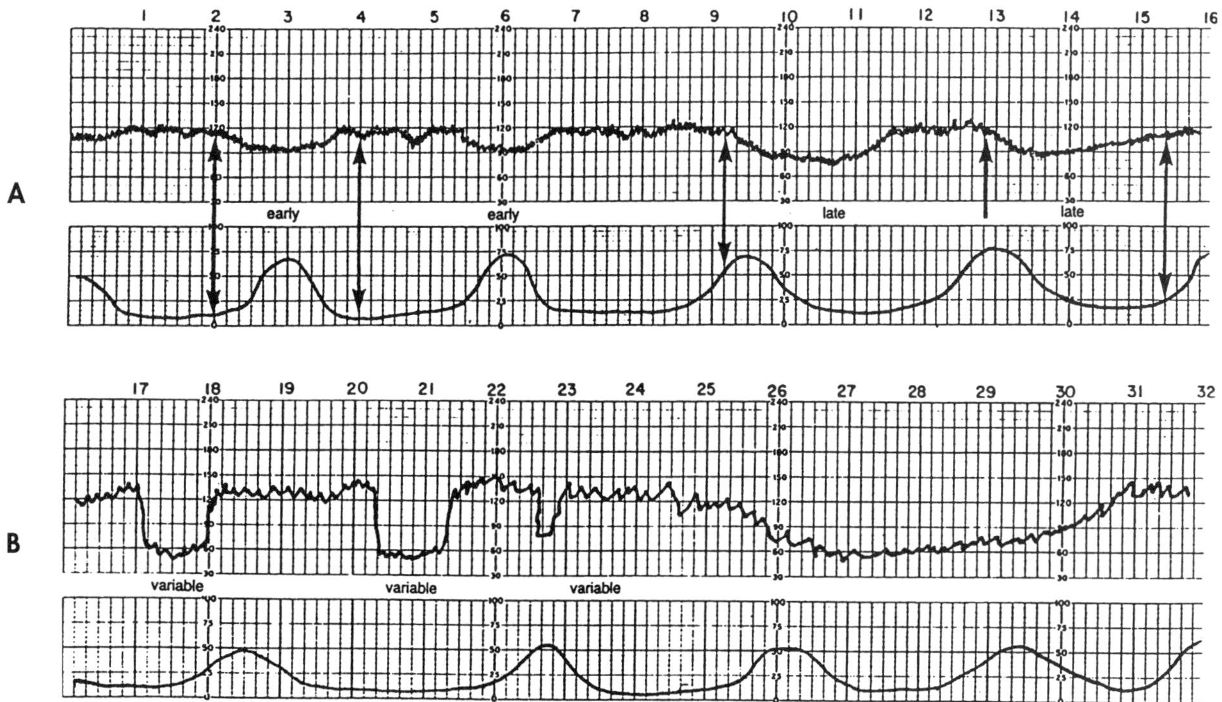

Figure 9-7. A. Schematic drawing of periodic changes. Although the shape and depth of early and late decelerations are similar, note the differences in the onset of the decelerations and the recovery time to the baseline rate. **B.** Schematic drawing of variable and prolonged decelerations. Note the abrupt drop in FHR in both types of decelerations. The variable decelerations return to baseline more quickly than the prolonged decelerations at 26.5 minutes, however.

From Afriat, C.I. (1989) Electronic fetal monitoring. Rockville, MD: Aspen.

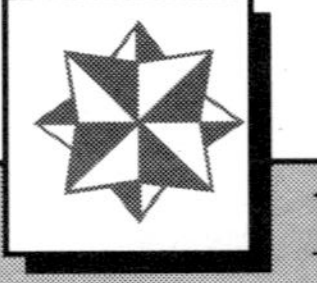

DISPLAY 9-6

Causes of Periodic Decelerations

Early Decelerations

Fetal Head Compression
- Vertex presentation
- Primigravidas
- Second stage of labor may appear to be variable)

Late Decelerations

Uteroplacental Insufficiency
- Maternal supine position
- Fetal and uterine compression of maternal inferior vena cava or aorta
- Decreased maternal blood flow to placenta
- Deteriorating placenta
- Uterine hyperstimulation with decreased placental blood flow

Variable Decelerations

Umbilical Cord Compression
- Decreased blood flow through cord to fetus causing
  - stimulation of baroreceptors
  - decreased oxygen flow to fetus
  - Increase in carbon dioxide
  - stimulation of chemoreceptors
  - complete cord occlusion

Head Compression (second stage of labor)
- Increased intracranial pressure causing
  - increased peripheral resistance
  - increased blood pressure
  - reflex (vagal) deceleration

Prolonged Decelerations

Umbilical Cord Compression (same mechanisms)

Decreased Uteroplacental Blood Flow (same mechanisms)

Vagal Response (head compression or cord compression)

Adapted from Afriat, C.I., (1989). Electronic fetal monitoring. Rockville, MD: Aspen.

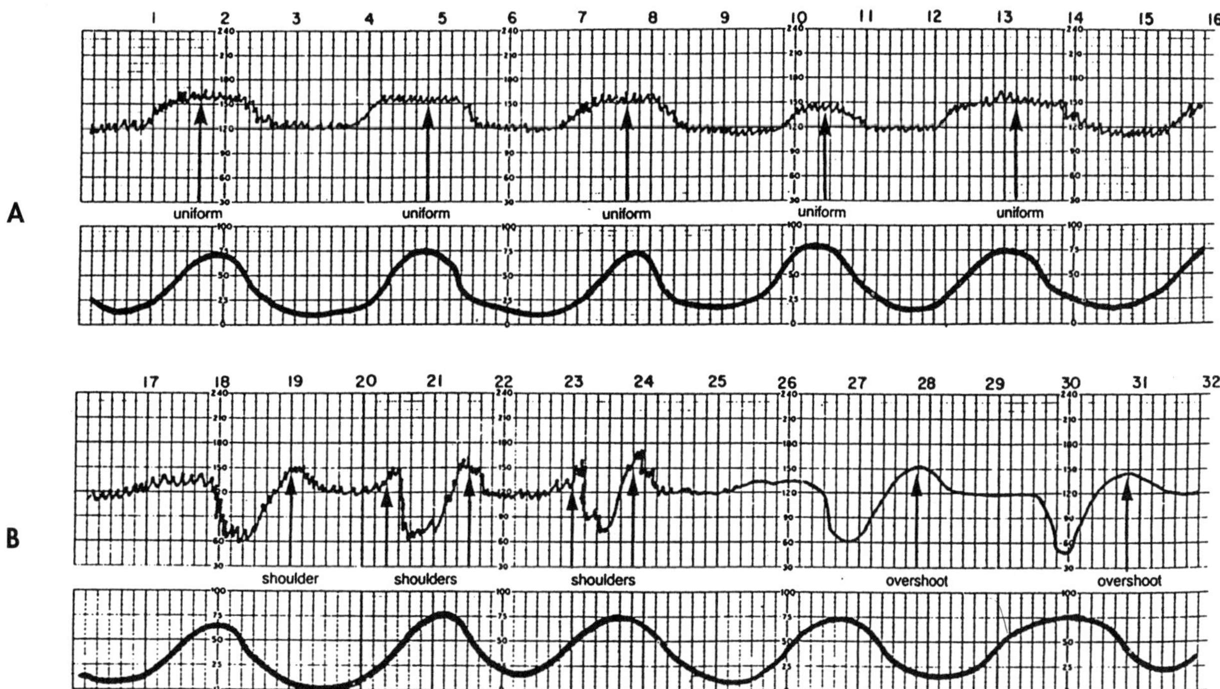

Figure 9-8. Schematic drawings of periodic accelerations. **A.** Uniform accelerations begin at the beginning of the contraction and return to baseline at the end of the contraction. **B.** Shoulders precede and follow variable decelerations with average short-term variability. Rebound overshoots only follow variable decelerations with absent or minimal short-term variability.

From Afriat, C.I. (1989). Electronic fetal monitoring. Rockville, MD: Aspen.

and accelerations warrant less concern than late decelerations in the presence of an abnormal baseline rate, decreased variability, and absence of accelerations. If late decelerations develop, the precipitating factor should be explored. If the FHR pattern had been reassuring prior to the onset of decelerations, an iatrogenic cause, such as maternal hypotension, frequently can be determined. Maternal history for risk factors for uteroplacental insufficiency and evaluation of the uterine activity pattern are essential (Display 9-7).

Management of late decelerations focuses on maximizing placental function by maintaining a lateral maternal position, increasing intravenous fluids to correct dehydration or volume depletion, discontinuation of oxytocin, and administration of oxygen by mask. Collectively, these interventions are sometimes referred to as intrauterine resuscitation. In addition, iatrogenic insults that may further compromise the placenta, such as hyperstimulation with oxytocin or maternal hypotension secondary to maternal supine position, should be avoided.

If the FHR pattern does not return to the previously reassuring tracing following interventions described above, tocolytics may be used to inhibit uterine activity. Usually this allows the fetus to recover (Figure 9-9). However, if tocolytics are used and birth follows quickly, the possibility of a postpartum hemorrhage secondary to uterine atony should be anticipated.

If the tracing never demonstrated any reassuring signs (such as average STV, a reactive FHR, or an adequate response to scalp stimulation) and late decelerations fail to respond to nonsurgical interventions, a fetal scalp blood gas sample assessment or cesarean birth may be indicated.

Variable Decelerations

The most frequently seen FHR deceleration pattern in labor is variable decelerations. Variable decelerations result from either umbilical cord compression or vagal stimulation. They are described as having a very abrupt drop in FHR. Variable decelerations are called "variables" because the characteristics may change. They vary in

A

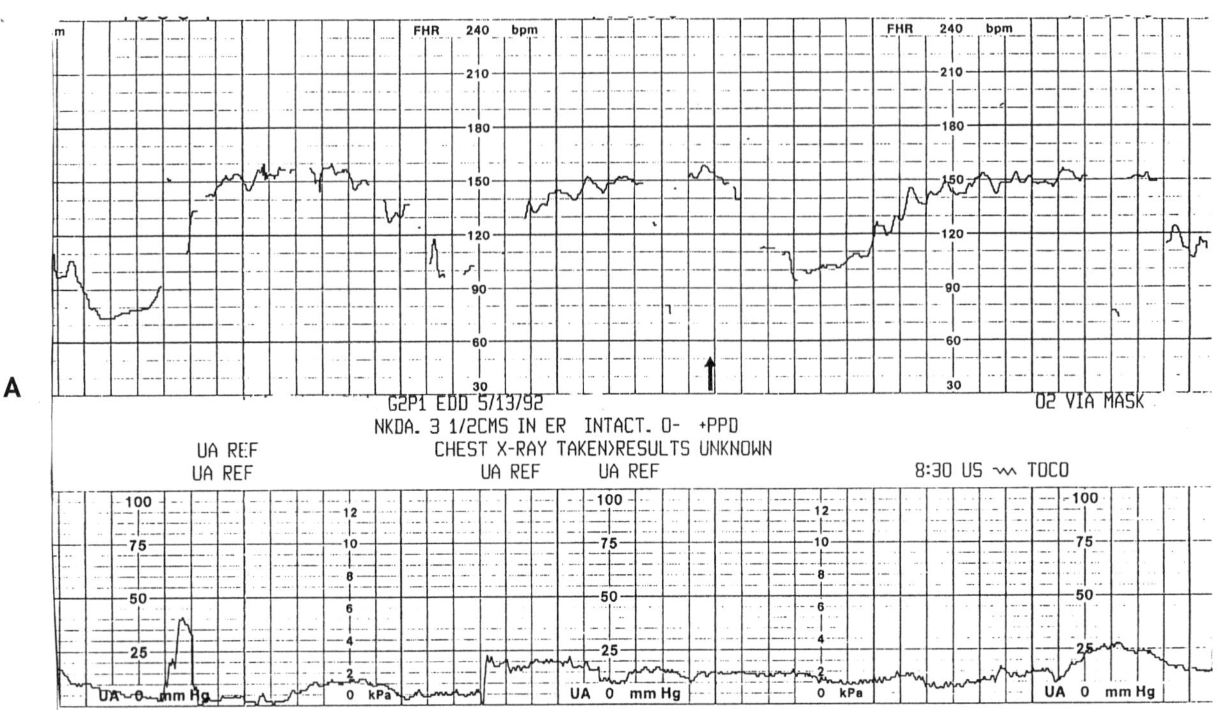

B

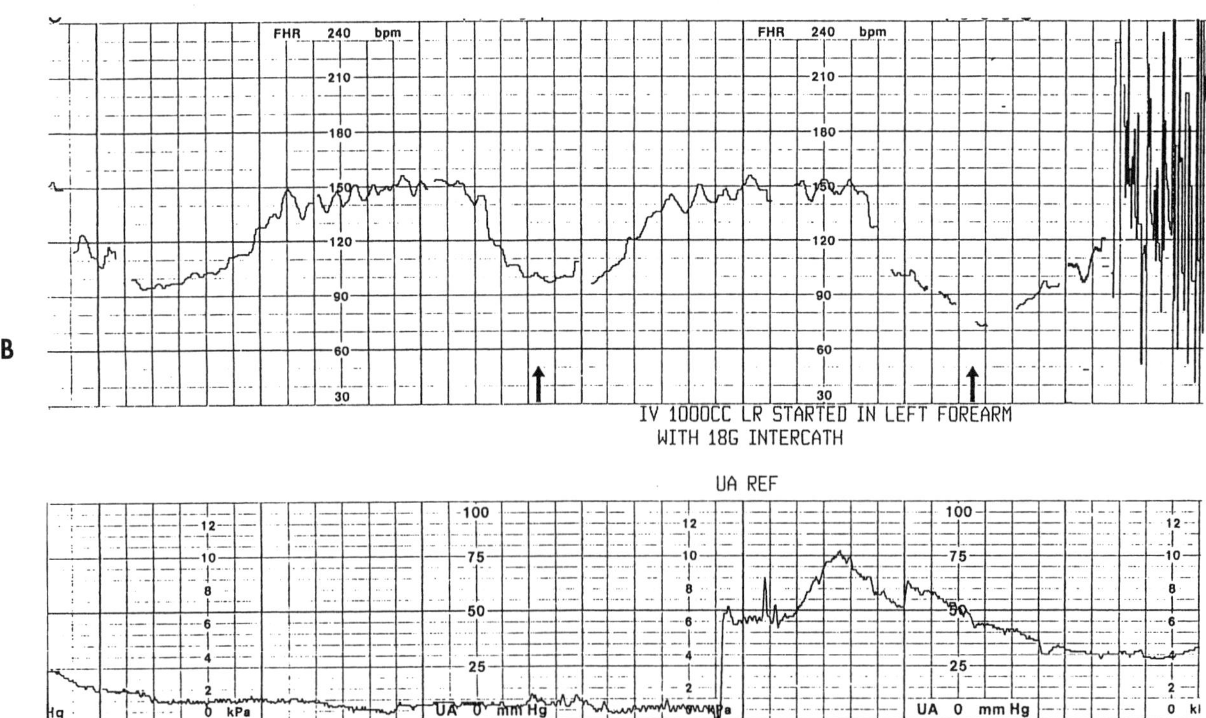

Figure 9-9. A,B, C, & D. Late decelerations, secondary to sponataneous uterine hypertonus were successfully treated with the administration of terbutaline. The fetal blood gas obtained at the end of the fourth panel on page 205 had a pH of 7.25 and B.E. −3.5. A vaginal birth occured with a normal cord blood gas.

Figure 9-9 (cont.)

C

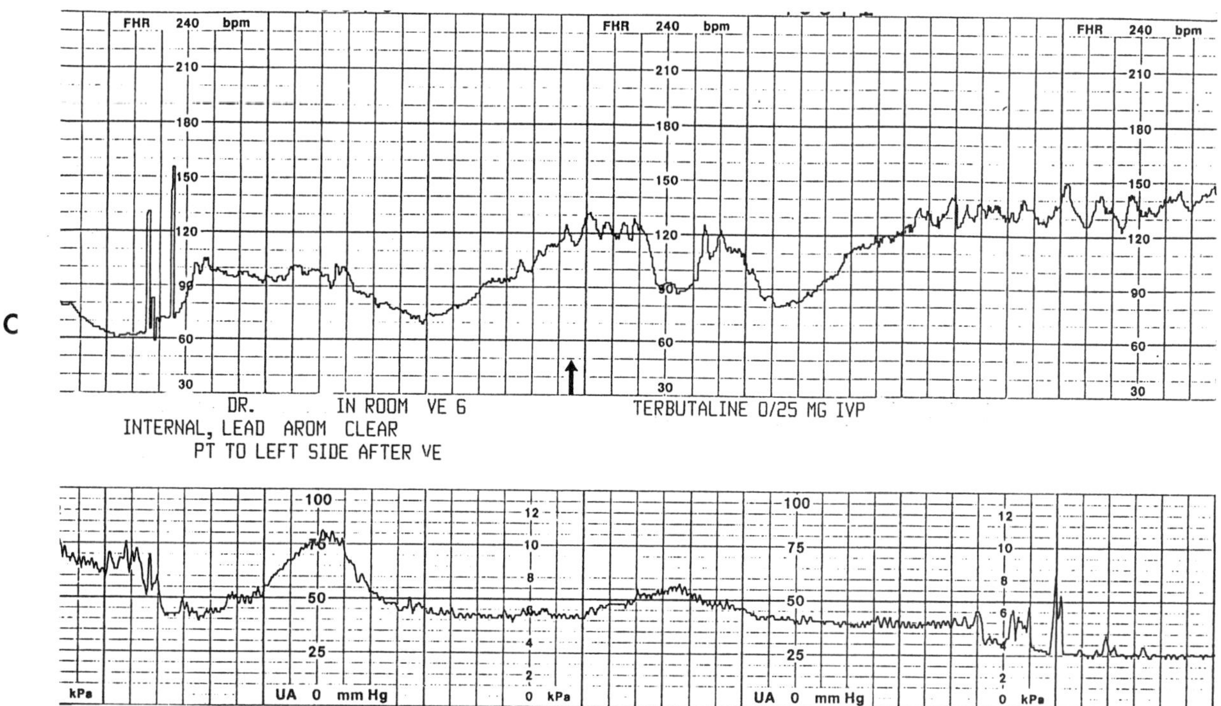

D

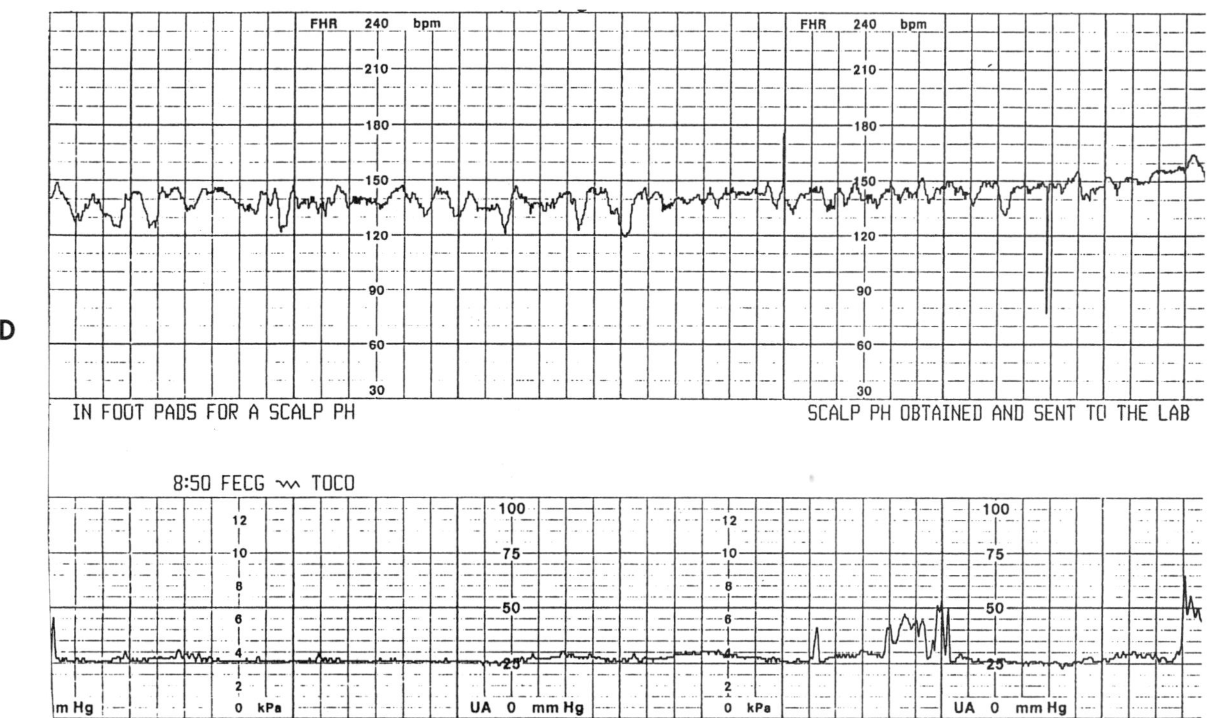

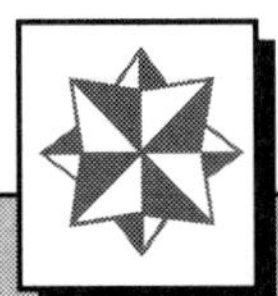

DISPLAY 9-7

Conditions Related to Late Decelerations in Fetal Heart Rate Pattern

Obstetric and Anesthetic Procedures

Uterine Hyperstimulation
Decreasing Uteroplacental Blood Flow
- Spontaneous uterine activity
- Oxytocin administration

Maternal Supine Position
Allowing Fetal and Uterine Compression of Maternal Inferior Vena Cava or Aorta
- Maternal position choice for comfort
- Nursing position choice for improvement of external monitoring tracing
- Position choice of anesthesiologist after epidural or spinal anesthesia
- Position choice of nurse-midwife, or obstetrician attending delivery

Spontaneous or Preexisting Conditions

Uterine Hyperstimulation
Decreasing Uteroplacental Blood Flow
- Placental abruption

Chronic Deterioration of Placenta
- Maternal preexisting disease such as diabetes, collagen disease, or chronic hypertension
- Maternal condition such as preeclampsia or pregnancy-induced hypertension
- Postdate pregnancy
- Maternal drug abuse
- Maternal smoking
- Poor maternal nutrition

Adapted from Afriat, C.I. (1989). Electronic fetal monitoring. Rockville, MD: Aspen.

their timing, shape, depth, and duration. Some last for brief seconds; others have very slow recoveries to the baseline rate. They may be caused by a uterine contraction pressing the cord against the fetus, by a short or nuchal cord, or by intense vagal stimulation in the second stage of labor (Display 9-6). If the cord is entrapped between the uterine wall and the fetus, the variable deceleration may be seen with every contraction. In the case of oligohydramnios, the cord may be compressed only during fetal movement, causing occasional variable decelerations. Therefore, variables have multiple appearances in all aspects except one; the initial FHR drop is abrupt.

Variable decelerations may also occur in the absence of uterine activity and are seen during antepartum testing. They may be referred to as "nonperiodic changes" or simply as variable decelerations. Their presence may indicate oligohydramnios or cord entanglement, placing the fetus at risk for cord compression. This FHR pattern requires further evaluation (e.g., ultrasound examination) to assess amniotic fluid volume and umbilical cord position if possible.

Much has been written about the different wave forms of variable decelerations. Some are shaped like a V or a W or a U. Thus far, the shape does not seem to provide necessary or consistent clinical data. Rather than quantifying variable decelerations in terms of shape and beats-per-minute drop in FHR, they can be systematically assessed in evaluation of the overall pattern displayed and determined to be either reassuring or nonreassuring. Reassuring variable decelerations last no more than 30 to 45 seconds, have a rapid return to baseline, and are accompanied by normal baseline rate and variability (Freeman, Garite, Nageotte, 1991). Nonreassuring variable decelerations are those with a prolonged return to baseline, with or without overshoots, a rising baseline, and absence of STV (Freeman et al., 1991)

Attempts to correct variable decelerations by alleviating the cord compression begin with changing the maternal position from lateral to lateral position, to release the cord from where it is entrapped. Oxygen can be administered by mask at 8–12 L/min. A vaginal examination may be done to palpate for a cord

A

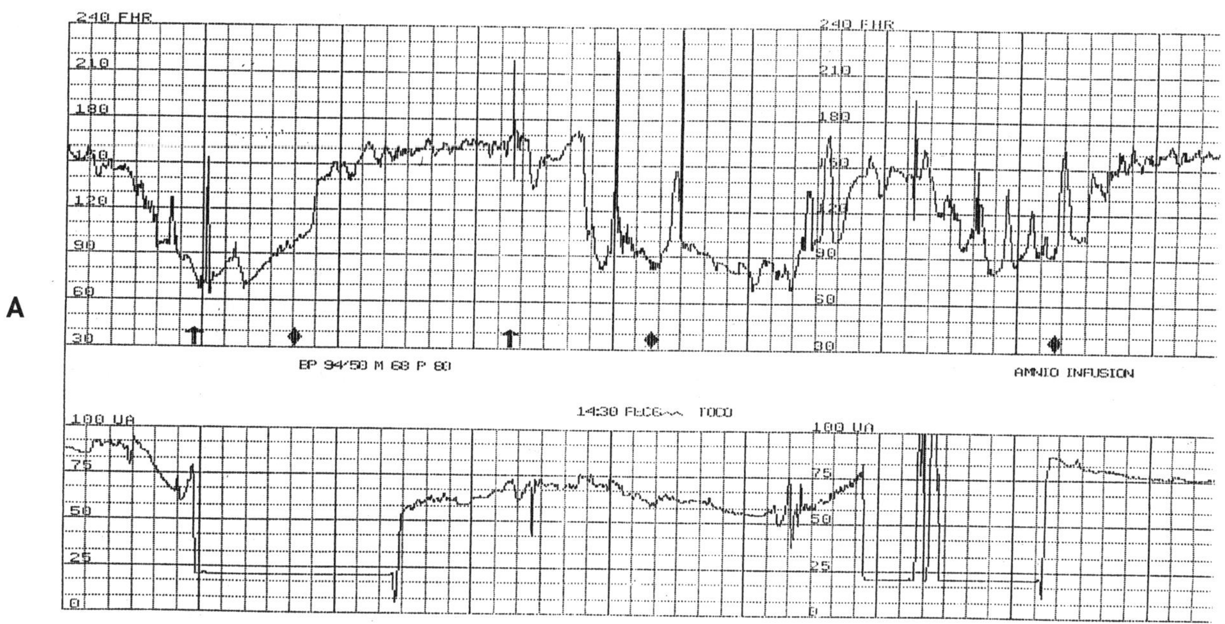

B

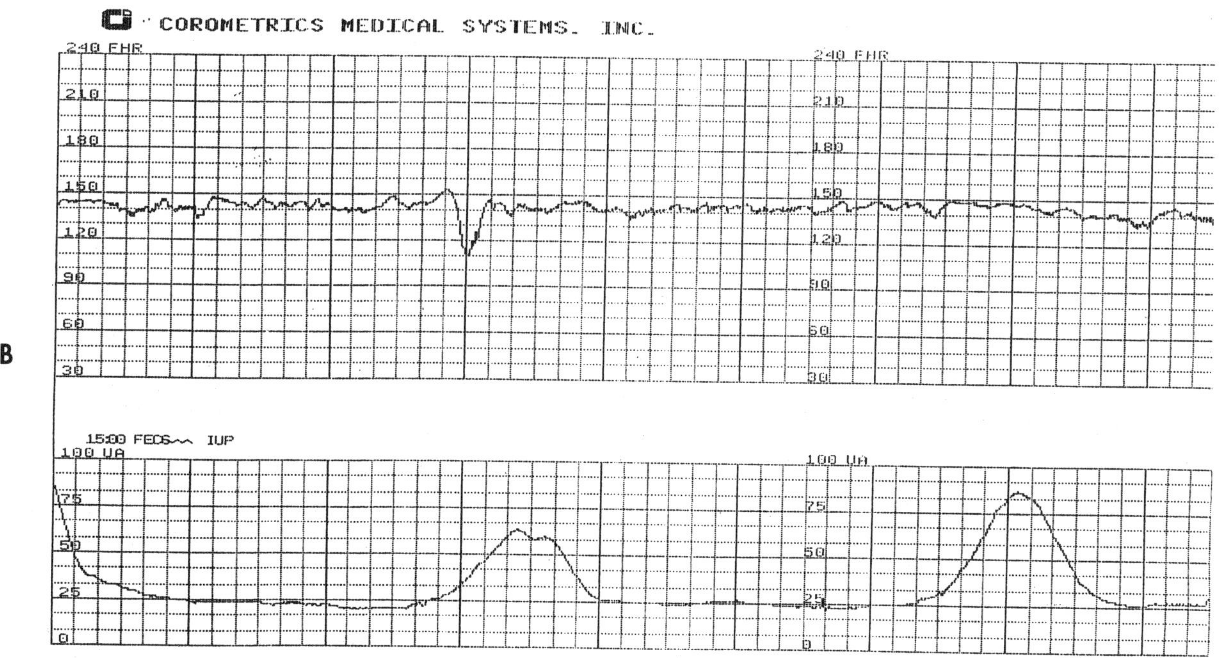

Figure 9-10. A & B. Prolonged decelerations successfully treated by an amnioinfusion, scalp pH 7.32 BE–1.0.

prolapse. The cord compression may be behind the fetus; therefore, the woman might be placed on her hands and knees. An IV should be started in the event that the pattern is not remediable. If oxytocin is infusing, it should be discontinued until recovery of the FHR is evident.

In some cases of severe variable decelerations, a vaginal examination may be done to gently elevate the presenting part. This would be successful if an occult prolapse of the cord had occurred. However, by elevating the presenting part, a risk of creating a true prolapse of the cord exists. When performing this maneuver, care must be taken to have the operating room prepared for an emergency cesarean birth.

In the event of known oligohydramnios, an amnioinfusion may be instituted by instilling either lactated Ringer's or normal saline solution into the uterus via an intrauterine catheter (Galvan, Van Mullen, & Boekhuizen, 1989; Knorr, 1989). However, recent data suggest prophylactic amnioinfusion for oligohydramnios without the presence of variable FHR decelerations does not improve perinatal outcomes (Ogundipe, Spong, & Ross, 1994). Amnioinfusion has also been used with severe variable FHR decelerations in the absence of oligohydramnios. Careful documentation of fluid infused is important to avoid iatrogenic polyhydramnios (Magann, Nolan, Hess, Martin, Whitworth, & Morrison, 1992) (Figure 9-10). (See Chapter 8 for a comprehensive discussion of amnioinfusion.)

Tocolytics may be given to stop uterine activity, even though the etiology is cord compression and not placental dysfunction. This is done to enhance blood flow through the placenta by inhibiting uterine contractility to supplement the loss of blood flow through the cord. Tocolytic administration is also helpful while waiting for the readiness of the operating room personnel, if a cesarean birth is deemed necessary.

Prolonged Decelerations

Prolonged decelerations are changes in the fetal heart rate that last longer than 2 to 3 minutes but fewer than 10 minutes. The heart rate drops abruptly and stays down for several minutes and is usually an isolated occurrence. It may occur in the presence or absence of contractions and may have either an abrupt or slow return to the baseline rate. Prolonged decelerations may be the result of an isolated episode of cord compression, maternal hypotension, excessive uterine activity, or vagal stimulation.

If the precise etiology is unknown, management of prolonged decelerations includes discontinuing oxytocin if infusing to improve uterine blood flow, increasing IV fluids to improve blood volume, vaginal examination to rule out prolapsed cord, and repositioning the woman to remove pressure from the umbilical cord. Tocolytics may also be administered (Figure 9-11). A summary of interventions for periodic heart rate changes is in Display 9-8.

PERIODIC ACCELERATIONS

Periodic accelerations are described as being uniform, variable, or rebound in shape (Display 9-9). Accelerations, per se, are not treated. The associated decelerations may be treated.

Uniform accelerations begin with the onset of the contraction, and the FHR returns to the baseline rate with the end of the contraction. The acceleration has a smooth rise and fall. They are believed to reflect presence of sympathetic stimulation and absence of parasympathetic stimulation. During a contraction, the head is pressed into the pelvis, stimulating the parasympathetic which lowers the heart rate. The fetal torso is stimulated simultaneously by the contraction which in turn triggers the sympathetic system causing the heart rate to increase. Therefore, the parasympathetic and sympathetic systems are counterbalanced and the FHR remains stable during the contraction. However, in the nonvertex presentation there is no parasympathetic stimulation so the FHR increases with the contraction, causing a uniform acceleration. Uniform accelerations are benign, requiring no treatment. They are more common in the nonvertex presentation so fetal presentation should be reevaluated in their presence (Schifrin, 1990).

Variable accelerations are also called "shoulders." Shoulders are brief accelerations of the FHR that may either precede or follow variable decelerations (Figure 9-8). During umbilical cord compression, the thin-walled vein is compressed first, resulting in decreased blood flow to the fetus. An acceleration of the FHR is seen as the fetus responds by increasing its heart rate to increase cardiac output. As the umbilical arteries are also compressed, fetal blood pressure increases, stimulating a vagal response and thus a decrease in the FHR. When the cord compression is alleviated and the arteries are released, the FHR increases toward the baseline. The umbilical vein is then released and the fetus may increase its heart rate again and then return to baseline.

A

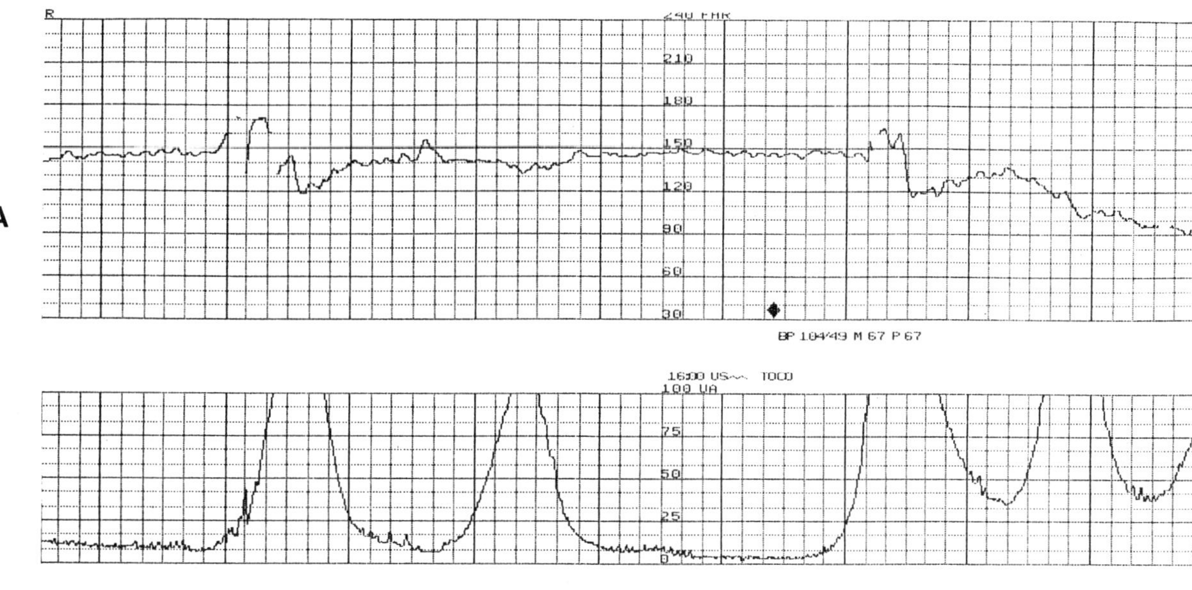

B

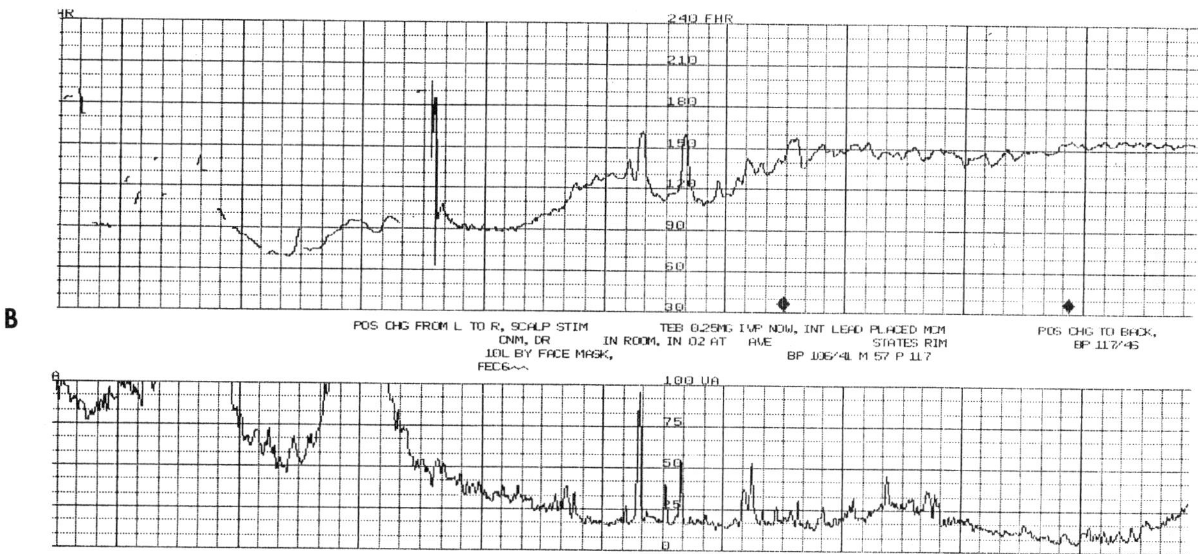

Figure 9-11. A & B. Prolonged deceleration secondary to hyperstimulation successfully treated with terbutaline. The cord blood gas had a pH of 7.385 and B.E. −5.3.

A

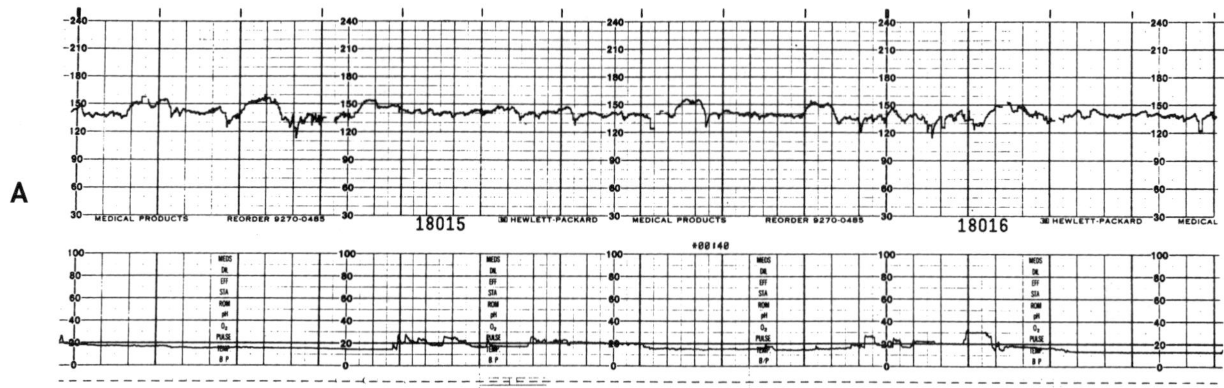

B

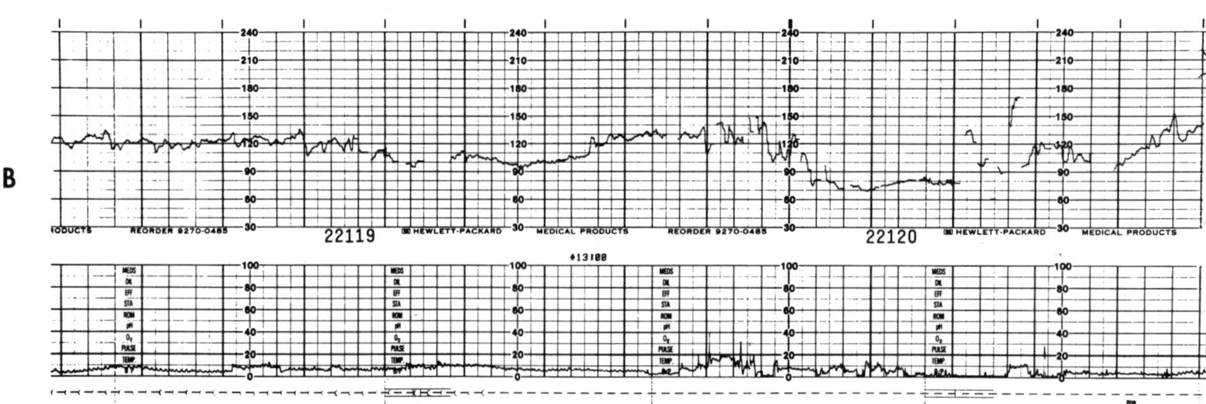

Figure 9-12. Nonperiodic changes are accelerations or decelerations that have no relationship to uterine activity. **A**: accelerations, **B**: decelerations.

Rebound overshoots are accelerations of the fetal heart rate following a variable deceleration of any size with absent baseline variability (Figure 9-8). These accelerations reflect an autonomic system imbalance secondary to fetal hypoxemia, medications, or prematurity. In the absence of medications and prematurity, these accelerations are considered to be nonreassuring and require immediate evaluation. Because of the importance in assessing variability to distinguish between shoulders and overshoots, a direct fetal electrode is indicated, if possible.

NONPERIODIC CHANGES

Nonperiodic changes in FHR indicate that the deceleration or acceleration occurs in the absence of uterine activity. They are isolated events. These include occasional variable decelerations, accelerations in response to fetal movement, and prolonged decelerations (Figure 9-12). Common causes are maternal position changes, vaginal examinations, or administration of anesthesia. Treatment of nonperiodic changes in the FHR are based on the causative factor.

UTERINE ACTIVITY ASSESSMENT

The FHR is evaluated in terms of response to uterine activity. Therefore, interpretation of FHR patterns includes a complete assessment of the frequency, duration, and intensity of contractions, and the uterine resting tone between contractions. Uterine activity is evaluated by direct palpation or application of the external or internal electronic monitor. Frequency is measured from the beginning of one contraction to

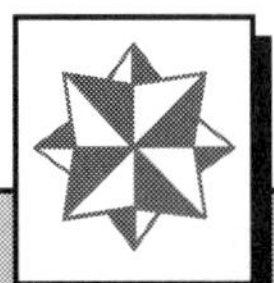

DISPLAY 9-8

Interventions for Fetal Heart Rate Periodic Changes

Cause	Intervention
Autonomic nervous system imbalance (overshoots)	Improve blood flow • Institute lateral position • Administer oxygen • Administer IV fluids as prescribed • Stop oxytocin administration • Notify appropriate personnel
Uteroplacental insufficiency	Determine cause Improve uteroplacental blood flow • Institute lateral position • Stop oxytocin administration • Increase IV fluids • Administer oxygen • Possibly obtain fetal blood sample for blood gas analysis • Notify appropriate personnel • Watch for rising baseline rate and loss of variability
Umbilical cord compression	Improve blood flow • Change maternal position to opposite side • Institute Trendelenburg's position • Perform vaginal examination for cord prolapse • Possibly administer oxygen • Watch for loss of variability and overshoots • Notify appropriate personnel • Possibly obtain fetal blood sample • Elevation of the presenting part by MD only

From Afriat, C.I. (1989) Electronic fetal monitoring. Rockville, MD: Aspen.

the beginning of the next and is described in minutes. Duration is the length of the contraction and is described in seconds. Intensity refers to the strength of the contraction. It is described as mild, moderate, or strong by palpation, or millimeters of mercury (mmHg) of intraamniotic pressure with an intrauterine pressure catheter (IUPC). Uterine resting tone is assessed in the absence of contractions. By direct palpation, resting tone is described as soft or rigid, and by IUPC in terms of mmHg of intraamniotic pressure. The external tocotransducer detects abdominal wall changes during contractions and uterine relaxation. This method provides information about frequency and duration; however, resting tone and intensity must be determined by palpation. Contraction frequency, duration, intensity, and uterine resting tone can be evaluated by both palpation and an IUPC. The IUPC is more accurate because direct measurement of intraamniotic pressure is recorded but requires ruptured membranes for insertion. As with any procedure, the least invasive approach is preferred unless maternal–fetal status indicates need for more objective data.

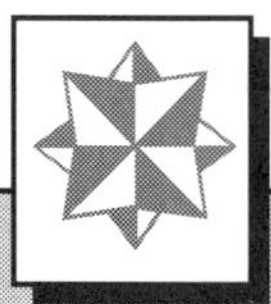

Display 9-9

Conditions Related to Periodic Accelerations in Fetal Heart Rate Pattern

Uniform Accelerations	Variable Accelerations (Shoulders)	Overshoots
Lack of Parasympathetic Stimulation • Nonvertex presentation (breech, transverse lie) • Unengaged vertex presentation	Umbilical Vein Compression • Decreased oxygen flow to fetus causing – increase in carbon dioxide – stimulation of chemoreceptors – acceleration of FHR • Preceding or following variable decelerations with average variability	Autonomic Nervous System Imbalance Secondary to Chronic Hypoxemia/ Hypoxia or Other Cause • Decreased oxygen flow to fetal central nervous system • Autonomic nervous system asphyxiation • Inability to regulate fetal heart rate • Rebound acceleration following variable decelerations with absent variability Expected Response in Normal Premature Fetus

Adapted from Afriat, C.I. (1989). Electronic fetal monitoring. Rockville, MD: Aspen.

Prolonged uterine contractions (hyperstimulation) or too frequent uterine contractions (tachysystole) can cause a decrease in placental blood flow and precipitate FHR decelerations. Normal contraction frequency during augmentation and induction is every 2–3 minutes; however, some fetal/placental units may be unable to tolerate this level of uterine activity and late decelerations may result. If decelerations occur during oxytocin administration, the infusion should be discontinued until the pattern is evaluated. Once FHR characteristics indicate fetal recovery, resuming the oxytocin at a lower rate of infusion may be all that is necessary to correct the pattern.

FETAL BLOOD FLOW

A prerequisite to pattern interpretation is understanding the etiology of pattern changes. Oxygenated blood is transferred to the fetus by uteroplacental blood flow through the umbilical cord. Blood flow that is impeded through either site lays the groundwork for potential fetal hypoxia and chronic asphyxia. It is not highly critical to know where the decreased blood flow originates, although the information will be useful. It is important, however, to recognize that the fetus is receiving an inadequate amount of oxygen-rich blood and to implement measures to improve the blood flow through *both* the cord and the placenta.

The shape or waveform of the deceleration is an indication of the etiology of the blood flow problem. Late decelerations indicate there is diminishment of blood across the placenta to the fetus. Variable decelerations indicate the blood flow impedance is through the cord. However, it is possible for there to be oddly shaped decelerations that make it difficult to ascertain the etiology of the blood flow problem. In this case, it is acceptable to describe the decelerations as "undefined"; and describe and document them in the record as such (Cohn, 1990). Treat it as a general fetal blood flow problem by attempting to maximize blood flow through both the cord and the placenta. There are at least seven different descriptions and names of various types of variable declarations (Krebs, Petres, & Dunn, 1983), all of which are indicative of cord blood flow impedance. Treatment for all of them is the same; maximize blood flow through the cord by correcting the cord compression.

Also of critical importance is maternal blood flow. It is not unusual for late decelerations to occur as a result of maternal hypotension. In the event of FHR decelerations, maternal blood pressure and pulse should be assessed and recorded. Simply turning the woman to a lateral position may be sufficient for improving maternal blood flow and thereby improving the fetal-placental blood flow.

FHR PATTERN INTERPRETATION

Reassuring Patterns

It has been well established that EFM's greatest contribution to fetal healthcare is the ability to predict normal outcomes (Schifrin, 1990). A reassuring fetal tracing virtually assures the perinatal team that, barring unforeseen acute insults such as abruptio placentae or cord prolapse, a well-oxygenated neonate will be born. A reassuring tracing (Figure 9-13a) may have the following characteristics: (1) on an external monitor, a reactive heart rate within the normal baseline range with the absence of decelerations, or (2) with a direct electrode, average STV, stable baseline rate and no decelerations.

Nonreassuring Patterns

Nonreassuring tracings fail to provide any of the reassuring characteristics listed above but do not necessarily indicate fetal compromise. If a tracing is nonreassuring, evaluation of the fetus before implementing any procedure that has potential for causing fetal compromise (e.g., administration of regional anesthetic agents or oxytocin) is warranted. When a nonreassuring tracing is noted, continuous monitoring with a direct electrode may be indicated because STV can be assessed.

One of the greatest criticisms of EFM is its inability to predict poor outcome (Ellison, Foster, Sheridan-Pereira, & MacDonald, 1991; Schifrin, 1990). When a tracing is interpreted to be nonreassuring or indicative of fetal stress, a well-oxygenated newborn is delivered at least 50% of the time. The low positive predictive value of EFM may also be related to pattern misinterpretation or a failure to fully understand which changes in FHR patterns indicate stress or distress.

A nonreassuring tracing indicates the need to further investigate fetal well-being, first with noninvasive interventions such as maternal position change, administration of oxygen, or intravenous fluids. Scalp stimulation may elicit an acceleration of the FHR. In the presence of an acceleration greater than 15 beats above the baseline lasting more than 15 seconds, the fetal condition is comparable to a fetal blood gas pH of 7.20 or greater and is considered reassuring (Clark, Gimovsky, & Miller, 1984). When noninvasive measures fail to provide a reassuring FHR, a direct electrode should be placed if cervical status allows. In some perinatal centers, fetal scalp blood gases may be obtained (Figure 9-13B). Depending on maternal-fetal status, cesarean birth may be indicated.

SYSTEMATIC ASSESSMENT AND MANAGEMENT STRATEGIES

A systematic, organized approach to interpreting the EFM pattern prevents misinterpretation and confusion. The deceleration in the middle of the tracing is eye catching and anxiety producing, but it is not the most important aspect of the tracing. The deceleration may be a symptom of a problem; it does not provide any clues as to the fetal condition prior to the deceleration nor the fetal response to the deceleration. It means that the fetus has an intact autonomic nervous system that allows it to accelerate and decelerate and that something has temporarily interfered with blood flow. Assessment of the entire strip, including uterine contractions and all procedures that transpired prior to the deceleration, is required.

Review of the maternal medical record is of critical importance. Assessment should include the following: (1) maternal/fetal risk for uteroplacental insufficiency, (2) administration of regional anesthesic, (3) maternal blood pressure, temperature, pulse, and respirations, (4) administration of medications, or maternal drug use, (5) oxytocin infusion, and (6) any other pertinent maternal/fetal information. Nearly everything occurring in the mother affects the fetus. Accurate FHR pattern interpretation is dependent on knowledge of maternal status.

After collecting all pertinent data, the pattern can be interpreted by the following:

1. Evaluate the baseline rate prior to and following the deceleration. If the FHR had risen but then returned to its prior baseline rate, the fetus successfully compensated by eliminating the excess carbon dioxide (CO_2). If the rate had risen and remained high, the compensatory mechanism failed and the pattern may indicate hypoxemia.
2. Evaluate the STV for changes prior to and following the deceleration. The STV may be diminished following the deceleration simply secondary to the rise in rate. When the baseline rate returns to the original rate, the STV should return to average.

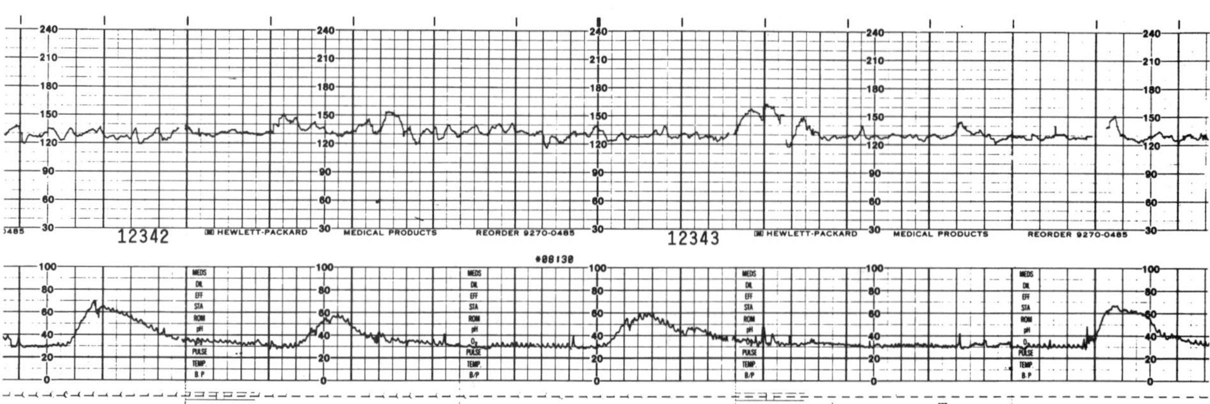

Figure 9-13 A. This tracing was obtained with an external ultrasound transducer. The presence of accelerations indicates a reassuring fetal heart rate pattern.

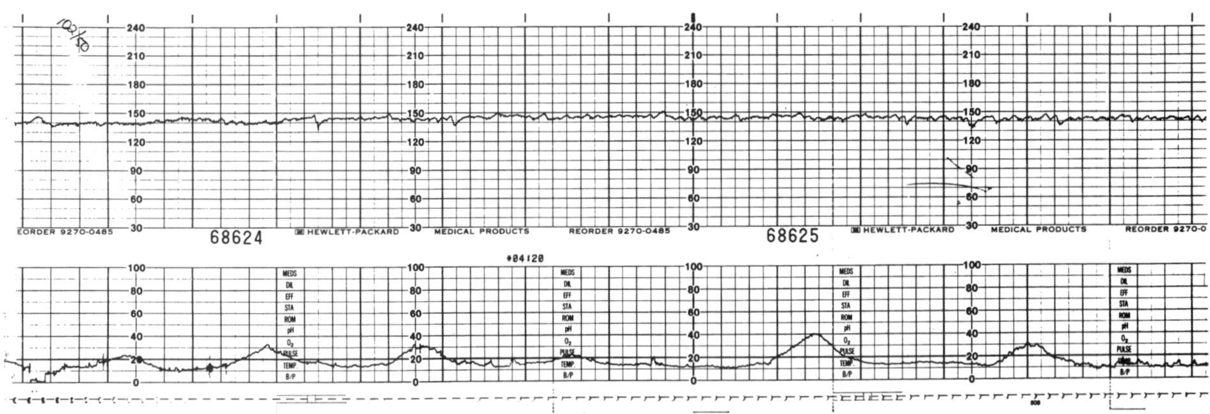

Figure 9-13 B. The absence of fetal accelerations may indicate a fetal sleep cycle or the potential of a nonreasssuring condition, thus warranting futher evaluation.

3. Evaluate uterine contractions for evidence of hyperstimulation.
4. Identify the precipitating event. Management of nonreassuring FHR patterns is based on the causative factor. Eliminating the cause (e.g., uterine hyperstimulation or maternal hypotension) usually results in the return of a reassuring FHR pattern.

FETAL BLOOD SAMPLING

In any situation in which fetal hypoxemia is suspected, scalp stimulation may be a component of assessment and management. If the FHR fails to respond to scalp stimulation, a fetal blood gas (FBG) from the presenting part may be obtained. The blood gas analysis consists of all of the parameters used in adult blood gas analysis; however, generally only the pH and base excess are used to evaluate fetal status (Display 9-10) (Mondanlou, 1991).

The base excess information differentiates between metabolic acidemia, a chronic, potentially damaging process, and respiratory acidemia, an acute, transitory state. Therefore, the pH may be in the acidotic range, but if the base excess is less than 10–15, the acidemia is most likely respiratory and may be corrected by maternal position changes. If the base excess is rising, the intrauterine environment may not be sufficiently supporting fetal oxygenation.

Both false normal and false abnormal results can occur secondary to prolonged exposure of the sample to air, protracted sampling time, inadequate temperature control, laboratory technique, timing of sampling relating to contractions, presence of caput succedaneum, or maternal factors such as fever, hypertension, acidemia, or the supine position. If a FBG result seems incongruent with the EFM tracing interpretation, the FBG may be in error and must be repeated (Figure 9-14). More than one FBG is indicated in all situations since it is the gas result *trend* that is predictive of outcome and not the result of a single sample.

Although fetal blood sampling (FBS) provides an adjunct measure to determine fetal status when a nonreassuring FHR is noted, thereby in theory eliminating the need for cesarean birth if results indicate a well-oxygenated fetus, there has been a trend away from use of FBS. Widespread use of FBS in tertiary centers in the late 1980s did not result in a significant decrease in the rate of cesarean births (Goodwin, Milner-Masterson, & Paul, 1994). The role of FBS in clinical practice is now being questioned. The majority of perinatal centers in the United States no longer use FBS or use it infrequently. Intrapartum fetal pulse oximetry, an alternative approach to assessing fetal oxygen status during labor, is currently under investigation. Preliminary research has shown promise in managing difficult cases where the FHR is nonreassuring or uninterpretable (Dildy, Loucks, & Clark, 1993). However, more data and improvements in technology are necessary to determine if fetal pulse oximetry will be a useful tool in clinical practice (Dildy et al., 1994).

Umbilical cord blood gases drawn at birth provide objective evidence confirming or refuting the presence of intrapartum acidemia. A normal cord blood gas can alleviate suspicion of intrapartum asphyxia, regardless of Apgar scores (Thorpe, Sampson, Parisi, & Creasy, 1989). In a study conducted by Johnson and Riley (1993), approximately one in four university hospitals surveyed obtained cord samples after all births. Most centers considered this test to be clinically useful and also of assistance in the reduction of medical-legal risks (Johnson & Riley).

Progression of Fetal Hypoxemia/Hypoxia

Fetal heart-rate patterns follow a fairly precise pattern in response to untreated chronic hypoxemia/hypoxia (Schifrin, 1990). If the etiology is placental in origin and remains uncorrected, the following may develop over an extended period of time: late decelerations, loss of reactivity, rise in baseline rate, and loss of STV. As the progressive hypoxia continues, ultimately the autonomic nervous system will no longer be able to respond with accelerations or decelerations. The late decelerations, therefore, will become progressively smaller until no decelerations are present. The baseline rate will return to a "normal" rate between 110 and 160 bpm with absent variability until death is imminent. Finally, a bradycardia occurs followed by death (Figure 9-15).

A similar series of events occurs if the decreased blood flow is due to cord compression. Initially, variable decelerations with average STV and a stable baseline are seen. Without treatment, the baseline rate rises, the STV becomes absent, and the variable decelerations become smaller. Rebound overshoots develop until, finally, the variable decelerations disappear. The FHR ultimately stabilizes within a normal baseline range, followed by a bradycardia and death.

In either situation, the EFM pattern becomes a flat, fixed pattern with absent variability. Scalp stimulation elicits no response. Most likely, the woman would indicate an absence of fetal movement. By auscultation, it is likely that one would hear a regular rate well with-in the normal range, thus providing false reassurance.

Understanding the progression of hypoxemia/hypoxia allows those interpreting the EFM tracings to observe for subtle changes in fetal condition. Women at risk of chronic placental blood flow problems are those with diabetes, hypertension, collagen vascular diseases, suspect IUGR, chemical dependency, and those with a history of viral diseases such as cytomegalovirus. A chronic umbilical cord compression problem may be the result of oligohydramnios, a short cord, true knot in the cord, a nuchal cord, or limb or body entanglement.

Acute Fetal Insults

Abrupt changes in fetal blood flow may also occur across both the placenta and cord, causing fetal hypoxemia. Acute placental changes may result from events such as placental abruption, uterine hyperstimulation, and maternal hypotension. Acute changes in umbilical cord blood flow may result from an occult or complete cord prolapse or cord entanglement. Acute changes may progress to chronic hypoxia if left untreated.

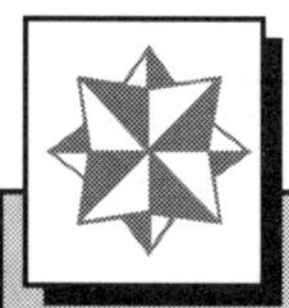

DISPLAY 9-10

Adult and Fetal Acid-Base Parameters

Subject	pH	Oxygen Pressure	Carbon Dioxide Pressure	Base Deficit
Nonpregnant adult	7.35–7.45	90–100 mmHg	32–42 mmHg	0
Pregnant adult	7.40–7.45	104–108 mmHg	27–32 mmHg	0
Fetus				
Scalp	7.25–7.40	18–22 mmHg	40–50 mmHg	0–10
Venous blood	7.35±0.05	29.2±5.9 mmHg	38.2±5.6 mmHg	
Arterial blood	7.28± 0.05	18±6.2 mmHg	49.2±8.4 mmHg	
Prepathologic	7.20–7.24			
Pathologic	<7.20			

Adapted from Afriat, C.I. (1989). Electronic fetal monitoring. Rockville, MD: Aspen.

Generally, if an acute insult occurs, the fetus will respond with a sudden prolonged deceleration or bradycardia. If the decreased blood flow is not corrected, the bradycardia will lead to death. If the blood flow is improved, the fetus will respond initially with a tachycardia to increase cardiac output and rid the blood of CO_2 prior to resuming its normal baseline rate. A well-oxygenated fetus can generally tolerate acute insults such as maternal hypotension or hyperstimulation and fully recover, but a compromised fetus with no reserve oxygen may not be able to tolerate any dramatic insults. Therefore, it is prudent to be assured that the fetal heart rate tracing is normal prior to the administration of regional anesthesia, analgesics, or oxytoxics (Figure 9-16).

UNUSUAL FHR PATTERNS

Whenever a strikingly unusal tracing is observed in the absence of any prior abnormal tracing, the possibility of a fetus with a congenital anomaly should be considered. Hydrocephalic and anencephalic fetuses may present with FHR patterns that do not fit any category or definition. If possible, an ultrasound examination may be performed to rule out gross anomalies as the cause of the pattern, although the results of the ultrasound examination may be inconclusive. An anomaly that effects the fetal central nervous system most likely will have an impact on the variability and/or the fetal cardiac system's ability to accelerate and decelerate. Unusual decelerations with a flat, fixed rate may be seen.

Another unusual pattern type is the sinusoidal tracing, first identified in the early 1970s during observation of Rh-sensitized fetuses (Rochard, Schifrin, Goupil, Legrand, Blottiere & Sureau, 1976). As severe fetal anemia developed, the FHR tracing became persistently rhythmic in an undulating fashion (Figure 9-17A) and remained so. A sinusoidal pattern caused by anemia will subside after a successful fetal transfusion, if detected in time.

A sinusoidal-appearing FHR tracing has been noted to follow the maternal administration of stadol, and some narcotics. This type of sinusoidal tracing resolves as the drug is excreted, thus giving it the name of "pseudosinusoidal or "drug-induced" sinusoidal. No treatment is indicated.

DYSRHYTHMIA DETECTION

Because the functioning of the electronic fetal monitor is based on its ability to accurately record from one fetal heart beat to the next, it is an excellent detector of irregularities of the fetal heart rate. The direct electrode has three leads which detect the PQRST complex. The filter within the electronics of

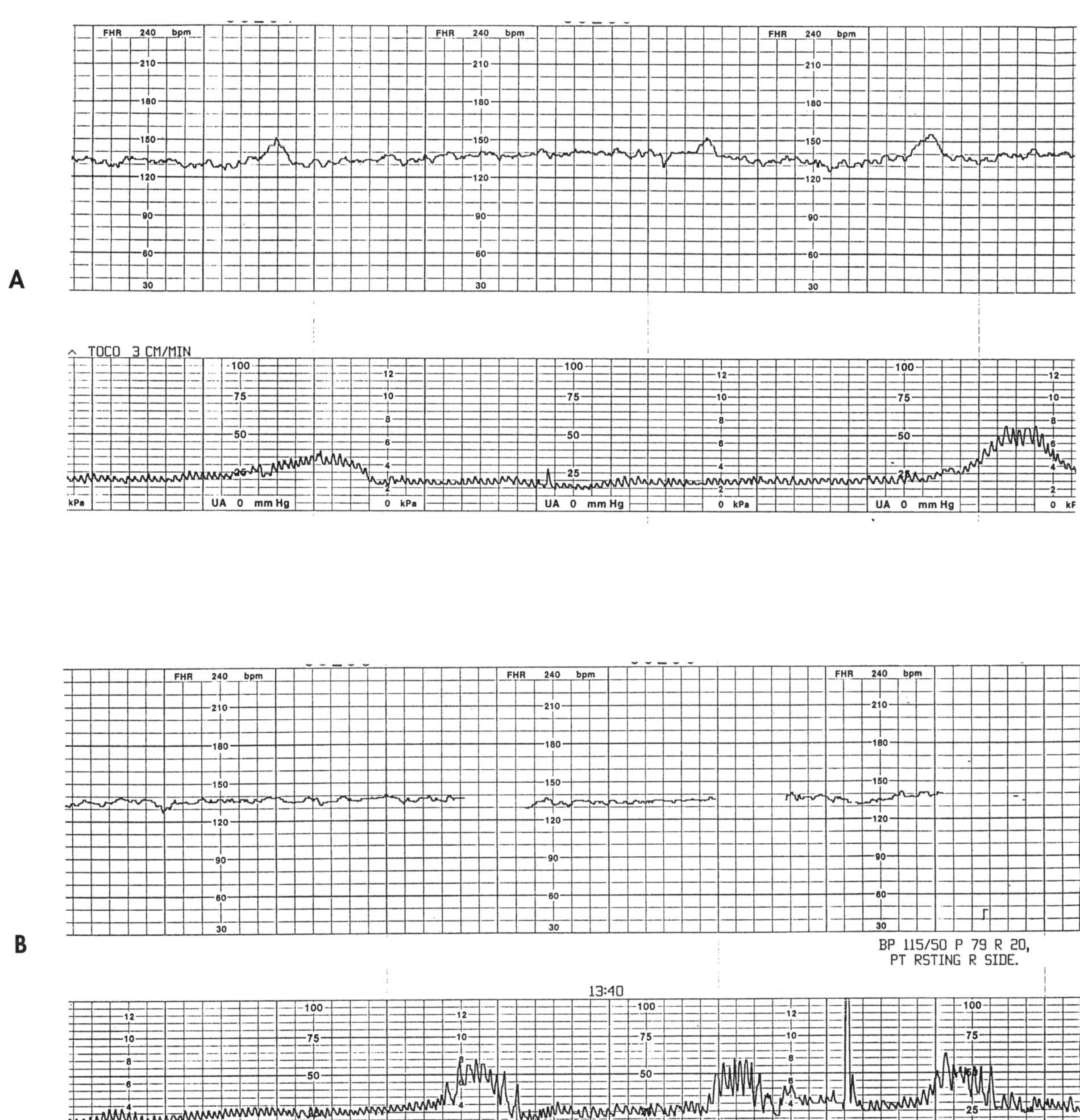

Figure 9-14. A indicates a reassuring tracing with FHR accelerations, a stable baseline rate and the absence of periodic decelerations. **B** occurred about one hour later. Although no other FHR changes occurred in the intervening time, a fetal blood sample was obtained with a pH of 6.87 and B.E. −25. An emergency cesarean section was performed with the cord blood gas pH 7.32 and B.E. −2.1. The first blood gas was a laboratory error. It should be noted that if the blood gas result seems inconsistent with the tracing, the fetal blood gas should be repeated.

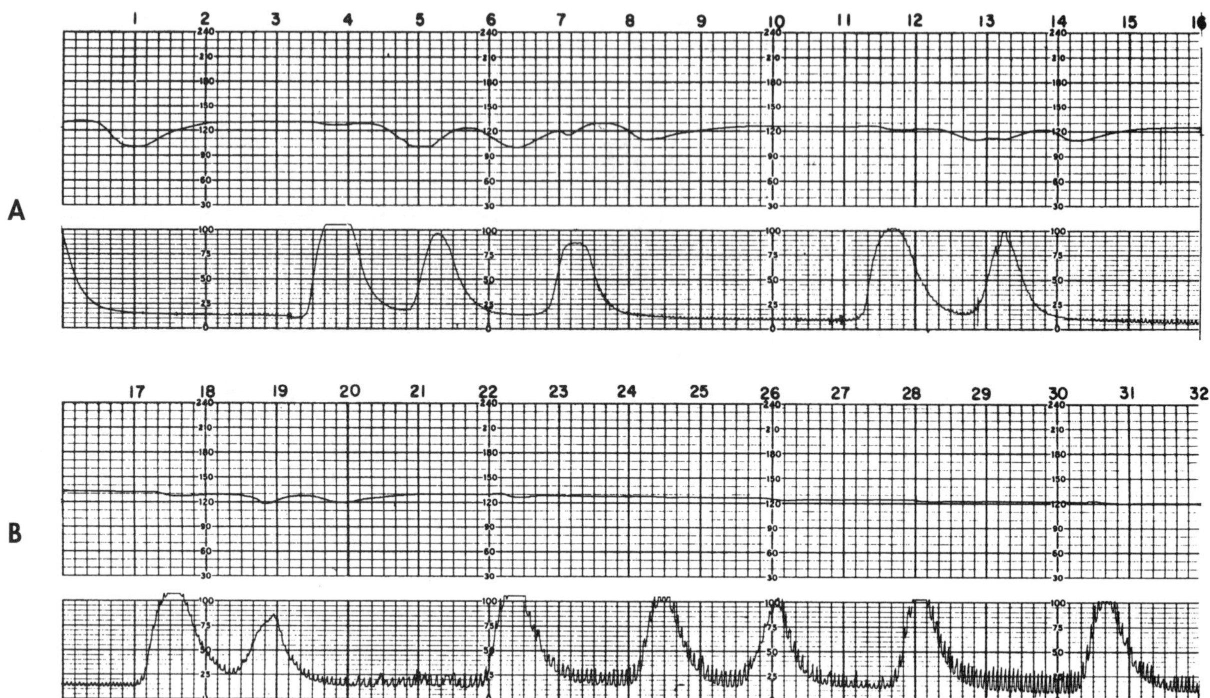

Figure 9-15. A & B. The tracing was obtained with a direct electrode. Late decelerations with absent variability are demonstrated, followed by the absence of decelerations and no return of short-term variability. This tracing is highly suspicious of progressive hypoxia secondary to uteroplacental insufficiency.

From Afriat, C.I. (1989). Electronic fetal monitoring. Rockville, MD: Aspen.

the machine removes all components except the R wave. The R wave then triggers the machine to count, it waits for a second complex, filters all but the R wave, and then calculates how much time elapsed from the first to the second R wave.

The elapsed time is then converted into bpm and the pen records that beat on the paper. The process repeats itself for every R wave. The electronic sophistication of counting each and every interval not only is the basis for recording STV but also the ability to detect fetal dysrhythmias (Figure 9-18).

Most fetal dysrhythmias are benign and require no intervention. However, one of the fetal dysrhythmias of concern is a supraventricular tachycardia. Rates greater than 240 bpm have been verified by simultaneous auscultation, fetal electrocardiogram, or M-mode ultrasound. The risk to the fetus is congestive heart failure and may, therefore, require medical intervention with medications or delivery.

Irregular FHRs, such as premature contractions (PVCs) or bigeminy (every other beat is a PVC) will be recorded accurately. Most irregularities in the FHR do have an organized appearance to them, differentiating them from artifact which appears haphazardly (Figure 9-19). Artifact is usually caused by a loose electrode and is easily corrected by changing the lead.

The presence of a dysrhythmia may be verified by auscultating the FHR and listening for the irregularity. Most will convert to normal sinus rhythm shortly after birth. However, an ultrasound examination of the fetus to evaluate for fetal or cardiac anomalies is indicated. Fetal echocardiography may also be obtained to further evaluate the fetal heart. In some instances, the neonatal resuscitation team may be requested to attend the birth.

EFM EDUCATION AND COMPETENCY VALIDATION

The level of responsibility perinatal nurses accept mandates that their skills in fetal assessment, whether by auscultation or electronic means, is based on thorough knowledge current with advancing and changing information. In addition, competency in

A

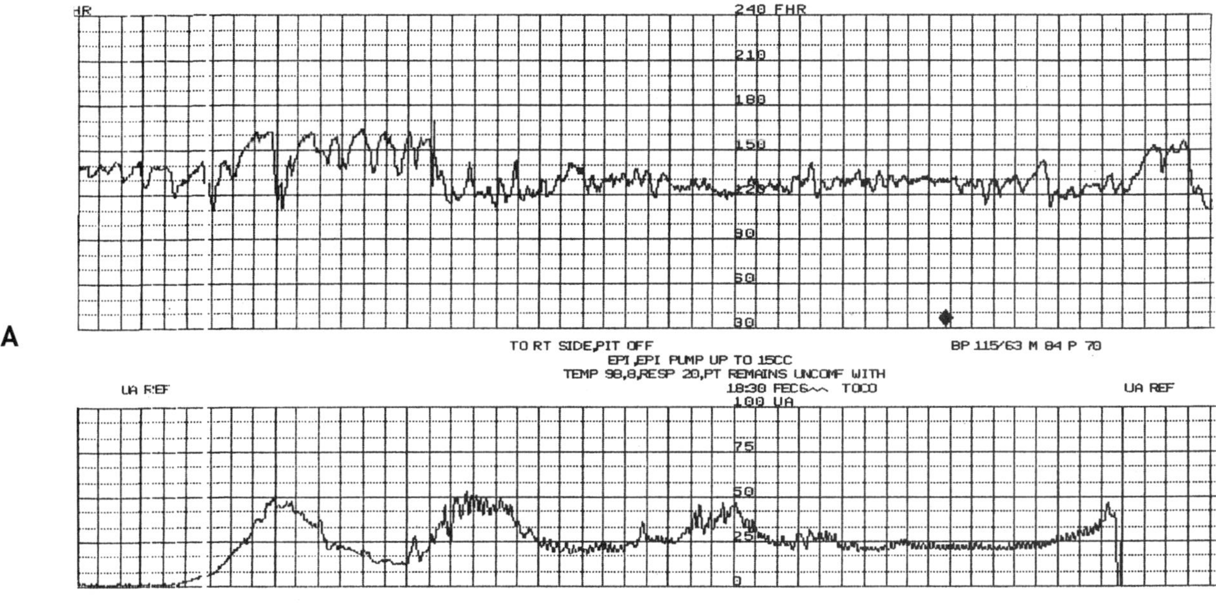

B

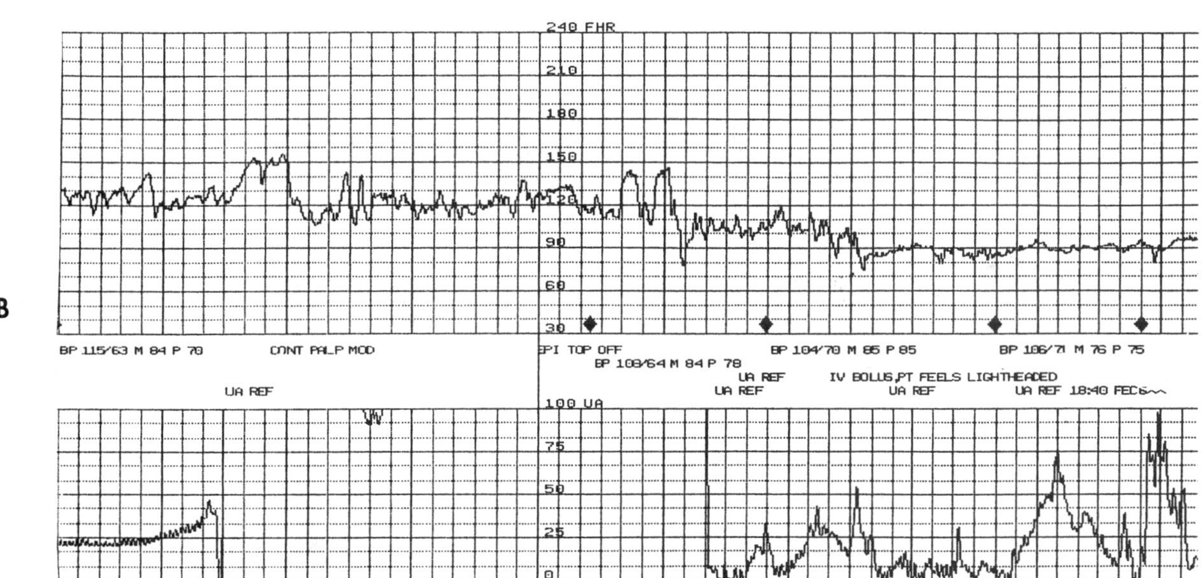

Figure 9-16. A, B, C. & D. The initial portion of the tracing which has been obtained by a direct electrode shows a stable baseline rate, average short-term variability and no periodic changes. An epidural is given at the first arrow on panel B followed by a prolonged decelerations. At the final arrow, the fetal heart rate has recovered and the short-term variability remains reassuring. This indicates a decrease in blood flow to the fetus secondary to iatrogenic causes (the epidural) followed by recovery.

Figure 9-16 (cont.)

C

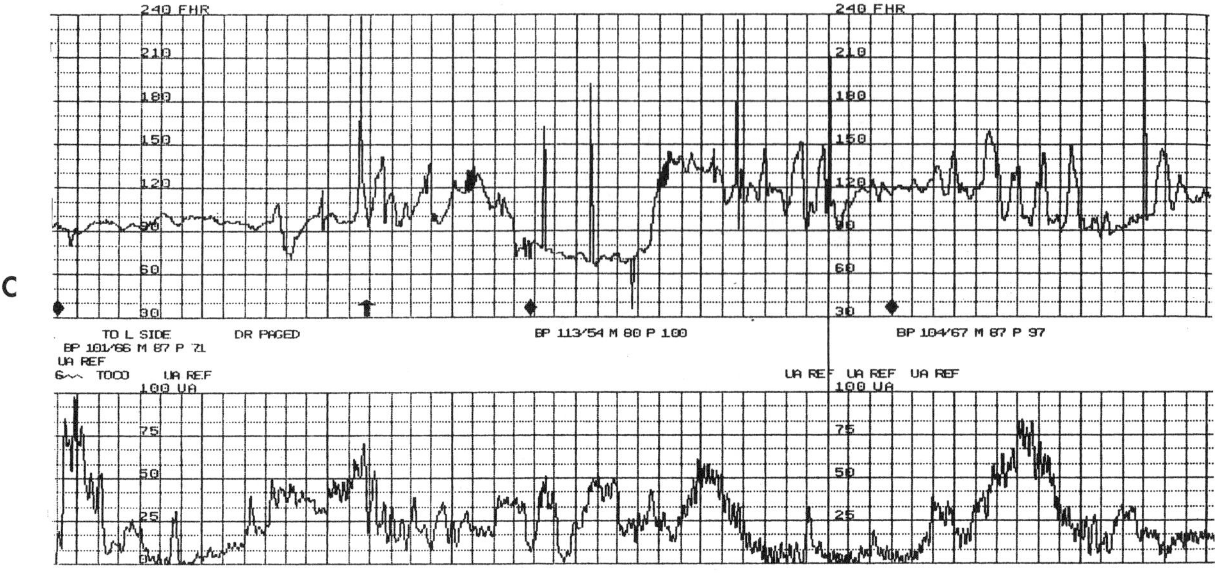

D

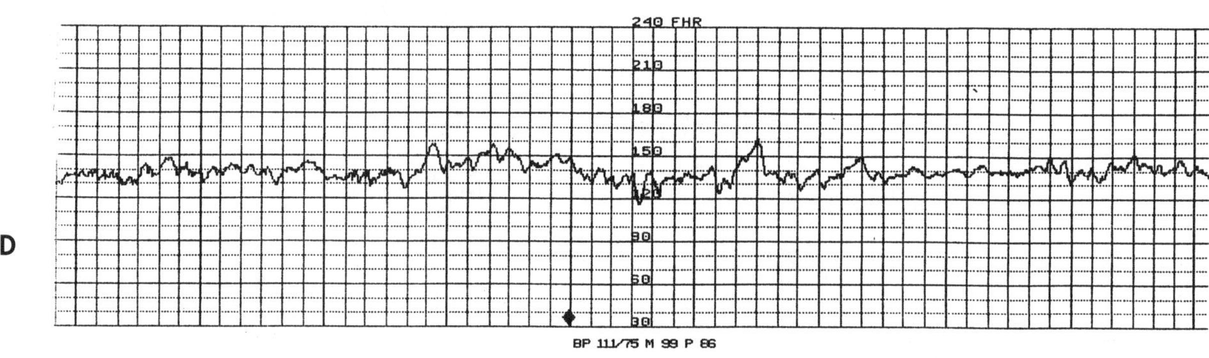

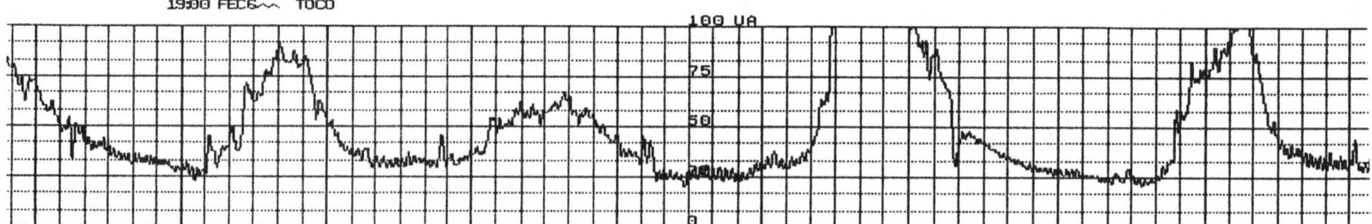

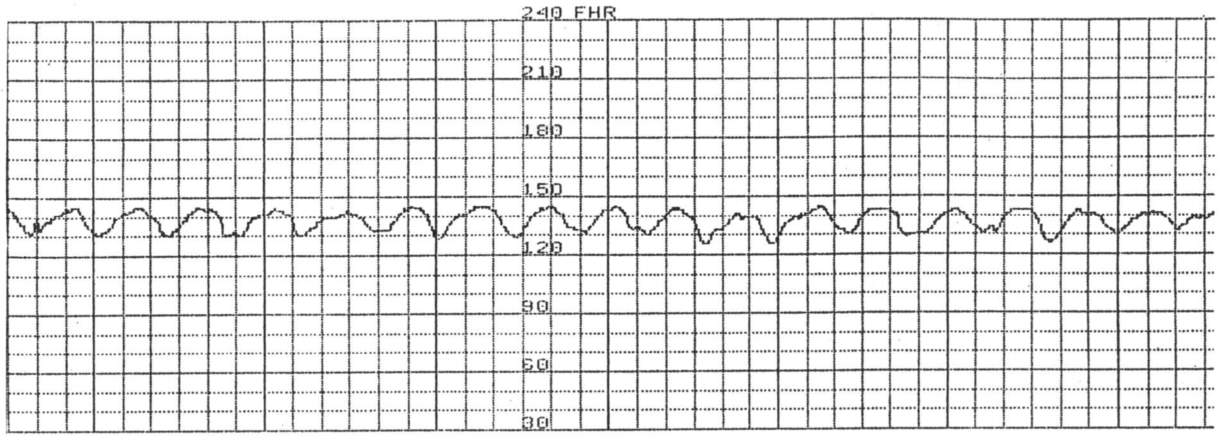

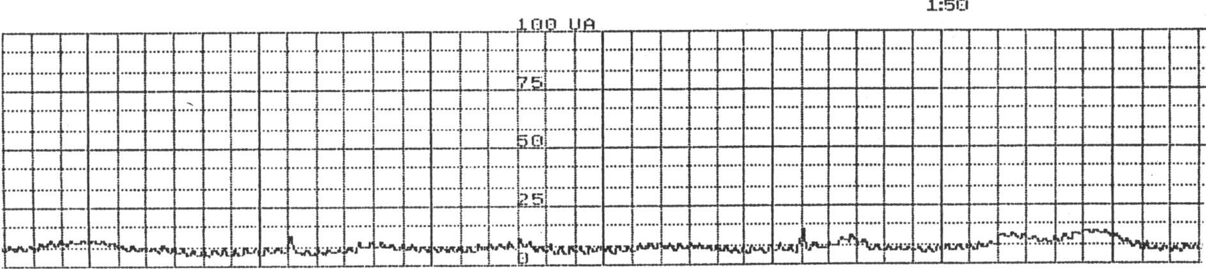

Figure 9-17 A sinusoidal tracing that was obtained from a fetus with severe anemia.

both auscultation evaluation and fetal monitoring pattern interpretation must be validated by written or verbal exercises prior to providing independent patient care (NAACOG, 1991).

Three major issues of concern regarding quality assurance in EFM are as follows: (1) acquisition of minimal level of competency, (2) competency validation, including knowledge-base evaluation and skills verification, and (3) maintenance of skill level. Methods of acquiring and maintaining competency in EFM pattern interpretation vary from institution to institution. A limited amount of didactic EFM education is taught in most undergraduate nursing programs. Orientation programs for new graduate nurses also vary among institutions with some providing a very basic introduction to EFM while others offer intensive training involving computer and video educational programs with didactic and clinical application (Eganhouse, 1991). Until recently, the majority of perinatal nurses acquired and maintained EFM skills by attending community, regional, and national conferences. More institutions are now taking responsibility for in-house education and competency validation. Specific educational standards and guidelines for minimal competency levels have been established (AWHONN, 1993b; NAACOG, 1991). Incorporating EFM competency validation into evaluation of all expected labor and delivery nursing knowledge and skills is important. Knowledge of the physiologic basis for FHR monitoring and interpretation of FHR patterns and appropriate nursing interventions are integral components of antepartum and intrapartum care and should be evaluated as such (Afriat, Simpson, Chez, & Miller, 1994).

The provision of basic EFM education has been difficult due to the lack of consensus in pattern identification, definitions, and implications. Recent malpractice litigations has focused attention on educational pitfalls. It is now clear that all perinatal nurses are responsible for pattern recognition, interpretation, nursing intervention, and documentation and for maintaining a current knowledge base (NAACOG,

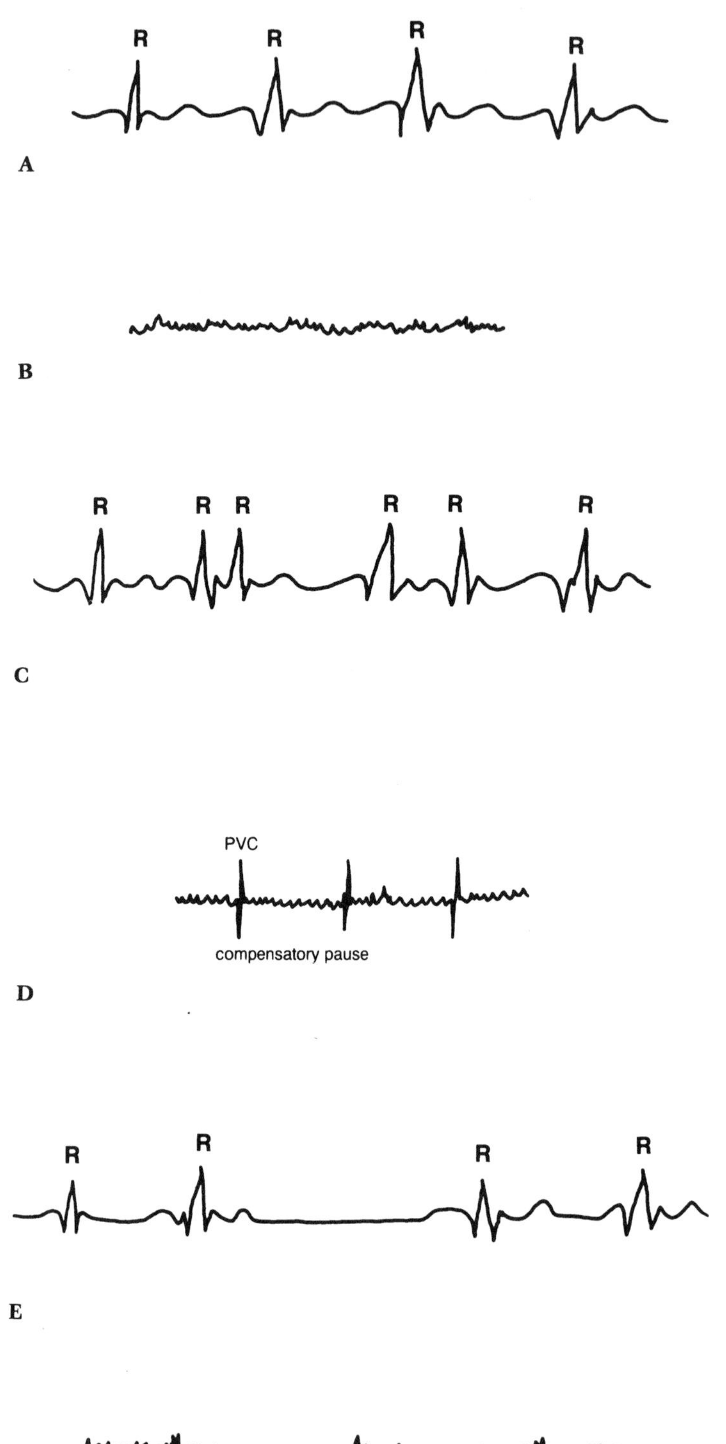

Figure 9-18. Fetal dysrhythmia detection. **A.** Appearance of R waves in a normal fetus. **B.** FHR pattern when each R-to-R interval is counted. **C.** An example of an irregular heart rhythm. There is an occasional premature ventricular contraction. (PVC) **D.** FHR pattern counting each interval between R waves of the irregular rhythm depicted in C. **E.** Another example of an irregular heart rate due to skipped or dropped beats. **F.** FHR pattern of the rhythm depicted in E.

From Afriat, C.I. (1989). Electronic fetal monitoring. Rockville, MD: Aspen.

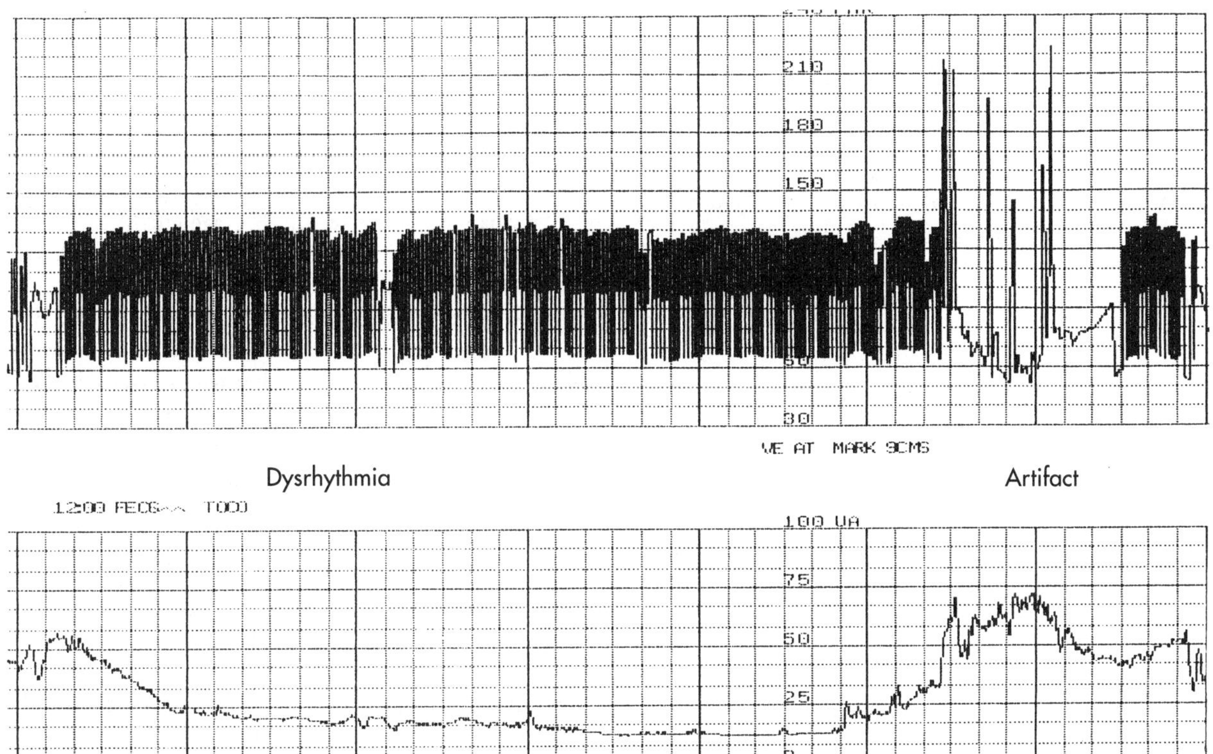

Figure 9-19. This tracing has both fetal dysrhythmias and artifact. Note the "randomness" of the artifactual information as compared to the "organization" of the dysrhythmias.

1992). Periodic competency validation and continuing education are measures to ensure quality in practice.

SUMMARY

The goal of perinatal healthcare providers is to facilitate a positive birth experience for all families. This includes using good judgment to ensure the best possible maternal-fetal outcome. Electronic fetal monitoring is one assessment tool that can be used to achieve this goal.

ACKNOWLEDGMENTS

The author would like to thank the excellent labor and delivery staff nurses at Women and Infants' Hospital in Providence, RI for their keen documentation on fetal heart rate tracing and for collecting tracings which provide educational opportunities for their colleagues nationwide and David Becker and Bradley Glaeser, Medical Photographers at St. John's Mercy Medical Center, St. Louis, MO.

REFERENCES

Afriat, C.I. (1989). Electronic fetal monitoring. Rockville, MD: Aspen.

Afriat, C.I., Simpson, K.R., Chez, B.F., & Miller, L.A. (1994). Electronic fetal monitoring competency—to validate or not to validate: The opinions of experts. Journal of Perinatal and Neonatal Nursing, 8(3), 1-16.

American Academy of Pediatrics & American College of Obstetricians and Gynecologists. (1992). Guidelines for perinatal care (3rd ed.). Washington, DC: Author.

American College of Obstetricians and Gynecologists. (1992). Human immunodeficiency virus infections (Technical Bulletin No. 169). Washington, DC: Author.

American College of Obstetricians and Gynecologists. (1995). Fetal heart rate patterns: Monitoring, interpretation, and management (Technical Bulletin No. 207). Washington, DC: Author.

Association of Women's Health, Obstetric, and Neonatal Nurses. (1993a). Fetal heart monitoring: Principles and practices. Washington, DC: Author.

Association of Women's Health, Obstetric, and Neonatal Nurses. (1993b). Didactic content and clinical skills verification for professional nurse providers of basic, high-risk and critical care intrapartum nursing. Washington, DC: Author.

Benson, R., Schubeck, F., Deutschberger, J., Weiss, W., & Berendes, H. (1968). Fetal heart rate as a predictor of fetal distress: A report from the collaborative project. Obstetrics and Gynecology, 32(2), 259-266.

Chez, B.F., & Harvey, C. (1994). Essentials of electronic fetal monitoring [Videotape Series (2nd ed.)]. Baltimore: Williams & Wilkins.

Clark, S.L., Gimovsky, M., & Miller, F. (1984). The scalp stimulations test: A clinical alternative to fetal scalp pH blood sampling. American Journal of Obstetrics and Gynecology, 148(3), 274-277.

Cohn, S.D. (1990). Malpractice and liability in clinical obstetrical nursing. Rockville, MD: Aspen.

Craven, D.E., Steger, K.A., & Jarek, C. (1994). Human immunodeficiency virus infection in pregnancy: Epidemiology and prevention of vertical transmission. Infection Control and Hospital Epidemiology, 15(1), 36-47.

Dildy, G.A., van den Berg, P.P., Katz, M., Clark, S.L., Jongsma, H.W., Nijhuis, J.G., & Loucks, C.A. (1994). Intrapartum fetal pulse oximetry: Fetal oxygen saturation trends during labor and relation to delivery outcome. American Journal of Obstetrics and Gynecology, 171(5), 679-684.

Dildy, G.A., Loucks, C.A., & Clark, S.L. (1993). Intrapartum fetal pulse oximetry in the presence of fetal cardiac arrhythmia. American Journal of Obstetrics and Gynecology, 169(6), 1609-1611.

Eganhouse, D.J. (1991). Electronic fetal monitoring, education and quality assurance. Journal of Obstetric, Gynecologic, and Neonatal Nursing, 20(1), 16-22.

Ellison, P.H., Foster, M., Sheridan-Pereira, M., MacDonald, D. (1991). Electronic fetal heart monitoring, auscultation, and neonatal outcome. American Journal of Obstetrics and Gynecology, 164, (5, Pt. 1), 1281-1289.

Fitzpatrick, E., Reeder, S.J., & Mastroianni, L. (1971). Maternity nursing (12th ed.). Philadelphia, J.B. Lippincott.

Freeman, R.K., Garite, T.J., & Nageotte, M.P. (1991). Fetal heart rate monitoring (2nd ed.). Baltimore: Williams & Wilkins.

Galvan, B., Van Mullem, C., & Boekhuizen, F.F. (1989). Using amnioinfusion for the relief of repetitive variable decelerations during labor. Journal of Obstetric, Gynecologic, and Neonatal Nursing, 18(3), 222-229.

Goodlin, R.C. (1979). History of fetal monitoring. American Journal of Obstetrics and Gynecology, 133(3), 323-352.

Goodwin, T.M., Milner-Masterson, L., & Paul, R.H. (1994). Elimination of fetal scalp blood sampling on a large clinical service. Obstetrics and Gynecology, 83(6), 971-974.

Hohn, A., & Stanton, R. (1992). The cardiovascular system. In A. Fanaroff & R. Martin (Eds.) Neonatal-perinatal medicine: Diseases of the fetus and infant (5th ed.). St. Louis MO: Mosby-Year Book.

Hon, E.H. (1958). The electronic evaluation of the fetal heart rate. American Journal of Obstetrics and Gynecology, 75(6), 1215-1230.

Johnson, J.W., & Riley, W. (1993). Cord blood gas studies: A survey. Clinical Obstetrics and Gynecology, 36(1), 99-101.

Knorr, L.J. (1989). Relieving fetal distress with amnioinfusion. American Journal of Maternal Child Nursing, 14(5), 346-350.

Krebs, H.B., Petres, R.E., & Dunn, L.J. (1983). Intrapartum fetal heart rate monitoring: VIII. Atypical variable decelerations. American Journal of Obstetrics and Gynecology, 145(3), 297-305.

Magann, E.F., Nolan, T.E., Hess, L.W., Martin, R.W., Whitworth, N.S., & Morrison, J.C. (1992). Measurement of amniotic fluid volume: Accuracy of ultrasonography techniques. American Journal of Obstetrics and Gynecology, 167(6), 1533-1537.

Mondanlou, H.D. (1991). Uses of biochemical profile of the fetus. Contemporary Obstetrics and Gynecology, 36(9) 69-85.

Munde, P. (1880). The diagnosis and treatment of obstetric cases by external abdominal examination and manipulation. New York: William Wood.

Nurses Association of the American College of Obstetricians and Gynecologists. (1990). Fetal heart rate auscultation (Practice Resource). Washington, DC: Author.

Nurses Association of the American College of Obstetricians and Gynecologists. (1991). Standards for the nursing care of women and newborns (4th ed.). Washington, DC: Author.

Nurses Association of the American College of Obstetricians and Gynecologists. (1991). Nursing practice competencies and educational guidelines, antepartum fetal surveillance and intrapartum fetal heart monitoring (2nd ed.). Washington, DC: Author.

Nurses Association of the American College of Obstetricians and Gynecologists. (1992). Nursing responsibilities in implementing intrapartum fetal heart rate monitoring (Position Statement). Washington, DC: Author.

Ocak, V., Sen, C., Demirkiran, F., Colgar, U., Ocer, F., & Kilavuz, U. (1992). FHR monitoring and perinatal mortality in high risk pregnancies. European Journal of Obstetrics, Gynecology, and Reproductive Biology, 44(1), 59-63.

Ogundipe, O.A., Spong, C.Y., & Ross, M.G. (1994). Prophylactic amnioinfusion for oligohydramnios: A reevaluation. Obstetrics and Gynecology, 84,(4, Pt. 1), 544-548.

Parer, J.T. (1983). Handbook of fetal heart rate monitoring. Philadelphia: W.B. Saunders.

Phelan, J. (1991). Was it intrapartum fetal distress? Contemporary Obstetrics and Gynecology, 32, 26-34.

Rochard, F., Schifrin, B.S., Goupil, F., Legrand, H., Blottiere, J., & Sureau, C. (1976). Nonstressed fetal heart monitoring in the antepartum period. American Journal of Obstetrics and Gynecology, 126(6), 699-706.

Schifrin, B.S. (1982). The fetal monitoring polcmic. Clinics in Perinatology, 9(2), 399-409.

Schifrin, B.S. (1990). Exercises in fetal monitoring. St. Louis MO: Mosby-Year Book.

Shy, K.K., Luthy, D.A., Bennett, F.C., Whitfield, M., Larson, E.E., van Belle, G., Hughes, J.P., & Stenchever, M.A. (1990). Effects of electronic fetal heart rate monitoring, as compared with periodic auscultation, on the neurologic development of premature infants. New England Journal of Medicine, 322(9), 588-593.

Thorpe, J.A., Sampson, J.E., Parisi, V.M., & Creasy, R.K. (1989). Routine umbilical cord blood gas determinations. American Journal of Obstetrics and Gynecology, 161, 600-605.

Tucker, S.M. (1996). Pocket guide to fetal monitoring (3rd ed.). St. Louis MO: Mosby-Year Book.

Pain Relief and Comfort Measures During Labor

Patricia A. Creehan

Pain management continues to be a challenge for perinatal nurses caring for women during the labor and birth process. Most pregnant women have concerns about their ability to handle painful contractions and maintain a sense of control. Labor coaches may also be worried about being able to support their partner in such a way as to minimize pain or discomfort. Nearly every woman in labor will experience some degree of discomfort. Pain is an individual, subjective experience that varies within the same person from one episode to the next (Bird, 1992). An appreciation of each women's unique experience of pain is possible when perinatal nurses understand the physiologic basis of pain, physiologic responses to pain, and psychosocial factors influencing pain perception.

During labor, responsibility for managing pain and providing comfort is shared by nurses, physicians, and labor-support persons. Interventions exist along a continuum, from noninvasive to invasive and from nonpharmacologic to pharmacologic. As healthcare professionals move along this continuum, potential for complications and side effects increase. This chapter discusses the physiologic basis for pain along with psychosocial factors influencing pain perception. Nonpharmacologic interventions are presented first since, in clinical practice, these are usually used prior to pharmacologic interventions.

PHYSIOLOGIC BASIS OF PAIN

Most pain during childbirth results from normal physiologic events. During the first stage of labor, uterine muscle hypoxia, lactic acid accumulation, cervical and lower uterine segment stretching, traction on ovaries, fallopian tubes, and uterine ligaments, and pressure on the bony pelvis cause afferent pain impulses to be carried along sympathetic nerve fibers entering the neuraxis between the 10th–12th thoracic and first lumbar spinal segment. During the second stage of labor, distention of pelvic floor muscles, vagina, perineum, and vulva, and pressure on the urethra, bladder, and rectum cause afferent pain impulses to be carried along sympathetic nerve fibers entering the neuraxis between the 2nd–4th sacral spinal segment (Oxone-Foote, 1986). Subjective descriptions of pain during the first and second stage of labor vary (Table 10-1). Some women describe a decrease in intensity during second stage, probably due to maternal focus on pushing. Others experience increased painful sensations, possibly due to the position of the fetus descending through the birth canal.

Gate-Control Theory

Gate-control theory is based on the premise that pain can be blocked by a "gating mechanism" (Melzack & Wall, 1965). McCaffery and Beebe (1993) developed a model based on gate-control theory which can be applied to pain management for childbearing women. Three physiologic processes have been identified as contributing to individual pain experience and provide a structure for categorizing various nonpharmacologic pain-management strategies (Table 10-2).

The first process is explained by the structure of the central nervous system, which is composed of large and small sensory nerve fibers. Impulses are carried via the spinal cord from the site of the stimuli to the cerebral cortex where impulses are interpreted. Small, thinly myelinated or unmyelinated fibers transport impulses such as pressure and pain from the uterus, cervix, and pelvic joints. Large myelinated fibers transport impulses from the skin. Since passage along large fibers occurs more quickly, it is possible for cutaneous stimulation to block or alter painful impulses. Based on this premise, tactile stimulation is used during labor.

The second process is stimulation of the reticular activating system located in the brain stem. The reticular activating system interprets auditory, visual, and painful sensory stimuli. When the cerebral cortex focuses on auditory or visual stimulation, painful stimulation is less able to pass through the "gate." Thus, many forms of distraction are used during labor to decrease pain perception.

TABLE 10-1. Verbal Descriptions of Pain During Labor and Birth

Sensory	Affective
First Stage of Labor	
Cramping, pulling, aching, heavy, sharp, stabbing, cutting intermittent, localized, global	Exciting, intense, tiring/exhausting, scary/frightening, bearable/unbearable distressing, horrible, agonizing, indescribable overwhelming, engulfing
Second Stage of Labor	
Painful pressure, burning, ripping, tearing, piercing, explosive, rending, localized	Exhausting, overwhelming, out-of-body feeling, inner focused/tunnel vision, exciting, horrible, excruciating, terrifying, less intense

From Mahlmeister, L. R. (1994a). Managing pain during the intrapartum and postpartum periods. In K. A. May, & L. R. Mahlmeister, Maternal and neonatal nursing: Family-centered care (3rd ed., p. 603). Philadelphia: J. B. Lippincott. Reprinted with permission.

The third process recognizes the impact of memory and cognitive processes on pain. Past experiences, cultural conditioning, level of anxiety, understanding of the labor process, and the meaning that the current situation has for the individual are used by the cerebral cortex to interpret a sensation as painful. Just as thoughts and emotions can increase pain, they can also increase feelings of confidence and control, thus decreasing painful sensations. Prenatal education and labor support can enhance maternal confidence and sense of control; therefore, they are effective pain management strategies.

Physiologic Responses To Pain

In addition to obvious physical discomfort, there are physiologic responses to pain over which women have little control. These physiologic responses may, over time, or in the context of other maternal or fetal conditions, have a negative impact on the fetus and the labor process.

In response to stress of labor, maternal catecholamine production increases, resulting in increased cardiac output and increased peripheral vascular resistance. Changes in maternal physiology include increased oxygen consumption, increased blood pressure, and decreased uterine blood flow. Lederman, Lederman, Work, & McCann (1985) demonstrated that catecholamines influence the labor process by reducing strength, duration, and coordination of uterine contractions and influence the fetus as demonstrated by nonreassuring changes in the fetal heart rate pattern.

TABLE 10-2. Using the Gate-Control Theory to Organize Nonpharmacologic Pain-Management Strategies

Use of cutaneous stimuli to relieve painful stimuli	Massage Touch Back-rub Counterpressure Movement Positioning Application of heat or cold Acupuncture Hydrotherapy Effleurage
Use of auditory or visual stimulation to block the transmission of the painful stimuli	Focal point Breathing techniques Attention focusing Distraction Hypnosis Music
Use of memory or cognitive processes to control the degree to which a sensation is interpreted as painful	Prenatal education Relaxation Labor support

PSYCHOSOCIAL FACTORS INFLUENCING PAIN PERCEPTION

Childbirth Preparation

There is a relationship between women's expectation of labor and their actual experience of labor (Green, 1993). Women who expect breathing and relaxation techniques to work find them helpful. Women who wish to avoid medications can be successful. Level of prenatal anxiety concerning pain in labor is inversely related to a woman's satisfaction with the birth experience (Green).

The basis of childbirth preparation is the belief that pain during childbirth is a cyclic process (Figure 10-1). As fear and anxiety heighten, muscle tension increases, inhibiting the effectiveness of contractions and increasing the experience of discomfort, thus further heightening fear and anxiety. The goal of childbirth education is to interrupt this cycle intellectually, with an understanding of what is occurring, and physiologically, with nonpharmacologic and pharmacologic pain-management strategies to use during labor. An awareness of the woman's childbirth preparation and skills that she and her partner are prepared to use is helpful when planning nursing support strategies during labor. Labor admission assessment should include questions related to type and amount of childbirth preparation (i.e., classes, reading, or video tape viewing). Knowledge and skills learned in childbirth preparation classes are enhanced when the nurse present during labor and birth believes in and actively supports the couple as they apply these principles.

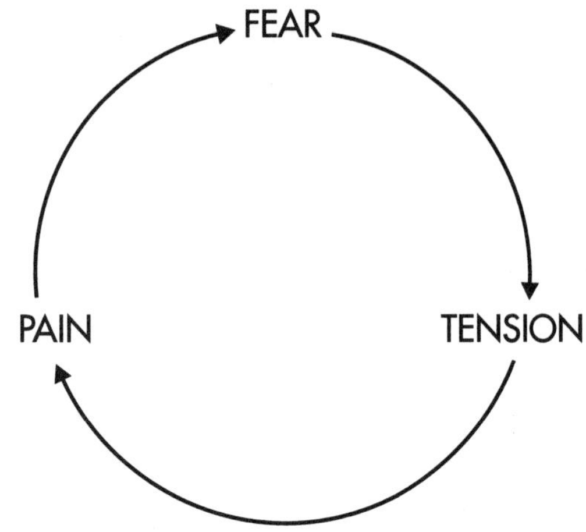

Figure 10-1. Fear-tension-pain cycle

From Jimenez, S. L. M. (1988). Supportive pain management strategies. In F. Nichols, & S. Humenick, Childbirth education: Practice, research, and theory (p. 104). Philadelphia: W. B. Saunders.

Characteristics of the Current Labor

Unique circumstances of every labor influence the experience of pain. Responsiveness of the cervix to uterine contractions is influenced by surgical or diagnostic procedures that compromise the integrity of the cervix. Prior procedures can result in incompetence and shorter labors or cause scarring and adhesions, resulting in failure to dilate and longer labors (Turley, 1993). Some medical and nursing procedures are uncomfortable. Interventions such as oxytocin administration, vaginal examinations performed in the supine position, bedrest, amniotomy, tight external electronic fetal monitor (EFM) belts, and enemas may change the character of labor contractions and increase discomfort. Length of labor does not necessarily correlate directly with a woman's perception of pain. A woman with short labors may experience very intense contractions. Women with a fetus in a persistent posterior position frequently report increased discomfort.

As duration of intense pain increases, discouragement and fatigue increase, decreasing ability to cope effectively with contractions. Fatigue may occur with a prolonged latent phase or be experienced by the woman who reports on admission that she has "not slept for 2 days."

Labor Support

Quality support during labor, whether offered by a partner, other family members, friends, or nursing personnel has a tremendous impact on a woman's perception of labor and ability to cope. Support influences use of analgesia and anesthesia (Hodnett & Osborn, 1989); duration of labor (Klaus, Kennell, Robertson, & Sosa, 1996; Pascoe, 1993); and maternal satisfaction with the labor and birth experience (Klein, Gist, Nicholson, & Standley, 1981; Oakley, 1983).

At the time of admission, the perinatal nurse identifies family members or friends who will act as labor-support persons. Fathers have an important role in providing physical and emotional support during childbirth. Chapman (1992) described three roles assumed by expectant fathers during labor:

Coach—actively assisted his partner, during and after labor contractions, with breathing and relaxation techniques. Men who assumed this role of coach led or directed their partners through labor and birth and viewed themselves as the managers or directors of the experience.

Teammate—assisted their partners throughout the experience of labor and birth by responding to requests for physical or emotional support or both. At times they would lead their partners, but their usual role was that of follower or helper.

Witness—viewed themselves primarily as companions, with emotional and moral support as their task. They were present during labor and birth to observe the process and to witness the birth of their child.

In this qualitative study, roles were developed by organizing behaviors observed during labor and described in interviews after birth. Contrary to commonly held perceptions of childbirth educators, consumers, and many nurses, the majority of men in the study adopted the role of witness rather than teammate or coach (Chapman, 1992).

As use of technology has expanded in obstetrics, the role of the intrapartum nurse has also changed, moving from providing hands-on comfort to relying on technology and pharmacologic interventions (Hodnett & Osborn, 1989). Emotional support behaviors, including giving praise, appearing calm and confident, assisting with breathing and relaxation, and treating women with respect are most helpful to laboring women (Bryanton, Fraser-Davey, & Sullivan, 1994).

Currently, there is increased interest in the role of professional and lay labor support in addition to support provided by the perinatal nurse. Labor support persons, doulas, or monitrices, with a variety of credentials and levels of education, are assisting women and their partners during labor (Simkin, 1992). Lay women can be trained to provide labor support. A monitrice is a registered nurse who performs assessments and provides nursing care in addition to labor support. A doula may be a nurse or lay person who provides emotional support and physical comfort measures during labor. The Doulas of North America and the American Society for Psychoprophylaxis in Obstetrics offer programs that prepare professionals and lay women to provide labor support. Services of a labor support person are arranged prior to labor by the expectant couple.

Healthcare Environment

Every perinatal unit has a unique approach to caring for laboring women. A culture develops, which over time, is accepted by most of those working within the department and is a reflection of their values and beliefs. Cultural differences may be as significant as the availability of labor, delivery, recovery, and postpartum rooms (LDRPs) or as subtle as the routine initiation of intravenous fluids upon admission. These practices reflect the evolution of intrapartum care within a particular institution. Unit culture extends to treatment of pain and has an impact on the woman's perception of pain. Nurses who value nonpharmacologic approaches to pain management use these techniques in clinical practice. Knowledge that woman gain in childbirth preparation classes is reinforced by the nurse during labor, in an attempt to disrupt the fear-tension-pain cycle.

Pain Tolerance

In labor, pain tolerance may be defined as duration or intensity of pain that a woman is able to endure without pharmacologic pain relief (Bird, 1992). Descriptive words such as mild, moderate, and severe do not provide a measure of pain tolerance since laboring women may describe pain as severe yet not request pain medication. A woman's pain tolerance or length of time she is able to go without medication may be increased by the use of nonpharmacologic pain-management techniques.

NONPHARMACOLOGIC PAIN-MANAGEMENT STRATEGIES

Nursing expertise in a variety of pain-management strategies is important. Not all nurses believe in or use nonpharmacologic approaches to pain relief when caring for laboring women. Possible reasons are lack of familiarity with alternative techniques or routine practices that tend to be pharmacologic. With increased popularity of epidural anesthesia use by both healthcare providers and consumers, many nurses new to the specialty have not had the opportunity to learn about or use pharmacologic measures. Pain-management strategies are chosen by nurses, based on what they have observed to work in practice, are personally comfortable with, or have used during their own labors.

Women choose pain-management strategies based on what they learned in prenatal classes, primary healthcare providers' recommendations, and listening to what worked for their family members and friends. Although few randomized, controlled, clinical trials exist supporting the effectiveness of specific nonpharmacologic techniques during labor, suggestion and initiation of any of these techniques are within the scope of perinatal nursing practice. For some women, multiple pain-management strategies may be necessary during the course of labor. Habituation may occur as the continued use of one technique becomes monotonous or offers insufficient stimuli to interfere with pain perception. As any technique becomes less of a distraction and thus less effective, perception of pain increases (Bird, 1992). Therefore, it is necessary for perinatal nurses to develop expertise in a variety of pain-management strategies.

Cognitive Techniques

Relaxation

Achieving a state of relaxation is the basis of all nonpharmacologic interventions during labor. Women benefit from a state of relaxation because it (1) conserves energy rather than creating fatigue from the prolonged tension of voluntary muscles, saving energy for second stage of labor, and (2) enhances the effectiveness of nonpharmacologic and pharmacologic pain-management strategies.

Relaxation is both a skill and a physical state. In childbirth classes, woman are introduced to the skill of relaxation. How well they learn this skill depends on quality of instruction, amount of time they practice, and their belief that this technique can be beneficial. Relaxation is as contagious as panic, tension, and feelings of being overwhelmed. Relaxation skills can not be taught during active labor, but an environment that promotes relaxation can be created by the perinatal nurse (Display 10-1). Women who learn relaxation techniques during childbirth classes benefit from reinforcement and encouragement.

Focusing

During early labor, distraction is an effective strategy. Walking in the hallway, sitting in a chair, talking with visitors, watching television, playing cards, and using the telephone keep laboring women occupied. Most women reach a point during labor when they no longer are able to talk comfortably through contractions. Labor is hard work requiring intense concentration necessary to maintain a sense of control. When this point is reached, laboring women should be encouraged to focus on an object in the room or a support person's face or eyes. Some women are able to increase their level of concentration by closing their eyes; however, during labor this is usually the exception rather than the rule.

Imagery

Imagery is simple daydreaming. Childbirth educators teach imagery as a skill, encouraging expectant women to focus on pleasant scenes or experiences to increase their level of relaxation. Nurses encourage women to use imagery when making statements such as "think of the baby moving through the birth canal," "think of the baby moving down and out," and "think about the cervix dilating." Imagery is used to keep women focused and to encourage them to work with their contractions.

Breathing Techniques

Breathing techniques are usually taught in prenatal classes and are used as a distraction during labor to decrease pain and promote relaxation. On admission, the perinatal nurse reviews with the woman and her support person specific techniques they were taught in prenatal class. If a woman has not attended class, early labor is the time to discuss and practice a slow, controlled breathing pattern. A deep breath at the beginning of a contraction stretches respiratory muscles. Exhaling this breath relaxes respiratory muscles as well as other voluntary muscles. At some point in labor, perinatal nurses may find it necessary to breathe with a couple through several contractions. Women are encouraged to breathe slowly except when attempting to control urge to push. In this case a rapid, shallow breathing pattern is more helpful.

Movement and Positioning

Women naturally choose positions of comfort and are more likely to change position during early labor (Carlson, et al., 1986). Modern technology (i.e., electronic fetal monitors [EFMs], intravenous lines, automatic blood pressure monitors, and fetal scalp electrodes) may interfere with a woman's ability to find a comfortable position and frequently restrict her to bed. Many nurses and physicians encourage bedrest

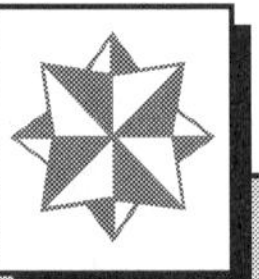

DISPLAY 10-1

Creating a Relaxed Environment During Labor

- Control the amount of light, noise, and interruptions
- Maintain an unhurried demeanor
- Use a calm, soft, slow, voice
- Recognize signs of tension – Changes in voice
Frowning
Clenched fists
Stiff, straight posture
Tense arms or legs
Stiff, raised shoulders
- Maintain eye contact, use touch or massage if this is acceptable to the woman
- Sit, rather than stand, next to the woman

for labor because they feel more in control of the situation and believe it may be safer for the woman and fetus. However, it is possible to use all of the technology without maintaining continuous bedrest. An upright position can be accomplished in a recliner, rocking chair, or birthing bed adjusted to a chair position. EFM telemetry units or intermittent auscultation of the fetal heart rate can be used to evaluate fetal response to labor while women are ambulating.

Women should be encouraged to change their position frequently during labor. Moving decreases muscle fatigue, alters the relationship between the fetus and pelvis, and facilitates the effectiveness of labor contractions (Fenwick & Simkin, 1987). Sensory stimulation resulting from movement competes with the discomfort of uterine contractions. A woman sitting in a chair can walk to the bathroom; a woman in bed can be assisted to different positions. Women unwilling or unable to walk in the hallway during labor can stand or lean on a support person, wall, or bed through several contractions or walk around in their room. Women may initially resist suggestions to change position or may find new positions uncomfortable. When encouraging a woman to change position, the nurse should suggest that she remain in the new position through several contractions before deciding whether or not it is comfortable.

Pillows are used generously to maintain positions and support extremities. When lying on her side, pillows should be placed behind the back and between the knees. In a semi-Fowler's position, pillows should be placed under her knees or arms. Shorter women, sitting in a chair, may find that a pillow or stool under their feet decreases stretching of leg muscles. Women who labor with the baby's head in an occiput posterior position find that being on their hands and knees relieves back pain (Mahlmeister, 1994a).

Superficial Heat and Cold

The exact mechanism of how heat and cold benefit women during labor is not fully understood. It is theorized that transmission of temperature sensations occurs along the same small, unmyelinated nerve fibers as painful stimuli, causing perception of pain to be interrupted (Simkin, 1989). Techniques to provide heat and cold during labor include hot water bottle, moist towels, electric heating unit, shower, Jacuzzi, ice pack, or chemical cooling unit.

Use of jet hydrotherapy (whirlpool tub) during labor has been found to increase relaxation, provide pain relief, reduce blood pressure, and increase diuresis (Church, 1989). Limited research supports the safety of immersion in a tub or whirlpool during labor (McCandlish & Renfrew, 1993). Perinatal nurses often share anecdotal reports of women who labored quite successfully for periods of time in the shower. Women progress through labor more rapidly and report being more comfortable. They are sometimes so comfortable that it may be difficult to entice them out of the tub or shower. Several reports note no increase in infection rate when women labored in a tub following rupture of membranes (Church, 1989; Waldenstrom & Nilsson, 1992). Using a shower eliminates potential for infection acquired from a tub or whirlpool. Aderhold and Perry (1991) developed a protocol based on their experience in a tertiary obstetrical unit for using a shower or tub during labor (Display 10-2). Women may at first seem embarrassed or express some inhibition about laboring in the shower; however, they quickly appreciate the relaxing qualities of warm water.

Touch

Perinatal nurses and others providing support during labor use touch both consciously and unconsciously throughout labor to communicate their support and presence, to relieve muscle tension, and to decrease the pain of labor. All forms of massage except effleurage are accomplished with moderate pressure, activating

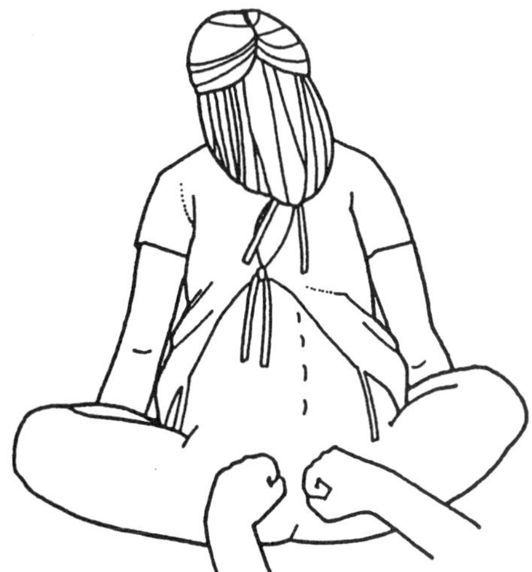

Figure 10-2. Firm counterpressure of the fists on the lower back.

From Bird, I. S. (1992). The nurses' contribution to pain relief during labor. In S. J. Reeder, L. L. Martin, & D. Koniak (Eds.), Maternity nursing family, newborn, and women's health care (17th ed., p. 528). Philadelphia: J. B. Lippincott.

large myelinated nerve fibers. Since habituation can occur, decreasing beneficial effects of massage, the type of stroke and location should be varied during labor.

Counterpressure

Counterpressure requires application of enough force to meet the intensity of pressure from the fetal occipital bone against the sacrum (Figure 10-2). Steady pressure from the heel of a support person's hand or another firm object counteracts the strain against the sacroiliac ligaments caused by the fetal occiput (Simkin, 1989). This technique moves the sacrum into normal alignment with the ilium, reducing the pain experienced by laboring women.

Effleurage

Effleurage is any light massage that glides over the skin but does not cause pressure or movement of deep muscle masses (Tappan, 1978). Effleurage is performed by the laboring woman drawing rhythmic circles or lines with finger tips on her abdomen or thighs, or by a support person using finger tips to gently rub up and down the woman's arm or leg (Figure 10-3).

Music

Music is used as a distraction in labor. Familiar music, associated with restful or pleasant recollections may be an adjunct to relaxation and imagery. Birthing rooms can be equipped with compact disc or cassette tape players, and women can be encouraged to bring their musical preferences. Music creates an atmosphere in the birthing room that also may change the approach of healthcare professionals to laboring women. Perinatal nurses and physicians become more relaxed, slow their activities, and respond with increased respect for the unique personal event in progress (DiFranco, 1988). When women use earphones or a headsets to listen to music, an auditory sensation is created that is difficult to ignore (Bird, 1992). Women should vary the type or style of music and use this technique intermittently to decrease the possibility of habituation.

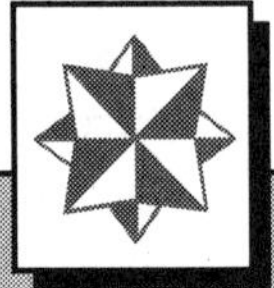

DISPLAY 10-2

Protocol for Using a Tub or Shower During Labor

- Establish fetal and maternal well-being by conducting a thorough assessment prior to using a tub or shower
- Use of intermittent fetal monitoring/auscultation
- Oral fluids to prevent dehydration
- Water temperature maintained at 96°–98° F
- At least 2 hours after last dose of Prostaglandin Gel
- Intact or ruptured membranes
- Contraindications– Thick meconium
Oxytocin infusion
Bleeding or large bloody show
- Continuous intravenous therapy or a heparin lock may be in place
- Stable maternal vital signs

Adapted from Aderhold, K., & Perry, L. (1991). Jet hydrotherapy for labor and postpartum pain relief. American Journal of Maternal Child Nursing, 16(2) 7.

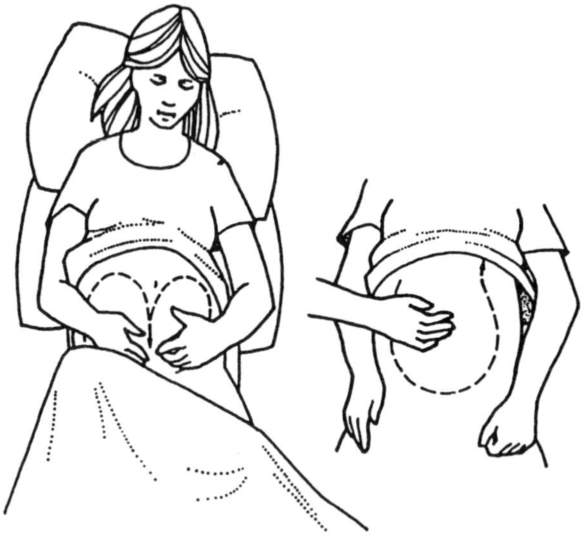

Figure 10-3. Two types of abdominal effleurage

From Bird, I. S. (1992). The nurses' contribution to pain relief during labor. In S. J. Reeder, L. L. Martin, & D. Koniak (Eds.), Maternity nursing family, newborn, and women's health care. (17th ed., p. 527). Philadelphia: J. B. Lippincott.

PHARMACOLOGIC PAIN-MANAGEMENT STRATEGIES

The perinatal nurse assesses preferences for pain management during labor at the time of admission and conducts ongoing assessments of factors influencing pain perception throughout labor. There will always be laboring women who need or desire pharmacologic agents. The decision to use medication should be made in collaboration with the woman and the physician/nurse midwife. Ideally the laboring woman should clearly understand benefits and potential maternal-fetal side effects. This information is best introduced during the prenatal period, rather than during the stress of labor. Pharmacologic pain management is divided into two categories: analgesia (use of a medication to decrease or alter the normal sensation of pain) and anesthesia (partial or complete loss of sensation with or without loss of consciousness).

Analgesics

Sedatives and Tranquilizers

Sedatives such as secobarbital sodium (Seconal) and pentobarbital (Nembutal) do not relieve pain. Traditionally they are given orally or as an intramuscular injection to induce sleep. During labor, sedatives decrease anxiety, inhibit uterine contractions, and allow for rest (Miller, DeVore, & Eisler, 1993). Women in prolonged early labor may benefit from a brief period of sleep, which is frequently followed by a more coordinated, effective contraction pattern. Since sedatives may have effects on the neonatal central nervous system, such as decreased responsiveness and ability to suck, their use is reserved for early labor when birth is unlikely for 12 to 24 hours (Levinson & Shnider, 1993).

Tranquilizers such as promethazine hydrochloride (Phenergan), hydroxyzine hydrochloride (Vistaril), and propiomazine (Largon) are frequently administered with narcotics during labor to relieve anxiety, increase sedation, and decrease nausea and vomiting. These drugs have traditionally been thought to potentiate the effects of narcotics; however, there is no objective evidence to support this belief (Wakefield, 1994). Prochlorperazine maleate (Compazine), chlorpromazine (Thorazine), and promazine (Sparine) are rarely used due to their α-adrenergic blocking properties, resulting in increased incidence of hypotension (Levinson & Shnider, 1993). While all tranquilizers have a sedative effect on the woman in labor, they do not appear to increase neonatal depression (Levinson & Shnider, 1993). Routes of administration and side effects for all tranquilizers are similar; however, promethazine causes respiratory depression and hydroxyzine is limited to IM use.

In the presence of pain, both sedatives and tranquilizers administered without IV opioids have an antianalgesic effect, increasing the perception of pain (Wakefield, 1994).

Parenteral Opioids

Opioids are the category of drugs most commonly administered parenterally during labor. Depending on the dose, route of administration, and stage of labor, they do not eliminate pain but instead cause a blunting effect, decreasing the perception of pain and allowing women to relax and rest between contractions (Table 10-3). Following administration of an opioid during early labor, frequency and duration of contractions and fetal heart rate variability may decrease (Wakefield, 1994). For this reason, opioids may not be administered until a labor pattern is well established. Effects of these medications cause some woman to doze between contractions. Coaching by a support person or nurse is important to help the woman anticipate and recognize the beginning of a contraction.

TABLE 10-3. Opioids and Agonist/Antagonists for Labor Analgesia

	Dosage	Onset of Action	Duration of Action
Meperidine (Demerol)	25 mg IV 50 mg IM	5–10 min IV 40–45 min IM	2–3 hr
Morphine	2–5 mg IV 10 mg IM	5 min IV 20–40 min IM	3–4 hr
Fentanyl	25–50 micrograms IV 100 micrograms IM	2–3 min IV 10 min IM	30–60 min
Nalbuphine (Nubain)	10–20 mg IV/IM	2–3 min IV 15 min IM/SQ	3–6 hr
Butorphanol (Stadol)	1–2 mg IV/IM	5–10 min IV/IM	3–4 hr
Pentazocine (Talwin)	20–40 mg IV/IM	2–3 min IV 15–20 min IM/SQ	2–3 hr

From Wakefield, M. L. (1994). Systemic analgesia: Opioids, ketamine, and inhalational agents. In D. Chestnut, Obstetric anesthesia: Principles and practice (p. 341). St. Louis: Mosby.

Opioids are administered IV or IM every 3 to 4 hours. Given IV, onset of action is quicker; however, medication effects do not last as long. IV-push medications are given slowly during a contraction to decrease transfer of the medication to the fetus. During the peak of a contraction, blood supply to the placenta essentially ceases. Administering the medication at this time allows for rapid distribution of the drug and decreased maternal plasma concentration to the placenta when circulation resumes (Spielman, 1987).

Neonatal side effects are related to dosage and timing of administration. Because of the potential for neonatal respiratory depression, the timing of administration relative to birth of the newborn is important. Ideally birth should occur within 1 hour or after 4 hours following administration (Wakefield, 1994). Kuhnert, Linn, and Kuhnert (1985), in a review of the literature, found that newborn behavioral responses may be altered for several days. Effects include decreased muscle tone and social responsiveness, ineffective suck, and abnormal reflexes.

Naloxone hydrochloride (Narcan), a narcotic antagonist, is administered to the newborn whose mother has received an opioid in labor if he fails to breath spontaneously, appears depressed, or requires prolonged resuscitative efforts.

Agonist/Antagonist

Medications such as nalbuphine (Nubain), butorphanol (Stadol), and pentazocine (Talwin) are classified as mixed agonist/antagonist (Table 10-3). They act as antagonists similar to naloxone, blocking receptors responsible for respiratory depression while stimulating receptors that block painful sensations. Quality of pain relief and potential for maternal and neonatal respiratory depression are equal to opioids. However, less maternal nausea and vomiting is observed. Unlike opioids, respiratory depression does not increase with increasing doses of medication (Wakefield, 1994).

Intravenous opioids or agonist/antagonists may be administered with local infiltration of the perineum during the second stage of labor for a difficult operative delivery when visualization of the cervix or upper vagina is required for a repair or for manual exploration of the uterus.

Regional Anesthesia

These medications provide almost immediate pain relief at the site of injection or to a large region of the body when injected in the epidural or subarachnoid space.

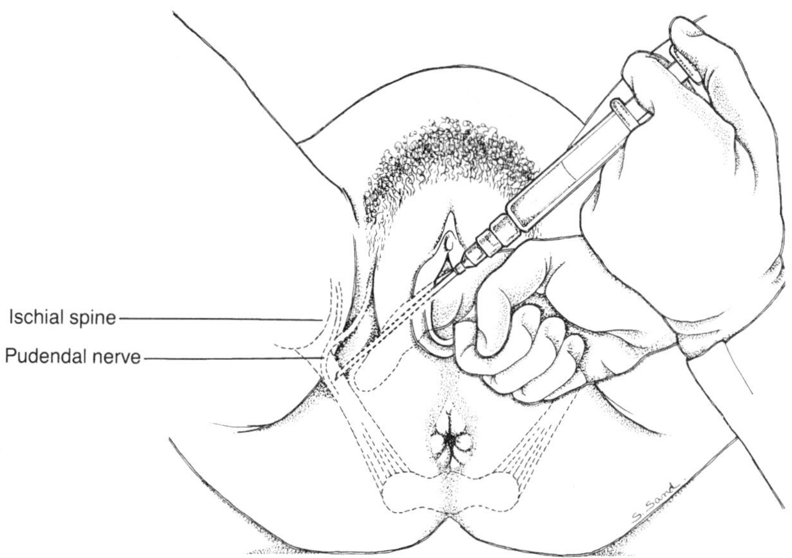

Figure 10-4. Procedure for administration of a pudendal block

From Waugaman, W. (1992). Analgesia and anesthesia during childbirth. In S. J. Reeder, L. L. Martin, & D. Koniak (Eds.), Maternity nursing family, newborn, and women's health care (17th ed., p. 551). Philadelphia: J. B. Lippincott.

Local Infiltration

During second stage of labor, a local anesthetic may be injected into the perineum and posterior vagina prior to performing an episiotomy. This area may be reinjected after delivery of the placenta in preparation for perineal repair.

Pudendal Block

A pudendal block, during second stage of labor, anesthetizes the lower vagina, vulva, and perineum. An anesthetic is injected through the lateral vaginal walls into the area of the pudendal nerve (Figure 10-4). This technique provides adequate anesthesia for vaginal birth, application of outlet forceps, and perineal repair. Since it is possible for a pudendal block to be ineffective, it is frequently combined with local infiltration of the perineum (Chestnut, 1994).

Epidural Anesthesia/Analgesia

Epidural anesthesia/analgesia for pain management during labor has become popular in many labor and delivery settings where 24-hour anesthesiology coverage is available. Although it is possible for an epidural to be ineffective or only partially effective, most women report adequate pain control using this technique.

For many years, epidural anesthesia was limited to local anesthetics such as lidocaine (Xylocaine), bupivacaine (Marcaine), and chloroprocaine (Nesacaine). These drugs act on nerve fibers as they cross the epidural space, causing sensory blockade. To obtain a therapeutic level of pain relief, the dose of local anesthetic resulted in loss of motor function. By using dilute concentrations of local anesthetic, such as bupivacaine 0.125% or 0.0625%, in combination with narcotics, such as fentanyl (Sublimaze), sufentanil (Sufenta), and alfentanil (Alfenta), via a continuous infusion pump, the goal of pain relief without significant motor block can be achieved. Epidural narcotics act by crossing the dura into the cerebral spinal fluid and binding to opiate receptors in the dorsal horn of the spinal cord. Adding a narcotic to the local anesthetic lessens the risk of toxicity by decreasing amount of local anesthetic needed, speeding onset of action, improving the quality of pain relief, and increasing duration of action (Wright, 1991). While narcotics alone may be effective in early labor, the combination of a local anesthetic and narcotic is frequently required to control pain as labor progresses. Adding epinephrine may prolong the effect of the anesthetic by decreasing absorption from the epidural space (Mahlmeister, 1994b). This effect also decreases the risk of systemic toxicity.

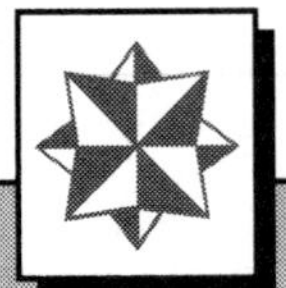

DISPLAY 10-3

Contraindications to Epidural Anesthesia/Analgesia

- Patient refusal
- Coagulation disorders
- Local infection at the site of injection
- Maternal hypotension and shock
- Nonreassuring FHR pattern requiring immediate birth

Procedure

The anesthesiologist/certified registered nurse anesthetist (CRNA) is responsible for identifying women with contraindications to the procedure (Display 10-3). During this meeting, the procedure and potential complications are discussed and questions answered. Some institutions provide the opportunity for women to meet with an anesthesiologist/CNRA prior to admission. Without this type of preparation, obtaining true informed consent from a woman in active labor is practically impossible.

After catheter placement in the epidural space between the 4th–5th lumbar vertebra, a test dose of a local anesthetic mixed with epinephrine may be injected to determine if the catheter is not in the epidural vein or the subarachnoid space (Figure 10-5). Injection into the epidural vein would result in tachycardia, palpitations, increased blood pressure, numbness of the tongue, lightheadedness, or tinnitus within 2 to 3 minutes. In some women, a test dose may not determine intravascular injection, either because there is existing baseline tachycardia or because it occurs too quickly to be noted. This supports incremental dosing rather than a bolus dose of medication and continued observation for side effects. Placement in the subarachnoid space causes immediate loss of sensation.

When the anesthesiologist/CRNA is satisfied that the catheter is properly placed, the anesthetic medication is injected. Depending on the specific medication used, women will begin to feel relief in 5 to 10 minutes. Complete block usually occurs in 15 to 20 minutes (Taylor, 1993).

Once the catheter is in place, epidural anesthesia/analgesia is administered intermittently or as a continuous infusion. Advantages of a continuous infusion include a consistent level of pain relief (Purdy, Currie, & Owen, 1987) and prevention of hemodynamic changes associated with the repeated occurrence of pain. Continuous flow through the catheter also stabilizes the catheter, decreasing the risk of migration into an epidural vein or through the dura into the subarachnoid space (MacDonald, 1992). Disadvantages of epidural anesthesia/analgesia include potential side effects, additional technology added to the birth experience, and in most institutions; bedrest restriction.

Historically, the use of epidural anesthesia/analgesia has been thought to increase the length of the first and second stage of labor. Research has been inconsistent regarding the influence of epidural anesthesia on length of labor. In a review of the literature, Miller et al. (1993) found that if hypotension does not occur and uterine displacement is maintained, length of labor is not affected by epidural anesthesia/analgesia. Furthermore, they suggested that any decrease in uterine activity may be related to the intravenous fluid

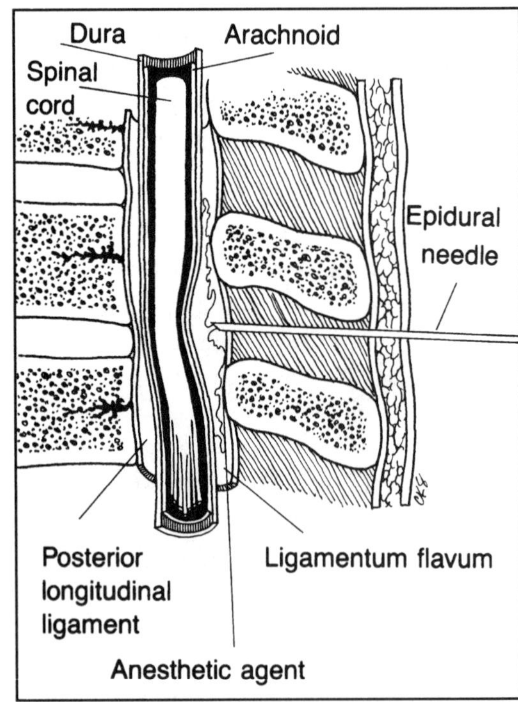

Figure 10-5. Epidural injection site

From Mahlmeister, L. R. (1993). Managing pain during the intrapartum and postpartum periods. In K. A. May, & L. R. Mahlmeister, Maternal and neonatal nursing: Family-centered care (3rd ed., p. 616). Philadelphia: J. B. Lippincott.

TABLE 10-4. Complications of Epidural Anesthesia

Cause	Symptom
Local anesthetic	Shivering Hypotension Increased incidence of operative birth Maternal pyrexia Neonatal hyperthermia Persistent occiput posterior Late decelerations Seizures
Narcotic	Respiratory depression Urinary retention Nausea and vomiting Sedation Pruritus
Result of actual procedure	Backache Inadvertent puncture of the dura Headache Unilateral block Migration of the catheter

bolus administered prior to placement of the catheter. Any change in uterine contractility is usually transient, lasting only 20 to 30 minutes (Miller, et al., 1993). Table 10-4 outlines potential side effects of epidural anesthesia/analgesia and their etiology.

Nursing Interventions

The Association of Women's Health, Obstetric, and Neonatal Nurses (AWHONN) has provided guidelines for practice for nurses caring for women receiving epidural anesthesia (Nurses' Association of the American College of Obstetricians and Gynecologists [NAACOG], 1991). Guidelines for Perinatal Care (American Academy of Pediatrics [AAP] and American College of Obstetricians and Gynecologists [ACOG], 1991) suggest 1:1 nurse-patient ratio for initiating epidural anesthesia. Perinatal nurses must be comfortable with operation of additional technology, be familiar with nursing care during all phases of the procedure, and be able to recognize potential complications. Continuous epidural anesthesia is always delivered through an infusion pump, and continuous EFM is the most frequently used method of fetal assessment. Depending on institutional practice or standards of care, women may also be monitored by a cardiac monitor, pulse oximeter, and automatic blood pressure devices.

Controversy exists in the literature and in clinical practice related to the frequency of maternal-fetal assessments during epidural anesthesia/analgesia for laboring women. While many perinatal units have policies that require blood pressure assessments every 15 to 30 minutes for women with epidurals, there are no published standards of care or practice guidelines from the American Society of Anesthesiologists (ASA), the American Association of Nurse Anesthetists (AANA), the American College of Obstetricians and Gynecologists (ACOG), or AWHONN that prescribe specific maternal blood pressure frequencies during epidural infusion for labor and delivery. The published standards are general. Display 10-4 shows the current published guidelines from these professional organizations related to maternal-fetal assessment frequencies during epidural anesthesia/analgesia in labor. Obstetric anesthesia textbooks (*Obstetric Anesthesia: Principles and Practice* [Chestnut, 1994] and *Anesthesia for Obstetrics* [Shnider & Levinson, 1993]) contain suggested protocols; however, while these textbooks provide valuable clinical information, they do not define standards of care. There are no research-based data to demonstrate optimal time intervals for maternal-fetal assessments during epidural infusion. The type and amount of medication used, the level of the block given, and maternal-fetal status should be considered when determining intensity of monitoring.

Another area of controversy in practice is the role of the registered nurse in management of analgesia by catheter techniques during labor and birth. In 1990, the American Nurses Association (ANA) facilitated the development of a position statement after representatives of state nurses associations and nursing specialty organizations sought clarification on registered nurses' roles and responsibilities while caring for patients receiving analgesia by catheter techniques. A year of discussion and consensus building followed, including meetings with members of the Nursing Organization Liaison Forum and the National Federation for Specialty Nursing Organizations, and draft copies were disseminated to state boards of nursing to allow input from all interested parties. This collaborative effort led to the 1991 *Position Statement on the Role of the Registered Nurse in the Management of Analgesia by Catheter*

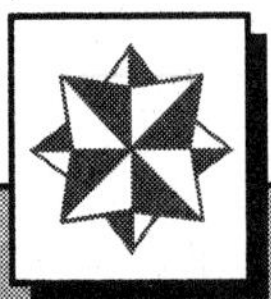

DISPLAY 10-4

Current Guidelines from Professional Organizations for Maternal Vital Signs and Fetal Heart Rate Assessment Frequencies during Epidural Anesthesia/Analgesia in Labor

Specific to Anesthesia/Analgesia

Guidelines for Regional Anesthesia in Obstetrics (ASA, 1991, p.1)

- During regional anesthesia for women in labor, "vital signs and FHR should be monitored and documented by a qualified individual".

Guidelines for Perinatal Care (AAP & ACOG, 1992, p. 74)

- "Maternal vital signs should be monitored at regular intervals by a qualified member of the healthcare team" during epidural anesthesia in labor.

Standards for the Nursing Care of Women and Newborns (NAACOG, 1991, p. 38)

- The nurse's responsibility is to "monitor and record maternal and/or fetal responses until stable and periodically thereafter, as indicated by protocol" during epidural anesthesia/analgesia during labor.

For all Women in Labor

Maternal Assessments

Guidelines for Perinatal Care, (AAP & ACOG, 1992, pp. 76)

- "Maternal temperature and pulse should be assessed at least every 4 hours or more often if indicated" and "maternal blood pressure should be taken and recorded regularly."

Fetal Assessments

Fetal Heart Rate Patterns: Monitoring, Interpretation, and Management, (ACOG, 1995, p. 2–3)

The intensity of FHR monitoring used during labor should be based on risk factors. When risk factors are present, the FHR should be assessed according to the following guidelines:

- "During the active phase of the first stage of labor, if auscultation is used, the FHR should be evaluated and recorded at least every 15 minutes after a uterine contraction. If continuous electronic monitoring is used, the tracing should be evaluated every 15 minutes."
- "During the second stage of labor, with auscultation, the FHR should be evaluated and recorded at least every 5 minutes. When electronic monitoring is used, the FHR should also be evaluated at least every 5 minutes."
- "In the absence of risk factors, the standard practice is to evaluate and record the FHR at least every 30 minutes during the active phase of the first stage of labor and at least every 15 minutes during the second stage of labor."

Source: Simpson, K.R. (1996).
(See also Display 8-3, page 159)

Techniques (Epidural, Intrathecal, Intrapleural, or Peripheral Nerve Catheters), which was endorsed by twenty-one professional nursing organizations, including AWHONN. According to this statement, registered nurses may monitor the mother and fetus, replace the empty infusion syringes or bags, stop the infusion, initiate emergency therapeutic measures if complications arise, and remove the catheter. It is also within the scope of practice for the registered nurse to manage the care of patients receiving analgesia by catheter if (1) the anesthesia provider is immediately available according to institutional policy, (2) management and monitoring of analgesia by catheter techniques, including reinjection and alteration of infusion rate by nonanesthetist registered nurses, is allowed by state laws and institutional policies, procedure, and protocol, (3) the attending physician or anesthesia provider orders the drugs, doses, and concentrations, and (4) guidelines for monitoring and drug administration and protocols for emergencies have been developed (American Association of Critical Care Nurses[AACN] et al., 1991). The registered nurse must also be able to meet the criteria of competency statements listed in the position statement. "For the woman in labor, only those registered nurses with education beyond licensure that is specific to obstetric analgesia may administer subsequent bolus doses and adjust infusion rates in compliance with the anesthesia provider's or physician's patient-specific written orders" (AACN et al., 1991).

Although this position statement requires that the registered nurse demonstrate knowledge and competency in all aspects of providing care to patients receiving analgesia by catheter or infusion device, the required education beyond licensure, how competencies will be evaluated, and how often this process should occur are not defined.

One professional nursing organization that did not endorse the 1991 (AACN et al.) position statement is the AANA. According to the AANA Position Statement, *Provision of Pain Relief by Medication Administered via Continuous Epidural, Intrathecal, Intrapleural, Peripheral Nerve Catheters or Other Pain Relief Devices* (1990), "...reinjection or continuous infusion of epidural catheters for anesthesia or analgesia for the obstetrical patient in labor may be performed *only* by a qualified/credentialed anaesthesia provider." Obstetrical laboring patients receiving epidural analgesia may be monitored by an obstetrical nurse appropriately trained in accordance with established guidelines provided an anesthesia provider is *immediately available* as defined by institutional policy, and this monitored care is to be done only following stabilization of vital signs after either bolus injection or establishment of continuous pump infusion" (American Association of Nurse Anesthetists [AANA], 1990).

Published standards and individual state nurse practice acts are inconsistent regarding the role of the nurse in caring for women in labor receiving anesthesia/analgesia and do not provide specific guidelines for how often and what type of monitoring will lead to optimal maternal-fetal outcomes. Therefore, perinatal nurses, in collaboration with obstetric and anesthesia providers in each institution must develop protocols that delineate responsibilities and care for women receiving epidural anesthesia/analgesia during labor and delivery.

Use of additional technology, bedrest restriction, and increased monitoring increases patient acuity. Contrary to the practice in most perinatal units, there is evidence to suggest that women receiving epidural analgesia with selected pharmacologic agents can safely ambulate during labor (Breen, Shapiro, Glass, Foster-Payne, & Oriol, 1993).

One advantage to this approach is that the woman is able to remain in an upright position, thus using the force of gravity to enhance labor progress. Advances in technology, such as mini-infusion pumps and EFM telemetry units, and increased knowledge of pharmacologic agents allowing medication dosages that provide effective analgesia without imparing motor function, have contributed to this practice. As data continue to emerge related to efficacy and safety, more women will have the benefit of ambulation in labor during epidural analgesia infusion. Table 10-5 contains a sample care plan for intrapartum use of epidural anesthesia/analgesia.

Additional Techniques

Two methods of regional anesthesia, paracervical block and saddle block, were once widely accepted techniques for relief of labor pain. Paracervical block is now rarely used due to potential fetal bradycardia caused by rapid absorption of local anesthetic from the paracervical space. Saddle block, injection of a local anesthetic into the subarachnoid space at L4–L5 at the onset of the second stage of labor, is also used infrequently because pain relief is generally so complete that women were unable to push effectively with their contractions,

TABLE 10-5. Nursing Care: Intrapartum Epidural Anesthesia/Analgesia

Nursing Diagnosis	Interventions	Scientific Rationale
Alteration in comfort related to positioning for placement of the epidural catheter	1. Explain procedure and the importance of remaining still during insertion of the catheter. 2. Assist the woman to maintain a side lying or sitting position. 3. Encourage use of Lamaze breathing techniques during procedure.	Avoid severe spinal flexion since this can decrease the epidural space and increase the possibility of puncturing the dura.
Alteration in comfort related to inadequate level of anesthesia/analgesia	1. Evaluate the effect of the epidural dose. Request that the anesthesiologist/CRNA redose the epidural as necessary, to provide effective pain relief.	Promotes spread of medication through epidural space.
	2. If pain continues to be felt on one side of the body, instruct the woman to lay on that side. 3. Assist the woman to change position at least q 1 hr.	Turning avoids continued pressure on one area of the body and decreases the risk of unilateral blocks.
Potential for maternal injury related to hemodynamic changes	1. Infuse IV bolus of 500–1,000 cc Ringer's lactate or normal saline solution 15–30 min prior to the procedure. 2. After catheter has been placed, maintain woman in a lateral tilt.	Avoid IV fluids containing glucose. These cause increased insulin production in the fetus and potential hypoglycemia after birth. Avoid rapidly infusing IV fluids into women with cardiac disease or severe preeclampsia without direct measurement of hemodynamic status.
	3. After each injection, monitor blood pressure, pulse, and respirations according to institutional protocol.	Since epidural anesthesia causes a sympathetic block and vasodilation, hydration and avoiding the supine position decreases the risk of maternal hypotension which can result in uteroplacental insufficiency.
	4. If hypotension occurs, increase IV fluids, maintain uterine displacement, administer oxygen, and administer Ephedrine as ordered.	Administering 2.5–5.0 mg IV Ephedrine promotes peripheral vasoconstriction without constricting the umbilical vessels and increases cardiac output.
	5. The nurse or anesthesia provider remains with the woman for the first 15 to 20 minutes following a bolus or initiation of a continuous infusion.	

TABLE 10-5. Cont.

Nursing Diagnosis	Interventions	Scientific Rationale
Potential for maternal injury related to placement of the catheter in the subarachnoid space or toxic response to anesthetic.	1. Oxygen and suction are set up and functioning prior to start of procedure. 2. Assess for symptoms of respiratory distress. 3. Crash cart with ambu bag and mask, laryngoscope and blades, and endotracheal tubes immediately available.	
Potential for migration of the catheter out of the epidural space	1. Assess the woman for lack of effect from the anesthetic. 2. Evaluate the woman for symptoms such as severe hypotension, motor block including the upper extremities, and respiratory or cardiac arrest.	These symptoms may indicate migration of the catheter into the subarachnoid space.
Potential for maternal injury related to late onset of respiratory depression	1. Respiratory rate should continue to be assessed frequently into the postpartum recovery period. When epidural morphine is used, respiratory rates are monitored according to institutional protocol. 2. Administer Naloxone if respiratory rate is <10.	Respiratory depression may occur 4–8 hr after the last narcotic dose.
Potential for fetal injury related to hemodynamic changes	1. Obtain a 20–30 min baseline EFM strip prior to initiation of the epidural, with continuous EFM for the duration of epidural infusion.	Maternal hypotension can decrease uteroplacental blood flow, adversely affecting fetal oxygenation which will be reflected in a nonreassuring FHR pattern.
Alteration in elimination related to decreased sensation of the bladder	1. Encourage the woman to void prior to the procedure and frequently during the infusion. 2. If the bladder is distended and the woman is unable to void, placement of an indwelling catheter eliminates the need for repeated catheterization.	Naloxone can also be used to reverse this effect on the bladder.
Potential pruritus related to epidural narcotic administration	1. Assess woman for complaints of itching.	Pruritus is most often seen with the administration of epidural morphine.

necessitating the application of forceps or vacuum extractor. Paracervical block and saddle block are uncommon in clinical obstetric practice today because of the popularity of epidural anesthesia.

SUMMARY

The ultimate goal is the birth of a healthy newborn to a healthy mother who is satisfied with her childbirth experience. Performing ongoing assessments, offering a variety of nonpharmacologic comfort measures, supporting woman receiving pharmacologic pain management, and recognizing when interventions are no longer effective or complications have developed are basic perinatal nursing practices.

Caring effectively for laboring women requires tremendous energy and commitment. Individual nurses and department managers have a responsibility to examine their own practices and the system as a whole. The challenge is to identify practices that have a positive impact on women's experiences and respond with flexibility to the opportunity to enhance perinatal nursing care related to pain management during labor and birth.

REFERENCES

Aderhold, K., & Perry, L. (1991). Jet hydrotherapy for labor and postpartum pain relief. American Journal of Maternal Child Nursing, 16(2), 97-99.

American Academy of Pediatrics & American College of Obstetricians and Gynecologists. (1991). Guidelines for perinatal care (3rd ed.). Elk Grove Village, Illinois: Author.

American Association of Nurse Anesthetists. (1990). Provision of relief by medication administered via continuous epidural, intrathecal, intrapleural, peripheral nerve catheters, or other pain relief devices (Position Statement). Park Ridge, IL; Author.

American College of Obstetricians and Gynecologists. (1995). Fetal heart rate patterns: Monitoring, interpretation, and management (Technical Bulletin No. 207), Washington, DC: Author.

American Association of Critical Care Nurses et al. (1991). The role of the registered nurse (RN) in the management of analgesia by catheter techniques (epidural, intrathecal, intrapleural, or peripheral nerve catheters (Position Statement). Washington, DC: AWHONN.

American Society of Anesthesiologists. (1993). Guidelines for regional anesthesia in obstetrics. In ASA standards, guidelines, and statements (pp. 22-23). Park Ridge, IL: Author.

Bird, I.S. (1992). The nurse's contribution to pain relief during labor. In S.J. Reeder, L.L. Martin, & D. Koniak (Eds.), Maternity nursing: Family, newborn, and women's health care (17th ed., pp. 507-536). Philadelphia: J. B. Lippincott.

Breen, T. W., Shapiro, T., Glass, B., Foster-Payne, D., & Oriol, N. (1993). Epidural anesthesia for labor in an ambulatory patient. Anesthesia and Analgesia, 77(5), 919-924.

Bryanton, J., Fraser-Davey, H., & Sullivan, P. (1994). Women's perceptions of nursing support during labor. Journal of Obstetric Gynecologic and Neonatal Nursing, 23(8), 638-644.

Carlson, J.M., Diehl, J.A., Sachtleben-Murray, M., McRae, M., Fenwick, L., & Friedman, E. A. (1986). Maternal position during parturition in normal labor. Obstetrics and Gynecology, 68(4), 443-447.

Chapman, L. (1992). Expectant fathers' roles during labor and birth. Journal of Obstetric, Gynecologic, and Neonatal Nursing, 21(2), 114-120.

Chestnut, D.H. (1994). Alternative regional anesthetic techniques: Paracervical block, lumbar sympathetic block, pudendal block, and perineal infiltration. In D.H. Chestnut, Obstetric anesthesia: Principles and practice (pp. 420-431). St. Louis: C.V. Mosby.

Church, L. K. (1989). Water birth: One birthing center's observations. Journal of Nurse Midwifery, 34(4), 165-170.

DiFranco, J. (1988). Relaxation: Music. In F. Nichols, & S.B. Humenick (Eds.), Childbirth education: Practice, research, and theory (pp. 201-215). Philadelphia: W.B. Saunders.

Fenwick, L., & Simkin, P. (1987). Maternal positioning to prevent or alleviate dystocia in labor. Clinical Obstetrics and Gynecology, 30(1), 83-89.

Green, J. (1993). Expectations and experiences of pain in labor: Findings from a large prospective study. Birth: Issues in Perinatal Care and Education, 20(2), 65-72.

Hodnett, E.D. & Osborn, R.W. (1989). A randomized trial of the effects of monitrice support during labor: Mothers' views two to four weeks postpartum. Birth: Issues in Perinatal Care and Education, 16(4), 177-183.

Jimenez, S.L.M. (1988). Supportive pain management strategies. In F. Nichols, & S.B. Humenick, Childbirth education: Practice, research, and theory (pp. 97-117). Philadelphia: W. B. Saunders.

Klaus, M.H., Kennell, J.H., Robertson, S.S., & Sosa, R. (1986). Effects of social support during parturition on maternal-infant morbidity. British Medical Journal, 293(6547), 585-587.

Klein, R., Gist, N., Nicholson, J., Standley, K. (1981). A study of father and nurse support during labor. Birth: Issues in Perinatal Care and Education, 8, 161-164.

Kuhnert, B.R., Linn, P.L., & Kuhnert, P.M. (1985). Obstetric medication and neonatal behavior. Clinics in Perinatology, 12(2), 423-440.

Lederman, R.P., Lederman, E., Work, B., & McCann, D.S. (1985). Anxiety and epinephrine in multiparous women in labor: Relationship to duration of labor and fetal heart rate pattern. American Journal of Obstetrics and Gynecology, 153(8), 870-871.

Levinson, G., & Shnider, S.M. (1993). Effects of anesthesia on uterine activity and labor. In S.M. Shnider, & G. Levinson (Eds.), Anesthesia for obstetrics (3rd ed., pp. 53-69). Baltimore: Williams & Wilkins.

Levinson, G., & Shnider, S.M. (1993). Systemic medication for labor and delivery. In S.M. Shnider, & G. Levinson (Eds.), Anesthesia for obstetrics (3rd ed., pp. 115-134). Baltimore: Williams & Wilkins.

MacDonald, R. (1992). Epidural analgesia for labor. Midwives Chronicle, 105(1251), 79-81.

Mahlmeister, L.R. (1994a). Managing pain during the intrapartum and postpartum periods. In K.A. May, & L.R. Mahlmeister, Maternal and neonatal nursing: Family-centered care (3rd ed., pp. 595-635). Philadelphia: J.B. Lippincott.

Mahlmeister, L.R. (1994b). Nursing care in normal labor. In K.A. May, & L.R. Mahlmeister (Eds.), Maternity and neonatal nursing; Family centered care (3rd ed., pp. 467-510). Philadelphia: J. B. Lippincott.

McCaffery, M., & Beebe, A. (1993). Pain: Clinical manual for nursing practice. St. Louis, MO: C.V. Mosby.

Melzack, R., & Wall, P. D. (1965). Pain mechanisms: A new theory. Science, 150, 971-979.

McCandlish, R., & Renfrew, M. (1993). Immersion in water during labor and birth: The need for evaluation. Birth: Issues in Perinatal Care and Education, 20(2), 79-85.

Miller, A.C., DeVore, J.S., & Eisler, E.A. (1993). Effects of anesthesia on uterine activity and labor. In S.M. Shnider & G. Levinson (Eds.), Anesthesia for obstetrics (3rd ed., pp. 53-70). Baltimore: Williams & Wilkins.

Nurses Associaton of the American College of Obstetricians and Gynecologists. (1991). NAACOG Standards for the nursing care of women and newborns. Washington, DC: Author.

Oakley, A. (1983). Social consequences of obstetric technology: The importance of measuring "soft" outcomes. Birth: Issues in Perinatal Care and Education, 10(2), 99-108.

Oxone-Foote, H. (1986). Human labor and birth (5th ed.). Norwalk,CT: Appleton-Century-Crofts.

Pascoe, J. (1993). Social support during labor and duration of labor: A community-based study. Public Health Nursing, 10(2), 97-99.

Purdy, G., Currie, J., & Owen, H. (1987). Continuous extradural analgesia in labor. Comparison between "on demand" and regular "top-up" injections. British Journal of Anaesthesia, 59(3), 319-324.

Shnider, S. & Levinson, G. (1993). Anesthesia for Obstetrics. Baltimore: Williams & Wilkins.

Simkin, P. (1989). Non-pharmacological methods of pain relief during labor. In I. Chalmers, M. Enkin, & M.J. N.C. Keirse (Eds.), Effective care in pregnancy and childbirth (pp. 893-912). Oxford: Oxford University Press.

Simkin, P. (1992). Labor support person. International Childbirth Education Association Journal, 16(1), 19-27.

Spielman, F.J. (1987). Systemic analgesics during labor. Clinical Obstetrics and Gynecology, 30(3), 495-504.

Tappan, F. (1978). Healing massage techniques. Reston, VA: Reston Publishing.

Taylor, T. (1993). Epidural anesthesia in the maternity patient. Journal of Maternal Child Nursing, 18(2), 86-93.

Turley, G.M. (1993). Essential forces and factors in labor. In S. Mattson, & J.E. Smith (Eds.), Core curriculum for maternal-newborn nursing (pp. 219-254). Philadelphia: W. B. Saunders.

Wakefield, M.L. (1994). Systemic analgesia: Opioids, detamine, and inhalational agents. In D.H. Chestnut, Obstetric anesthesia: Principles and practice (pp. 340-353). St. Louis, MO: C.V. Mosby.

Waldenstrom, U., & Nilsson, C. (1992). Warm tub bath after spontaneous rupture of the membranes. Birth: Issues in Perinatal Care and Education, 19(2), (57-63).

Waugaman, W. (1992). Analgesia and anesthesia during childbirth. In S.J. Reeder, L.L. Martin, & D. Koniak (Eds.), Maternity nursing: Family, newborn, and women's health care (17th ed., pp. 537-560). Philadelphia: J. B. Lippincott.

Wilson, S.J., Errick, J.K., & Balkon, J. (1986). Pharmacokinetics of nalbuphine during parturition. American Journal of Obstetrics and Gynecology, 155(2), 340-344.

Wright, W. (1991). Continuous epidural block for OB anesthesia. Contemporary Obstetrics and Gynecology, 36(11), 89-98.

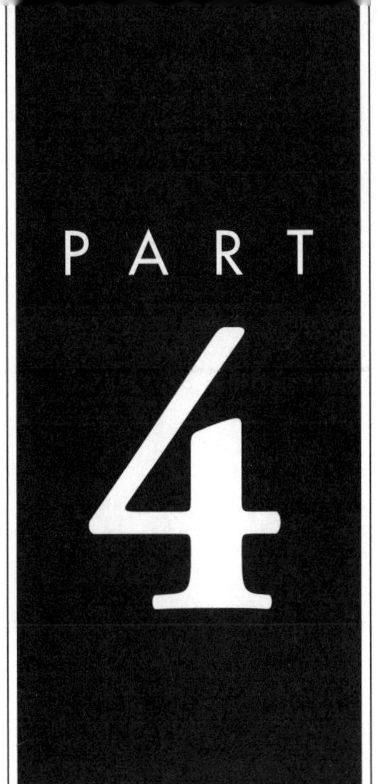

PART 4 Postpartum

Postpartum Care

Joy Grohar

The postpartum period is a time of transition. Physiologic changes occur, the woman adapts to the mothering role, and the family system is altered by the addition of the newborn. An arbitrary time frame divides the period into the immediate postpartum (first 24 hours), early postpartum (first week), and late postpartum (up to 90 days). This chapter begins with a discussion of physiologic changes during the postpartum period. Nursing care during the immediate postpartum period in the inpatient setting, including physical assessment and common complications, is also included. Care beyond the inpatient experience is covered in Chapter 18. Selected topics for patient education are presented. Teaching strategies for new mothers and general maternal-newborn learning needs are included in Chapter 17.

GUIDELINES FOR CARE

A woman experiences significant changes in physical and psychosocial status following childbirth. The woman's perception of care received during childbirth and the postpartum period has the potential to affect her self-concept and mothering abilities. Nurses, as well as other healthcare providers, have a unique opportunity to facilitate maternal and family adaptation by integrating the following guidelines into care:

1. Respect each woman for who she is, because she is the central focus of all care. Her permission, after discussion, is essential for simple procedures such as fundal assessment and perineal care. All women must be treated with respect, not just those who are "likable" or those who are "like us." The intrinsic worth of each human is tied to self-esteem. Caregivers have the opportunity to nurture a woman's core self-esteem with unconditional acceptance (e.g., "no matter how the world may judge you, I accept you as yourself"). The childbearing experience, including interactions with caregivers, may dominate the woman's adult life and the parenting of her child (Steinem, 1992). Self-awareness of attitudes and beliefs is crucial for nurses in order to provide respectful care because interactions with women and families are based on the nurse's view of the world. Consider that alternative paradigms exist.
2. Provide emotional and physical support. Women want to know their needs will be met and that caregivers will respond in a supportive and caring way. "Being there" is reassuring to both the woman and her family.
3. Include the woman's family and friends. Provide information, support, and access to food, telephones, and sleeping facilities, if necessary.
4. Encourage interaction with the newborn. Unless the woman requests otherwise or the newborn is clinically unstable, the newborn should remain with his or her parents. This is an ideal time to promote attachment and begin teaching the parents about normal newborn appearance and behavioral cues. The goal is to guide the family toward integration and health promotion while respecting family wishes.
5. Use technology appropriately. Try the most natural approach before moving to more invasive therapies. For example, to increase the normal newborn's temperature after drying him or her and applying a prewarmed stockinette hat, try maternal-infant skin-to-skin contact or double wrapping before removing the baby from the mother and placing him or her in a warmer (Vaughans, 1990).
6. Question policies and routines. Is the care woman- and family-based? If not, adjust it to that focus. Nurses can use creativity and problem-solving skills to meet various women's and families' needs.
7. Maintain collegial relationships among healthcare providers. Each caregiver is an essential partner in supporting the woman, newborn, and family

during this transition period. The feeling and ambiance created by a collegial working relationship is different from a traditional hierarchical relationship. It provides a satisfying and respectful working environment that is evident to the family and contributes to a quality outcome (Dwinell, 1992).

ANATOMIC AND PHYSIOLOGIC CHANGES DURING THE POSTPARTUM PERIOD

Uterus

Involution occurs primarily as a result of decreased myometrial cell size. Immediately after birth, uterine weight is approximately 1,000 g; at 6 weeks postpartum, it weighs less than 100 g. Observed changes are related to changes in uterine length as the decidua sloughs off in lochia. Beginning on postpartum day 2 or 3, the usual progression of uterine descent into the pelvis is 1 cm/day (Table 11-1). Multiparity, multiple gestation, and bladder distention can influence uterine size and the progression of uterine involution.

Cervix, Vagina, and Pelvic Floor

The cervix and lower uterine segment are thin and flaccid immediately postpartum. Cervical lacerations can occur during any birth; however, women with precipitous labor and operative procedures are at increased risk for lacerations. By the end of 1 week, the cervix narrows to a 1-cm diameter. It remains wider than its pregravid appearance, and depressions are noted at the site of lacerations. Cervical edema may persist for several months (Bowes, 1991). Rugae appear in the distended vagina by the third week. The voluntary muscles and supports of the pelvic floor gradually regain tone during the first 6 weeks postpartum.

TABLE 11-1. Uterine Involution

Immediately		PP	At the level of the umbilicus
1–2	hr	PP	Midline, midway between umbilicus and symphysis
12	hr	PP	1 cm above umbilicus
24	hr	PP	1 cm below umbilicus
3	days	PP	3 cm below umbilicus
7	days	PP	Just palpable at symphysis
14	days	PP	Not palpable

Placental Site and Lochia

Immediately after delivery of the placenta, the placental site contracts to a size less than one half that of its original diameter. Exfoliation over the first 8 days after birth occurs by necrotic sloughing of the infarcted superficial tissues. A reparative process follows in which marginal and decidual endometrium regenerates. The process of endometrial restoration occurs by day 16 after birth in all but the placental site. At 7 to 14 days postpartum, the eschar over the site of placental attachment sloughs. The woman may notice an episode of increased vaginal bleeding, usually self-limited in nature. Bleeding lasting more than 1 to 2 hours should be evaluated for late postpartum hemorrhage. Ultrasonography can be useful in determining the presence of retained placental tissue (Bowes, 1991).

Lochia is the postpartum uterine discharge. Initially, lochia is a flow of blood that lasts several hours. It rapidly diminishes to lochia rubra, a reddish-brown discharge lasting 3 to 4 days. Up to 15% of women will continue to experience lochia serosa, a mucopurulent discharge, at 6 weeks postpartum (Oppenheimer, Sherriff, Goodman, Shah, & James, 1986). Lochia alba, a yellow-white discharge, follows lochia serosa (Display 11-1). Choice of method of feeding the baby and the use of oral contraceptives do not affect duration of lochia (Bowes, 1991)

Ovarian Function

Estrogen and progesterone levels decrease suddenly following placental delivery. Estrogen reaches follicular phase levels by 3 weeks after birth in women who are not lactating. Ovulation can occur as early as 27 days after birth. Mean time for return of ovulation is 70 to 75 days postpartum for women who are not lactating and approximately 190 days postpartum for women who are breastfeeding (Bowes, 1991).

Return of Menses

The first menstrual period occurs about 3 months postpartum. Women who are nursing maintain depressed estrogen levels and begin to menstruate approximately 8 months after giving birth, but individual return to menses varies widely. Breastfeeding does not prevent pregnancy. Teaching for all women, whatever method of feeding the newborn is chosen, should include information prior to and after birth regarding family planning.

Metabolic Changes

Prolactin levels decrease with placental delivery. By the third week postpartum, the prolactin level returns to normal in women who formula feed their infants. For those who breastfeed, elevated prolactin levels persist for 6 weeks postpartum (Bowes, 1991).

Thyroid function returns to prepregnant levels within 4 to 6 weeks after birth. Because immunosuppression is a normal physiologic consequence of pregnancy, there is an increased risk of developing autoimmune thyroiditis, followed by hypothyroidism. There is a slightly increased risk of recurrence of autoimmune hypothyroidism or hyperthyroidism postpartum (Bowes, 1991; Novy, 1991).

Glucose levels are low after birth, because placental lactogen and growth hormone are absent after delivery of the placenta. As a result, women with insulin-dependent diabetes usually need less insulin after birth. Breastfeeding may precipitate hypoglycemia in women with insulin-dependent diabetes. Women with gestational diabetes often have normal glucose levels immediately postpartum.

The first 2 hours postpartum, plasma renin and angiotensin II levels (involved in blood pressure maintenance) fall to normal, nonpregnant levels (Novy, 1991). Blood pressure should remain stable during the postpartum period. Orthostatic hypotension may occur when a woman moves from the supine to a sitting position as a result of the low vascular resistance in the pelvis. An increase in blood pressure of 30 mmHg systolic or 15 mmHg diastolic, especially if accompanied by headache or visual changes, may indicate postpartum preeclampsia (Roberts, 1994).

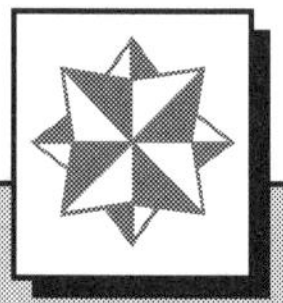

DISPLAY 11-1

Lochia Characteristics

Rubra: Blood-tinged uterine discharge containing shreds of tissue and decidua. Flow of blood lasts several hours, diminishing rapidly to a reddish-brown discharge through the third to fourth day PP.

Serosa: Pink to brownish discharge with a mucopurulent quality and fleshy odor. Usually lasts 4–10 days, but may last longer (15% of women have serosa at 6 week examination).

Alba: Yellowish-white discharge experienced by the majority of women. Usually lasts between 7–10 days.

Kidneys and Bladder

Mild proteinuria may exist for 1 to 2 days after birth in up to 50% of women (Novy, 1991). Glycosuria of pregnancy disappears, and creatinine clearance is usually normal by 1 week postpartum. By the end of the first week postpartum, the blood urea nitrogen level rises to values of 20 mg/dl compared with 15 mg/dl in the late third trimester (Novy).

Spontaneous voiding should resume by 6 to 8 hours after birth, and bladder tone usually returns 5 to 7 days later. Edema, hyperemia, and submucous extravasation of blood are evident in the bladder postpartum. The bladder has an increased capacity and decreased sensitivity to fullness. As a result, overdistention and incomplete emptying may occur. Other factors include the numbing effect of anesthesia and the temporary neural dysfunction of the traumatized bladder (Bowes, 1991).

Signs of bladder distention include uterine atony reflected in increased lochia, displacement of the uterus to the right and significantly above the umbilicus, decreased urine output compared to oral and intravenous (IV) intake, and a "soft fullness," sometimes with a palpable margin, in the suprapubic area. Women may report an urge but inability to urinate. Avoid rapid emptying if catheterization is performed. No more than 800 cc should be removed to avoid a precipitous drop in intraabdominal pressure, which may lead to splanchnic engorgement resulting in hypotension.

Stress Incontinence

Many women report transient stress incontinence during the first 6 weeks postpartum. Persistent stress incontinence has been thought to correlate to obstetric factors such as operative delivery, high neonatal weight, and perineal tissue damage (Allen, Hosker, Smith, & Warrell, 1990). However, over time, influence of obstetric factors diminish, and it is difficult to identify women at risk for developing persistent stress incontinence (Viktrup, Lose, Rolff, & Barfoed, 1992). Duration of the second stage of labor is an obstetric factor that does correlate with the development of stress incontinence (Viktrup & Lose, 1993). Epidural anesthesia has been thought to protect against this complication (Schuessler, Hesse, Dimpfl, & Anthuber, 1988); however, recent data suggest that epidural anesthesia is not a significant protective factor (Viktrup & Lose, 1993). Knowledge of clinical factors implicated in stress incontinence allows anticipatory guidance for women at risk.

Fluid Balance and Electrolytes

Excretion of extra fluid and electrolytes as a result of normal physiologic changes of pregnancy contributes to a postpartum net fluid loss of 4 kg (Novy, 1991). At least 2 L is lost during the first week, mostly as excretion of maternal extracellular fluid. Fluid loss is larger in women who have experienced preeclampsia-eclampsia. By the third postpartum day, resolution of the vasoconstriction and additional extracellular fluid of pregnancy-induced hypertension (PIH) contribute to significant expansion of the vascular volume (Novy).

Neurologic Changes

Discomfort and fatigue are common concerns after birth. Afterpains; discomfort associated with episiotomy, incisions, lacerations, or tears; muscle aches; and breast engorgement may contribute to a woman's discomfort. Neurologic changes related to anesthesia and analgesia are transient and require attention to the woman's safety while they are present. Deep tendon reflexes remain normal. Sleep disturbances contributing to fatigue are related to both discomfort and the demands of newborn care. If the woman has other children or a lack of social support, or both, time for rest may be limited. Natural or pharmacologic comfort measures should be offered. Psychosocial support is necessary, and referral to home-care nursing may be appropriate.

Headaches may result from fluid shifts in the first week after birth. Postpuncture headaches following regional anesthesia may occur. Assessment and appropriate intervention are required. Postpartum eclampsia (seizures beginning > 48 hours and < 4 weeks after birth) is frequently preceded by severe headache or visual disturbances. Women may have a postpartum eclampsic seizure without having been diagnosed as having preeclampsia or hypertension during pregnancy. Because women may experience prodromal signs and symptoms after discharge from the hospital, information should be provided about these subjective signs and symptoms, which include severe persistent occipital headache, scotomata (spots before the eyes), blurred vision, photophobia, and epigastric or right upper quadrant pain. Women should be encouraged to notify their primary healthcare provider if any of these symptoms develop, to facilitate immediate evaluation. Close attention to prodromal symptoms may prevent seizure onset and allow time for prophylactic interventions (Lubarsky et al., 1994).

Hemodynamic Changes

Cardiac output (CO) peaks immediately after birth to approximately 80% above the prelabor value in women who have received only local anesthesia (Bowes, 1991). After reaching a maximum value at 10 to 15 minutes after birth, CO begins to decline, reaching prelabor values approximately 1 hour postpartum (Duvekot & Peeters, 1994). CO after birth is dependent on use and choice of anesthesia or analgesia, mode of delivery, blood loss, and maternal position. An important factor is the autotransfusion that occurs as a result of elimination of blood flow to the placenta. The 500 to 750 ml per minute blood flow to the uteroplacental unit at term is diverted to maternal systemic venous circulation immediately after birth.

CO remains elevated for at least 48 hours after birth, decreases rapidly in the first 2 weeks postpartum, and returns to prepregnant levels by 24 weeks postpartum (Creasy & Resnik, 1994; Duvekot & Peeters, 1994; Novy, 1991). Plasma volume is diminished by approximately 1,000 ml as a result of blood loss and diuresis. Thus, most of the blood volume increase of 1,000 to 1,500 ml during pregnancy is eliminated within the first 2 weeks after birth, with return to preconception values over the course of the first 6 months postpartum (Duvekot & Peeters, 1994).

Heart rate remains stable or decreases slightly after birth, depending on maternal position (Duvekot & Peeters, 1994). By 10 days postpartum, heart rate returns to prepregnant values. When measured with the woman in the left lateral position, blood pressure decreases during the first 2 days postpartum to levels prior to labor, suggesting a transient blood pressure elevation during the intrapartum period (Duvekot & Peeters, 1994). Orthostatic hypotension may occur when a woman sits up from a reclining position. Preeclampsia should be suspected if blood pressure values increase by 30 mmHg systolic or 15 mmHg diastolic. Breastfeeding does not affect maternal hemodynamic status.

Cesarean birth prior to labor onset avoids the hemodynamic effect of contractions but not the rise in CO immediately postpartum. It is thought that epidural anesthesia during labor modifies the increase in CO after birth by decreasing pain and anxiety (Novy, 1991).

Balanced general anesthesia or subarachnoid block causes major fluctuations in blood pressure, CO, heart rate, and stroke volume. The preferred method of pain management for women with cardiac disease is epidural anesthetic without epinephrine. This anesthetic approach provides hemodynamic stability during cesarean birth and only a small rise in CO after birth (Novy, 1991).

Hematologic and Liver Changes

A 1-g drop in hemoglobin or 4-point decrease in hematocrit reflects up to a 500-ml blood loss during the intrapartum period. However, accurate blood loss results are not reflected in a hematocrit drawn earlier than 48 hours posthemorrhage. As extracellular fluid enters the vascular system, hemodilution occurs in women who have lost 20% of their circulating blood volume during delivery. Hemoconcentration may occur if a woman loses minimal blood, especially if she has preexisting polycythemia (Novy, 1991). Blood volume changes (16% decline) are the same regardless of the method of birth. Women who give birth vaginally may have a 5% increase in hematocrit, whereas cesarean birth usually decreases hematocrit by 6% (Ueland, 1976).

Leukocytosis from the stress of labor and birth extends into the postpartum period, contributing to a normal white blood cell (WBC) count of up to 25,000/uL with an increased number of granulocytes.

Normal serum iron levels are regained by the second week postpartum, when there is a relative erythrocytosis in those women who have an average blood loss and who have had iron supplementation during pregnancy. Approximately 84% of women are iron deficient at term if iron supplements were not taken during pregnancy (Graf & McPherson-Smith, 1991). Women who have experienced excessive blood loss or were anemic during pregnancy have a greater potential risk of infection. Serum ferretin concentration is the most reliable predictor of iron-deficiency anemia (Graf & McPherson-Smith, 1991). Fibrinolytic activity increases in the first 4 days after birth. Numbers of platelets and fibrinogen increase, as do other clotting factors.

Liver enzymes and lipids are normal within 10 to 14 days postpartum. Alkaline phosphatase may remain elevated for 6 weeks. The previously atonic gallbladder demonstrates increased contractility (Blackburn & Loper, 1992).

Respiratory and Acid-Base Changes

Vital capacity, inspiratory capacity, and maximum breathing capacity decrease after birth. Response to exercise may therefore be affected in the early postpartum weeks. Chest wall compliance increases to allow relief of dyspnea experienced during pregnancy.

Length and severity of the second stage of labor appear to contribute to an "oxygen debt" that extends into the immediate postpartum period (Bowes, 1991). The basal metabolic rate remains elevated for 7 to 14 days into the postpartum period and is attributable to mild anemia, lactation, and psychologic factors (Display 11-2).

PCO_2 rises to the normal prepregnant values (35 to 40 mmHg) within a few days after birth. Normal levels of pH and base excess gradually return by approximately 3 weeks' postpartum.

Skin, Muscle, and Weight Changes

Overdistention of the abdominal wall as a result of pregnancy can cause rupture of the collagen fibers of the dermis, resulting in striae, which can occur also on the breasts, buttocks, and thighs. Striae eventually become irregular white lines. Diastasis (separation) of the rectus muscles is common and usually is reapproximated by the late postpartum period (Novy, 1991).

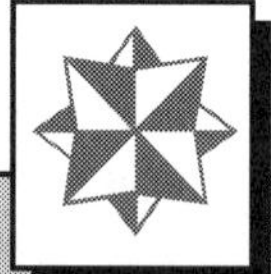

DISPLAY 11-2

Respiratory and Acid/Base Findings During the Postpartum Period

- PaO_2 (arterial oxygen saturation) 95% on day 1 PP
- Hypocapnia (< 30 mmHg)
- Elevated blood lactate
- Decreased pH
- Increased PCO_2
- Increased base excess
- Increased plasma bicarbonate

Evidence of diastasis can be assessed by asking the woman to lift her head while lying in a supine position. If diastasis has occurred, a "tent-like" protrusion in the lower abdomen will be noticeable.

Gastrointestinal Changes

Constipation may result from hemorrhoids, perineal trauma, dehydration, pain, fear of having a bowel movement, immobility, and medication (e.g., magnesium sulfate antenatally for tocolysis, iron supplementation, codeine for pain, anesthetics during labor or surgery).

Hernias and Anal Sphincter Damage

Overstretching or tearing of the muscles or fascia during delivery predisposes to genital hernias (cystocele, rectocele, uterine prolapse, enterocele). Disruptions in the anal sphincter, most often associated with episiotomy and forceps, occur in up to 24 percent (average 1 to 5 percent) of vaginal births. Vacuum extraction is associated with fewer third-degree tears than forceps delivery. Episiotomy does not always prevent a third-degree tear, and one half of women with third-degree tears experience anal incontinence associated with persistent mechanical sphincter disruption (not pudendal nerve damage) (DeLancy, 1993).

To prevent damage, attention should be directed toward preventing tears. However, ideal anal sphincter repair techniques have not been identified, nor has ideal management in subsequent deliveries of women with previous third-degree tears been prospectively established (Sultan, Kamm, Hudson, & Bartram, 1994).

Disturbances in bowel function (i.e., fecal urgency and anal incontinence of stool and flatus) from mechanical or neurologic injury to the anal sphincter during vaginal birth may also be the result of damage from the large size of the baby's head in relation to the vaginal opening (Sultan, Kamm, Hudson, Thomas, & Bartram, 1993). In one study, external sphincter defects occured in 90 percent and internal sphincter defects in 65 percent of 62 women (Burnett et al., 1991). Women who experienced a third- or fourth-degree perineal laceration reported a 6-times-greater incidence of incontinence of flatus than those without anal sphincter rupture (Crawford, Quint, Pearl, & DeLancey, 1991). Women with a long second stage of labor, a large newborn, or both have the most evidence of nerve damage (Allen, Hosker, Smith, & Warrell, 1990).

Controversy continues to exist regarding the use of episiotomy. Some practitioners recommend minimizing the use of midline episiotomy and using mediolateral episiotomy when the risk for extension is increased (e.g., macrosomia, shallow perineal body, instrumental delivery) (Crawford et al., 1991; Shiono, Klebanoff, & Carey, 1990).

Women do not generally report symptoms of anal sphincter damage spontaneously (47% did not offer the information in one study), and symptoms may disappear or worsen with time (Bek & Laurberg, 1992). An accurate history is essential so that women with major sphincter defects can be offered a cesarean delivery when appropriate (Sultan, Kamm, Bartram, & Hudson, 1994). Peak incidence of fecal incontinence among women occurs in the fifth and sixth decades of life (Laurberg and Swash, 1989). Aging, menopause, progression of neuropathy, and effects of subsequent births may contribute to sphincter weakness in the long term (Sultan, Kamm, Hudson, Thomas, & Bartram, 1993).

Weight Loss

Breastfeeding women have a steady, gradual, weight loss after birth if they return to prepregnancy caloric requirements and include foods from all of the food groups. Women who choose formula feeding can expect a 0.5- to 1-kg-per-week loss when eating a balanced diet containing slightly fewer calories than their usual daily expenditure. In a recent study, women who breastfed their newborns exclusively experienced significantly larger reductions in hip circumference and were less likely to be above their prepregnancy weight at 1 month postpartum than mothers who fed their newborns formula exclusively (Kramer, Stunkard, Marshall, McKinney, & Liebschutz, 1993). This research suggests that choice of infant-feeding practice temporarily influences postpartum anthropomorphic changes (Kramer et al., 1993).

Fluid and Nutritional Needs

Oral fluid administration, or intravenous fluid administration when indicated, help restore the balance altered by fluid loss during the labor and birth process. Women should be encouraged to drink 3,000 ml of water and other liquids every 24 hours. Most women have a hearty appetite after vaginal birth. Encourage healthy food choices with respect for ethnic background. Snack trays should be available for women who give birth at times when food service is unavailable. Women are usually able to have ice chips soon after cesarean birth. Diet progression varies by institutional protocol; however, women are able to advance to a regular diet after passing flatus. Nutrition counseling for women who breastfeed should include a recommendation for 500 calories greater than prepregnancy caloric demands.

NURSING ASSESSMENT AND INTERVENTIONS

Initial Postpartum Assessment

1. Assess vital signs every 15 minutes for 1 hour, (more frequently if condition warrants), then as per institutional protocol (AAP & ACOG, 1992)
2. Palpate fundus for uterine tone and position and assess lochia every 15 minutes for 1 hour; then every 4 hours, or more frequently if indicated, for 12 to 24 hours or per institutional protocol

Uterine massage is indicated if the uterus does not remain firmly contracted. Support the lower uterine segment during massage to prevent uterine prolapse or inversion (Figure 11-1). Uterine inversion is an obstetric emergency associated with hemorrhage and shock.

Pain Management

The uterus can be extremely tender after birth. Encouraging slow deep breaths, keeping the woman informed of the rationale for uterine massage and when touch can be anticipated, as well as gentle palpation with warm hands will enhance comfort and encourage participation in the procedure. Medication should be administered appropriately.

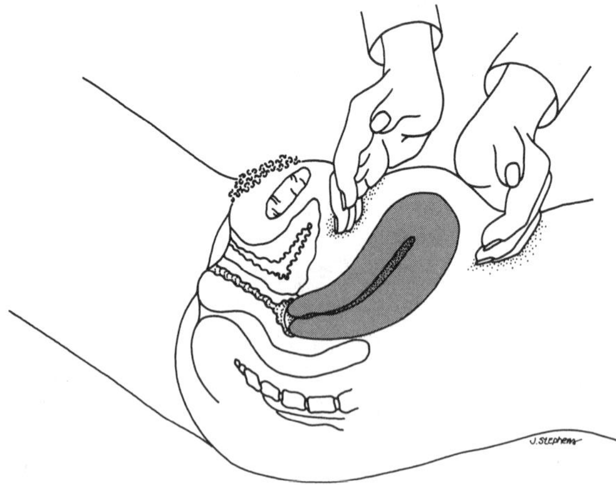

Figure 11-1. Fundal massage. The nurse uses two hands for fundal massage. One hand anchors the lower uterine segment just above the symphysis. The other gently massages the fundal area.

From May, K.A., & Mahlmeister, L.R. (1994). Maternal and Neonatal Nursing (3rd ed., p. 533). Philadelphia: J.B. Lippincott.

Women who have experienced cesarean birth may or may not require uterine massage to stimulate uterine contraction. If lochia indicates excessive bleeding, use palpation and pain-management measures. If pain management is inadequate, give additional pain medication, elicit the woman's participation, provide reassurance, and employ comfort measures after the procedure.

Continuing Assessments

1. Emotional status, interaction with newborn, fatigue level, and amount of social support
2. Breasts for redness, pain, engorgement, and if nursing, correct latch-on and removal of newborn from the breast
3. Uterus and lochia as described previously. Assess for foul-smelling lochia
4. Bladder fullness before and after voiding. Measure at least the first void
5. Abdominal muscle tone and incision if present. Assess bowel sounds
6. Perineum, labia, and anus for edema, redness, pain, bruising, and hematoma. Assess episiotomy or abdominal incision for approximation and drainage. Assess dietary intake and elimination patterns
7. Legs and feet for edema and varicosities. Assess Homan's sign and measure width of calf if thrombophlebitis is suspected. Assess activity tolerance
8. Comfort level and response to pain medication
9. Breath sounds if the woman has received magnesium sulfate, other tocolytics, been on bedrest, has an infection, or has experienced a multiple birth, because these women are at greater risk for pulmonary edema, especially if they have received large amounts of intravenous therapy (e.g., surgery)
10. Teaching needs based on interview and observation (see Chapter 17). Every interaction with a woman, beginning at the first prenatal visit and continuing through the postpartum visit at 6 weeks, offers a potential teaching "moment." For example, fundal assessment is an ideal time to provide information about involution, and bathing the newborn at the woman's bedside is an opportunity to discuss various aspects of newborn care

A helpful acronym to remember general aspects of the postpartum assessment is BUBBLERS: B, breasts; U, uterus; B, bladder; B, bowel; L, lochia; E, episiotomy/incision; R, emotional response; S, Homan's sign.

COMPLICATIONS DURING THE POSTPARTUM PERIOD

Postpartum Hemorrhage

Postpartum hemorrhage is potentially lethal. It can occur early (first 24 hours) or late (after 24 hours and less than 6 weeks after birth). (See Display 11-3 for causes of postpartum hemorrhage.) The greatest risk for postpartum hemorrhage is during the first hour after birth, because large venous areas are exposed following placental separation (Prichard, 1965). Therefore, ensuring uterine contraction by using fundal massage and intravenous oxytocin administration is critical. Blood loss during and after birth is often underestimated. Actual blood loss after uncomplicated birth may be 600 to 700 ml (Kapernick, 1991), although estimates in clinical practice vary widely. Nonetheless, 500 ml remains the accepted limit for "normal" blood loss after vaginal birth, and a blood loss of 1,000-1,200 ml is considered normal after cesarean birth.

Hemorrhage is defined objectively as a decrease in hematocrit of at least 10% or need for blood cell transfusion (Combs, Murphy, & Laros, 1991). The hemoglobin value will decrease 1 to 1.5 g/dl and the hematocrit will decrease 2 to 4 percent for each 450 to 500 ml of blood loss (Varney, 1987). Eighty to ninety percent of immediate postpartum hemorrhage results from uterine atony, reported as complicating 1 in 20 births (Dildy & Clark, 1993). Lack of clotting indicates a coagulation defect.

Assessment of Postpartum Hemorrhage

1. Assess for history of
    - previous postpartum hemorrhage
    - rapid or prolonged labor
    - uterine overdistention (macrosomia, multiple gestation, or polyhydramnios)
    - use of tocolytic or halogenated anesthetic agents
    - operative birth
    - high parity
    - chorioamnionitis/intraamniotic infection
    - placental abnormality (succenturiate lobe or hydatidiform mole)
    - previous uterine surgery

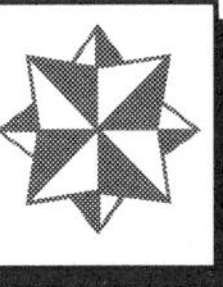

DISPLAY 11-3

Causes of Postpartum Hemorrhage

Uterine Atony

- Trauma/lacerations/hematoma of cervix and/or birth canal
- Difficult third stage (e.g., use of aggressive fundal manipulation or cord traction)
- Retained placenta
- Placenta Accreta
- Bleeding disorders [e.g. disseminated intravascular coagulation (DIC)]
- Uterine Inversion
- Drugs (large dosages of oxytocin; magnesium sulfate; beta-adrenergic tocolytic agents; Diazoxide, [a potent antihypertensive agent]; calcium channel blockers, such as nifedipine; and Halothane, [an anesthetic agent] (Arias, 1993)

Late Postpartum Hemorrhage

- Infection
- Subinvolution (delayed healing of placental site)
- Retained placenta

2. Assess blood loss.
   - weigh pads or chux (1 g = 1 ml). Keep a gram scale on unit.
3. Assess vital signs at least every 15 minutes. Mean arterial pressure (MAP) should be assessed because the first blood pressure response to hypovolemia may be a pulse pressure decreased to 30 mmHg or less (Cunningham, MacDonald, Gant, Leveno, & Gilstap, 1993). Normal vital signs do not necessarily mean that woman is not in shock. Vasoconstriction shunts available blood to vital organs during the initial phase of hypovolemic shock (Luegenbiehl, 1991).
4. Take accurate measurements of intake and output. Ringer's lactate solution, other plasma expanders, or blood components are usually given in amounts necessary to counteract hypovolemia. These amounts should produce at least 30 ml/hr (60 ml preferred) of urine output and hematocrit values of ≥ 30 percent (Cunningham et al., 1993)
5. Plan care. The ability to react promptly is enhanced when there is a unit management plan to treat potential complications. Early recognition minimizes blood loss and potential sequelae such as anemia, puerperal infection, thromboembolism, and necrosis of the anterior pituitary (Sheehan's syndrome). The nurse-patient ratio should be 1:1 (Hayashi & Castillo, 1993) (see Display 11-4, Management of Postpartum Hemorrhage).

Nursing Interventions

1. Ensure large-bore needle intravenous access.
2. Draw blood for hemoglobin and hematocrit, type and crossmatch, coagulation studies (fibrinogen, prothrombin time, partial thromboplastin time, fibrin split products, and fibrin degradation products), and blood chemistry. Arterial blood gases may be drawn. Urine should be sent to the laboratory as indicated.
3. Apply correct uterine massage to avoid ligament damage and potential uterine inversion (Figure 11-1). Place one hand pointing toward the woman's head with thumb resting on one side of the uterus and fingers along the other side. Use other hand to massage with *only the force needed to effect contraction or expulsion of clots* (Wheeler, 1991). Anticipate pain-management needs for fundal massage and uterotonic medications for treatment of hemorrhage. Overaggressive uterine massage can be detrimental, because constant stimulation may tire muscle fibers and contribute to further atony.
4. Insert Foley catheter to empty bladder and allow accurate measurement of output.
5. Administer intravenous fluids (e.g., rapid volume expanders, blood products).
6. Administer prescribed drugs (e.g., oxytocin IV infusion, methlergonovine IM, prostaglandin 15 methyl F_2 IM).
7. Apply pulse oximeter and administer oxygen, per protocol.
8. Avoid the Trendelenburg position (unless specific physician order), because it has been reported to interfere with cardiac and respiratory function by increasing pressure on chemoreceptors and baroreceptors and decreasing the area for lung expansion. Elevate the legs to a 20° to 30° angle to increase venous return.
9. Provide emotional support for the woman and her family.

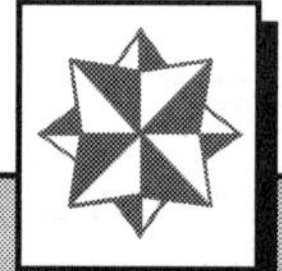

DISPLAY 11-4

Management of Postpartum Hemorrhage

GOAL: Correct hypovolemia and establish homeostasis

- Identify women at risk →
- Recognize early →
- Promptly initiate treatment →
- Treat underlying cause →
- If unresponsive to therapy, anticipate →
- Medical intervention: medication and/or mast trousers
- Surgical intervention: Uterine packing, curettage, ligation of uterine/ovarian/hypogastric artery(s), arterial embolization, hysterectomy, umbrella pack (Dildy & Clark, 1993)

Postpartum Infections

Endometritis

In the 1930s, the Joint Commission on Maternal Welfare defined puerperal infection and morbidity as an oral temperature of 38°C (100°F) or higher occurring on any 2 of the first 10 days postpartum, exclusive of the first 24 hours (Easterling, 1982). This definition is still used (Kapernick, 1991). Postpartum uterine infection, termed endometritis, endomyometritis, or endomyoparametritis, depending on the extent of the disease, is the most commonly identified cause of puerperal morbidity. Cesarean birth presents a twentyfold to thirtyfold relative risk for postpartum endometritis (10–50%) compared to vaginal birth (1–3%) (ACOG & AAP, 1992; Arias, 1993; Gibbs, 1989). The most effective method of prevention of infection is handwashing.

The most common cause of uterine infection tends to be polymicrobial, including aerobic and anaerobic organisms that have ascended to the uterus from the lower genital tract. Isolated organisms include *streptococci A and B, enterococci, Staphlococcus aureus, Gardnerella vaginalis, Escherichia coli, Enterobacter, Proteus mirabilis, Klebsiella, Bacteroides* species, *Peptostreptococci* species, *Ureaplasma urealyticum, Mycoplasma hominie* and *Chlamydia trachomatis* (Arias, 1993; Rosene, Eschenbach, Tompkins, Kenny, & Watkins, 1986). *Chlamydia trachomatis* has been specifically associated with late-onset postpartum endometritis (Hoyme, Kiviat, & Eschenbach, 1986).

Other causes of postpartum infection include wound and urinary tract infections, pneumonia (usually related to general anesthesia), mastitis, pelvic thrombophlebitis, and necrotizing fasciitis, an uncommon but serious localized infection of the deep soft tissues.

Assessment for Endometritis

1. History of pyelonephritis, cesarean birth, hemorrhage, prolonged labor, prolonged rupture of membranes, use of invasive procedures (e.g., internal monitoring, amnioinfusion, fetal scalp sampling, multiple pelvic examinations)
2. Evidence of socioeconomic and nutritional factors compromising host defense mechanisms and anemia and systemic illness that increase risk. Teenagers appear to be at greater risk for post-cesarean endometritis than older mothers (Magee, Blanco, Graham, Rayburn, & Prien, 1994).
3. Physical and laboratory findings, which may include the following:
   - Fever
   - Malaise
   - Lower abdominal pain
   - Foul-smelling lochia
   - Urinalysis to rule out urinary tract infections (UTI)
   - Leukocytosis (WBC count > 20,000/mm^3 with increased neutrophils or polymorphonuclear leukocytes)
   - Blood culture results, which can influence type and duration of antibiotic therapy
   - Endometrial cultures may have limited value, because of cervicovaginal contamination of the specimen, yet they may provide useful information if the woman does not respond to initial antibiotic therapy

Management of Postpartum Endometritis

Administration of a single dose of ampicillin or cephalosporin after cord clamping, has been shown to be effective prophylaxis following nonelective (e.g., after rupture of membranes) cesarean birth (AAP & ACOG, 1992).

Broad-spectrum antibiotic therapy is promptly initiated when postpartum endometritis is diagnosed. Treatment continues until the woman has been afebrile for 48 hours. A common treatment regimen is a combination of clindamycin 900-mg IV every 8 hours and gentamicin 2 mg/kg IV initial dose followed by 1.5 mg/kg every 8 hours. Maintenance is based on peak and trough levels. Clindamycin/gentamicin treatment is successful in only 75 to 92 percent of patients and is associated with a risk of renal toxicity. This treatment is not effective against enterococci. Women who do not respond to therapy are given ampicillin (Monga & Oshiro, 1993).

Women usually respond rapidly to antibiotic therapy. Occasional complications include pelvic abcesses, septic pelvic thrombophlebitis, persistent fever, and retained infected placenta (AAP & ACOG, 1992).

Nursing Interventions

1. Increase fluid intake and encourage adequate nutrition. Ensure adequate output, because renal toxicity can occur with antibiotic therapy.
2. Provide comfort through meeting the woman's personal hygiene needs. Cool compresses, linen

changes, massage, and positioning may enhance comfort.

3. Assess vital signs every 4 hours
4. Observe for signs of septic shock: tachycardia > 120; hypotension; tachypnea; changes in sensorium; and decreased urine output (Lagana, 1994). If septic shock develops, frequency of vital signs and other assessments are increased, dependending on the clinical situation.

Other Infections During the Postpartum Period

Wound Infections

Wound infections are more common in women with a history of chorioamnionitis, intraamniotic infection, hemorrhage, obesity, and underlying medical problems such as diabetes and malnutrition. Multiple vaginal examinations also increase the risk of wound infection (Monga & Oshiro, 1993). Assessment reveals wound erythema, swelling, tenderness, and discharge. Cultures should be performed, followed by drainage, irrigation, and occasionally, debridement. Closure is by secondary intention (Monga & Oshiro, 1993). The wound may be packed, and dressing changes may be very stressful. Ensuring pain management and adequate room ventilation, prior to dressing changes, will enhance comfort. Continued hospitalization or readmission may be required. Reassurance, encouragement, and frequent visits by the family may reduce anxiety. If the woman is breastfeeding, the nurse can assist with pumping or lactation suppression. Antibiotic therapy and frequent dressing changes may be continued after discharge. Postpartum follow-up visits by homecare nurses can reduce anxiety and incidence of rehospitalization by allowing early identification and treatment of infections.

Episiotomy infection is uncommon, but incontinence of stool and flatus may be the presenting symptom prior to wound breakdown (Kapernick, 1991). Treatment is directed toward cleaning the wound and promoting granulation. Sitz baths, frequent peripad changes, and pain medication may provide increased comfort.

Necrotizing fasciitis is a severe infection characterized by erythema, discharge, and severe pain. Surgical debridement is performed, and treatment with broad-spectrum antibiotics is initiated (Monga & Oshiro, 1993). Secondary healing may take 6 to 12 weeks.

Mastitis

Mastitis, both congestive and infectious, is more commonly seen in primigravidas and in nursing mothers. Nipple trauma has been implicated in development of mastitis. Trauma from incorrect latch-on or removal of the newborn from the breast allow the introduction of organisms from the newborn to the mother's breast. *Staphylococcus aureus* is the most common causative organism. Administration of penicillinase-resistant antibiotics such as dicloxacillin for 10 days is recommended.

Clinical presentation of mastitis is fever, localized tenderness, chills, and a palpable hard mass (Lagana, 1994; Monga & Oshiro, 1993). Nursing interventions include teaching preventive measures such as handwashing, breast cleanliness, frequent breast-pad change, exposure of the nipples to air, and correct infant latch-on and removal from the breast. If mastitis occurs, the woman should be taught comfort measures such as warm or cold compresses, wearing a supportive bra, the importance of completing the full regimen of antibiotic therapy, and increasing fluid intake to 2 to 2.5 L per day. Massage, positioning the newborn in the direction of the site, and frequent breastfeeding promotes milk flow. Many women find use of ice packs to be helpful in decreasing swelling and pain.

If a breast abcess develops, antibiotics and incision and drainage are indicated. The decision to continue breastfeeding should be made jointly by the woman and the healthcare provider. If breastfeeding is delayed while purulent drainage continues, the woman may need assistance with breast pumping to reestablish lactation. If advised to discontinue breastfeeding, emotional support, reassurance, and comfort measures are important. Lactation consultant referral is indicated when these services are available.

Urinary Tract Infections

UTI can occur following birth as a result of hypotonia of the bladder and lower urinary tract, birth trauma, anesthesia, frequent pelvic examinations, and catheterization. Dysuria, frequency, urgency, and low-grade fever may be the presenting symptoms. Occasionally an elevated temperature is the only presenting sign. Pyelonephritis may be accompanied by fever, costovertebral angle tenderness, chills, malaise, hematuria, and nausea and vomiting (Kapernick, 1991). Laboratory findings reveal increased WBCs, protein, or blood in the urine. *Escherichia coli* is the most commonly isolated causative organism.

The primary treatment is antibiotic therapy appropriate to the organism. IV antibiotic therapy is continued until the woman has been afebrile for 48 hours. Oral antibiotic therapy may follow for 10 to 14 days. Sulfa antibiotics are used for breastfeeding women. Nursing interventions include vital signs every 4 hours; encouraging increased oral fluid intake of water and cranberry juice (fluid total should be at least 1,000 ml/day); encouraging rest, adequate diet, and frequent voiding; and teaching the importance of wiping front to back and wearing cotton underclothing.

If readmission is necessary, reassurance and family support is essential. Separation from the newborn is distressing to the mother and child. If the woman has been breastfeeding, interventions such as pumping and newborn visits will help to maintain lactation after antibiotic therapy has been initiated. If breastfeeding is temporarily contraindicated, the nurse can provide emotional support and offer strategies to maintain lactation until breastfeeding can be resumed.

Thrombophlebitis and Thromboembolism

Risk factors for development of thrombophlebitis and thromboembolism include normal changes in coagulation status during pregnancy, cesarean birth, use of forceps, blood vessel and tissue trauma, previous history of thromboembolic disease or varicosities, obesity, age older than 40 years, sepsis, and immobility associated with antepartum bedrest (Bowes, 1991).

Diagnosis is based on objective and subjective signs and symptoms. Homan's sign may elicit pain as the calf muscle compresses the affected vein. Comparison of pulses in both extremities may reveal decreased venous flow to the affected area. Serial measurements of the suspected extremity allow for assessment of increased diameter caused by venous inflammation and engorgement. The affected leg circumference should be more than 2 cm larger than the contralateral leg at the same level for diagnosis, because Homan's sign is neither sensitive nor specific as a diagnostic tool for deep vein thrombosis (DVT). Women with DVT may have normal venography (Cranley, Canos, & Sull, 1976). Doppler flow studies and impedance plethysmography (IPG) are more accurate tools for diagnosing thrombophlebitis (Lagana, 1994).

Nursing interventions for superficial venous thrombophlebitis include assessment of vital signs and affected extremity for swelling and pain every 4 hours, application of antiembolic support stockings, application of warm packs to the affected area, slight elevation of the involved leg, and ambulation as indicated. Heparin anticoagulation therapy may be ordered. Nursing interventions for DVT include all of the previously described care measures plus anticoagulation therapy with IV heparin, monitoring coagulation laboratory values, and careful assessment of unusual bleeding. Heavy vaginal bleeding, generalized petechiae, bleeding from the mucous membranes, hematuria, or oozing from venipuncture sites should be reported to the physician. The heparin antidote protamine sulfate should be readily available.

Pulmonary Embolism

Deep vein thrombosis and septic pelvic thromboemboli predispose a woman to pulmonary embolization. Chills, hypotension, fever, and abdominal pain may accompany the most common signs of pulmonary embolism (i.e., dyspnea and chest pain). Diagnosis may be verified by ventilation/perfusion (V/Q) scan, blood gas studies, x-ray films, pulmonary angiogram, or a combination of these (Lagana, 1994). Pulmonary embolism should be treated as a life-threatening event; interruption of blood flow to the pulmonary bed can result in cardiovascular collapse and death.

Nursing interventions include elevation of the head of bed to facilitate breathing, oxygen administration at 8 to 10 L by tight face mask, IV fluids, pulse oximetry, frequent assessment of vital signs, arterial blood gases, and initiation of IV heparin. Dopamine for pressor support, morphine for analgesia, and other emergency drugs may be used. A pulmonary artery catheter may be placed. Staff who have completed an Advanced Cardiac Life Support course should be available for full resuscitation support, if needed. Women with a pulmonary embolism require critical-care-nursing skills. Ideally, care should be provided in an obstetrics-intensive care unit (OB-ICU); however, most perinatal centers do not have the volume of critically ill obstetric patients to warrant an OB-ICU. In this case, collaboration between the ICU staff and perinatal staff is essential. Maternal transport should be considered if the level of care and supportive staff necessary is unavailable. (See Chapter 7 for maternal transport guidelines.)

In addition to the common complications during the postpartum period previously discussed, see Display 11-5 for clinical signs and symptoms that should be reported to the primary healthcare provider.

INDIVIDUALIZING CARE FOR WOMEN WITH SPECIAL NEEDS

Cesarean Birth

The cesarean birth rate in the United States in 1993 was approximately 22.8 per 100 births (Centers for Disease Control and Prevention, 1995). In the 1970s and 1980s women discussed the extreme emotional distress experienced after cesarean birth. As a result of the normalization of cesarean birth, women seem to experience less negative reactions to a cesarean today (Reichert, Baron, & Fawcett, 1993). Today, the predominant reactions to cesarean birth are "happiness and excitement" about a health baby but disappointment about having a cesarean birth (Reichert et al., 1993). Women want information, caring, and "supportive words and actions" from nurses and physicians (Reichert et al.). Other helpful interventions during the childbirth experience include having the partner available and liberal visiting hours for family (Reichert et al.).

Cesarean birth adds stressors beyond those of the woman experiencing vaginal birth. Of 106 women delivering full-term infants via cesarean at a large urban hospital, physiologic concerns declined markedly from 2 to 8 weeks after birth. However, the number of psychologic and life-style concerns did not decrease during that time frame. Researchers suggest that, in this time of early hospital discharge, anticipatory guidance and teaching should include information on arranging for additional help at home; frequent rest periods, adequate nutrition and fluids; and differentiation of postpartum blues from depression. Also suggested is several scheduled postpartum visits over 8 to 12 weeks instead of the usual one visit 2 to 3 days after discharge (Miovech et al., 1994).

Implications of Antepartum Bedrest on Postpartum Recovery

Postpartum effects of bedrest have received little attention in the obstetric nursing and medical literature until recently. Despite lack of evidence to support

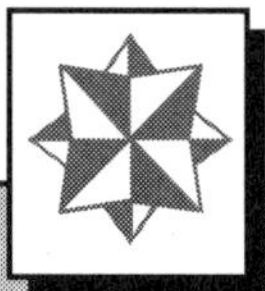

DISPLAY 11-5

Report the Following to the Physician or Nurse-midwife

- Uterine atony or large/excessive clots; passage of placental tissue
- Excessive bleeding (one peripad saturated with blood in 15 minutes or less) (Poole, 1993)
- Continued bleeding in the presence of a firm uterus (suggestive of laceration)
- Pain greater than expected (suggestive of hematoma)
- Foul-smelling lochia (suggestive of endometritis)
- Temperature elevated to >100°F (38°C) (suggestive of dehydration during first 24 hours; thereafter, elevation to this level signifies puerperal infection, most likely in the genitourinary tract. Mastitis, thrombophlebitis, or systemic infection may also be the cause) (Cunningham, MacDonald, Gant, Leveno, & Gilstrap, 1993).
- Bladder distention with inability to void
- Diminished urinary output (less than 30 cc/hr)
- Enlarging hematomas
- Restlessness; pallor of skin or mucous membranes; cool, clammy skin; tachycardia; thready pulse; fearfulness; vertigo; shaking; visual disturbances; (symptoms of shock)
- Pain, redness, warmth, firm area in the calf area (although pain may be absent in DVT)
- Dyspnea, tachypnea, tachycardia, chest pain, cough, apprehension, hemoptysis, change in skin/mucous membrane color (paleness and/or cyanosis): symptoms of pulmonary embolism or amniotic embolism (if immediately after birth)

bedrest therapy as contributing to positive outcomes (Maloni et al., 1993), it has been prescribed routinely for women with high-risk pregnancies. Approximately 18.2% of pregnant women who delivered after 20 weeks' gestation in 1988 in the United States were prescribed at least 1 week of bedrest therapy for various complications, including bleeding, preterm contractions, edema, and hypertension (Goldenberg et al., 1994).

Within 6 hours of bedrest, skeletal muscle atrophy begins (Maloni et al., 1993). Other physiologic and psychosocial changes include continued muscle loss, especially in the gastrocnemius muscle (used in ambulation); diuresis; weight loss; bone demineralization; increased heart rate and blood coagulation; heartburn and reflux; constipation; glucose intolerance; and sensory disturbances, including depression, fatigue, and inability to concentrate (Maloni et al., 1993).

Nursing implications: Isometric and isotonic conditioning exercises and range-of-motion movements are often used in the hospital antepartum setting for the woman on bedrest (Mayberry, Smith, & Gill, 1992). Deep breathing and coughing are added to exercise abdominal muscles and promote venous return (Mayberry et al., 1992). Physical therapy consultations can be initiated early in the hospital stay to decrease the detrimental effects of bedrest. Anticipatory guidance by healthcare providers, physical therapy interventions while on bedrest, and encouragement after birth can facilitate adaptation to the sequelae of antepartum bedrest.

After birth, the woman will need additional time, support, and education to prepare for safe and progressive levels of activity. Postpartum recovery may be prolonged and variable. The first several periods of ambulation after weeks of lying in bed require continued presence of the perinatal nurse. The woman should be informed that weakness, dizziness, and muscle soreness are normal physiologic consequences of prolonged bedrest. Depending on the length and degree of bedrest, nurses can adapt postpartum interventions to address leg muscle soreness, difficulty with stairs and other ambulation activities, shortness of breath on exertion, dizziness, and delayed return to common activities of daily living (Maloni et al., 1993).

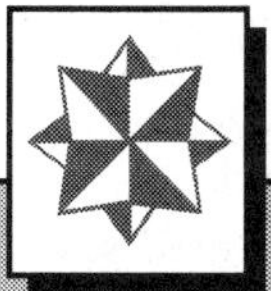

DISPLAY 11-6

Factors Contributing to Decline in Sexual Interest/Activity During the Postpartum Period

- Fatigue
- Fear of not hearing the infant
- Fear of pregnancy
- Emotional distress on a continuum from blues to psychosis
- Adjustments to role change
- Hormonal changes
- Physical discomfort related to changes of vulva, vagina, perineum, and breasts
- Breastfeeding
- Decreased sense of attractiveness

POSTPARTUM LEARNING-NEEDS ASSESSMENT AND EDUCATION

Access, availability, and acceptability are the critical issues when determining the best methods for providing postpartum education. Whatever the setting, each educational program approach must include the woman's and the family's goals in the assessment of specific learning needs and the identification of support structures to assist in meeting those needs. Asking a woman, "What is your greatest concern today?" will provide a starting point and show that the nurse is willing to adjust her teaching agenda to exactly what the woman sees as her first priority. (See Chapter 17 for a comprehensive discussion of maternal-newborn learning-needs assessment and teaching strategies.)

SELECTED POSTPARTUM TEACHING TOPICS

Pelvic-Floor Exercises

Patient education for all women should include pelvic-muscle (Kegel) exercises, per institutional protocol. A graduated training protocol begins with 15 moderate contractions per day and increases by five more each week, increasing in intensity. The program culminates with a strength-building prescription of 40 high-intensity contractions per day (DeLancey, Sampselle, & Punch, 1993). Once conditioned, as few as four to five contractions per day will maintain optimum muscle strength (Graves et al., 1988).

Women should be cautioned that some muscle discomfort may accompany increased muscle use and that overexertion of the levator ani muscle may cause dyspareunia (DeLancey, Sampselle, & Punch, 1993). Simple rest will relieve the pain, and gradual reintroduction of a moderate program will allow progression to an optimal level (DeLancey et al., 1993).

Postpartum Exercise

Exercise has benefits beyond the positive effects on mood, self-image, and energy level. Exercise also improves or maintains endurance, strength, and muscle tone (Mittelmark, Wiswell, & Drinkwater, 1991). Safety considerations are important when advising a home exercise program for women in the postpartum period. Special back exercises such as the "pelvic tilt" strengthen the abdomen and, in conjunction with other strengthening and stretching exercises for the back, abdomen and legs, can be included in a daily program during the postpartum period. *Exercise in Pregnancy* provides exercise and heart rate guidelines for postpartum exercise (Mittelmark et al., 1991).

Vigorous exercises are not recommended until the reproductive organs have returned to their "normal" state at 6 to 7 weeks postpartum and lochia has ceased (Chapman, 1994; Novy, 1991). Women who wish to begin gentle exercises in the early postpartum period can begin abdominal breathing exercises, arm raises, short walks, or other appropriate exercises per primary healthcare-provider protocol. Discharge instructions should include written information regarding activity, rest, and exercise, both for women who have given birth vaginally and by cesarean. Women who have been on antepartum bedrest should have special guidance regarding resumption of activities of daily living. A general rule for any exercise or activity is to listen to one's body and avoid fatigue and pain.

An exercise videotape entitled *Exercise During Pregnancy and the Postnatal Period* is available from the American College of Obstetricians and Gynecologists (ACOG; 1985), Washington, DC. Other commercial videotapes, books, and pamphlets are available as well.

Physical therapists specially trained to evaluate genital muscle tone and ensure correct use of Kegel and other appropriate exercises are available for referral in some regions (American Physical Therapy Association, Section on Obstetrics and Gynecology, 1-800-999-2782, 1111 N. Fairfax St., Alexandria, VA 22314). Kegel exercises improperly performed may be harmful (Kotarinos, personal communication, October 1994).

Women with third- or fourth-degree lacerations, a long second stage of labor, a large newborn, or a combination of these should be taught to report potential anal sphincter symptoms, such as incontinence of flatus or stool, to the primary healthcare provider.

Sexuality

Sexuality is one of the least understood and most superficially discussed topics by healthcare providers during a woman's postpartum experience. Sexuality encompasses physical capacity for sexual arousal and pleasure (libido), personalized and shared social meanings attached to sexual behavior and formation of sexual and gender identities. It is "biology transposed by culture" (Dixon-Mueller, 1993). Sexuality and gender attitudes and behaviors carry profound significance for women and men in every society.

Sexuality is a vital component of physical and emotional well-being for men and women. For a man, sexual functioning is close to the core of his self-esteem. Women may experience decreased interest, frequency, desire, and enjoyment of sex for up to 2 years after childbirth (Cowan et al., 1985; Guana-Trujillo & Grant-Higgins, 1987). In one study, 20 percent of women had little interest in sexual activity 3 months after birth, and an additional 21% had complete loss of desire or aversion to sex (Reamy & White, 1985). (See Display 11-6 for factors contributing to decline in sexual interest during the postpartum period.)

If potentially 40% of women have altered sexual interest after birth, and many men find the change in their partner's sexual feelings particularly distressing (May, 1987), nurses must assume responsibility for anticipatory guidance, reassurance, and counseling or referral. Information can be provided to the couple, both prenatally and after birth. Knowledge of normal physiologic and emotional changes allows the couple to discuss coping mechanisms and alternate means of maintaining intimacy during this challenging period. Teaching considerations for sexual activity during the postpartum period are presented in Display 11-7.

Contraception

Two factors influence women's choice and timing of postpartum contraception; infant feeding method and the involution process (Sweezy, 1992). Ideally, the primary healthcare provider discusses choice and use of contraceptive methods with both partners.

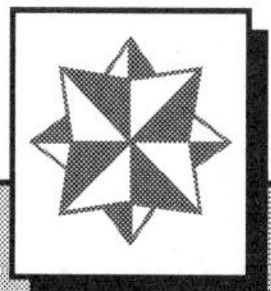

Display 11-7

Teaching Considerations for Postpartum Sexual Activity

The nurse can use the following points in teaching the postpartum couple:

- Sexual intercourse may be resumed around 2 to 4 weeks after both vaginal and cesarean births.
- Sexual intercourse should not be resumed until vaginal bleeding has stopped, to prevent introduction of infection at the placental site.
- Healing of episiotomy and perineum may be checked gently by inserting a finger into the vagina.
- Sexual arousal may cause milk to leak from the breasks. (Nursing the neonate before sexual activity or wearing a bra with absorbent pads during lovemaking may help this problem.)
- Contraceptive cream or a natural vegetable oil (safflower or soy, for example) may be used if additional lubrication is necessary. (K-Y jelly drys out rapidly.)
- Longer periods of foreplay will encourage lubrication.
- Couple should communicate openly.
- Alternate forms of sexual expression may be used.
- Kegel exercises may be used immediately after birth, whenever urinating, and frequently during the day.
- Sitz baths 3 times a day help heal the episiotomy.
- The perineum is examined with a good light and mirror within a few days of delivery and then again 3 weeks later to reassure yourself that it is healing. If something doesn't look right, contact a physician.
- Intercourse and your body do return to "normal."
- A bra is worn 24 hours a day as soon as possible after birth to help decrease engorgement.
- Partner is advised not to put pressure on breasts while they're sensitive, especially during the night when the infant is sleeping for longer periods without feeding.
- Realistic priorities are set. (Arrange schedule so that you nap when the infant does.)
- Nap or lie down and get off your feet at least 30 minutes every day.
- If you're depressed, help from friends and family is necessary. (Get further help if the depression lasts longer than 3 days.)
- When the infant is weaned, your sex drive will usually return to normal.

Adapted from May, K.A., & Mahlmeister, L.R. (1994). Maternal and Neonatal Nursing (3rd ed., p. 833). Philadelphia: J.B. Lippincott.

This approach allows sharing of responsibility, an opportunity to discuss advantages and disadvantages of methods, clarification of misconceptions, and discussion of prevention of sexually transmitted diseases (STDs) (Sweezy, 1992).

A key rule in providing education to women is to ensure that healthcare providers avoid personal biases in giving information. Decision-making should include factors regarding effectiveness, acceptability, and safety (King, 1992). Currently available options for women and their partners are described below.

Depo-Provera was approved by the U.S. Food and Drug Administration (FDA) in 1992 and provides long-acting nonintercourse-related contraception. Failure rates average 0.3%. Management includes counseling regarding the nonreversible aspects of the injection, which is given every 12 weeks. Weight change, menstrual changes, pregnancy symptoms, and osteoporosis in susceptible women are a few of the potential side effects (Policar, 1993). Barring contraindications, Depo-Provera may be given to women during the postpartum period prior to discharge.

Norplant is a subdermal implant inserted surgically that provides up to 5 years of contraception with an accidental pregnancy rate of 0.2% (King, 1992). Women must be advised that menstrual irregularities are a common side effect and that the implants must be surgically removed.

"New" oral contraceptives (OCs) containing 19-nortestosterone progestins have approval or are pending approval from the FDA. Failure rates are less than 1%. There may be confusion if women have previously taken older preparations of OCs. OCs are restricted for certain women, especially those who are older than 35 years of age and smoke more than 15 cigarettes a day (Sweezy, 1992). The use of combination pills (containing estrogen and progestin) in the first 6 to 8 weeks postpartum in women who are breastfeeding, is associated with increased risk of thromboembolic disease (World Health Organization Task Force on Contraceptives, 1987). There may be effects on breast milk with OCs. Women need individualized information and management regarding appropriate oral contraception. As discussion continues regarding over-the-counter availability of OCs, nurses can play an important role in education and follow-up.

Depo-Provera, OCs, and Norplant offer no protection from STDs. Women and their partners need to use other protective methods for this purpose.

Barrier methods are used alone for prevention of pregnancy, STDs, or both. They are used in combination with spermicides to achieve maximal protection against both pregnancy and STDs. Newer male condoms have various lengths, shapes, and adhesives. Tactylon (approved by the FDA in 1991) is a hypoallergenic, synthetic polymer that is impervious to sperm and virus and is not degraded by oxidation or oil-based lubricants.

The Reality vaginal pouch (approved by the FDA in 1992) is a female condom with two rings connected by a polyurethane sheath. The inner ring is fitted like a diaphragm; the outer ring protects the vulva and prevents slipping. Other types of female condoms are in clinical trials (Bikini and Women's Choice Condomme). The failure rate of these devices is similar to that for other female barrier methods.

Other barrier methods include the cervical cap and diaphragm. Chemical methods such as spermicidal creams, jellies, foams, suppositories, and vaginal film contain nonoxynol-9 as the sperm-inhibiting agent. Creams and jellies increase the effectiveness of diaphragms or cervical caps. The lubricating effect of creams and jellies may benefit the breastfeeding woman who experiences vaginal dryness.

Intrauterine devices (IUDs) can be used for postpartum and breastfeeding women. Their effectiveness is equivalent to that for OCs. Women with a history of pelvic inflammatory disease or STDs are not candidates for IUDs. The individual inserting the IUD must be skilled to prevent complications such as uterine or cervical perforation, which is estimated to occur in 1 in 2,500 users. Cramping, pain, and bleeding are side effects that should be evaluated. IUDs allow long-term and continuous use requiring minimal effort on the woman's part.

Postpartum tubal ligation (sterilization) is an option provided in some institutions for women who do not wish to become pregnant again. Appropriate counseling regarding risks of failure, surgical risk, potential psychosocial reactions to the procedure, and signed consent forms per institutional protocol should precede surgery. Postpartum sterilization may be delayed if women experience psychosocial, medical, or obstetric complications or if the neonatal outcome is in doubt (ACOG, 1992).

Natural family planning relies on fertility awareness and abstinence during the fertile portion of a woman's menstrual cycle. Methods include calendar rhythm, basal body temperature, and symptothermal techniques. The method may be difficult to implement until lochia ceases and an ovulatory pattern is reestablished. Lactation also may delay menses, and women must be aware that ovulation can occur without established menses.

Additional nursing interventions include (1) providing information on methods available, following exploration of the couple's needs, wants, and desires; (2) support for decisions; (3) clarification of areas of potential confusion and misconception; and (4) timing teaching to best meet the needs of the woman and her partner.

WOMEN'S PERSPECTIVES ON THE TRANSITION TO PARENTHOOD

Fatigue

For most women, the 6 weeks after giving birth are a time of change and adjustment. A major issue identified during the first 2 weeks postpartum in women identified as low-risk is underlying fatigue. Fatigue has an impact on emotional adjustment and feelings of inadequacy, in meeting the needs of other family members, and in assuming household responsibilities (Ruchala & Halstead, 1994). Anticipatory guidance is essential so the new mother is aware that fatigue is normal and plans can be made for her to get adequate rest. Together, the nurse and woman can develop strategies to ask for help with newborn care, household chores, and sibling care and to nap when the newborn is sleeping. Ideally, family members and friends are available to provide support.

Additional Stressors

Several stressors, in addition to fatigue, have been identified as contributing to difficulty in adapting to the postpartum period. Stressors include physical changes and complications, role conflict, newborn needs, and changes in the parents' relationship (Evans, 1991). First-time mothers cite lack of experience with newborns and amount of time and work involved with newborn care as concerns, yet most have positive feelings about motherhood. Experienced mothers have a greater sense of well-being in caring for their newborns (Ruchala & Halstead, 1994).

Postpartum Blues and Depression

Childbirth is typically a joyous event, yet up to 75 percent of new mothers are at risk for mental or emotional problems after delivery (Kumar, 1990). Ten to fifteen percent of women experience clinical depression in the 3 months after giving birth, yet one half of these women are not recognized by healthcare providers as being depressed (Kumar). There are many opportunities for preventive care in perinatal settings because pregnant women usually have repeated contact with healthcare providers. In Western society, however, the psychological well-being of the postpartum woman is considered of secondary importance. If perinatal care providers are sensitive to the woman's psychological well-being, prospects for early identification are enhanced, and crises may be prevented.

Transient emotional disturbances or "baby blues," usually occur around 3 to 5 days postpartum and last no more than several days. Fatigue, anger, psychic anxiety, and worry were the most frequently reported depressive symptoms in a study of 224 healthy women with uncomplicated pregnancies (Affonso et al., 1992). First-time mothers are most at risk for postpartum psychosis, which usually occurs within a few weeks to 3 months after giving birth (Kumar, 1990). Efficient methods for prediction and prevention of postpartum psychosis have yet to be developed. Mother-baby psychiatric units, supervised home care, "drop-in centers," and facilities to provide support and counseling during well-child visits should be available for women (Kumar). (See Chapter 5 for a discussion of postpartum psychological issues.)

FAMILY TRANSITION TO PARENTHOOD

Parental responsibilities and restrictions, gratifications, and marital intimacy and stability are multidimensional components involved in the transition to parenthood (Belsky & Pensky, 1988; Worthington & Buston, 1986). Marital satisfaction can be significantly influenced as couples experience a "baby honeymoon" just prior to birth and for a short time thereafter. This period is followed by a decline in marital satisfaction that lingers into the second year (Gjerdingen & Fontaine, 1991). There are conflicting data concerning whether wives have a more pronounced decline in marital satisfaction than husbands (Cowan et al., 1985). Couples with a support group appear to have higher levels of marital satisfaction from 6 to 18 months postpartum than do couples without a support group. Effects of new parenthood on unmarried partners and nontraditional family units are areas for further research.

In addition to an overall decline in marital satisfaction after childbirth, couples experience a more traditional division of household labor, less frequent leisure activities, fewer positive interactions, and an increase in conflict (Belsky & Pensky, 1988). Mothers felt more positive about the postpartum transition to parenting roles when there were nontraditional gender-role attitudes and greater father involvement in infant care (Belsky & Pensky, 1988).

The greatest factor influencing a woman's transition to the stressful role of motherhood seems to be the help she receives following childbirth (Romito, 1989). Child-development research suggests that fathers' involvement with their children and affectionate support of their wives enhance maternal competence and enjoyment of newborn care. A happy, confident, and competent mother has a positive influence on the cognitive and social development of her newborn (Romito).

Taking time to listen to women as they discuss their social circumstances and to explore with them a more realistic view of early parenthood is a primary nursing role (Romito, 1989). Strategies to deal with potential problem areas can then discussed before they become major issues. Primary prevention programs to provide information on coping with symptoms, involving support systems and self-surveillance activities, are not consistently available. However, perinatal nurses in the inpatient setting have a significant opportunity to influence positive outcomes for women and families by addressing these needs.

SUMMARY

Women need individualized care, support, and education as they adapt to physiologic and psychosocial changes during the postpartum period. The transition to new motherhood is both exciting and stressful. Using creativity, flexibility, and collaboration with other healthcare providers, perinatal nurses can make a significant difference in enhancing successful family-newborn integration.

REFERENCES

Affonso, D.D., Lovett, S., Paul, S., Sheptek, S., Nussbaum, R., Newman, L., & Johnson, B. (1992). Dysphoric distress in childbearing women. Journal of Perinatology, 12(4), 325-332.

American Academy of Pediatrics, & American College of Obstetricians and Gynecologists. (1992). Guidelines for Perinatal Care (3rd ed.). Washington, DC: Author.

Arias, F. (1993). Practical guide to high-risk pregnancy & delivery (2nd ed.). St. Louis, MO: Mosby-Year Book.

Bek, K.M., & Laurberg, S. (1992). Risks of anal incontinence from subsequent vaginal delivery after a complete obstetric anal sphincter tear. British Journal of Obstetrics and Gynacology, 99(9), 724-726.

Belsky, J., & Pensky, E. (1988). Marital change across the transition to parenthood. Marriage and Family Review, 3(4), 133-156.

Blackburn, S.T., & Loper, D.L. (1992). Maternal, fetal, and neonatal physiology. Philadelphia: W.B. Saunders.

Bowes, W.A. (1991). Postpartum care. In S.G. Gabbe (Ed.), Obstetrics: Normal and problem pregnancies (2nd ed., pp. 753-779). New York: Churchill Livingstone.

Burnett, S.J., Spence-Jones, C., Speakman, C.T., Kamm, M.A., Hudson, C.N., & Bartram, C.I. (1991). Unsuspected sphincter damage following childbirth revealed by anal endosonography. British Journal of Radiology, 64(759), 225-227.

Chapman, L.L. (1994). Nursing care of the family in the postpartum period. In K.A. May, & L.R. Mahlmeister (Eds.), Maternal & neonatal nursing: Family-centered care (pp. 783-836). Philadelphia: J.B. Lippincott.

Combs, C.A., Murphy, E.L., & Laros, R.K. (1991). Factors associated with postpartum hemorrhage with vaginal birth. Obstetrics and Gynecology, 77(1), 69-76.

Cowan, C.P., Cowan, P.A., Heming, G., Garrett, E., Coysh, W.S., Curtis, B.H., & Boyles, A.J. (1985). Transitions to parenthood: His, hers, and theirs. Journal of Family Issues, 6(4), 451-481.

Cranley, J.J., Canos, A.J., & Sull, W.J. (1976). The diagnosis of deep venous thrombosis: Fallibility of clinical symptoms and signs. Archives of Surgery, 111(1) 34-36.

Crawford, L.A., Quint, E.H., Pearl, M.L., & DeLancey, J.O. (1991). Incontinence following rupture of the anal sphincter during delivery. Obstetrics and Gynecology, 82 (4, Pt. 1), 527-531.

Creasy, R.K., & Resnik, R. (1994). Maternal-fetal medicine: Principles and practice (2nd ed.). Philadelphia: W.B. Saunders.

Cunningham, F.G., MacDonald, P., Gant, N., Leveno, K., & Gilstrap, L. (1993). The puerperium. In Williams obstetrics (19th ed., pp. 459-473). Norwalk, CT: Appleton & Lange.

DeLancey, J.O. (1993). Childbirth, continence, and the pelvic floor. New England Journal of Medicine, 329(26), 1956-1957.

DeLancey, J.O., Sampselle, C.M., & Punch, M.R. (1993). Kegel dyspareunia: Levator ani myalgia caused by overexertion. Obstetrics and Gynecology, 82 (4, Pt. 2 Suppl.), 658-659.

Dildy, G.A., & Clark, S.L. (1993). OB emergencies. Contemporary Obstetrics and Gynecology, 38(5), 21-29.

Dixon-Mueller, R. (1993). The sexuality connection in reproductive health. Studies in Family Planning, 24(5), 269-282.

Duvekot, J.J., & Peeters, L.L. (1994). Maternal cardiovascular hemodynamic adaptation to pregnancy. Obstetrical and Gynecological Survey, 49(Suppl. 12), S1-S14.

Dwinell, J. (1992). Birth stories: Mystery, power, and creation. Westport, CT: Bergin & Garvey.

Easterling, H.W. (1982). The puerperium. In D.N. Danforth (Ed.), Obstetrics and gynecology (4th ed.). Hagerstown, MD: Harper & Rowe.

Evans, C.J. (1991). Description of a home follow-up program for childbearing families. Journal of Obstetric, Gynecologic, and Neonatal Nursing, 20(2), 113-118.

Gibbs, R.S. (1989). Severe infections in pregnancy. Medical Clinics of North America, 73(3), 713-721.

Gjerdingen, D.K., & Fontaine, P. (1991). Family-centered postpartum care. Family Medicine, 23(3), 189-193.

Goldenberg, R.L., Cliver, S.P., Bronstein, J., Cutter, G., Andrews, W., & Mennenmeyer, S. (1994). Bed rest in pregnancy. Obstetrics and Gynecology, 84(1), 131-136.

Graf, L.A., & McPherson-Smith, L. (1991). Nongenetic perinatal anemias: Conventional, herbal, and homeopathic treatments. NAACOG's Clinical Issues in Perinatal and Women's Health Nursing, 2(3), 357-363.

Graves, J.E., Pollock, M.L., Leggett, S.H., Braith, R.W., Carpenter, D.M., & Bishop, L.E. (1988). Effect of reduced training frequency on muscular strength. International Journal of Sport Medicine, 9(5), 316-319.

Guana-Trujillo, B., & Grant-Higgins, P.G. (1987). Sexual intercourse and pregnancy. Health Care for Women International, 8(5/6), 339-348.

Hayashi, R.H., & Castillo, M.S. (1993). Bleeding in pregnancy. In R. Knuppel & J. Drukker, (Eds.). High-risk pregnancy: A team approach (2nd ed., pp. 539-560). Philadelphia: W.B. Saunders.

Hoyme, U.B., Kiviat, N., & Eschenbach, D.A. (1986). Microbiology and treatment of late postpartum endometritis. Obstetrics and Gynecology, 68(2), 226-232.

Kapernick, P. (1991) Postpartum hemorrhage and the abnormal puerperium. In M.L. Pernoll (Ed.), Current obstetric & gynecologic diagnosis & treatment (7th ed., pp. 568-588). Norwalk, CT: Appleton & Lange.

King, J. (1992). Helping patients choose an appropriate method of birth control. MCN: American Journal of Maternal Child Nursing, 17(2), 91-95.

Kramer, R.M., Stunkard, A.J., Marshall, K.A., McKinney, S., Liebschutz, J. (1993). Breastfeeding reduces maternal lower-body fat. Journal of the American Dietetic Association, 93(4), 429-433.

Kumar, R. (1990). An overview of postpartum psychiatric disorders. NAACOG's Clinical Issues in Perinatal and Women's Health Nursing, 1(3), 351-358.

Lagana, K. (1994). Postpartum complications. In K.A. May & L.R. Mahlmeister (Eds.), Maternal and neonatal nursing: Family-centered care (pp. 837-876). Philadelphia: J.B. Lippincott.

Laurberg, S., & Swash, M. (1989). Effects of aging on the anorectal sphincters and their innervation. Diseases of the Colon and Rectum, 32(9), 737-742.

Lubarsky, S.L., Barton, J.R., Friedman, S.A., Nasreddine, S., Ramadan, M.K., & Sibai, B.M. (1994). Late postpartum eclampsia revisited. Obstetrics and Gynecology, 83(4), 502-505.

Luegenbiehl, D.L. (1991). Postpartum bleeding. NAACOG's Clinical Issues in Perinatal and Women's Health Nursing, 2(3), 402-409.

Magee, K.P., Blanco, J.D., Graham, J.M., Rayburn, C., & Prien, S. (1994). Endometritis after cesarean: The effect of age. American Journal of Perinatology, 11(1), 24-26.

Maloni, J.A., Chance, B., Zhang, C., Cohen, A.W., Betts, D., & Gange, S.J. (1993). Physical and psychosocial side effects of antepartum hospital bed rest. Nursing Research, 42(4), 197-203.

May, K.A. (1987). Men's sexuality during the childbearing year: Implications of recent research findings. Holistic Nursing Practice, 1(4), 60-66.

May, K.A., & Mahlmeister, L.R. (Eds.) (1994). Maternal and neonatal nursing: Family centered care (3rd ed.). Philadelphia: J.B. Lippincott.

Mayberry, L.J., Smith, M., & Gill, P. (1992). Effect of exercise on uterine activity in the patient in preterm labor. Journal of Perinatology, 12(4), 354-358.

Miovech, S.M., Knapp, H., Borucki, L., Roncoli, M., Arnold, L., & Brooten, D. (1994). Major concerns of women after cesarean delivery. Journal of Obstetric, Gynecologic, and Neonatal Nursing, 23(1), 53-59.

Mittelmark, R.A., Wiswell, R.A., & Drinkwater, B.L. (1991). Exercise in Pregnancy (2nd ed.). Baltimore: Williams & Wilkins.

Monga, M., & Oshiro, B.T. (1993). Puerperal infections. Seminars in Perinatology, 17(6), 426-431.

Novy, M. (1991). The normal puerperium. In M.L. Pernoll (Ed.), Current obstetric and gynecologic diagnosis and treatment (pp. 237-268). Norwalk, CT: Appleton & Lange.

Oppenheimer, L.W., Sherriff, E.A., & Goodman, J.D., Shah, D., & James, C.E. (1986). The duration of lochia. British Journal of Obstetrics and Gynaecology, 93(7), 754-757.

Policar, M. (1993). Contraception: Perspectives and prospects. Presentation at the 17th Annual OB/GYN Nurse Practitioner Conference, Philadelphia.

Poole, J.H. (1993). Maternal hemorrhagic disorders. In I.M. Bobak & M.D. Jensen (Eds.), Maternity and gynecologic care: The nurse and the family (5th ed.). St. Louis, MO: C.V. Mosby.

Pritchard, J.A. (1965). Changes in the blood volume during pregnancy and delivery. Anesthesiology, 26, 393-399.

Reamy, K., & White, S.E. (1985). Sexuality in pregnancy and the puerperium: A review. Obstetrical and Gynecological Survey, 40(1), 1-13.

Reichert, J.A., Baron, M., & Fawcett, J. (1993). Changes in attitudes toward cesarean birth. Journal of Obstetric, Gynecologic, and Neonatal Nursing, 22(2), 159-167.

Roberts, J. (1994). Current perspectives on preeclampsia. Journal of Nurse-Midwifery, 39(2), 70-90.

Rosene, K., Eschenbach, D.A., Tompkins, L.S., Kenny, G.E., Watkins, H. (1986). Polymicrobial early postpartum endometritis with faculative and anaerobic bacteria, genital mycoplasmas and chlamydia trachomatis: Treatment with piperacillin or cefoxitin. Journal of Infectious Diseases, 153(6), 1028-1037.

Romito, P. (1989). Unhappiness after childbirth. In I. Chalmers, M. Enkin & M.J. Keirse (Eds.), Effective care in pregnancy and childbirth (Vol. 1, pp. 1433-1446). Oxford: Oxford University.

Ruchala, P.L., & Halstead, L. (1994). The postpartum experience of low-risk women: A time of adjustment and change. Maternal-Child Nursing Journal, 22(3), 83-89.

Schuessler, B., Hesse, U., Dimpfl, T., & Anthuber, C. (1988). Epidural anaesthesia and avoidance of postpartum stress urinary incontinence [Letter]. Lancet, 1(8588):762.

Shiono, P.H., Klebanoff, M.A., & Carey, J.C. (1990). Midline episiotomies: More harm than good. Obstetrics and Gynecology, 75(5), 765-770.

Steinem, G. (1992). Revolution from within: A book of self-esteem. Boston: Little, Brown.

Sultan, A.H., Kamm, M.A., Hudson, C.N., Thomas, J.M., & Bartram, C.I. (1993). Anal-sphincter disruption during vaginal delivery. New England Journal of Medicine, 329(26), 1905-1911.

Sultan, A.H., Kamm, M.A., Hudson, C.N., & Bartram, C.I. (1994). Third degree obstetric anal sphincter tears: Risk factors and outcome of primary repair. British Medical Journal, 308(6933), 887-891.

Sultan, A.H., Kamm, M.A., Bartram, C.N., & Hudson, C.J. (1994). Perineal damage at delivery. Contemporary Review in Obstetrics and Gynecology, 6(1), 18-24.

Sweezy, S.R. (1992). Contraception for the postpartum woman. NAACOG's clinical issues in perinatal and women's health nursing: Contraception, 3(2), 209-225.

Ueland, K. (1976). Maternal cardiovascular dynamics. VII. Intrapartum blood volume changes. American Journal of Obstetrics and Gynecology, 126(6), 671-677.

Varney, H. (1987). Nurse-midwifery (2nd ed.). Boston, MA: Blackwell Scientific.

Vaughans, B. (1990). Early maternal-infant contact and neonatal thermoregulation. Neonatal Network, 8(5), 19-21.

Viktrup, L., & Lose, G. (1993). Epidural anesthesia during labor and stress incontinence after delivery. Obstetrics and Gynecology, 82(6), 984-986.

Viktrup, L., Lose, G., Rolff, M., & Barfoed, K. (1992). The symptoms of stress incontinence caused by pregnancy or delivery in primiparas. Obstetrics and Gynecology, 79(6) 945-949.

Wheeler, D.G. (1991). Intrapartum bleeding. NAACOG's clinical issues in perinatal and women's health nursing: Bleeding in women, 2(3), 381-384.

World Health Organization Task Force on Contraception. (1987). Contraception during the postpartum period and during lactation: The effects on women's health. International Journal of Gynaecology and Obstetrics, 25 (Suppl: 13-26).

Worthington, E.L., & Buston, B.G. (1986). The marriage relationship during the transition to parenthood: A review and model. Journal of Family Issues, 7(4), 443-473.

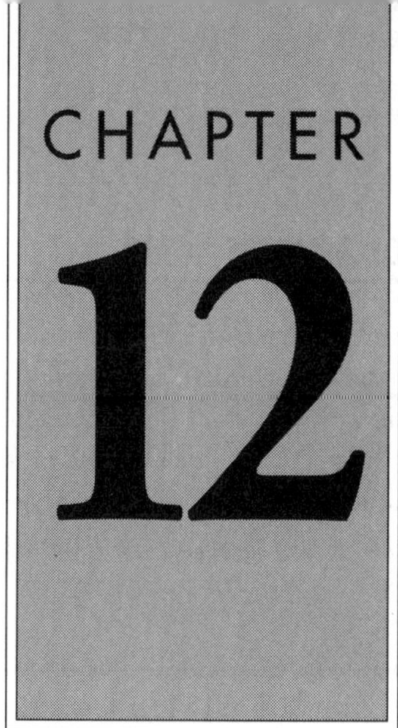

Loss and Bereavement: Psychological, Sociological, Spiritual, and Ontological Perspectives

Karren Kowalski

Philosophically, when one human being dies everyone is diminished (Irion, 1976). Any death can initiate a grief response. In one sense each person grieves for his or her own death; in another sense death creates conflict. Humans function in relationships with the belief that there is always more time: time to correct misunderstandings, time to love someone, time to hold them, and time to communicate innermost thoughts and feelings (Lattanzi, 1983). Perinatal death is unique because it is out of sequence, outside the normal life cycle. It is a reminder of human vulnerability. There is no time to hold or communicate or even to love.

While American culture has focused on the successful pursuit of happiness and the American dream, mourning and bereavement in Western culture has become equated with failure. Losses are somehow translated into road blocks and obstacles; they are not to be discussed. This cultural shift has influenced all aspects of our daily lives and particularly the reproductive cycle which deals with birth *and* death.

The study of loss and bereavement is an evolving process. In the 1960s and 1970s loss and bereavement were confined to a medical model. The model had multiple categories in which one could fit a particular patient—thus, enhancing the ability to refer for therapy. Professionals did not understand that healing comes from within, that families have choices, or that societal normative behavior might cause problems. It was more acceptable to diagnose and refer for therapy than to acknowledge the pain and be with the patient in that pain.

Many professionals have yet to differentiate between supportive caring for the bereaved and "fixing" people and situations. Consequently, when a death occurs, some nurses view the event as a personal and professional failure. Their professional image is called into question. A sense of failure is magnified if even one aspect of the medical or nursing care was questionable or in error. If no aspects of care are questionable or in error, nurses frequently manufacture a reason.

This chapter explores experiences of loss and bereavement related to women, their families, reproduction, and nursing care. Loss and bereavement are studied from perspectives of phenomenology, psychology, sociology, ontology, and spirituality.

THE PHENOMENOLOGY OF LOSS

Losses take many different forms; they may be anticipated or unexpected, instant or gradual, traumatic or nontraumatic. The classic work of Peretz (1970b) identifies four key types of loss: (1) loss of a significant person, (2) loss of some aspect of self, (3) loss of an external object, and (4) loss of stages of growth and development. These losses, how they occur, and examples are given in Table 12-1.

Two additional reproduction-oriented categories have been identified by Kowalski (1987): loss of a dream and loss of creation.

Loss of a Dream

Because of the complete dependency of the growing fetus and the newborn on the parents, a unique attachment or bond is created. Much has been written about bonding and attachment. The desire to have children is associated with many factors such as

TABLE 12-1. Types of Loss

Loss	How They Occur	Reproductive Examples
Loss of significant person	Through death, separation, rejection, or divorce	Stillbirth Infant that dies Maternal death Gynecologic death, (i.e., oncology: breast, uterine, ovarian) Relinquishment
Loss of some aspect of self	Self equates to an overall mental image that each has of themselves, ideas and feelings about worth, attractiveness, normalcy, lovability, or body functioning.	Structural losses such as hysterectomy or mastectomy; infants with anomalies Functional losses such as infertility or complications of pregnancy–a bodily misfunction–wrong sex infant Psychological loss as in self-esteem, status, role of parent
Loss of external objects	Loss of possessions; material objects, money, property	Loss of a child as a possession– "our child" Loss or giving up of associated objects– furniture, clothes, toys, etc,. are packed away
Loss of stages of growth and development	Naturally occurring developmental loss as the person progresses through the stages/phases of life. There is no developmental growth of the ego without loss and letting go.	Children lose or relinquish the breast for solid food. Adults relinquish the "single life" when they form long-term relationships or marry. They give up duality when they have a baby.

perpetuating the family name and traditions, a parental attempt to resolve an unhappy childhood of their own, and hope that the child will succeed where the parent has failed. Although it is too early for the developing fetus or newborn to demonstrate personality, the parents focus their hopes, dreams, and aspirations on the child. When the child dies, these hopes and dreams are extinguished. The parents experience a sadness for what might have been. Consequently, as each life transition occurs, as each developmental stage progresses (e.g., the first day of school, obtaining a driver's license, graduation from high school, marriage, etc.), the parents again grieve the loss and their inability to share that life experience with the child.

Loss of Creation

An artist whose painting is vandalized or destroyed suffers great anguish over loss of control and powerlessness to protect his or her creation. Likewise, human beings create progeny. This creation is an extension of themselves and that specific relationship. The parents usually invest time, energy, and emotions in the creation of this new life. It is nurtured in the woman's body. As it progresses from embryo to fetus to newborn it is continually with the mother, a part of her, yet separate. When this creation dies, she experiences an event over which she has no control, a process she can not stop. The narcissistic blow to her self-image can be terrible. Additionally, the father feels out of control because he is unable to protect his spouse or to provide whatever could have saved the child.

Perceptions of Loss

Peretz (1970a) emphasized that any kind of loss is simultaneously a reality and a perceptual or symbolic event. Even perceptual or symbolic events can produce intense reactions. For example, some women who experience a cesarean birth rather than a vaginal birth react to this process as a loss. They perceive that they have lost the experience they desired. Somehow they have failed in actualizing this event called childbearing, and they grieve for this loss or assault to their self-esteem. In contrast, women who experience a perinatal loss would give anything to have been able to deliver a live, healthy infant, even by cesarean birth. Consequently, grieving about a cesarean birth is incomprehensible to them. It is all in one's perceptions. Each of us chooses how we perceive a given event, based on past experience.

Types of Perinatal Loss

Perinatal loss can be divided into two major types: death of the fetus or newborn or birth of a less than perfect child. Because the perinatal period represents the total embryonic, fetal, and neonatal life span and because there is greater danger to life during this period than at any other time during the life cycle, adverse outcomes can be expected.

Five types of loss are discussed here: miscarriage, fetal and neonatal demise, sudden infant death syndrome (SIDS), anomalies, and adoption. These losses reflect the two major outcomes.

Miscarriage

Over the last two decades, knowledge has expanded about miscarriage, also known as spontaneous abortion. Previously viewed as benign, miscarriage affects one in every five pregnancies. Swanson-Kaufman's (1983) early work identified areas of support needed by a bereaved parent:

- understanding of this personal experience
- empathy
- support for the grieving process
- attendance to physical needs
- identification of normalcy of the response to the event

Hutti (1992) further identified areas in which parents need support. These areas are: the reality of the pregnancy, recognition that something was wrong, acknowledgement of miscarriage as an actual event, appropriate and sensitive medical intervention, and concern for the ability to produce a subsequent normal, healthy child. It is clear that parents, particularly women, respond to miscarriage with intense emotional reactions. These can be predicted, based on how the event is defined and what coping styles have been adopted by the couple. For instance, when an ectopic pregnancy occurs, multiple aspects are involved: there is loss of pregnancy, serious threat to the life of the mother, and serious threat to opportunities for future pregnancies.

Fetal and Neonatal Demise

Death occurring prior to the onset of labor is referred to as fetal death, while neonatal death occurs anytime from birth to 28 days of life. In fetal demise, parents often have knowledge that something is not right. There may be no fetal movement or medical tests may show adverse results. These indications provide time for "anticipatory grief." The parents begin the bereavement process prior to the event. There are many commonalities in fetal and neonatal losses. One key difference, however, relates to the length of time the neonate lives. If the fetus dies prior to birth, the woman is often the only person who has bonded to the child. In contrast, if the neonate survives several days, people other than the mother have an opportunity to become attached to the newborn. For instance, the father and grandparents also feel a tremendous loss.

Sudden Infant Death Syndrome (SIDS)

SIDS refers to any infant death that is unexpected and in which a thorough postmortem examination and case study fail to demonstrate a cause. The cause of SIDS remains speculative in spite of extensive research. Parents do not cope well when no cause, no opportunity for prevention, and no hope for cure are combined. When death is sudden, unexpected, and premature, parents have no opportunity to evoke appropriate coping mechanisms. Thus, the personal search for cause and meaning is particularly anguishing. The guilt associated with SIDS seems overwhelming. The parents agonize over what they might have done or should have done to prevent the death. Such situations can become even more complicated if the event occurred while a sitter or other responsible adult was caring for the child.

The "Imperfect" Child

Bereavement is not limited to death or lost pregnancies. There are several instances of what can be called "the less than perfect child or birth." In such situations parents did not produce the full-term or perfectly formed newborn they had expected. When a newborn is seriously ill, parents grieve the loss of the fantasized "perfect" newborn, thus creating difficulties in the attachment process. Parents apparently have difficulty attaching to a newborn until there is evidence that the newborn will survive. It is important for nurses to understand this process and to support parents until they are able to attach to a sick newborn.

A similar process occurs when a newborn has anomalies. There is a period of denial, the initial phase of the bereavement response. There is an adjustment phase in which there is developing awareness, characterized

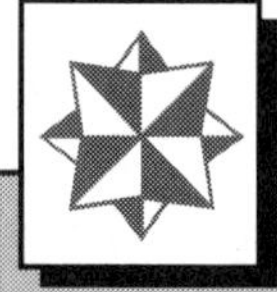

Display 12-1

Stages of Normal Bereavement

- Shock and denial. A period of time lasting as much as 72 hours or more in which the bereaved believe that they are experiencing a bad dream and that they will wake up and everything will be okay.
- Acute grief work. This includes varying manifestations of the behaviors described in Table II .
- Disintegration. There is a general downward spiral or sense of disintegration that overlaps with this acute bereavement process. Families describe the process as being on a roller coaster. Anytime they begin to feel better, physically or emotionally, they then feel guilty about feeling better and this drives the cycle of helplessness downward. During this time, bereaved families, particularly the parents of stillborns and newborns that die, seem quite surprised at the depth of their feelings. The mothers feel a strong sense of responsibility and guilt while the fathers appear to deal with these feelings more quickly by focusing on their careers or work.
- Reintegration. A sense of continuity and reintegration is established as the bereaved gradually relinquish parts of their relationship with the dead loved one and reestablish their definition of the meaning of life separately from the dead infant. In this way grief is mastered not by ceasing to care for the dead, but by abstracting the essence of the relationship and reintegrating it to fit a future in which the deceased will not share. This becomes more complicated in perinatal losses due to two additional aspects that are frequently not involved in other types of loss such as that of a parent, a spouse, or a close friend—loss of creation and loss of a dream.

by the parents feeling helpless, hopeless, and anxious. They are sad, and they experience severe psychological pain, anger, and guilt. Frequently, extended periods of chronic bereavement occur in which parents function in either adaptive or maladaptive ways. In extreme maladaptive instances, the family becomes dysfunctional. They may experience a failed marriage, unemployment, and separation from friends and relatives. It is extremely difficult for them to live each day with what they consider is obvious failure.

It is not uncommon for parents to have definite ideas and fantasies about the preferred sex of their child. For example, the ideal middle class American family consists of one boy and one girl. In some ethnic groups, it is essential to produce male children. Thus, when a child of the "wrong" sex is delivered, parents may require considerable time adjusting; in fact, some parents become permanently estranged from the child, creating significant psychological problems. When professionals assess that the sex of the child is a critical issue, they need to create possibilities in which parents become involved in the birth and caretaking. By demonstrating her acceptance, a nurse can promote attitudinal changes in acceptance of the child. Not all situations can be corrected, but most can be improved.

Considerable time and energy are invested in pregnancy and birth. When discrepancies occur between reality and the idealized perfect birth experience, a sense of loss arises. The ultimate in a wrong delivery method is a cesarean birth. This is especially true if the woman was committed to a normal vaginal birth. If expectations and reality do not coincide, parents need time to adjust.

Adoption

Giving up a neonate for adoption involves issues of loss and bereavement. This process, called "relinquishment", contains aspects of the general bereavement process as well as chronic grief. Women need to be assured that their newborn is healthy and will be happy and that adoption is an appropriate decision. When adoption was finally recognized as a cause for bereavement rather than a punishment for immoral sexual behavior, nursing management changed from a judgmental to an educational and supportive focus. If good nursing care is available, women who choose adoption are able to sort through feelings and find meaning in the relinquishment of their child.

PSYCHOLOGICAL PERSPECTIVE OF GRIEF

Historical Development of the Understanding of Grief

Psychological explanations of grief originated in the work of Freud (1937) and his classic paper, "Mourning and Melancholia." He emphasized the painful psychological processes involved in relinquishing or letting go of a loved person or object. Freud was most interested in the pathological clinical manifestations or aberrations of the grief process.

It was another 15 years before Lindemann (1944) described patterns of "normal" bereavement. He was convinced that pathological grief was merely an exaggeration or distortion of the normal bereavement process. To recognize the pathology it is imperative to know the normal process. Lindemann identified the acute phase of bereavement which he called "acute grief work." His conclusions, based on extensive interviews and treatment of bereaved individuals, were that the normal grief behaviors are those listed in Table 12-2.

These are the behaviors that nurses witness on a daily basis in families whose loved ones die. Professionals have long attempted to protect patients from the pain of bereavement, primarily as a way to protect themselves. Lindemann (1944) was the first person to identify that the "no tears, stiff upper lip" approach to bereavement was in fact an aberration of the normal bereavement process. Table 12-2 relates normal grief behaviors to the manifestations of the symptoms and appropriate nursing care.

The original work of Lindemann was expanded and clarified by such researchers as Parks (1970) and Bowlby (1980) who primarily studied widows and widowers. They determined the stages or phases of normal bereavement as summarized in Display 12-1.

Maris (1974) stated that grief work does not necessarily focus on the loss of the loved one. Rather, he believed the fundamental crisis of grief comes from the loss of self rather than the loss of others. It is as though the bereaved mourn their own death. The loss of a key person in one's life translates as a loss of structure that has held the bereaved's life together. Consequently, their life's purpose is in question and the bereaved feel helpless.

TABLE 12-2. Nursing Care in Acute Grief Work

Acute symptom	Manifestations of Symptom	Nursing care
Somatic distress	Intense sadness demonstrated by tears, sobbing, questions about "why did this happen," loss of appetite, sighing respirations, exhaustion, sleep loss.	Do not give sleeping medication (these only delay acute grief work until after discharge so that professionals do not have to deal with it).
		Listen and provide comfort. Answer as many questions as possible, saying "I don't know" when appropriate.
Preoccupation with image of the deceased	Desire of parents to see and hold infant and have family members see.	Show infants, even tiny infants.
	Without an image of the infant acute grief work is difficult to accomplish. The loss is unreal and transfer of emotional investment from the deceased to another child cannot be completed.	Provide mementos and pictures to make experiences real.
Guilt	A search through the pregnancy for evidence of failure to do "the right thing" to have prevented the loss.	Assure parents these feelings are normal.
	Parents find negligence and exaggerate minor omissions or problems such as "old wives tales" that have been violated.	Review these fears and guilt systematically.
	The father may feel he did not provide for or protect his wife.	Support parents to see that these ideas have no basis in realistic facts.
Irritability or anger	Can be seen as a desire to be left alone when friends/relatives make an effort to maintain relationships.	Listen. Do not personalize the behavior, realize it is driven by grief.
	Overt anger focused on healthcare professionals who are seen as "responsible" or not helping enough.	Co-create plan with parents to meet their needs.
	Anger about relationships or systems seen as impersonal or dehumanizing.	Apologize for any problems or misunderstandings or inability of personnel to meet parents' needs.
	Anger at God.	Listen and refer to a spiritual counsellor if person desires.
Inability to maintain organized patterns of activity	Common tasks undertaken as if *only* going through the motions and simple tasks require enormous energy.	Provide bereavement education and information sheets (focus on normalcy of these responses).

TABLE 12-2. Cont.

Acute symptom	Manifestations of Symptom	Nursing care
	Bereaved mother home alone has difficulty structuring time or accomplishing common tasks (i.e., meal preparation).	Provide bereavement education and information sheets.
	Father has difficulty concentrating on specific tasks.	Recommend support group of other bereaved parents. Recommend books for bereaved parents.

Types of Grief

Anticipatory Grief

Lindemann (1944) and others first observed anticipatory grief as a process in families of the terminally ill. During the illness, family members were observed to be depressed, feel concern for the ill family member, and rehearse the death in an attempt to adjust to the consequences. Therefore, at the time of the actual death, they might not exhibit acute grief work behaviors as they had been moving in and out of these behaviors throughout the duration of the illness. The process of anticipatory grieving may also occur in the following instances:

- when a fetus dies prior to the onset of labor or when there is a diagnosis of a condition incompatible with life
- when there is selective termination of the pregnancy
- when the newborn is diagnosed as extremely ill, possibly terminally ill.

In the latter situation the parents frequently experience the initial acute grief work prior to the actual death. Consequently, when the fetus or newborn expires, the parents may experience a low-grief response, causing the staff some initial concerns. Families need to be supported throughout the process and their attempts to deal with the loss recognized.

Chronic Grief

Some very low-birth-weight newborns or those that have serious physical anomalies do not die at birth. Yet the parents of these newborns experience all the stages of initial acute grief work. The mother's worst fear, that of giving birth to a sick or deformed child, has been actualized and the initial grief response begins. In actuality she is grieving the wished for, fantasized, or perfect child. Even after they have moved through most of the bereavement process, parents still have a less than perfect child. Many parents suffer intense guilt, which places increased stress on the adult relationship.

They are reminded every day that they have failed to fulfill societal expectations of producing a normal, healthy child. Chronic grief is prolonged and recurrent because parents experience and reexperience the acute grief process with each major crisis surrounding the defective child, such as major illnesses, intense physical care demands, growth and developmental problems, and ongoing battles with health care systems and school systems to receive services required in caretaking of the child (Kowalski, 1985).

While chronic sorrow is evident with severely physically and mentally disabled children, it also occurs for children with less obvious problems such as learning disabilities. Parents experiencing chronic grief need support from other parents and from the professional community. They need accurate and complete information about resources and they need help in planning realistic coping strategies that encompass the needs of all the family members.

Grief Resolution: Fact or Fantasy

One of the perceptions prevalent in the psychologic perspective of grief is that to be normal one must be "resolved." When bereaved parents are asked about the issue of resolution they are quick to tell any listener that there is no resolution—the loss of their child only becomes "less all-consuming." Although some professionals refer to a concept called grief resolution, there is little evidence in the literature to validate such a phenomenon.

Some women are able to conceive again soon after the loss, while others choose to wait several months or even question ever getting pregnant again. When women have great difficulty in conceiving following a perinatal loss, it is possible that they are not able to withdraw emotional investment in the lost child (Kowalski, 1987). The emotion, the spirit, and the mind have a considerable influence over the process of fertility.

Parks (1970), in his study of widows, found that such events as anniversary dates, unexpected visits from old friends, or the chance discovery of old photographs activated acute pining and sadness, resulting in a miniature bereavement.

Bittersweet Grief

Kowalski (1984) reported that the mothers in her study, all of whom were 18 months to 3 years post-loss, believed that the feelings they had for their infants would always be present. Peppers and Knapp (1980) called this "shadow grief." They believed that shadow grief was a burden a parent would have for the rest of their lives. However, they suggested that parents would not have to experience this process with the proper psychological interventions.

Kowalski (1984), on the other hand, denies that what she calls "bittersweet grief" is a burden. She found that parents had no wish to relinquish the sadness and longing. The parents found a certain bittersweet pleasure in the memories and the few occasions they found to talk about the child. She further believes that, with the love and support of family and friends, the parents who have coped well with the perinatal death will still experience this gentle sadness, embrace it, and know how very special it is to always love this child who lived for so brief a time.

Duration of Normal Grief

It is difficult to predict the length, duration, or depth of the bereavement process because it depends on factors such as the following:

- the relationship of the couple,
- the circumstances surrounding the death,
- the process of bereavement,
- the support of friends, family and professionals
- the inner-resources of the bereaved

The process is highly individualized and differs with each family. Pincus (1974) believed there could be no norm for grief or for adaptation just as there is no time limit imposed on the process. Consequently, it is inappropriate for parents to be labeled or placed in categories according to their progress through the grieving process.

Pincus (1974) reduced the thought process around pathological grieving to its lowest common denominator when he declared that the inability to cope with life was the only valid indication of pathological grief. This view represents a general trend that is reluctant to attach pathological labels to various grief experiences. Grief requires time for healing, and the bereavement process vacilates between traditionally normal and pathological behaviors. Those people whose behaviors seem to be the most "unique" often find it very difficult to conform to society's inappropriate definition of bereavement behavior.

SOCIOLOGICAL PERSPECTIVE OF BEREAVEMENT

Rites of Passage

Transitional phases in human lives are acknowledged and celebrated. Society focuses attention on these important events through the use of symbols and accompanying rituals referred to as "rites of passage." Rites of passage prescribe what gifts are given, what words are spoken, and what behaviors are exhibited. The rites of greatest interest in perinatal care are those of pregnancy, birth, and death.

The transition rights of pregnancy are for the benefit of the parents and their relationship to the social group rather than for the fetus. Rites of passage such as christening and dedication of infants are often performed even though parents and family members are not particularly religious. The symbolism of these acts notes acceptance into the social group.

The funeral ceremony is part of the rite of passage for death. It is personal in its focus and societal in its consequences. The body is disposed of and the bereaved are helped through their personal shock and social reorientation and reincorporation. The entire societal group is provided with a method of readjusting, following the loss of a member. In effect, funeral rites tie people together through mutual support and comfort. This experience is shared and a bond is enhanced among members of the social network.

When death occurs near the time of birth but prior to the community's initiation or recognition of this new life, there is no rending of the social fabric. Society has not recognized the child and, therefore, there is no recognition of death. From the studies of

Parks (1970) Kowalski (1984) and others, it is evident that many bereaved individuals in Western societies are forced to accomplish the life/death transition with only private symbols to assist them. A significant problem in Western society is the factor of time. The transition from bereavement to resumption of normal life in the case of perinatal loss often lasts only a couple of weeks. Friends and family no longer ask about the welfare of the bereaved couple, nor do they demonstrate a willingness to talk about the deceased fetus.

When grief work is done without the support of the social network, it can be so painful that the bereaved feel that they are losing contact with reality. Support that is provided to the bereaved is the key measure of a society's attitude about death (Stevenson, 1980). In Western societies, isolation from and lack of involvement with the bereaved are major problems.

Bereaved parents need emotional support from members within their social network. They need assurance that their feelings are understood and normal, under the circumstances. If the network is to be supportive, there must be congruency in perception of the loss. When there is incongruency or lack of common experience, for example, when no one within the network has had an infant die or knows anyone who has, the network may be unable to provide the needed support. When members of the social network are confronted with this situation for which they have no prior experience, they often inquire within the network to discover if others have experience. Oftentimes, as bereaved parents search for someone with common experience, new social relationships occur. For example, a healthcare professional might recommend parents to a support group; parents might search out such groups through newspaper articles or contact from a support group member. Although more research is needed to determine what motivates the bereaved to come into groups of strangers to talk about their experience, this may occur because existing networks of the bereaved couple refuse to support the necessary healing process. It has been speculated that failure to receive appropriate support results in pathological avoidance of the intense emotions of acute grief. Consequently, establishment of new contacts within a social network can be positive and healthy and can facilitate integration of the loss experience into a bereaved couple's lives.

Mourning

Mourning behaviors may have an evolutionary function which ensures group cohesiveness in species for which social bonding is necessary for survival. Averill (1975) indicated that the pain of separation from the social network creates stress that, in turn leads to efforts to reconnect with the network. Social acts that lead to reconnection were described by Darwin (1864), who observed that the outward signs of adult grief such as facial expressions or sadness and crying resemble the behavior of an abandoned child trying to attract the mother's attention. Just as a mother is attracted by this behavior in a child some members of a social network are attracted to bereaved persons who demonstrate sadness and crying. Consequently, the social actions that result from this attraction serve to reinforce the social group and the bond that binds its members together.

Kowalski (1984) found that one of the most powerful factors supporting parents working through the bereavement process was a social network that perceived the perinatal death in the same way as the parents and went out of its way to help the bereaved parents. Some parents who do not have this type of social network appear to create one by involving themselves in bereaved parent support groups. They search for others who understand what they are experiencing and who are unafraid to talk about fetal or neonatal death. Parents who choose not to seek out support are those who seem to have the most difficulty in working through the bereavement process; they appear to be the same families who experience psychological sequelae.

Sometimes the bereaved parents can be supported by reading about people in a similar situation. Several suggestions for reading material are listed at the end of the chapter.

SPIRITUAL PERSPECTIVE OF BEREAVEMENT

There is variety in the spiritual perspective of bereavement. As discussed above, it is critical to have congruency between the grieving parents and their social network. In fundamental religious groups, where spiritual convictions are congruent between the bereaved couple and their primary social network, the bereaved parents progress through the process in a constructive way. Many spiritual and religious systems also support the concept of an afterlife that holds the hope and the possibility of being reunited with the deceased.

Other spiritual belief systems hold possibilities for grieving families. An example of such a system is demonstrated by Dr. Steven Sunderland, who works with grieving children at Fernside Center (Warrick, 1993). Sunderland studied and uses teachings in Native American spirituality. Many Native Americans (e.g., the Ojibwa elders in Canada) describe a source of healing within each person. Sunderland uses these spiritual belief systems to provide techniques for expressing fear and loss. The premise of this approach is based in Native American spirituality which reports that everyone has "medicine." In other words, inside of every person is a healing energy that is always available and accessible. Because of these spiritual components, Sunderland perceives a grief counselor as a friend whose function is to remind the bereaved of the good in his or her own heart and to help that person bring it forth. Sunderland now opens meetings with a prayer for the release of healing energy. He then asks participants and group members to consider whatever will bring them out of their pain.

This kind of spiritual approach is all-encompassing, more so than many of the more structured religious doctrines in this country. But its empowering aspects suggest that all of us can choose how we proceed through our life experiences.

ONTOLOGICAL PERSPECTIVE OF BEREAVEMENT

An ontological approach believes that human beings create their own reality and that reality is defined as "what is." Ontology is the science of "being." "Being" is the quality or state of having existence, something that actually is. It is required of beings that they are "in the present moment"—that they spend time in the present without judgement but focused on possibilities.

Much of the science of being focuses on people's choices. We choose our responses to any given situation; this includes perinatal loss and bereavement. Most professionals have seen families who spiral downward due to their negative attitude, whereas other families choose to create as much of a positive approach to the tragedy as they possibly can. In working with the bereaved from an ontological perspective, one can educate about choices, about reality, about acceptance, about pain and suffering, and about forgiveness of self and others.

Such a bereavement support model, based on an ontology model, exists in Reno, Nevada. Its course outline is given in the accompanying display (Display 12-2). It appears to be the next step beyond "support." Healthcare professionals can permit people to remain stuck in their suffering, anger, and acting-out behavior or people can be given support to move their lives forward. Classes in the bereavement support model in Reno are limited to 8 participants in the children's group and 15 in the adult group. Adult classes meet for 2 hours and the children's group meets for an hour and a half. The focus is on using the bereavement process as a facilitative event to promote personal growth in one's life. While bereavement groups do not work for everyone, they are exceedingly helpful for many parents. Research is needed to indicate who uses support groups and why they are supportive.

NURSING MANAGEMENT

A desire to "fix" things, so prevalent in the nursing profession, can originate from a genuine desire to alleviate pain and suffering. It can also emanate from a desire to alleviate discomfort over situations beyond one's control. "Fixing" things often gains peoples' acknowledgement and approval. Whatever the motivating factor, in instances of perinatal loss and bereavement, the only thing that will "fix it" is for the baby to be alive and healthy (Kowalski, 1991). This is impossible and so it is essential to support parents through the bereavement experience. Actions are useless unless the nurse is willing to share herself or himself with the bereaved parents at a deep, interpersonal level. This is accomplished not only by spending time with parents, but also through the nurse giving them full attention and listening to their story.

Nursing Assessment

A general assessment of the individual's bereavement state includes recognition and identification of acute grief work behaviors. Other assessments which prove invaluable in determining the nursing diagnosis and a plan for intervention are as follows:

- forewarning of problems
- wanted versus unwanted pregnancy
- multiple losses
- religious belief systems
- social network

The information one hopes to attain from these areas of investigation include the amount of advanced

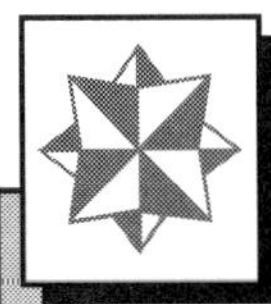

DISPLAY 12-2

Course Outline for Bereavement Support Group

Class 1:	Introduction which includes sharing about each other. Discussion of a concept called acceptance. Understanding that the participants are in a process. The process requires work. It's not easy and they will be in it until they decide not to be. These concepts in some form or another are reviewed each week. A distinction is made between pain and suffering. • Suffering: getting stuck in an emotion and having that emotion dominate your life. • Pain which is actually being in the process and suddenly becoming tearful. The concept of judgement is discussed. Participants are discouraged from judging themselves or others.
Class 2:	The focus is on shock and denial about the loss and the processes involved. Discussion focuses on what it was like at the time of the event and where each participant might still be experiencing denial.
Class 3 & 4:	The focus is on anger. For example, there is a homework assignment in which participants are asked to define what anger is for them, what loss is to them, and to examine the interrelationships between the two. Participants are asked to observe how they express anger, do they do it in healthy ways? In the fourth class, examples are given of ways to deal with anger appropriately. Vocal and physical methods of reaching past the anger to the pain are explored.
Class 5:	Guilt. A distinction is made between shame and guilt. The "could have," "should have," and "would have's" are discussed.
Class 6:	Depression. The occurrence of depression is acknowledged and the distinction between clinical depression and the depression occurring as part of the bereavement process are reviewed. The concept of accepting depression and its benefit rather than resisting is presented. It can be looked at as a "time out".
Class 7:	Powerlessness. The group looks at what parts of their experience had them feel most out of control. Ways to empower themselves are then discussed.
Class 8:	The last class is a summary and closing which includes reconstruction and review. The participants look at the progress made in 8 weeks and examine aspects that are easier for them now. They also look at a life without the deceased person.

From Higgins, P. Reno Bereavement Support Group.

warning which parents had about the death of the infant. Was the pregnancy desired or planned? Have there been other losses in the family in the last 12 to 24 months? What are the religious structures that support the family unit and are they perceived as helpful and an intimate support system? What are the size and types of connections within the social network? Are there key people who are supportive and with whom the parents feel connected?

Nursing Intervention

After careful assessment of the parents' needs and strengths, nursing diagnoses and planning will help to establish priority in nursing interventions. Physical comfort and physical support measures are necessary through the pregnancy and birth experience. Psychological support is given by the nursing staff with support for the processes through which the woman and her family are proceeding. The more families know, the better they are able to cope. Support can be given by allowing the parents to see and hold the dead infant, if they so desire. On the other hand, they are not forced into situations that they desire to avoid. Mementos of the child help in the grieving process. Allowing the parents to know that they can make choices is beneficial to them. It may be helpful for the nurse to discuss with the parents how they will inform other family members, other children, or friends. Follow-up care should be planned carefully so that the parents are not forgotten or lost in the process. Goals and nursing intervention are outlined in Table 12-3. Nursing care in acute grief work was summarized in Table 12-2 earlier in the chapter.

Parent Support Groups

Due to the dichotomy between the reality of the parental experience and the societal behavior of family and friends, parents often feel a need to find support elsewhere. Consequently, in the last 15 years groups focusing specifically on bereavement support have sprung up across the United States. Examples include hospital-based support groups, Compassionate Friends, community-based grief institutes, and Resolve Through Sharing. Parents find in these groups that which they could not find elsewhere—a supportive social network.

Two distinct types of support groups exist. One is an ongoing group, in which bereaved parents may enter or leave the group at will. The second type is a structured group in which a specific number of formal classes are conducted (Display 12-2). In addition to these two types, there are a variety of structures within groups themselves. These less formal groups can be facilitated by parents or professionals. If professionals are involved, the groups can be either informal and focus on facilitation or formal and focus on therapeutic interventions. In the early days of bereavement support, there was much more focus on informal groups with professionals as facilitators rather than therapists.

Originally, the more informal support group participants worked very hard to improve the way health care was provided for bereaved parents. They produced pamphlets about issues confronting the newly bereaved, attended hospital physician and nurse staff meetings to educate professionals about the process of bereavement, and distributed information to the community. These efforts frequently added meaning to the parent's lives and created something positive out of a tragedy.

HEALING THE HEALER

It takes great stamina and peace of mind to be a professional caring for families experiencing perinatal loss. This is particularly true in face of the professional's personal responses to bereavement. Frequently, healthcare professionals are reminded not only of their own future demise, but also of other losses that have occurred in their lives. Feelings of sadness and grief over personal and professional losses are often repressed. Nurses and other healthcare professionals often do what society suggests—they "get on with their lives." When losses go unacknowledged and the grief process is denied, losses begin to stack one on top of the other. Consequently, when some nurses are confronted with death, their unacknowledged feelings of failure and their unprocessed and unacknowledged losses rise to the conscience level. It is not unusual to respond by feeling out of control, tearful, and focused on issues of self. Professionals are not unique in these feelings and responses; the family and friends of the grieving parents are often in similar positions.

In the process of healing themselves, professionals begin at their own level of awareness of past losses and past behavior. Usually, they make conscious decisions to add value to their own lives and to the lives of bereaved parents by focusing on growth and functioning at a higher level. Professionals commit time and energy to reading, learning, and acknowledging their own processes of loss and bereavement as well as acquiring skills and tools to better support the bereaved. In acquiring such skills they provide support to colleagues by demonstrating role-modeling behavior with the bereaved. They help inexperienced nurses and physicians in understanding their own feelings and how to work with parents. Novice care providers should not be expected to work with these very complex situations without prior experience, direction, and role models.

Professionals can gain more experience and understanding by attending workshops on bereavement support and death and dying. Grief institutes and other relevant workshops and learning experiences focus on adult growth and development. Additional insights into human behavior can support new attitudes and belief systems about involvement with the bereaved. Nurses working in complex bereavement situations in pediatric intensive care, neonatal intensive care, and high-risk obstetrics can be helped by skilled members of the chaplaincy corps, social work department, or

TABLE 12-3. Nursing Interventions with Grieving Families

Goals	Purpose	Action
Provide psychological support	• To develop a trust relationship	• be warm and caring • listen attentively • exhibit unconditional positive regard • respond truthfully • keep parents informed • minimize number of caregivers for continuity
Keep families together	• To assess all members • To provide support	• teach about bereavement process • answer questions • teach specific interventions for supporting the bereaved
Give opportunity to see and hold deceased child	• To create a memory so that a clear connection is made to the family • The death is a reality	• encourage (not force) seeing and holding • describe infant prior to event–prepare for viewing by changing and wrapping in blanket • dress infant if possible to "normalize" (volunteer department/church groups make beautiful outfits) • ensure support (nurse will stay with parents while infant is with them) • show all infants (even with anomalies) • identify familiar characteristics
Provide photographs and other mementos	• To facilitate integration of experience into life	• support other family members to see • have polaroid camera to take photos • include anything that touched infant • use 35mm camera to increase clarity or 1st photo camera • take one photo of infant being held by parents if possible • save mementos in permanent file if parents say they don't want them (most claim them within 12 months) • provide any of the usual hospital keepsakes: ID bracelet, footprint record, lock of hair

TABLE 12-3. Cont.

Goals	Purpose	Action
Provide choices	• To give parents a sense of some control over a situation that feels out of control	• identify choices and options: –what unit they want to be on –funeral and/or memorial service –by whom and where infant will be seen by others –choice to bathe infant with nurse's assistance
Participate in hospital paperwork	• To prepare parents for decisions to be made	• Discuss autopsy • Give death certificate information including name • Discuss funeral arrangements and memorial service
Informing family and friends	• To provide choices for dealing with shock and surprise of friends	• have a resource book in OB/Neonatal areas that supports off-shift personnel in working with families
Develop method to tell other siblings	• To support parents in thinking through how they want to inform other children	• encourage parents to be open and direct with children. Do not say, "The baby went to sleep," or "God took the baby" • Encourage parents to acknowledge feelings of sadness and fear–baby will be missed just as other children would be • Help parents place and express the death within the families' religious belief • Assure other children they in no way caused the baby's death
Provide bereavement education	• To teach families the normal process so that behavioral expectations will be "normal"	• identify four phases of grief • use Parks symptomatology of loss • include list of area parent support groups • discuss the emotional roller coaster • discuss length of grieving: normal time can last 12 months or more • tell parents they can choose how they respond to the event –make reading/book referrals –alert parents to thoughtless things people will say to them

TABLE 12-3. Cont.

Goals	Purpose	Action
Give follow-up care	• To ensure ongoing assessment and support posthospital discharge	• schedule physician visits for last appointment of day—so they can ask questions and don't feel rushed • ask to go in on gyn day • be sure to inform office staff of infant death when making an appointment over the phone • can schedule support group discussion during wait in physician office • use all available resources, i.e., chaplain, social worker, public health nurse, etc. • provide community health nurse referral • prepare parents for fact that final autopsy report takes 3 months to receive • connect parents with a support group
Prepare for subsequent pregnancy	• To make concerned recommendations for further attempts to conceive	• suggest parents wait 6 months to attempt to conceive—for psychologic and bereavement process reasons • Discuss fact that mother needs as much emotional healing as possible prior to conceiving so her perception of subsequent pregnancy can be "normal".

psychiatric department. This kind of support for the nursing staff can truly facilitate nurses in their own healing.

SUMMARY

The nurse is the pivotal care provider with families who experience perinatal loss and bereavement. When the nurse intervenes using knowledge and skills from psychologic, sociologic, spiritual and ontologic perspectives, parents feel cared for, understood, and supported.

Recommended reading for bereaved parents

Berezin, N. (1982). After a loss in pregnancy. New York: Simon & Schuster.

Borg, S., & Lasker, J. (1981). When pregnancy fails. Boston: Beacon.

Ewy, D., & Ewy, R. (1984). Death of a dream. New York: Dutton

Nouwen, H. (1974). Out of solitude. South Bend, IN: Ave Maria.

Viorst, J. (1986). Necessary losses. New York: Simon & Schuster.

References

Averill, J. (1975). Grief: Its nature and experience. Chapel Hill, NC: Health Sciences.

Bowlby, J. (1980). Attachment and loss (Vol. 2). New York: Basic Books.

Darwin, C. (1864). A concordance to Darwin's: The expression of the emotions in man and animals'. Barret, NY: Cornell University.

Freud, S. (1937). Mourning and melancholia. In The standard edition of the complete psychological works of Sigmund Freud (Vol. 14). London: Hogarth.

Hutti, M.H. (1992). Parents' perceptions of the miscarriage experience. Death Studies, 16, 401-415.

Irion, P.E. (1976). The mourning of the caring professional. Ethicon, 13(2), 8-9.

Kowalski, K.E.M. (1984). Perinatal death: An ethnomethodological study of factors influencing parental bereavement. Doctoral dissertation, University of Colorado, Boulder.

Kowalski, K. (1987). Perinatal loss and bereavement. In L. Sonstegard, K. Kowalski, & B. Jennings (Eds.), Women's health: Crisis and illness in child bearing. Orlando, FL: Grune & Stratton.

Kowalski, K. (1991). No happy ending: Pregnancy loss and bereavement. NAACOG's Clinical Issues in Perinatal and Women's Health Issues, 2(3), 368-380.

Kowalski, K. (1985). The impact of chronic grief. American Journal of Nursing, 85(4), 398-399.

Lattanzi, M.E. (1983). Professional stress: Adaptation, coping and meaning. In J.C. Hansen & T.T. Frantz (Eds.), Death and grief in the family. Rockvillé, MD: Aspen Systems.

Lindemann, E. (1944). Symptomatology and management of acute grief. American Journal of Psychiatry, 101, 141-148.

Maris, P. (1974). Loss and change. New York: Pantheon.

Parkes, C.M. (1970). The first year of bereavement: A longitudinal study of the reaction of London widows to the death of their husbands. Psychiatry, 33(4), 444-467.

Peppers, L.G., & Knapp, R.S. (1980). Motherhood and mourning: Perinatal death. New York: Praeger.

Peretz, D. (1970a). Development, object-relationships and loss. In B. Schoenberg, A.C. Karr, D. Peretz, & A.H. Kutscher (Eds.), Loss and grief: Psychological management in medical practice. New York: Columbia University.

Peretz, D. (1970b). Reaction to loss. In B. Schoenberg, A.C. Karr, D. Peretz, & A.H. Kutscher (Eds.), Loss and grief: Psychological management in medical practice. New York: Columbia University.

Pincus, L. (1974). Death and the family: The importance of mourning. New York: Pantheon.

Stevenson, K.M. (1980). Parental utilization and perceptions of helpful social networks following a sudden infant death. Doctoral dissertation, University of Washington, Seattle.

Swanson-Kauffman, K. (1983). The unborn one: A profile of human experience of miscarriage. Doctoral dissertation, University of Colorado, Denver.

Warrick, C. (1993, March 16). Healing Native American spirituality helps kids deal with grief: Interview with Steve Sunderland. Cincinnati Post, p. 1b.

PART 5

The Newborn

Newborn Adapation to Extrauterine Life

Dawn Reimann
Mary Coughlin

Transition from fetal to newborn life is a critical period involving diverse physiologic changes. Hemodynamic and thermoregulatory mechanisms function to assure successful adaptation to the extrauterine environment. This chapter focuses on maternal history influencing adaptation and physiologic changes during the early newborn period. Nursing assessment and interventions during transition such as resuscitative needs and interventions facilitating maternal/newborn attachment are also presented.

INFLUENCE OF MATERNAL HISTORY

Maternal medical and obstetric conditions influence newborn adaptation to extrauterine life; therefore, a thorough review of the mother's prenatal and intrapartum history is essential to identify factors with the potential to compromise successful transition. See Table 13-1 for maternal risk factors and associated fetal and neonatal complications. In addition to identification of current pregnancy complications, it is important to review prior obstetrical history. Conditions that predispose the newborn to risk may recur in subsequent pregnancies (Display 13-1). Intrapartum risk factors may also influence adaptation (Table 13-2). Intrapartum fetal assessment provides important data about fetal response to labor. Electronic fetal heart rate (FHR) monitoring allows continuous documentation of fetal well-being. Requisite perinatal nursing skills include knowledge of the physiologic basis for monitoring, FHR patterns and the initiation of appropriate nursing interventions based on data from the monitor. The fetal monitor strip illustrates fetal response to labor. The perinatal nurse focuses on discriminating between reassuring and nonreassuring patterns. If the FHR pattern is nonreassuring, intrauterine resuscitation procedures such as maternal position change, oxygen therapy, and intravenous fluids are initiated. Safe passage through the labor and birth process sets the stage for successful transition to extrauterine life.

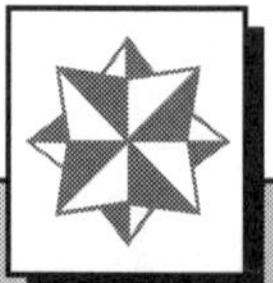

DISPLAY 13-1

Previous Pregnancy Complications Which May Reoccur in Subsequent Pregnancies

Fetal loss over 28 weeks of gestation
Preterm Birth
Abnormal fetal position/presentation
Bleeding in second or third trimester
Rh sensitization
Fetal compromise of unknown origin
Birth of newborn with anomalies
Birth of newborn over 10 lb
Birth of postterm newborn
Neonatal death

PHYSIOLOGIC CHANGES DURING TRANSITION

The respiratory, cardiovascular, thermoregulatory, and immunologic systems undergo significant physiologic changes and adaptations during the transition from fetal to neonatal life. Successful transition requires a complex interaction between these systems.

Respiratory Adaptations

Critical to the neonate's transition to extrauterine life is the establishment of respirations, as lungs become the organ of gas exchange after separation from maternal uteroplacental circulation. Initiation of breathing is a complex phenomena dependent on chemical, thermal, and sensory stimulation of the respiratory center in the brain, and mechanical stimulation of the lung. Pulmonary blood flow, surfactant production, and respiratory musculature are additional factors influencing respiratory adaptation to extrauterine life. Establishment of independent breathing and oxygen/carbon dioxide exchange is dependent on these physiologic factors.

Chemical Stimuli

Mild, transitory physiologic stress is experienced by the fetus during labor and birth. This normal response occurs due to temporary interruption in umbilical blood flow during uterine contractions and ultimately when the umbilical cord is clamped. Decreased oxygen concentration, increased carbon dioxide concentration, and decreased pH stimulate fetal aortic and carotid chemoreceptors, triggering the respiratory center in the medulla to initiate respiration (Nelson, 1994).

TABLE 13-1. Maternal Risk Factors and Potential Fetal and Neonatal Complications

Risk Factors	Potential Complications
Maternal Substance Abuse	
Drug addiction	Small for gestational age (SGA); neonatal abstinence syndrome; neonatal human immunodeficiency virus (HIV)
Alcoholism	Fetal alcohol syndrome
Smoking	SGA; polycythemia
Maternal Nutritional Status	
Maternal weight <100 lbs	SGA
Maternal weight >200 lbs	SGA; Large for gestational age (LGA)
Maternal Medical Complication	
Hereditary CNS disorders	Inherited central nervous system (CNS) disorder
Seizure disorders requiring medication	Congenital anomalies (result of medication [Dilantin] use)
Chronic hypertension	Intrauterine growth restriction (IUGR); asphyxia; SGA
Congenital heart disease with congestive heart failure	Preterm birth; inhereted cardiac defects
Anemia <10 g	Preterm birth; low birth weight
Sickle cell disease	IUGR; fetal demise
Hemoglobinopathies	IUGR; inherited hemoglobinopathies
Idiopathic thrombocytopenic purpura (ITP)	Transient ITP
Chronic glomerulonephritis; Renal insufficiency	IUGR; SGA; preterm birth; asphyxia
Recurrent urinary tract infection	Preterm birth
Uterine malformation	Preterm birth; fetal malposition
Cervical incompetence	Preterm birth
Diabetes	LGA; hypoglycemia & hypocalcemia; anomalies; respiratory distress syndrome
Thyroid disease	Hypothyroidism; CNS defects; Hyperthyroidism; goiter
Current Pregnancy Complications	
Pregnancy induced hypertension	IUGR; SGA
TORCH infections	IUGR; SGA; active infection; anomalies
Sexuality transmitted diseases	Opthalmia neonatorum; congenital syphilis
Hepatitis	Hepatitis
AIDS or HIV seropositive	Neonatal HIV
Multiple gestation	Preterm birth; asphyxia; IUGR; SGA
Fetal Malposition	Prolapsed cord; asphyxia; birth trauma
Rh sensitization	Erythroblastosis fetalis
Prolonged pregnancy	Postmaturity; meconium aspiration; IUGR; asphyxia
Intraamniotic infection	Newborn sepsis; preterm birth
+ Group B-strep	Newborn sepsis; preterm birth

Adapted from Maternal and Neonatal Nursing: Family-Centered Care (3rd ed., pp. 962-963), by K.A. May and L.R. Mahlmeister, 1994b, Philadelphia: J.B. Lippincott.

TABLE 13-2. Intrapartum Risk Factors and Potential Fetal and Neonatal Complications

Risk Factors	Potential Complications
Umbilical Cord	
Prolapsed umbilical cord	Asphyxia
True knot in cord	Asphyxia
Velamentous insertion	Intrauterine blood loss; shock; anemia
Vasa previa	Intrauterine blood loss; shock; anemia
Rupture or tearing of cord	Blood loss; shock; anemia
Membranes	
Premature rupture of membranes	Infection; respiratory distress syndrome; prolapsed cord; asphyxia
Prolonged rupture of membranes	Infection
Amnionitis	Infection
Amniotic Fluid	
Oligohydramnios	Congenital anomalies
Polyhydramnios	Congenital anomalies; prolapsed cord
Meconium-stained fluid	Asphyxia; meconium aspiration syndrome
Placenta	
Placenta previa	Preterm birth; asphyxia
Abruptio placenta	Preterm birth; asphyxia
Placental insufficiency	IUGR; SGA; asphyxia
Abnormal Fetal Presentations	
Breech birth	Asphyxia; birth injuries (CNS, Skeletal)
Face or brow presentation	Asphyxia; facial trauma
Transverse lie cord prolapse	Asphyxia; birth injuries; cesarean birth; umbilical
Birth Complications	
Forceps-assisted birth	CNS trauma; cephalhematoma; asphyxia; facial trauma
Vacuum extraction	Cephalhematoma
Manual version or extraction	Asphyxia; birth trauma; prolapsed cord
Shoulder dystocia	Asphyxia; brachial plexus injury; fractured clavicle
Precipitous birth	Asphyxia; birth trauma (CNS)
Undiagnosed multiple gestation	Asphyxia; birth trauma
Administration of Drugs	
Oxytocin	Complications of uterine hyperstimulation (asphyxia)
Magnesium sulfate	Hypermagnesemia; CNS depression
Analgesics	CNS and respiratory depression
Anesthetics	CNS and respiratory depression; bradycardia

Adapted from *Maternal and Neonatal Nursing: Family-Centered Care* (3rd ed., p. 964), by K.A. May and L.R. Mahlmeister, 1994a), Philadelphia: J.B. Lippincott.

Mechanical Stimulation

In utero, fetal lungs are filled with fluid. Mechanical compression of the chest during vaginal birth forces approximately 1/3 of this fluid out of fetal lungs. As the chest is delivered through the birth canal, it reexpands creating negative pressure and drawing air into the lungs. This passive inspiration of air replaces fluid that previously filled alveoli. Further expansion and distribution of air throughout the alveoli occurs when the infant cries. Crying creates a positive intrathoracic pressure keeping alveoli open, and forcing remaining fetal lung fluid into pulmonary capillaries and lymphatic circulation.

Thermal Stimuli

Cold stress also stimulates breathing. After birth when the newborn is exposed to a much cooler environmental temperature than in utero (98.6°F compared with 70-72°F), thermal receptors in the skin trigger the respiratory center to initiate breathing. (Mahlmeister, 1994b). Care is taken to prevent excessive chilling, since hypothermia may cause respiratory compromise by increasing metabolic rate, increasing oxygen consumption, decreasing surfactant production, and increasing glucose metabolism.

Sensory Stimuli

The newborn is exposed to numerous tactile, visual, auditory, and olfactory stimuli during and immediately after birth. Tactile stimulation begins in utero as the fetus experiences uterine contractions and descent through the pelvis and birth canal. Stimulation to initiate breathing continues after birth as the neonate is exposed to stimuli such as light, sound, touch, smell, and pain. Vigorously drying the newborn immediately after birth is a significant tactile stimulation.

Contributing Factors

Maturation of alveoli. Newborn lungs contain approximately 20-24 million alveoli. These terminal air sacs grow in size and number reaching 296-300 million during childhood or early adult years (Blackburn, 1992). Structural characteristics of alveoli unique to the newborn period influence oxygenation and carbon dioxide transport. During the newborn period, small size and limited number of alveoli decrease alveolar surface area available for gas exchange. Also, the alveolar wall is thick, making the movement of oxygen and carbon dioxide across the membrane difficult (Blackburn, 1992).

Pulmonary blood flow. In utero, the placenta is the organ of gas exchange for the fetus. Oxygenated blood is delivered from the placenta via the umbilical vein through the inferior vena cava, ductus venosus, superior vena cava, and ultimately to the right side of the fetal heart. Oxygenated blood is diverted from pulmonary circulation in utero and instead flows through the ductus arteriosus to the fetal body. Constriction of pulmonary arterioles, creating high pulmonary vascular resistance (PVR), results in decreased pulmonary blood flow. Fetal pulmonary arterioles have thick musculature due to low oxygen tension in utero (Blackburn & Loper, 1992). After birth, pulmonary blood flow is established as PVR decreases with normal changes in arterial PO_2, alveolar PO_2, acid/base status, and absence of vasoactive substances such as prostaglandin and bradykinin (Blackburn, 1992).

The fluid-filled lungs of the fetus create a state of alveolar hypoxia (Hazinski, 1992). After birth, following onset of breathing, fluid in the lungs is replaced by air. Since oxygen is a potent vasodilator, pulmonary vasodilation occurs. Adequate pulmonary blood flow is crucial for newborn gas exchange.

Surfactant production. Pulmonary surfactant is necessary to maintain expanded alveoli. Surfactant lowers surface tension preventing alveolar collapse during inspiration and expiration. By approximately 34 to 35 weeks of gestation there is adequate surfactant production to support respiration and protect against development of respiratory distress syndrome (Hagedorn, Gardner & Abman, 1993). Surfactant deficiency increases risk of atelactasis and requires greater than normal breathing efforts. Oxygen and metabolic needs increase as the newborn must use more energy to maintain respirations. Preterm newborns are at high risk for surfactant deficiency which may significantly jeopardize respiratory adaptation to extrauterine life.

Respiratory musculature. Intercostal muscles support the rib cage and assist with inspiration by creating negative intrathoracic pressure. Intercostal muscles may not be fully developed at birth, thus increasing risk of respiratory compromise by increasing breathing effort.

Cardiovascular Adaptations

Transition from fetal to neonatal circulation is a major cardiovascular change and occurs simultaneously with respiratory system adaptation. To appreciate hemodynamic changes, an understanding of structural and blood-flow differences between fetal and neonatal

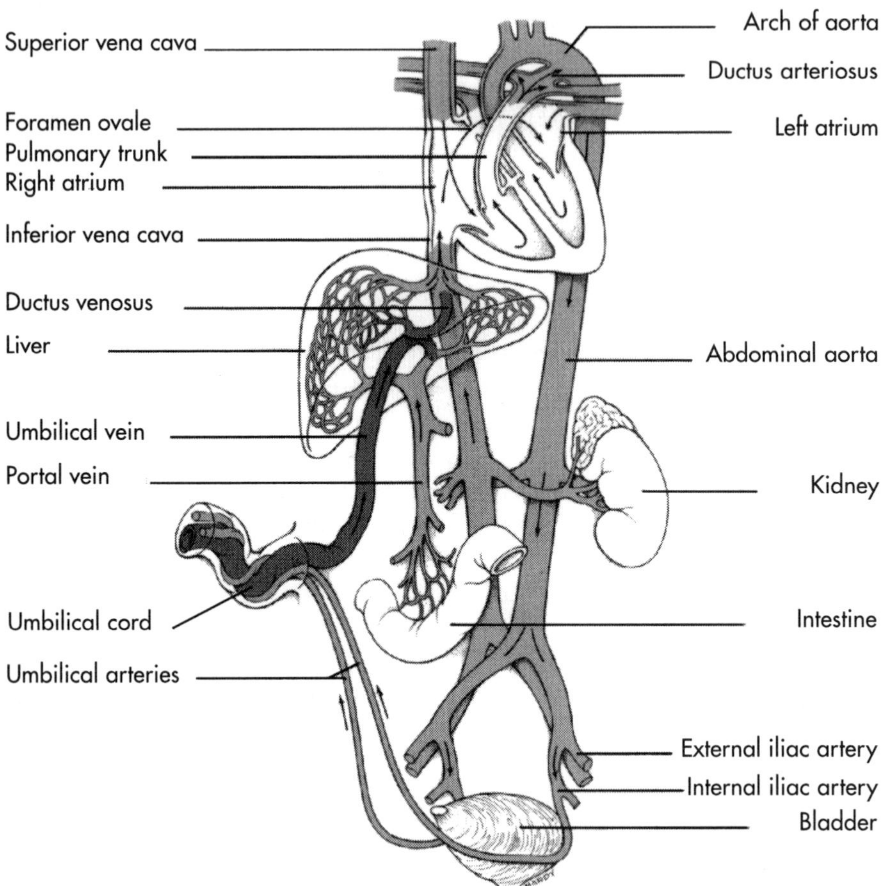

Figure 13–1. Fetal Circulation.

Adapted from Maternal and Neonatal Nursing: Family–Centered Care (3rd ed., p. 264), by K.A. May and L.R. Mahlmeister, 1994, Philadelphia: J.B. Lippincott.

circulation is necessary. Figure 13-1 illustrates fetal circulation. Also influencing the cardiovascular system are physiologic changes in the vasculature. Decreased PVR, resulting in increased pulmonary blood flow and increased systemic vascular resistance (SVR), controls cardiovascular changes.

Fetal Circulation

In utero, oxygenated blood flows to the fetus from the placenta through the umbilical vein. Although a small amount of oxygenated blood is delivered to the liver, the majority bypasses the hepatic system through the ductus venosus. The ductus venosus is a vascular structure that forms a connection between the umbilical vein and the inferior vena cava. Oxygenated blood from the vena cava enters the right atrium and most is directed through the foramen ovale to the left atrium, to the left ventricle, and on to the aorta. Foramen ovale is a flap-like structure located between the right and left atrium. Blood flows through the foramen ovale because pressure in the right atrium is greater than the left atrium, due to high PVR.

Superior vena cava drains deoxygenated blood from the head and upper extremities into the right atrium, where it mixes with oxygenated blood. Because of increased PVR, only a small amount of blood in the right atrium is directed into the right ventricle and pulmonary artery. This blood circulates to lung tissue, to meet metabolic needs. Because PVR is high, most is diverted through the ductus arteriosus, a vascular connection between the pulmonary artery and the aorta. This mixture of oxygenated and deoxygenated blood continues through the descending aorta and eventually drains back to the placenta via the umbilical arteries.

Neonatal Circulation

During fetal life, the placenta is an organ of low vascular resistance. Clamping the umbilical cord at birth eliminates the placenta as a reservoir for blood, causing a rise in blood pressure and SVR. Blood returns to the heart via the inferior and superior vena cava. It enters the right atrium to right ventricle and travels through the pulmonary artery to the pulmonary vascular bed. Oxygenated blood returns through pulmonary veins to the left atrium, left ventricle, and through the aorta to systemic circulation. For successful transition from fetal to newborn circulation, structures specific to fetal circulation must cease functioning.

At birth, when the pulmonary vascular bed dilates, there is increased blood flow to the lungs, and pressure in the right atrium falls. Additionally, there is increased pulmonary venous return to the left atrium, causing increased left atrial pressure and closure of the foramen ovale (Bloom, 1992). Blood is directed from the right atrium to the right ventricle, rather than through the foramen ovale.

In utero, shunting of blood from the pulmonary artery through the ductus arteriosus to the aorta occurs as a result of high PVR. After birth, SVR rises and PVR falls, causing a reversal of blood flow through the ductus. The major contributing factor to closure of the ductus arteriosus is sensitivity to rising arterial oxygen concentrations in the blood (Bloom, 1992). As the PaO_2 level increases after birth, the ductus arteriosus begins to constrict (Nelson, 1994). In utero, elevated prostaglandin levels helped maintain ductal patency. Removal of the placenta decreases prostaglandin levels, further influencing closure (Nelson, 1994).

Constriction of the ductus arteriosus is a gradual process, permitting bidirectional shunting of blood after birth. PVR may be higher than the SVR, allowing some degree of right to left shunting, until the SVR rises above PVR and blood flow is directed left to right. In healthy, full-term newborns, right to left shunting can persist for up to 12 hours of life; most will have a closed or closing ductus arteriosus by 24 hours of life (Walther, Benders & Leighton, 1993). Permanent anatomic closure of the ductus arteriosus occurs within 3 weeks to 3 months of age. Any clinical situation that causes hypoxia, with pulmonary vasoconstriction and subsequent increased PVR, will potentiate right-to-left shunting (Lott, 1993).

When the umbilical cord is clamped, blood flow through the umbilical vein to the ductus venosus ceases. Systemic venous blood flow is now directed, through the portal system for hepatic circulation. Umbilical vessels constrict, with functional closure occurring immediately (Zabloudil, 1993). Fibrous infiltration occurs at about 1 to 2 weeks of life leading to anatomical closure (Lott, 1993).

Relationship Between Respiratory and Cardiovascular Adaptation

Successful initiation of respirations and transition from fetal to neonatal circulation is essential to maintain life after birth. Conditions that lead to sustained high PVR such as hypoxia, acidosis, or congenital heart defects can interrupt the normal sequence of events. Closure of fetal shunts is dependent on oxygenation and pressure changes within the cardiovascular system. Closure of these shunts occurs only if PVR drops with the onset of respiration and subsequent oxygenation. The pulmonary vascular bed is very reactive to low oxygen levels. If the neonate experiences significant hypoxia, PVR with resultant decreased pulmonary blood flow and right-to-left shunting across the foramen ovale and ductus arteriosus may occur. These events potentiate an hypoxic state, as deoxygenated blood bypasses the lungs through the patent fetal shunts to be mixed with oxygenated blood entering the systemic circulation. A vicious cycle results, necessitating aggressive cardiorespiratory support.

Thermoregulation

The newborn's ability to maintain temperature control after birth is limited by external environmental factors and internal physiologic processes. Characteristics of newborns that predispose them to heat loss include a large body area in relation to body mass and a limited amount of subcutaneous fat. Newborns attempt to regulate body temperature by nonshivering thermogenesis, increased metabolic rate, and increased muscle activity. Peripheral vasoconstriction also decreases heat loss to the skin surface. Mechanisms of heat-loss evaporation, conduction, convection, and radiation play an integral part in newborn adaptation to extrauterine life. Nursing care is critical in supporting thermoregulation through ongoing assessments and environmental interventions to decrease heat loss.

Mechanisms of Heat Production

Nonshivering thermogenesis. Newborns generate heat through nonshivering thermogenesis. Heat is produced by metabolism of brown fat, a unique process present only in newborns. This highly vascular adipose tissue is located in the neck, scapula, axilla, mediastinum, and around kidneys and adrenal gland. Production of brown fat begins around 26 to 28 weeks of gestation and continues for 3 to 5 weeks after birth (Thomas, 1994). When exposed to cold stress, thermal receptors in skin transmit messages to the central nervous system, activating the sympathetic nervous system and triggering metabolism of brown fat (Gerds, 1992). Preterm newborns, with smaller brown-fat stores, have decreased ability to generate heat. Instead, they rely on increased oxygen consumption and muscle activity to increase metabolic rate and produce heat (Roncoli & Medoff-Cooper, 1992).

Voluntary muscle activity. Heat produced through voluntary muscle activity is minimal in the newborn. Flexion of the extremities and maintaining a fetal position decreases heat loss to the environment. Term newborns have the ability to maintain this flexed posture, while preterm and compromised newborns may lack the muscle tone for this posturing, making them more vulnerable to cold stress (Brueggemeyer, 1993).

Mechanisms of Heat Loss

Evaporation. Evaporation and heat loss occur as water (amniotic fluid) on skin is converted to a vapor. Drying the newborn immediately after birth and removing wet blankets decreases evaporative losses and prevents further cooling of the skin. Amount of insensible water loss from the skin is inversely related to gestational age. Skin of a preterm newborn is more susceptible to evaporative losses, because the keratin layer of the skin has not matured. Absence or greater permeability of this skin layer allows for increased water loss (Thomas, 1994). The larger the surface area, the greater the evaporative losses and the more heat which is lost. Since the newborn's head is the largest surface area of the body, covering the head with a knit cap after birth when not under the radiant warmer greatly conserves heat. Adding humidity to the environment may also decrease evaporative heat loss.

Conduction. Conductive heat loss occurs when two solid objects of differing temperatures come in contact. Heat loss occurs if the newborn is placed in direct contact with a cold scale, mattress, x-ray plate, or if cold blankets are used. Mechanisms for preventing conductive heat loss in the birthing room and immediately after birth include using a preheated radiant warmer, warm blankets for drying, and warm blankets covering scales and x-ray plates. Preheating the radiant warmer is necessary, since it may take 15-30 minutes to warm the mattress.

Providing skin-to-skin contact between mother and newborn after birth helps prevent conductive heat loss and enhances maternal-infant attachment. Newborns who experience extended periods of skin-to-skin contact, beginning soon after birth, demonstrate heart rates, respiratory rates, and oxygen saturation levels within normal limits (Ludington-Hoe et al., 1993). Preterm newborns provided with opportunities for skin-to-skin contact with their mothers maintained their temperature; demonstrated normal vital signs; had increased episodes of deep sleep and alert inactivity; had less crying, no increase in infection rates, greater weight gain, longer breastfeeding periods, and earlier discharge (Anderson, 1991). Axillary temperatures of full-term newborns placed under a radiant heat source or on their mother's abdomen do not differ significantly within 10 minutes of birth (Vaughans, 1990).

Convection. Convection is the transfer of heat from a solid object to surrounding air. Heat is lost from newborn skin as cooler air passes over it. Convection heat loss is dependent on amount of exposed skin surface, temperature of air, and amount of air turbulence created by drafts (Thomas, 1994). Interventions which prevent convection heat loss in the newborn include clothing, eliminating source of drafts, and when necessary, providing heated, humidified oxygen through face mask or hood.

Radiation. Radiation heat loss occurs when heat is transferred from two objects not in contact with each other. The newborn loses heat by radiation to cooler surfaces in close proximity such as cold crib or isolette walls, cold windows, or cold objects. Some of the more common and efficient methods for preventing radiant heat loss are use of a radiant warmer after birth, moving crib or isolette away from a cold window, and use of a heat shield inside an incubator (for small, preterm infants) creating an additional warmer barrier between skin and incubator wall.

Effects of Cold Stress

Thermal management of the newborn during the first few hours of life is critical to prevent detrimental effects of cold stress and hypothermia. Table 13-3 summarizes nursing interventions that support the newborn and

TABLE 13-3. Mechanisms of Heat Loss and Nursing Interventions That Prevent Heat Loss

Evaporation	Dry infant thoroughly
	Remove wet linen
	Place knit cap on head when not under radiant warmer
	Bathe under radiant heat source after temperature stabilizes
Convection	Move away from drafts, open windows, vents, traffic patterns
	When necessary use humidified, warmed oxygen
	Move infant in transport isolette
Conduction	Preheat radiant warmer
	Use warmed blanket
	Place cover between newborn and metal scale, x-ray plate
Radiation	Place stabilizing unit on an interior wall of the birthing room (away from cold windows)
	Preheat radiant warmer, transport isolette

prevent cold stress. Since heat production requires oxygen consumption and glucose utilization, persistent hypothermia may deplete these stores leading to metabolic acidosis, hypoglycemia, decreased surfactant production, and increased caloric requirements (Mahlmeister, 1994b). This process is illustrated in Figure 13-2.

Immune System Adaptation

Newborns are vulnerable to infection because of their immature immune system and lack of exposure to organisms. Neonates are dependent on passive immunity acquired from their mother transplacentally through active transport of IgG during the third trimester (Bellanti, Pung & Zeligs, 1994). Preterm infants are at greater risk for infection because they may not have received this passive immunity and because their immune mechanisms are overall more immature (Blackburn & Loper, 1992).

Immunity is conferred through immunoglobulins, antibodies secreted by lymphocytes and plasma cells. There are three main classes of immunoglobulins responsible for immunity, IgG, IgA, and IgM. Because of small molecular size, only IgG antibodies are capable of crossing the placenta. Maternally, transmitted IgG provide protection for the newborn against bacterial and viral infections for which the mother already has antibodies (e.g., diptheria, tetanus, small pox, measles, mumps, and poliomyelitis).

IgM and IgA immunoglobulins do not cross the placenta. If elevated levels of IgM are found in the newborn, it may indicate the presence of an intrauterine infection such as one of the TORCH agents. IgA, found in colostrum, is thought to contribute to passive immunity for newborns who are breast fed (Riordan, 1993).

Immature leukocyte function in the newborn inhibits ability to destroy pathogens. Deficiency in response prevents mature processes of chemotaxis (movement of leukocytes toward site of infection), opsonization (altering or preparing the cells for ingestion), and phagocytosis (ingestion of cells) from occurring. Low levels of immunoglobulins and complement components (plasma proteins that assist the immune system) leaves newborns, especially preterm newborns, vulnerable to infection (Blackburn & Loper, 1992).

Lymphocytes are responsible for the specific response in the immune system that involves antibody production. When lymphocytes are exposed to pathogens, they become sensitized to them. If repeated exposure occurs, lymphocytes will attempt to destroy the pathogen. Since newborns lack exposure to most common organisms, any action by lymphocytes is delayed.

Weak newborn defenses against infection make it imperative for the perinatal nurse and anyone coming in contact with newborns to follow careful hand-washing practices and use of aseptic technique. Promoting skin integrity is of primary importance in preventing neonatal infections. Newborn skin is thin and delicate,

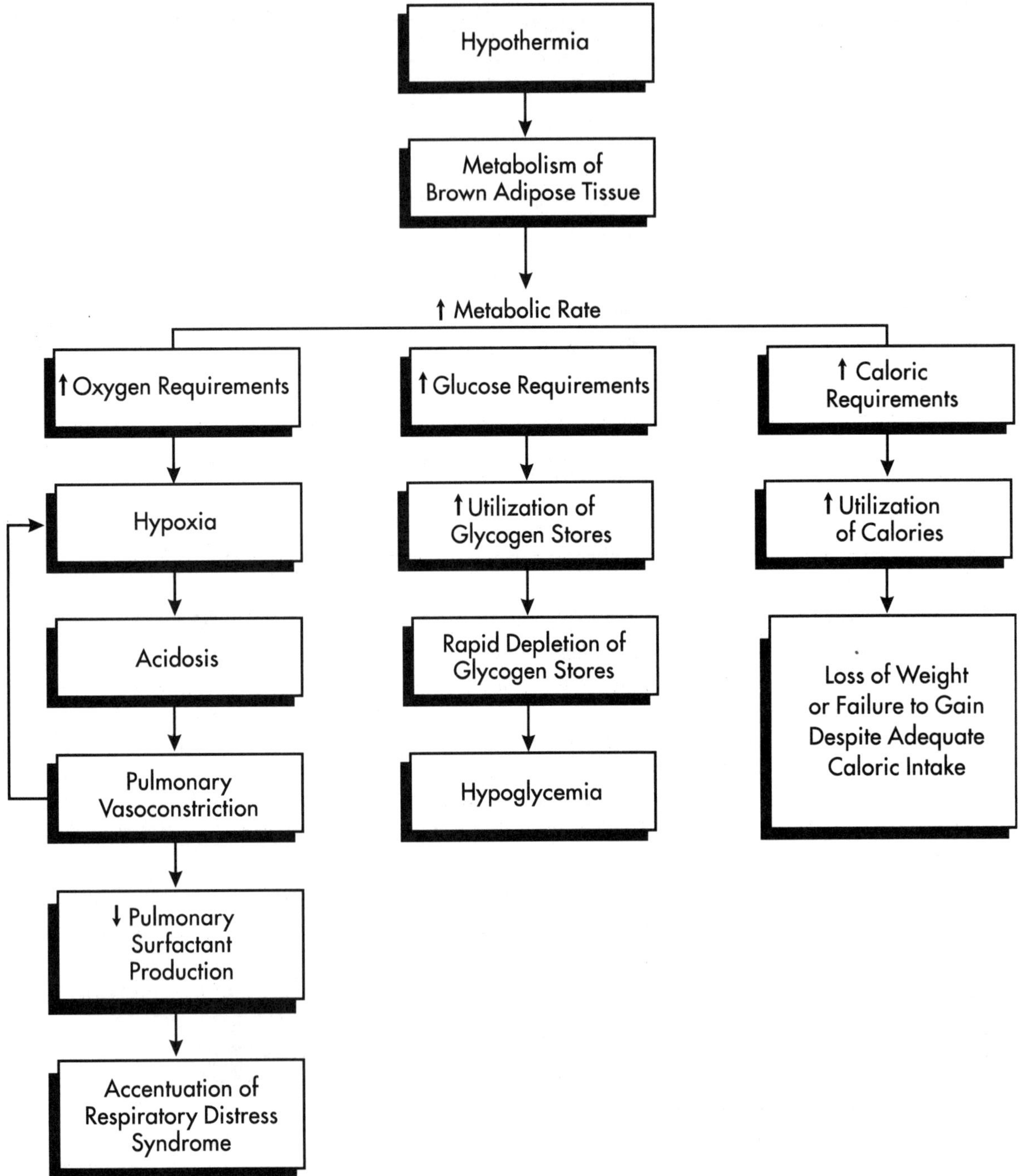

Figure 13–2. Effects of Hypothermia in the Newborn.

Adapted from High–Risk Neonatal Care (p. 101), by N. Streeter, 1986, Rockville, MD: Aspen.

making it susceptible to alteration in integrity. Fetal scalp electrodes, fetal scalp pH sampling, and skin abrasions create portals for entry of organisms. Umbilical cord and circumcision site are also potential sites of infection.

Preterm newborns, with even more fragile skin, are at a greater risk for infection. Invasive procedures, performed during the early hours after birth, further challenge the immune system. Treatments such as vitamin K injection, suctioning, and heelstick blood samples predispose newborns to infection, if proper aseptic technique is not maintained.

STABILIZATION AND RESUSCITATION OF THE NEWBORN

While most births result in a healthy newborn who is able to transition to extrauterine life without difficulty, perinatal nurses must anticipate and prepare for complications. This includes ensuring immediate availability of functioning resuscitation equipment and knowledge of equipment operation. Display 13-2 identifies equipment that should be available in every birthing room.

The Neonatal Resuscitation program developed by the American Heart Association (AHA) and American Academy of Pediatrics (AAP) (1994) has become the standard for educating health care providers involved in newborn stabilization. Using an algorithm, assessments and interventions during newborn resuscitation are clearly outlined. Figure 13-3 illustrates steps used to evaluate and establish airway, breathing, and circulation as a basis for stabilization of the newborn, immediately after birth. While most newborns will respond successfully to oral suctioning and tactile stimulation, some may require additional interventions including ventilation by bag/mask or endotracheal intubation, chest compressions, and administration of resuscitative medications.

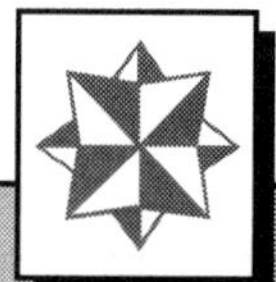

DISPLAY 13-2

Equipment Needed for Neonatal Resuscitation

Clock with second hand
Preheated radiant warmer
Warmed blankets
Neonatal stethoscope
Bulb syringe
Mechanical suction with manometer
Oxygen source, flowmeter, tubing
Resuscitation bag capable of delivering 100% oxygen and pressure gauge
Face masks (newborn and preemie size)
Laryngoscope with size 0 and 1 blades (extra batteries and bulbs)
Endotracheal tubes (sizes 2.5, 3.0, 3.5, and 4.0)
Suction catheters (sizes 5 Fr, 8 Fr, and 10 Fr)
Meconium aspirator device
8 Fr feeding tube
Syringes (Sizes 1 cc, 3 cc, 5 cc, 10 cc, and 20 cc)
Cord clamp
Tape
Resuscitative drugs

- Epinephrine 1:10,000 concentration
- Sodium bicarbonate 4.2%
- Naloxone hydrochloride (1 mg/ ml or 0.4 mg/ml)
- Volume expanders: 5% Albumin
Normal saline
Ringer's lactate

INITIAL ASSESSMENT OF THE NEWBORN

In addition to undergoing dramatic physical changes to adapt to extrauterine life, newborns must handle the events and procedures they are subjected to after birth. Once airway, breathing, and circulation have been established, a thorough assessment of the newborn is performed. This assessment includes Apgar scoring, evaluation of vital signs, physical examination, and measurements. Ideally, all aspects of transitional assessments and care are performed in the presence of parents in the birthing room. Only if maternal or newborn complications occur are parents and newborns separated.

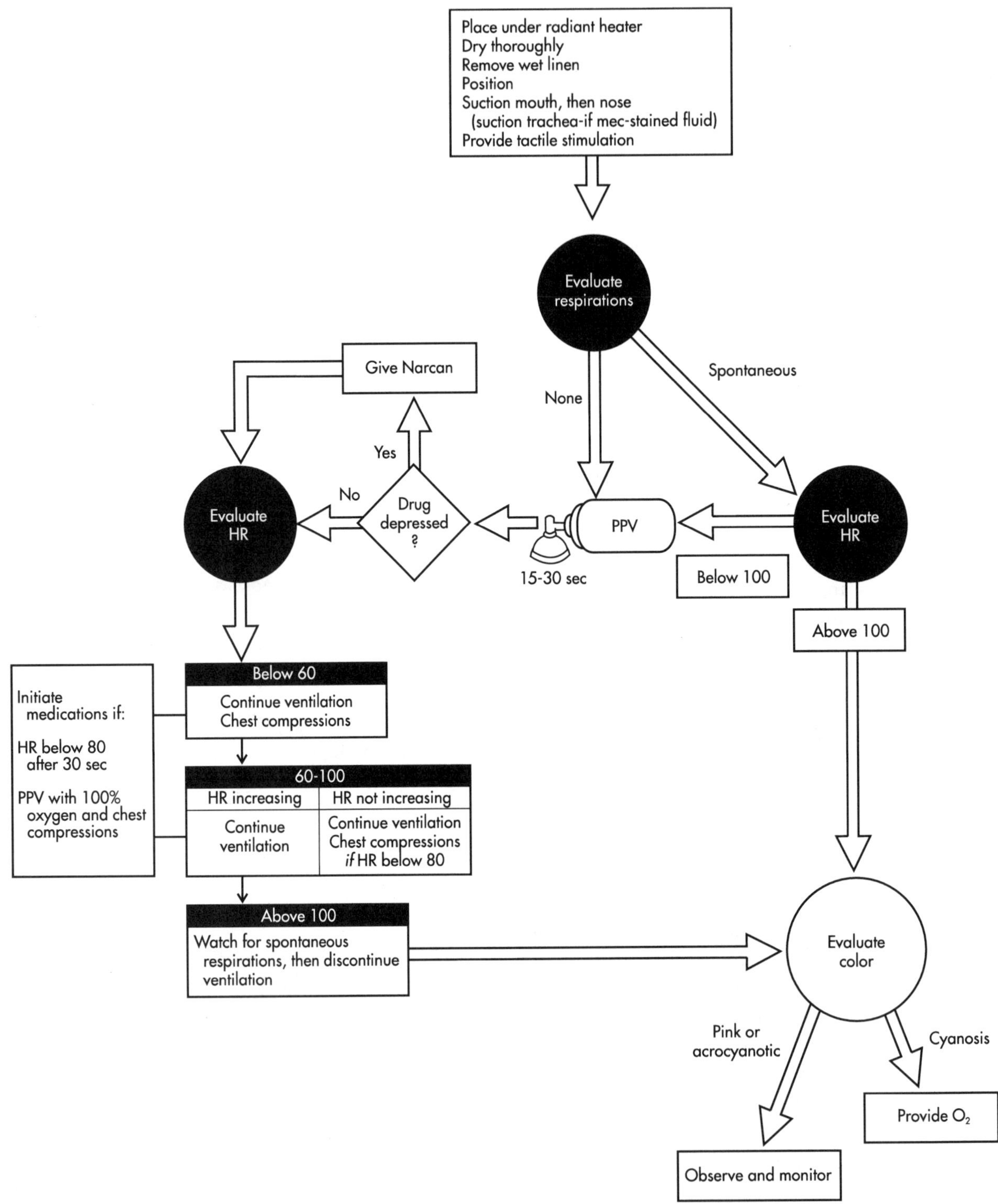

Figure 13–3. Steps for performing neonatal resuscitation

Adapted from Essentials of Maternity Nursing (p. 383), By L.L Martin & S.J. Reeder, 1991, Philadelphia: J.B. Lippincott.

Apgar Score

Introduced in 1952 by Virginia Apgar, M.D., the apgar score provides a simple method to evaluate the condition of the newborn at 1 and 5 minutes after life (Apgar & James, 1962). Five categories (heart rate, respiratory rate, muscle tone, reflex irritability, and color) are each scored from 0-2. Highest total possible score is 10. The AAP and American College of Obstetricians and Gynecologists (ACOG) (1992) recommend a 10-minute apgar score, if earlier scores are less than 7. If the 5-minute apgar score is less than 7, the apgar score should be reevaluated every 5 minutes until 20 minutes have passed or until two successive scores greater than or equal to 7 are obtained. When used to evaluate preterm newborns, the apgar score may have less validity. Findings common in the preterm newborn such as irregular respirations, decreased muscle tone, and decreased reflex irritability will affect the overall score (Paxton & Harrell, 1991). Apgar score should not be used as an indication for resuscitation. (AHA/AAP, 1994).

Initial Physical Assessment

A thorough physical assessment is performed soon after birth. This examination gives the perinatal nurse opportunity to evaluate overall newborn well-being and transition to extrauterine life. Chapter 15 presents a discussion of a comprehensive physical examination including normal and abnormal findings. During the initial examination in the birthing room, all systems are evaluated using inspection, auscultation, and palpation. Figure 13-4 provides an example of a checklist format for documenting the initial newborn physical assessment. During the transitional period after birth, temperature, heart rate, rate and character of respirations, skin color, level of consciousness, muscle tone, and activity level are evaluated and documented at least once every 30 minutes until the newborn's condition has remained stable for 2 hours (AAP & ACOG, 1992).

Skin

An overall visual assessment of the newborn is performed noting any obvious defects (neural tube defects, abdominal wall defects, extra digits, etc.) or trauma (bruising, petechiae, puncture wound from fetal scalp electrode, etc.). Skin is observed for color, texture, birth marks, rashes, and meconium staining. The newborn's back is inspected for presence of a closed vertebral column, masses, and dimple or tuft of hair at the base.

Head and neck

Symmetry of the head and face is noted as well as presence of molding, caput succedaneum, and bruising. Fontanels are palpated. While it is not uncommon for eye lids to be edematous, presence of drainage from the eye or subconjunctival hemorrhage would not be normal during this period. The neck is palpated for masses and full range of motion. Position of ears and presence of skin tags or sinus on or around the ears is noted. While assessing the mucus membrane of the mouth for normal pink color, lips and palate are inspected for presence of a cleft.

Respiratory

Inspection of the chest includes observing shape, symmetry, and equality of chest movement. Asymmetry in chest movement may indicate pneumothorax or congenital defect. Respirations are unlabored at a rate of 30-60 breaths/minute. Retractions, grunting, and nasal flaring are abnormal findings indicating respiratory distress. Breath sounds should be equal bilaterally. Initially, moist sounds may be heard as fluid is cleared from the lungs by absorption through pulmonary capillaries and by drainage through the nose and mouth.

Special attention is paid to newborns, when thick meconium-stained amniotic fluid is present. Since meconium aspiration is a risk, careful assessment of respiratory rate, quality of breath sounds, and color determines need for interventions such as suctioning and chest physiotherapy (CPT). In the absence of thick meconium-stained amniotic fluid, the newborn's mouth and nose are suctioned with a bulb syringe. Use of CPT may facilitate removal of respiratory secretions. Ventilation and oxygenation may improve as a result of postural drainage, percussion, and vibration of the chest. Specific orders are usually written for type and frequency of CPT. Some institutions have standing orders for performing CPT on newborns meeting certain criteria. Oxygen levels may decrease during CPT especially in preterm and low- or very low-birth-weight newborns (Cheng & Williams, 1989). Continuous evaluation of the newborn should occur prior to and while performing CPT .

INITIAL ASSESSMENT

DOB ______________________ Initial Bath: ______________ (Time/Initials) Length: ________ cm. ________ in.

TIME ______________________ Triple Dye to Cord ______________ (Time/Initials) Head: ________ cm. ________ in.

TRANSITIONAL CARE ADMINISTERED IN: Infant Removed from Radiant Warmer: Chest: ________ cm. ________ in.

☐ LDRP ☐ Special Care Nursery Date: __________ Time: __________ Abdomen: ________ cm. ________ in.

Weight: _____ gms. lbs. _____ oz. _____

Time	Radiant Warmer Temp	Temp	Pulse	Resp.	Breath Sounds	B/P	Color	Activity	Muscle Tone	SILVERMAN Upper Chest	Lower Chest	Xiphoid	Flare	Grunt	Total	Chest PT	Initials

COLOR
Pink, Pale, Dusky, Jaundiced, Plethoric, Mottled, Cyanosis, Acrocyanosis

✓ = chest PT

MUSCLE TONE
Normal flexion, Flaccidity, Spasticity

ACTIVITY
Active, Active With Stimulation, Quiet, alert, Irritable, Lethargic, Hyperactive, Tremors, Sleeping

BREATH SOUNDS
Equal, Rales, Clear, Diminished, Rhonchi

SKIN
_____ Pink _____ Acrocyanosis
_____ Central cyanosis _____ Dusky
_____ Pale _____ Plethoric
_____ Mottled _____ Jaundice
_____ Abrasions ______________
_____ Birthmarks ______________
_____ Dry _____ Meconium stained
_____ Ecchymosis ______________
_____ Lacerations ______________
_____ Milia _____ Peeling
_____ Mongolian spots ______________
_____ Petechiae _____ Pustules
_____ Rash ______________
_____ Skin tags ______________
_____ Vesicles

CHEST
_____ Symmetrical _____ Asymmetrical
_____ Barrel chest
_____ Breast engorgement
_____ Supranummary nipples
_____ Breast discharge

RESPIRATIONS
_____ Normal _____ Labored
_____ Apnea _____ Grunting
Length ______________

BREATH SOUNDS
_____ Equal _____ Clear
_____ Rales _____ Rhonchi

CLAVICLES
_____ Straight _____ Smooth
_____ Crepitus ___ Rt ___ Lt

REFLEXES
_____ Moro _____ Suck _____ Grasp

CRY
_____ Normal _____ Weak _____ Shrill
_____ No cry, quiet, alert

HEAD
_____ Symmetrical _____ Molding
_____ Caput ______________
_____ Cephalohematoma ___ Lt ___ Rt
_____ Forcep marks ______________
_____ Fontanels normal

FACE
_____ Symmetrical _____ Asymmetrical

EYES
_____ Clear _____ Discharge
_____ Lid edema
_____ Subconjunctival hemmorhage

NECK
_____ Full ROM _____ Limited ROM

HEART
_____ Regular _____ Irregular
_____ Murmur _____ Abnormal PMI
Location: ______________

FEMORAL PULSES
_____ Equal _____ Unequal

EXTREMITIES
_____ Symmetrical _____ Asymmetrical
_____ Normal ROM _____ Limited ROM
_____ Hipclicks ___ Rt ___ Lt
_____ Polydactylism _____ Syndactylism
_____ Abnormal foot position

FEMALE GENITALIA
_____ Normal _____ Discharge
_____ Vaginal skin tag

MALE GENITALIA
_____ Normal
_____ Epispadias
_____ Hypospadias
_____ Undecended testicle
___ Rt ___ Lt
_____ Hydrocele

EARS
_____ Normal _____ Low set
_____ Sinus _____ Skin tags

NOSE
_____ Normal _____ Discharge

MOUTH
_____ Clear

MUCUS MEMBRANE
_____ Pink _____ Cyanosis _____ Thrush
_____ Cleft palate _____ Cleft lip
_____ Hard _____ Soft

CORD
_____ 3 vessels _____ 2 vessels
_____ Meconium stained

ABDOMEN
_____ Symmetrical _____ Asymmetrical
_____ Flat _____ Scaphoid
_____ Rounded _____ Distended
_____ Soft _____ Hard

BOWEL SOUNDS
_____ Present _____ Absent

RECTUM
_____ Patent

SPINE
_____ Closed vertebral column
_____ Asymmetry _____ Mass
_____ Dimple _____ Tuft of hair

Initials ________ **Date/Time** ________

PALOS COMMUNITY HOSPITAL
PALOS HEIGHTS, ILLINOIS

P-768
91480
Rev. 6/94

NEWBORN CARE RECORD

Figure 13–4. Documentation of Initial Newborn Assessment

Cardiovascular

Inspection of the cardiovascular system includes observation of color of the skin and mucous membranes and location of the point of maximal impulse (PMI). While acrocyanosis is a normal finding, central cyanosis indicates inadequate oxygenation and the need for supplemental oxygen. Heart rate, rhythm, presence of normal heart sounds, and murmurs are best identified when auscultated using a newborn stethoscope.

Cardiovascular assessment also includes palpation for presence and equality of femoral pulses. Pulses should be equal and nonbounding. Bounding pulses may indicate patent ductus arteriosus, while absent or decreased pulses may be present with coarctation of the aorta (Vargo, 1993). A single baseline blood pressure (B/P) may be recorded. Taking the B/P in all four extremities is usually reserved for newborn showing signs of distress. Routine blood pressure screening for newborns in the absence of risk factors and without complications is no longer recommended by AAP (1993).

Abdomen

Shape, symmetry, and consistence of the abdomen is noted. The umbilical cord stump is inspected for presence of three vessels (two arteries, one vein). The umbilical cord of newborns exposed to meconium in utero, for extended periods of time, will have a yellowish-brown discoloration. The abdomen is auscultated for presence of bowel sounds.

Musculoskeletal

Extremities are assessed for symmetry, range of motion, and the presence of extra or missing digits. While moving the newborn's arm, clavicles are palpated for crepitus which may indicate presence of a fracture. The newborn's hips are evaluated for presence of "clicks" which may indicate dislocation. Normal muscle tone is noted during this part of the examination as well as while evaluating Apgar Score.

Genitalia

Presence of normal male or female genitalia is evaluated. Male newborns are assessed for location of the urethral meatus and presence of a hydrocele. The scrotum is palpated for presence of testis.

Neurologic

A complete neurological assessment is usually reserved for newborns who are born with or develop complications. A brief neurological assessment is performed by evaluating the presence of reflexes such as moro, grasp, and suck. These reflexes are usually vary obvious and easy to illicit.

PROCEDURES PERFORMED IN THE BIRTHING ROOM

In addition to ongoing physical assessments of the newborn, procedures such as newborn identification, instillation of eye prophylaxis, administration of vitamin K, and cord care are performed soon after birth. Ideally each perinatal unit develops policies and procedures outlining expected newborn care. *Guidelines for Perinatal Care*, (AAP & ACOG, 1992) is a resource for developing unit standards.

Newborn Identification

One of the first procedures after birth is newborn identification. It is imperative that perinatal nurses are meticulous when recording the identification band number and applying identification bands to mothers and newborns (AAP & ACOG, 1992). Some hospitals use a four band system that includes a band for the support person or father of the baby, in addition to the band for the mother and two bands for the newborns ankle and wrist. Infant footprinting and fingerprinting are not adequate methods of identification (AAP & ACOG, 1992). Some hospitals have abandoned footprinting and fingerprinting altogether, while others continue to do so, but give the prints to the parents as a birth souvenir. According to the National Center for Missing and Exploited Children, 12 to 18 infants are abducted from hospitals each year (Beachy & Deacon, 1992). Infant safety and security, including unit visiting policies should be discussed with parents and family members. Parents should be made aware of what the hospital is doing to ensure the safety of every newborn as well as understand what they can do to increase safety. An important part of any infant security program is a discussion with the parents including directions not to leave their newborn unattended and information about identification of caregivers who may transport the newborn to and from the nursery. The efficacy of electronic infant security systems in preventing newborns abductions remains controversial. Other security programs as described above may be equally effective and much less expensive than electronic systems. No one method is superior; the key issue is that there must be some systematic program in place known to both the parents and perinatal healthcare providers to decrease the risk of newborn abduction.

Vitamin K

Approximately 0.5%-1% of newborns develop hemorrhagic disease characterized by bleeding from the gastrointestinal (GI) tract, umbilical cord, circumcision site, or venipuncture site (Mosijczuk & Ellis-Vaiani, 1994). During the first week of life, newborns are at risk for bleeding disorders because of an immature liver that is unable to produce several coagulation factors and a sterile GI tract which has not begun producing vitamin K. Consumption of breast milk and formula causes colonization of bacteria in the GI tract, which is necessary for vitamin K production. Vitamin K stimulates the liver to synthesize coagulation factors II, VII, IX, and X (Blackburn & Loper, 1992). A single dose of 0.5 mg for newborns <1.5 kg and 1 mg for newborns >1.5 kg is administered intramuscularly within the first hour of life (AAP & ACOG, 1992).

Eye Prophylaxis

Most states in the United States mandate that every infant receives prophylaxis against eye infections. Erythromycin ointment is the drug of choice because of its effectiveness against both gonococcal and chlamydia infections. Some evidence suggests that when the pregnant woman has received ongoing prenatal care and been screened for sexually transmitted diseases, the decision to use eye prophylaxis can be left up to parents (Bell et al., 1993). Once the agent for prophylaxis is chosen, care should be taken to instill the ointment throughout the conjunctival sac within 1 hour of birth. Excessive medication can be wiped away with a sterile cotton ball 1 minute after instillation (AAP & ACOG, 1992).

Umbilical Cord Care

The umbilical cord is examined for the presence of two arteries and a vein. Since a moist cord is vulnerable to pathogens, alcohol is applied to facilitate drying and decrease risk of infection. Use of alcohol has been associated with shorter separation time than triple dye (Schuman & Oksol, 1985).

Promoting Family-Newborn Attachment

After addressing physiological adaptation to extrauterine life, the focus of nursing interventions is psychological adaptation. Perinatal nurses are in a position to promote early maternal-newborn attachment. Early and extended contact between mother and newborn facilitates development of a positive relationship (Szymanski, 1992). The perinatal nurse assists in the attachment process by encouraging parents to see, touch, and hold their newborn. Providing uninterrupted time for them to be together gives parents the opportunity to recognize and identify unique behavioral and physical characteristics of their newborn.

It should be stressed that practices used to promote attachment usually do not interfere with transition to extrauterine life. The perinatal nurse can make a positive contribution to enhancing the attachment process by modifying practices which separate mothers and newborns immediately after birth. Treatments performed on the baby can be done within the birthing room, decreasing separation time between mother and baby. Providing that the newborn is dried and covered, the mother may immediately hold him/her without inhibiting neonatal thermoregulation. Application of opthalmic antibiotics may safely occur within the first hour of life, enhancing maternal-infant eye contact (Symanski, 1992). Providing the opportunity to breastfeed soon after birth supports the attachment process. Breastfeeding is more than a feeding method; it is an intimate relationship between a mother and her newborn (Driscoll, 1992). Early suckling and opportunities for uninterrupted contact between mother and newborn increases breastfeeding duration (Righard & Alade, 1990).

CONCLUSION

The majority of newborns need minimal support to make the transition to extrauterine life. Diverse and complex system adaptations make it a critical time for newborns. Strong desires to interact with their newborn make this a significant time for parents. The perinatal nurse must be knowledgeable about normal physiologic changes during the period of newborn transition from extrauterine life. Caring for newborns during this time requires the ability to recognize alterations from normal and becoming proficient at the psychomotor skills necessary for conducting a newborn resuscitation.

References

American Academy of Pediatrics & American College of Obstetricians and Gynecologists. (1992). Guidelines for perinatal care (3rd ed.). Elk Grove Village, IL: American Academy of Pediatrics.

American Academy of Pediatrics Committee on Fetus and Newborn. (1993). Routine evaluation of blood pressure, hematocrit, and glucose in newborns. Pediatrics, 92(3), 474-476.

American Heart Association, & American Academy of Pediatrics. (1994). Textbook of Neonatal Resuscitation. Elk Grove Village, IL: American Heart Association.

Anderson, G.G. (1991). Current knowledge about skin-to-skin (kangaroo) care for preterm infants. Journal of Perinatology, 11 (3), 216-226.

Apgar, V. & James, L.S. (1962). Further observations on the newborn scoring system. American Journal of Diseases of Children, 104, 419-428.

Beachy, P., & Deacon J. (1992). Preventing neonatal kidnapping. Journal of Obstetric, Gynecologic, and Neonatal Nursing, 21(1), 12-16.

Bell, T.A., Grayston, J.T., Krohn, M.A., & Kronmal, R.A. (1993). Randomized trial of silver nitrate, erythromycin, and no eye prophylaxis for the prevention of conjunctivitis among newborns not at risk for gonococcal opthalmitis. Eye Prophylaxis Study Group Pediatrics, 92(6), 755-760.

Bellatni, J.A., Pung, Y., & Zeligs, B.J. (1994). Immunology. In G.B. Avery, M.A. Fletcher, & M.G. MacDonald (Eds.), Neonatology: Pathophysiology and management of the newborn (4th ed.) (pp. 1000-1028). Philadelphia: J.B. Lippincott.

Blackburn, S. (1992). Alterations of the respiratory system in the neonate: Implications for clinical practice. Journal of Perinatal and Neonatal Nursing, 6(2), 46-58.

Blackburn, S.T., & Loper, D.L. (1992). Maternal, fetal and neonatal physiology: A clinical perspective. Philadelphia: W.B. Saunders.

Bloom, R.S. (1992). Delivery room resuscitation of the newborn. In A.A. Fanaroff, & R.J. Martin (Eds.). Neonatal perinatal medicine: Diseases of the fetus & newborn (5th ed.,) (pp. 301-324). St. Louis: Mosby-Year Book.

Brueggemeyer, A. (1993). Neonatal thermoregulation. In C. Kenner, A. Brueggemeyer, & L.P. Gunderson (Eds.). Comprehensive neonatal nursing: A physiologic perspective (pp. 247-262). Philadelphia: W.B. Saunders.

Cheng, M., & Williams, P.D. (1989). Oxygenation during chest physiotherapy of very-low birth-weight infants: relations among fraction of inspired oxygen levels, number of hand ventilations, and transcutaneous oxygen pressure. Journal of Pediatric Nursing, 4(6), 411-418.

Driscoll, J.W. (1992). Breastfeeding success and failure: Implications for nurses. NAACOG'S Clinical Issues in Perinatal and Women's Health Nursing, 3(4), 565-569.

Gerds, R. (1992). Assessment of the newborn. In S.J. Reeder, L.L. Martin, & D. Koniak, Maternity Nursing: Family, newborn, and women's health care (17th ed.,) (pp. 641-680). Philadelphia: J.B. Lippincott.

Hagedorn, M.I., Gardner, S.L., & Abman, S.H. (1993). Respiratory diseases. In G.B. Merenstein, & S.L. Gardner (Eds.), Handbook of neonatal intensive care (pp. 311-313). St. Louis: Mosby-Year Book.

Hazinski, M.F. (1992). Cardiovascular disorders. In M.F. Hazinski (Ed.), Nursing care of the critically ill child (pp. 117-394). St. Louis: Mosby-Year Book.

Lott, J.W. (1993). Assessment and management of cardiovascular dysfunction. In C. Kenner, A. Brueggemeyer, & L.P. Gunderson (Eds.), Comprehensive neonatal nursing: A physiologic perspective (pp. 355-391). Philadelphia: W.B. Saunders.

Ludington-Hoe, S.M., Anderson, G.C., S., Hollingsead, A., Argote, L.A., Medellin, G., & Roy, H. (1993). Skin-to-skin contact beginning in the delivery room for Colombian mothers and their preterm infants. Journal of Human Lactation, 9(4), 241-242.

Mahlmeister, L.R. (1994a). Assessment of the at-risk neonate. In K.A. May, & L.R. Mahlmeister (Eds.), Maternal and neonatal nursing: Family-centered care (3rd ed., pp. 961-985). Philadelphia: J.B. Lippincott.

Mahlmeister, L.R. (1994b). Assessment of the neonate. In K.A. May, & L.R. Mahlmeister (Eds.), Maternal and neonatal nursing: Family-centered care (3rd ed., pp. 877-922). Philadelphia: J.B. Lippincott.

Martin, L.L., & Reeder, S.J. (1991). Essentials of maternity nursing: Family centered care. Philadelphia: J.B. Lippincott.

Mosijczuk, A.D., & Ellis-Vaiani, C. (1993). Hematologic diseases. In G.B. Merenstein, & S.L. Gardner, Handbook of neonatal intensive care (pp. 247-271). St. Louis, Mosby-Year Book.

Nelson, N. (1994). Physiology of transition. In G.B. Avery, M.A. Fletcher, & M.G. MacDonald (eds.), Neonatology: Pathophysiology and management of the newborn (4th ed., pp. 223-247). Philadelphia: J.B. Lippincott.

Paxton, J.M., & Harrell, H. (1991). Delivery room management of the asphyxiated neonate. NAACOG'S Clinical Issues in Perinatal and Women's Health Nursing, 2(1), 35-47.

Pletch, P. (1994). The genetic code and fetal development. In K.A. May, & L.R. Mahlmeister, Maternal and neonatal nursing: Family-centered care (3rd ed., pp. 251-274). Philadelphia: J.B. Lippincott.

Righard, L., & Alade, M.O. (1990). Effect of delivery room routines on success of first breast-feed. Lancet, 336(8723), 1105-1107.

Riordan, J. (1993). The biologic specificity of breastmilk. In J. Riordan, & K.G. Auerbach, Breastfeeding and human lactation (pp. 105-134). Boston: Jones and Bartlett.

Roncoli, M., & Medoff-Cooper, B. (1992). Thermoregulation in low-birth weight infants. NAACOG'S Clinical Issues in Perinatal and Women's Health Nursing, 3(1), 25-33.

Schuman, A.J., & Oksol, B.A. (1985). The effect of isopropyl alcohol and triple dye on umbilical cord separation time. Military Medicine, 150(1), 49-50.

Streeter, N. (1986). High-risk neonatal care. Rockville, MD: Aspen.

Symanski, M.E. (1992). Maternal-infant bonding: Practice issues for the 1990's. Journal of Nurse Midwifery, 37(2 Suppl.), 67S-73S.

Thomas, K. (1994). Thermoregulation in neonates. Neonatal Network, 13(2), 15-22.

Vargo, L. (1993). Cardiovascular assessment of the newborn. In E.P. Tappero & M.E. Honeyfield (Eds.), Physical Assessment of the Newborn (pp. 67–80). Petaluma, CA: NICU INK.

Vaughans, B. (1990). Early maternal-infant contact and neonatal thermoregulation. Neonatal Network, 8(5), 19-21.

Walther, F.J., Benders, M.J., & Leighton, J.O. (1993). Early change in the neonatal circulatory transition. Journal of Pediatrics, 123 (4), 625-632.

CHAPTER

14

Newborn Physical Assessment

Alison Benzies Miklos
Patricia A. Creehan

Perinatal nurses frequently perform the first head-to-toe physical assessment on the newborn. Ideally this examination occurs in the birthing room or labor, delivery, recovery, and postpartum room (LDRP) in the presence of the parents. Conducting the examination while parents observe allows the nurse to use this time to identify and discuss normal newborn characteristics and note variations. It also provides an opportunity for parents to ask questions about the newborn's physical appearance and condition.

Physical assessment skills of inspection, palpation, auscultation, and percussion are used throughout the examination. When performing a physical assessment, the following equipment should be available: scale, tape measure, tongue blades, stethoscope with neonatal diaphragm, and ophthalmoscope. A preheated radiant warmer is used to avoid cold stress. Adequate lighting is essential.

The sequence in which the nurse conducts the physical assessment is a matter of personal preference. Many nurses perform the assessment in a cephalocaudal

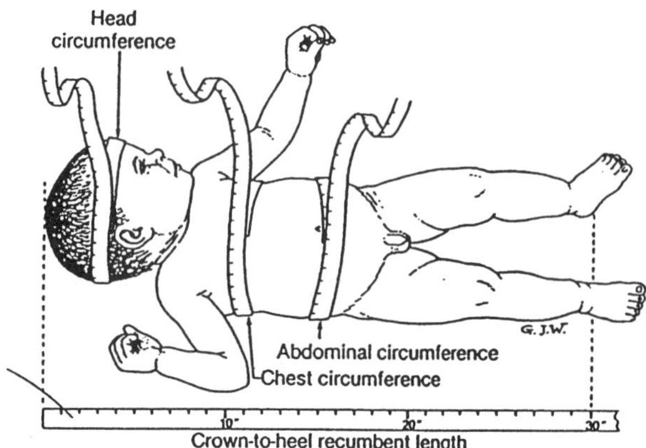

Figure 14-1. Newborn Measurements

From Nursing Care of Infants and Children (5th ed.) by L.F. Whaley and D.L. Wong, 1995, St. Louis, MO: Mosby-Year Book. Copyright 1995 by Mosby-Year Book. Reprinted with permission.

fashion, while others prefer to examine the newborn system by system. It is important however to begin the assessment by observing the newborn in a quiet, alert state. Note breathing pattern, overall skin color, posture, and muscle tone. The newborn is then weighed and measured. Ninety-five percent of full-term newborns weigh between 2,500 and 4,250 g (5 lb, 8 oz to 9 lb, 6 oz) (Mahlmeister, 1994b). Average length of full-term newborns is 48-53 cm (19-21 in) (Gerds, 1992). Figure 14-1 illustrates the technique for accurate measurements.

GESTATIONAL AGE ASSESSMENT

A gestational age assessment, evaluating physical and neuromuscular characteristics, is usually performed as part of the initial physical examination. In some perinatal centers, gestational age assessment of all newborns is routine practice. In other institutions criteria for performing gestational age assessment may include birth weight <2500 grams or >4082 grams, suspected intrauterine growth restriction, <37 weeks gestation, and cesarean birth. An indepth discussion of gestational age assessment techniques can be found in most basic maternal-newborn nursing texts and thus will not be covered here. Data from this comprehensive assessment are helpful in identifying newborns who are preterm, term, or post-term, and those who are small for gestational age (SGA), appropriate for gestational age (AGA), or large for gestational age (LGA). These classifications are important components of the initial examination because the likelihood of early identification and timely interventions for potential complications related to birth weight and gestational age during the immediate newborn period is enhanced. Most institutions use the Ballard form, a modified version of the original work of Dubowitz (Ballard, Novack, & Driver, 1979). In 1991 the Ballard Maturational Score was reevaluated and expanded resulting in the development of a New Ballard Score (Figure 14-2). Criteria were broadened to provide greater accuracy when evaluating extremely premature neonates. Controversy exists about the timing of this assessment. Endo and Nishioka (1993) suggest that the tool is accurate up to 5 days of life, at which time changes in physical characteristics make the evaluation less valuable.

The physical examination can either preceed or follow the gestational age assessment. Normal findings, common variations, and abnormal findings are identified and documented for each body system. Within this chapter the normal findings and common variations for each system are reviewed. Tables are included describing these pathological findings and their causes.

INTEGUMENT

Newborn skin is assessed using inspection and palpation. Color, birth marks, rashes, skin lesions, texture, and turgor are noted. At birth, newborns are covered with vernix, an odorless, white, cheesy, protective coating produced by sebaceous glands. Vernix develops during the third trimester and increases with gestational age. At term, the amount of vernix begins to decrease.

Color

Skin color reflects general health. Color is best observed when the newborn is quiet. At birth, color ranges from pale to plethoric, varying with ethnic origin. Skin pigmentation deepens over time. Caucasian newborns have pinkish-red skin tones a few hours after birth while African American newborns have a reddish-brown skin color. Hispanic newborns have an olive or yellowish skin tone. Changes in skin color may be the first sign of sepsis, cardiopulmonary, or hematologic diseases. Variations in skin color indicating illness may be more difficult to evaluate in African American and Asian newborns.

Cyanosis

Acrocyanosis, the bluish discoloration of newborn hands and feet, is seen in the first 24 to 48 hours of life and may last up to 10 days. Usually a benign

Neuromuscular Maturity

	-1	0	1	2	3	4	5
Posture							
Square Window (wrist)	>90°	90°	60°	45°	30°	0°	
Arm Recoil		180°	140°-180°	110°-140°	90°-110°	<90°	
Popliteal Angle	180°	160°	140°	120°	100°	90°	<90°
Scarf Sign							
Heel to Ear							

Physical Maturity

Skin	sticky iriable transparent	gelatinous red, translucent	smooth pink visible veins	superficial peeling &/or rash few veins	cracking pale areas rare veins	parchment deep cracking no vessels	leathery cracked wrinkled
Lanugo	none	sparse	abundant	thinning	bald areas	mostly bald	
Plantar Surface	heel-toe 40-50 mm:-1 < 40 mm:-2	>50mm no crease	faint red marks	anterior transverse crease only	creases ant. 2/3	creases over entire sole	
Breast	imperceptible	barely perceptilble	flat areola no bud	slippled areola 1-2mm bud	raised areola 3-4mm bud	full areloa 5-10 mm bud	
Eye/Ear	lids fused loosely:-1 tightly:-2	lids open pinna flat stays folded	sl. curved pinna; soft; slow recoil	well-curved pinna: soft but ready recoil	formed & firm instant recoil	thick cartillage ear stiff	
Genitals male	scrotum flat, smooth	scrotum empty faint rugae	testes in upper canal rare rugae	testes descending few rugae	testes down good rugae	testes pendulous deep rugae	
Genitals female	clitoris prominent labia flat	prominent clitoris small labia minora	prominent clitoris enlarging minora	majora & minora equally prominent	majora large minora small	majora cover clitoris & minora	

Maturity Rating

score	weeks
-10	20
-5	22
-0	24
5	26
10	28
15	30
20	32
25	34
30	36
35	38
40	40
45	42
50	44

Figure 14-2. Gestational Age Assessment.

From "New Ballard Score, expanded to include extremely premature infants," by J.L. Ballard, J.C. Khoury, K. Wedig, L. Wang, B.L. Ellers–Walsman, and R. Lipp, 1991, Journal of Pediatrics, 119, p. 418. Copyright 1991.

condition, it is related to poor peripheral circulation and tends to worsen if the newborn becomes chilled.

Jaundice

Jaundice, a yellow discoloration of the skin, is due to deposits of unconjugated bilirubin. Fifty percent of newborns develop jaundice during the first 3-4 days of life; however, it is considered an abnormal finding in the first 24 hours of life (Jackson & Saunders, 1993). Jaundice is visible when indirect bilirubin levels rise to 6-7 mg/dl (Frank, Turner, & Merenstein, 1993). It appears first on the head and face, progressing downward to the truck and extremities, and finally to the sclera of the eye. Jaundice is observed by blanching skin over the bridge of the nose; skin blanches a yellowish hue when jaundice is present. In dark-skinned newborns, jaundice is more easily observed in the sclera and buccal mucosa.

Bruising

Ecchymosis may occur over the head or buttocks if forceps or vacuum extractor were applied or following a breech or face presentation. Petechiae is common over the presenting part.

Variations Related to Vasomotor Instability

Cutis marmorate, mottling, or "lace-like" pattern on the skin is a vasomotor response to chilling, stress, or over stimulation. Harlequin's sign occurs when some newborns are positioned on their side. The dependent side of the body becomes pink, while the upper half of their body is pale. Color change lasts 1 to 30 minutes, disappearing gradually when the infant is placed on their abdomen or back (Witt, 1993).

Capillary Hemangiomas

Telangiectatic nevi, or a "stork bite," is a pink macular lesion. This lesion blanches with pressure and becomes darker when the newborn cries. Lesions may last 1-2 years or persist into adulthood. Stork bites are most often seen at the back of the neck, forehead, eyelids, bridge of the nose, and over the base of the occipital bones. Nevus flammeus, "port wine stain," is a red-to-purple macular lesion that results from dilated capillaries below the epidermis. Nevus flammeus is present at birth. Location and size are variable. The lesion is permanent and does not blanch to pressure. Nevus vasculosus, "strawberry mark," is elevated, rough, and bright or dark red. It may be present at birth or develop and become larger over the first 6 months of life. Most strawberry marks, but not all, will disappear over several years. Cavernous hemangioma is a soft compressible swelling of veins present at birth or soon after. The swelling appears bluish to red in color and is usually located on the head. It increases in size between 6-12 months and disappears spontaneously.

Other Normal Variations

Mongolian spots are macular blue lesions located over the sacral area (Figure 14-3). They are most common in African American and Asian newborns and are caused by infiltration of melanin-forming cells into the dermal skin layer. Mongolian spots decrease in intensity by 1 year of age and disappear or fade in early childhood. Erythema toxicum, "newborn rash," is a generalized, blotchy rash on the face, shoulders, and buttocks. It appears in the first few days of life as small yellow vesicles surrounded by an erythematous area. Erythema toxicum usually disappears in a day or two, but it may continue to appear for 7-10 days. Milia, clogged sebaceous glands, appear as small, white, firm lesions. The lesions are usually present over the chin, forehead, and bridge of the nose, disappearing during the first 2 weeks of life.

Texture

Skin is evaluated for texture and presence of lanugo during the physical examination and as part of the gestational age assessment. Texture ranges from smooth to superficial peeling. At birth, most term infants have dry, flaky skin with peeling of their hands and feet. Excessive peeling and leathery skin with deep cracks may indicate postmaturity.

Lanugo, a fine, downy hair which covers the body, is seen in abundance on premature infants and rarely on infants greater than 42 weeks' gestation. At term, lanugo is confined to the shoulders, ears, and forehead.

Turgor

Skin turgor is the natural rebound elasticity of the skin. It can be assessed anywhere on the body by pinching the skin between the thumb and index finger, and quickly releasing it. Ideally this is best assessed on the abdomen. Healthy, elastic tissue rapidly resumes its normal position without creases or tenting. If skin remains tented, this is indicative of poor hydration and nutritional status. Table 14-1 identifies skin findings during the physical assessment that are abnormal and their related pathology.

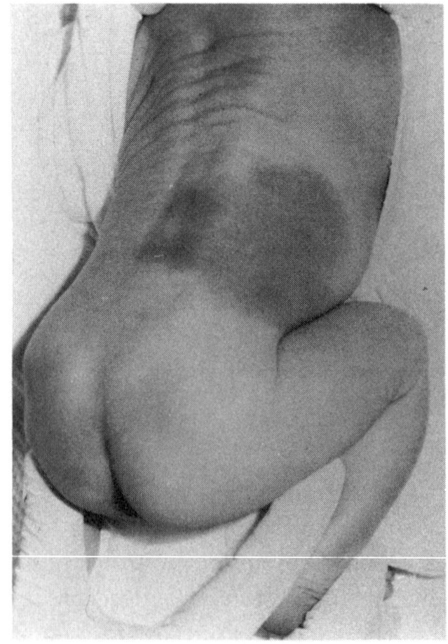

Figure 14-3. Mongolian Spots.

From Principles and Practice of Pediatrics (p. 899), by F. Oski, 1994, Philadelphia: J.B. Lippincott. Copyright 1994 by J.B. Lippincott.

HEAD

The newborn head is examined using inspection and palpation. The head is assessed for size, shape, and symmetry. The head of a full term, average for gestational age newborn has a circumference between 32 cm and 37 cm (12.5 in. and 14.5in.) and comprises approximately 25% of the total body size (Lepley, Gardner & Lubchenco, 1993). To measure the newborn's head, a tape measure is placed slightly above the eyebrows and continues around to the occipital prominence at the back of the skull (Figure 14-1). Vaginal birth may cause the cranial bones to overlap, as the fetus descends through the birth canal, giving the head an elongated appearance (Figure 14-4). The cranial bones can be palpated overlapping each other along the suture lines, giving the head an asymmetrical shape. Molding may last several days and cause the head circumference to be smaller immediately after birth. Circumference returns to normal within 2 to 3 days after birth. Newborns delivered by cesarean section will have a more rounded, symmetrical head. Caput succedaneum, edema over the presenting part of the newborn's head, is caused by pressure of the scalp against the mothers cervix during labor. Caput feels soft and spongy, crosses suture lines, and resolves within a few days. See Figure 14-5 for a comparison of caput succedaneum and cephalhematoma, an abnormal condition discussed in Table 14-2.

The skull is palpated for masses and craniotabes, a softening of cranial bones caused by pressure of the fetal skull against the bony pelvis. When pressure is exerted with the examiner's fingers at the margins of the parietal or occipital bones, a popping sensation similar to indenting a ping-pong ball is felt. Craniotabes is primarily seen in breech presentations and usually disappears in 1-2 months (Jackson & Saunders, 1993).

Anterior and posterior fontanels, soft membranous coverings where two sutures meet, are palpated and measured (Figure 14-6). Fontanels are measured diagonally from bone to bone rather than from suture to suture. The anterior fontanel is diamond shaped, 4-5 cm, and closes around 18 months of age. The posterior fontanel is triangular in shape, 0.5-1 cm and closes between 2-4 months. Fontanels are best palpated when the infant is quiet. The area is soft, depressed slightly, and may bulge when the infant cries. Arterial pulsations may be felt over the anterior fontanel. Molding may make it impossible to palpate fontanels.

TABLE 14-1. Integument

Assessment	Pathology
Pallor	Anemia Asphyxia Shock Sepsis Hypothermia Twin-to-twin transfusion Cardiac disease
Central cyanosis	Hypothermia Sepsis Hypoglycemia Cardiac disease Respiratory disorder
Plethora	Polycythemia
Grey	Poor perfusion Sepsis
Jaundice within 24 hours of birth	Liver disease Blood incompatibilities Sepsis Maternal ingestion of drugs (i.e., aspirin)
Generalized petechiae	Clotting disorders Sepsis
Pustules	Staphylococcal infection β-hemolytic streptococcal infection
Greenish, yellow vernix	Meconium staining
Foul smelling vernix	Intrauterine infection
Generalized edema	Erythroblastosis fetalis Cardiac failure Renal failure
Bright-red erythematous area with small white or yellow pustules	Candida albicans

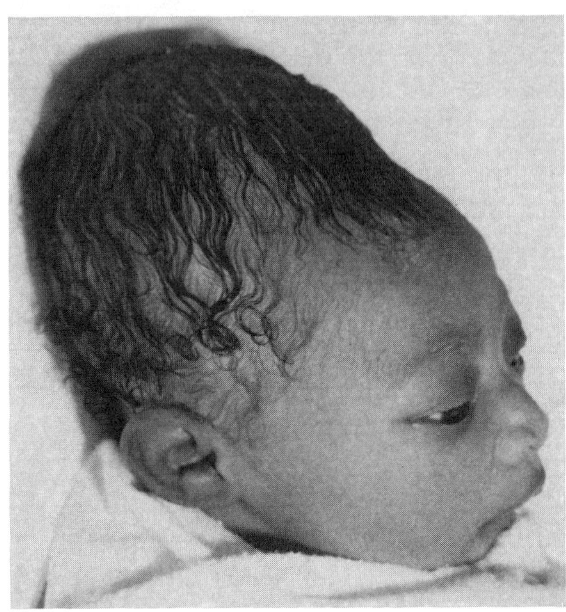

Figure 14-4. Molding.

From Maternity Nursing: Family, Newborn and Women's Health (17th ed., p. 653), by S.J. Reeder, L.L. Martin and D. Koniak, 1992, Philadelphia: J.B. Lippincott. Copyright 1992 by J.b. Lippincott.

The scalp is examined for distribution, amount, and texture of hair. Hair is silky and may be straight, curly, or kinky depending on ethnic origin. Bruising, lacerations, and bleeding are frequently seen following the application of a scalp electrode or vacuum extractor. Table 14-2 identifies findings during the physical assessment of the head that are abnormal and their related pathology.

EYE

The newborn's eyes are assessed using inspection and an ophthalmoscope. This can be done early in the examination, as part of assessment of the head, or whenever the newborn opens his eyes. Eyes should be symmetrical in size and shape. Lids may be edematous and puffy at birth.

The color of eye structures are observed. The iris is usually slate grey, brown, or dark blue. Eye color becomes permanent at about 6 months of age. The normally bluish-white sclera is examined. It is not uncommon to observe subconjunctival hemorrhages, the

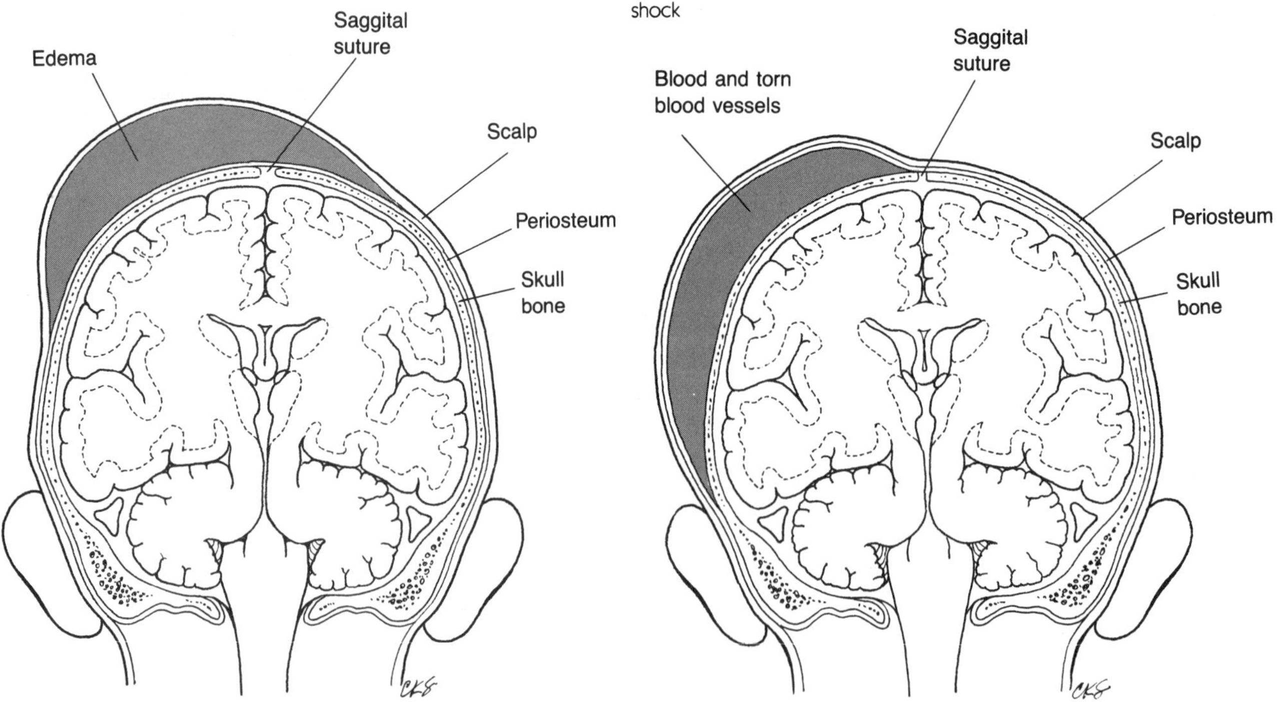

Figure 14-5. Comparison of Caput Succedaneum (left) and Cephalhematoma (right).

From Maternal and Neonatal Nursing: Family-Centered Care (3rd ed., p. 905), by K.A. May and L.R. Mahlmeister, 1994, Philadelphia: J.B. Lippincott. Copyright 1994 by J.B. Lippincott.

result of ruptured capillaries in the eye that occured during the birth process. Subconjunctival hemorrhages usually resolve within a week. A yellow sclera indicates hyperbilirubinemia. If silver nitrate is used as prophylaxis against ophthalmia neonatorum, conjunctiva may appear inflamed. Ilotycin does not generally cause this complication.

Tears are usually absent in the newborn until the lacrimal duct becomes fully patent at about 4-6 months of age. Prominent epicanthal folds (Mongolian slant) is a normal finding in Asian infants but may suggest Down Syndrome in other ethnic groups.

Blink reflex, size, and reactivity of pupils are evaluated in a darkened room with a pen light. Pupils are equal and reactive to light (PERL). When a light is shined at an angle toward the eye, the lens should be clear. Presence and clarity of the red reflex indicates an intact lens and is assessed using an ophthalmoscope.

Movement of the eye is observed. Strabismus, a crossed-eyes appearance, is often seen in newborns due to weak eye musculature and lack of coordination. Nystagmus, constant, rapid, involuntary movement of the eye, may also be present and usually disappears by 4 months of age. Newborns are nearsighted at birth and have visual acuity of 20/500 (Jackson & Saunders, 1993). They will respond to bright or primary colors and to contrast between colors such as black and white. They see objects clearly 8-10 inches in front of them. Table 14-3 identifies findings during the physical assessment of the eye that are abnormal and their related pathology.

TABLE 14-2. Head

Assessment	Pathology
Sutures separated more than 1 cm may indicate increased intracranial pressure (Johnson, 1993)	Hydrocephalus
Fusion of sutures (craniosynostosis)	Genetic disorder
Large anterior fontanel (Jones 1988)	Metabolic disorder
Bulging, tense fontanel	Hypothyroidism
	Hydrocephalus
	Tumor
	Meningitis
Head circumference below 10th percentile for gestational age (Johnson, 1993)	Intracranial hemorrhage
	Genetic disorder
	Congenital infection
Depressed fontanel	Maternal drug or alcohol ingestion
Cephalhematoma–swelling due to bleeding between periosteum and skull bone; does not cross suture line; may not be evident until one day after birth and take several weeks to resolve (Figure 14-5)	Dehydration Head trauma during delivery
Texture of hair is fine, woolly, sparse, coarse, brittle	
	Prematurity
	Endocrine disorder
Increased quantity of hair, low set hairline	Genetic disorder
	Genetic disorder

EAR

The newborn ear is assessed by inspection and palpation. External structures are examined for position and consistency of the cartilage. By 38-40 weeks' gestation, the pinna is firm and well formed and incurving exists over two thirds of the ear (Green, 1992). The pinna lies on or above an imaginary line drawn straight from the inner to the outer canthus of the eye, back toward the ear (Figure 14-7). A soft pinna lacking cartilage is seen in premature infants. Temporary asymmetry of the ears can result from intrauterine position.

Use of the otoscope is limited because the neonate's eustachian tubes contain vernix, mucus, and cellular debris. The ear canals clear spontaneously several days after birth. At this time, the tympanic membrane is visualized by pulling the pinna back and down. The tympanic membrane appears grayish white and highly vascular. If an infection is suspected, an otoscopic examination of the newborn is indicated.

Although hearing is well developed at birth, it becomes more acute as the eustachian tubes clear. The newborn responds to high-pitched vocal sounds and the familiar voice of his mother. Hearing acuity is difficult to evaluate. Since a sudden, loud sound may

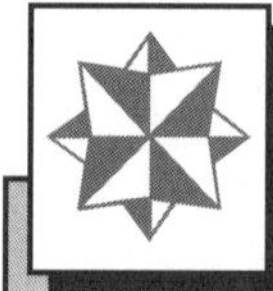

Display 14-1

Perinatal and Neonatal Complications Associated with Hearing Loss

Prenatal viral infection–rubella
cytomegalovirus
Sepsis
Neonatal hyperbilirubinemia
Persistent fetal circulation
Fetal alcohol syndrome
Cleft palate
Poorly or abnormally formed external ear
Perinatal hypoxia
Birth weight less than 1,500 grams
Atresia of the external auditory canal
Ototoxic drugs–kanamycin, gentamicin

Adapted from Pediatric diagnosis: Interpretation of symptoms & signs in infants, children, and adolescents (pp. 37-38), by M. Green, 1992, Philadelphia: W. B. Saunders.

A

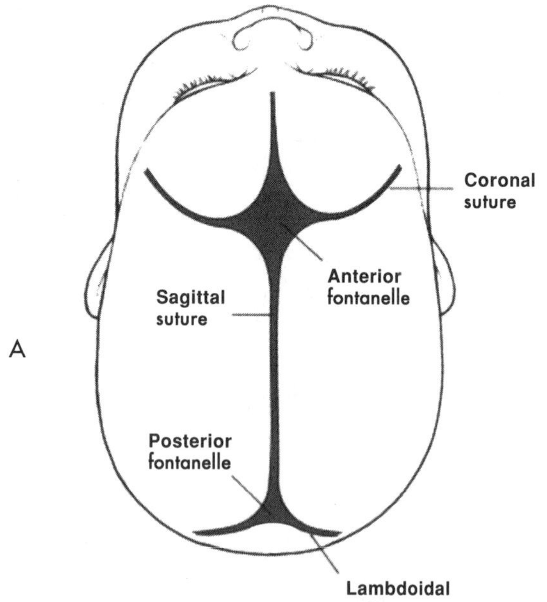

B

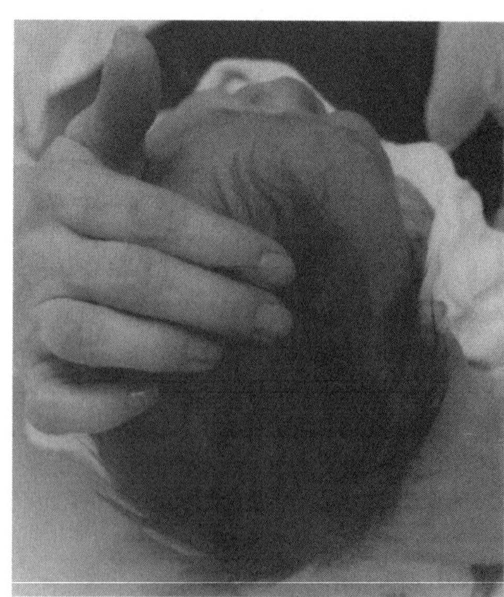

Figure 14-6. Palpating the Fontanelles.

From Health Assessment: A Nursing Approach (2nd ed., p.572), by Fuller and Schaller-Ayers, 1994, Philadelphia: J.B. Lippincott.

TABLE 14-3. Eye

Assessment	Pathology
Persistent purulent discharge	Ophthalmia neonatorum
	Chlamydia conjunctivitis
	Blocked lacrimal duct (dacryocystitis)
Inner canthal space greater than 2.5 cm (hypertelorism) (Endo & Nishioka, 1993)	Genetic disorder
Prominent epicanthal folds in the presence of other characteristics	Genetic disorder
Blue sclera	Osteogenesis imperfecta
Sclera visible above iris (Sunset eyes)	Hydrocephalus
Absent red reflex	Congenital cataracts the result of genetic disorder or intrauterine infection
	Retinoblastoma
	Glaucoma
	Retinal hemorrhage
White clouding of lens	Congenital cataracts
Black or white spots on periphery of iris (Brushfield spots)	Benign or associated with Down syndrome
Pupils not equal, nonreactive, fixed	Neurological insult

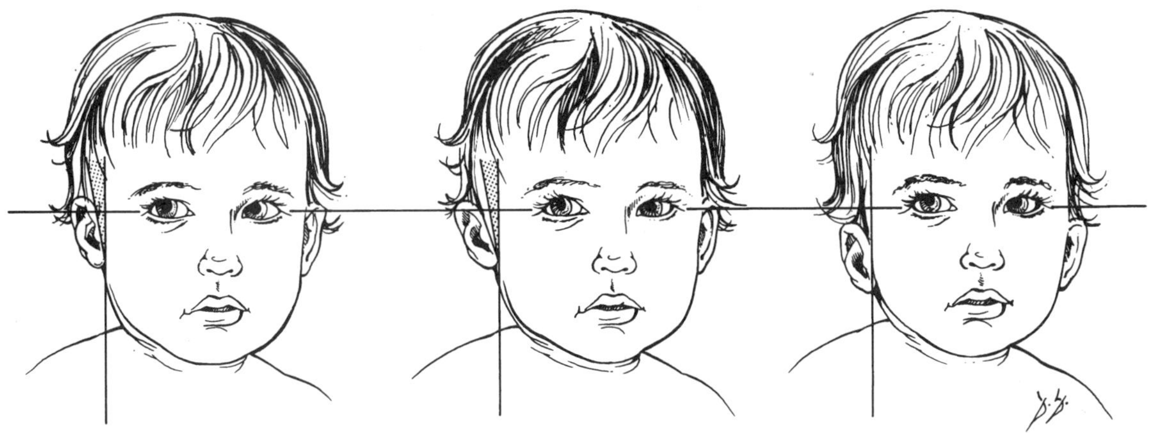

Figure 14-7. (A) Normal ear. (B) Abnormally angled ear. (C) Low set ear.

From Maternity Nursing: Family, Newborn and Women's Health (17th ed., p. 657), by S.J. Reeder, L.L. Martin and D. Koniak, 1992, Philadelphia: J.B. Lippincott. Copyright 1992 by J.B. Lippincott.

TABLE 14-4. Ear

Assessment	Pathology
Low set ears	Genetic disorder
	Kidney abnormality
Poorly formed external ear	Genetic disorder
Small skin tags Figure (14-8)	Familial variation
	Alteration in normal embryologic development
	Genetic disorder
Preauricular sinus "pits" located in front of the ear, may be closed or extend to the internal ear or brain (Figure 14-9)	Familial variation
	Alteration in normal embryologic development
	Genetic disorder (Brachial-Oto-Renal syndrome)
Absence of Moro reflex in response to loud noise	Hearing loss

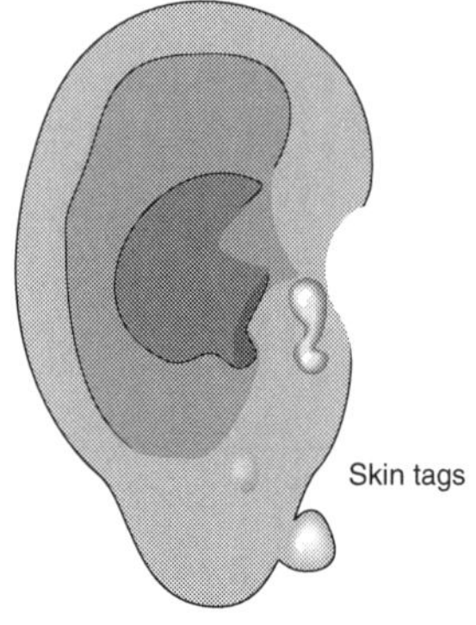

Figure 14-8. Preauricular skin tags.

From A Guide to Physical Examination and History Taking (5th ed., p. 219), by Bates, Philadelphia: J.B. Lippincott.

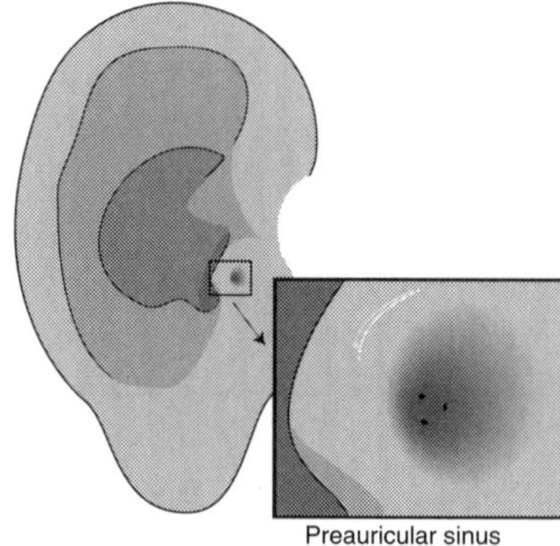

Figure 14-9. Preauricular sinus.

From A Guide to Physical Examination and History Taking (5th ed., p. 219), by Bates, Philadelphia: J.B. Lippincott.

elicit a startle reflex or crying, in response to the sound or to the vibration of air, hearing is more accurately assessed with the newborn in a quiet, alert state. With the examiner's mouth about 6-10 inches from the ear, movement towards a high pitched voice of normal intensity is observed. Hearing loss is associated with many genetic disorders. Display 14-1 describes complications that may result in hearing loss. These occur or are identified during the prenatal and neonatal periods but are not genetic. All indicate a need for a hearing evaluation. Table 14-4 identifies findings during the physical assessment of the ear that are abnormal and their related pathology.

NOSE

The newborn's nose is assessed using inspection. The nose should be symmetrical and midline. The nose may be misshapened at birth, due to the neonate's positioning in utero. If the septum cannot be easily straightened and the nose remains asymmetrical, treatment may be required. A flattened or bruised nose may result from passage through the birth canal.

Since newborns primarily breathe through their nose, it is imperative to check the nasal canals for patency. Patency is assessed in one of two ways. A small soft catheter may be passed down each nares to check

TABLE 14-5. Nose

Assessment	Pathology
Flat nasal bridge	Down syndrome
Pink when crying, chest retractions and cyanosis at rest, difficulty feeding	Choanal atresia
Stuffy nose & thin watery discharge	Neonatal drug withdrawal
"Sniffles" persistent, profuse mucopurulent or bloody discharge (Green, 1992)	Congenital syphilis

for an obstruction, or with the newborn's mouth closed, apply gentle alternating pressure on the nares. Assess newborn's ability to breathe by noting the air passage through the naris not occluded. If the infant exhibits any difficulty in breathing, these finding are reported immediately to a nurse practitioner/physician.

Nasal stuffiness and thin white mucous is not an uncommon finding immediately after birth. Newborn's sneeze to clear their upper respiratory tract. Nasal flaring, widening of the nares, is a compensatory mechanism that decreases upper airway resistance, allowing more air to enter the nasal passages. Nasal flaring is abnormal and one of the first symptoms observed when respiratory distress occurs. Table 14-5 identifies findings during the physical assessment of the nose that are abnormal and their related pathology.

MOUTH

The newborn mouth is assessed using inspection and palpation. In the sequence of the total examination, this assessment is frequently left until last. If the newborn's mouth is forced open, crying may result, altering aspects of the respiratory or cardiac assessments. The lips are observed for location, color, and symmetry. The mouth should be centrally located along the midline. At rest the lips appear symmetrical. Depending on skin color, the lips are pink or more darkly pigmented. Sucking blisters, centrally located on the upper lip, may be filled with fluid or have the consistency of a callous. Callouses may also be found on the hand resulting from vigorous sucking in utero or after birth. Muscle weakness or facial paralysis is best observed when the infant is sucking or crying; both conditions may be missed altogether if the infant is only observed in a quiet, alert state. (Figure 14-10). The presence of rooting, suck, and gag reflexes are evaluated during this portion of the examination or during feeding.

The mucus membrane and internal structures of the mouth are inspected. If the mouth does not open spontaneously while the newborn cries, it can be gently opened by a downward pressure on the chin or with a pediatric tongue blade. In a healthy newborn the mucous membrane is pink. Increased amounts of

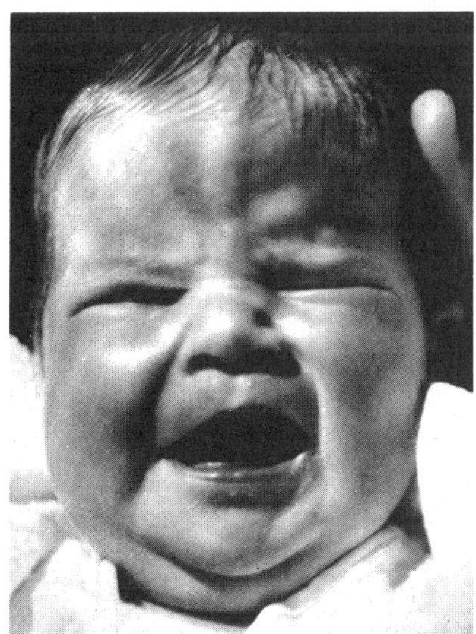

Figure 14-10. Facial nerve paralysis. Note the asymmetry of the mouth during crying.

From Maternity Nursing: Family Newborn, and Women's Health (17th ed., p. 1203), by S.J. Reeder, L.L. Martin and D. Koniak, 1992, Philadelphia: J.B. Lippincott.

TABLE 14-6. Mouth

Assessment	Pathology
Mucous membranes dry	Dehydration
Cyanotic mucous membranes	Poor oxygenation
Asymmetrical movement of mouth	Facial nerve injury
Cleft lip and/or palate (Figure 14-11)	Teratogenic injury
	Genetic disorder
	Multifactorial inheritance
Hypertrophied tongue	Down syndrome
	Beckwith syndrome
	Hypothyroidism
Protrusion of tongue	Genetic disorder
Weak, uncoordinated suck and swallow	Prematurity
	Neuromuscular disorder
	Asphyxia
	Maternal analgesia during labor
	Inborn error of metabolism
Frantic sucking	Infant of drug-addicted mother
Excessive drooling and salivating; unable to pass a naso-gastric tube	Esophageal atresia
Circumoral cyanosis	Respiratory distress
Thin upper lip	Fetal alcohol syndrome
Smooth philtrum	
Short palpebral fissures	
Translucent, bluish, swelling on either side of the frenulum under the tongue	Mucous or salivary gland retention cyst
Bifid uvula	Genetic disorder
Small lower jaw (micrognathia)	Pierre Robin syndrome
	Treacher Collins syndrome
	DeLanges syndrome

mucus during the first 1–2 days of life are removed with a bulb syringe. This is especially common in newborns born by cesarean section, since they do not benefit from compression of the thorax through the birth canal during delivery. The tongue is mobile and prominent within the mouth. Occasionally the frenulum is short causing a notch at the tip of the tongue. True congenital ankyloglossia (tongue tie) is rare (Green, 1992).

Using adequate lighting, the hard and soft palate are examined. The uvula is midline located at the posterior soft palate. Some practitioners use their index finger to palpate the hard and soft palate for the presence of clefts. Whitish yellow cysts (Epstein's pearls) containing epithelial cells may be present on the hard palate at birth, but disappear within a few weeks. Some newborns are born with one or two natal teeth. These

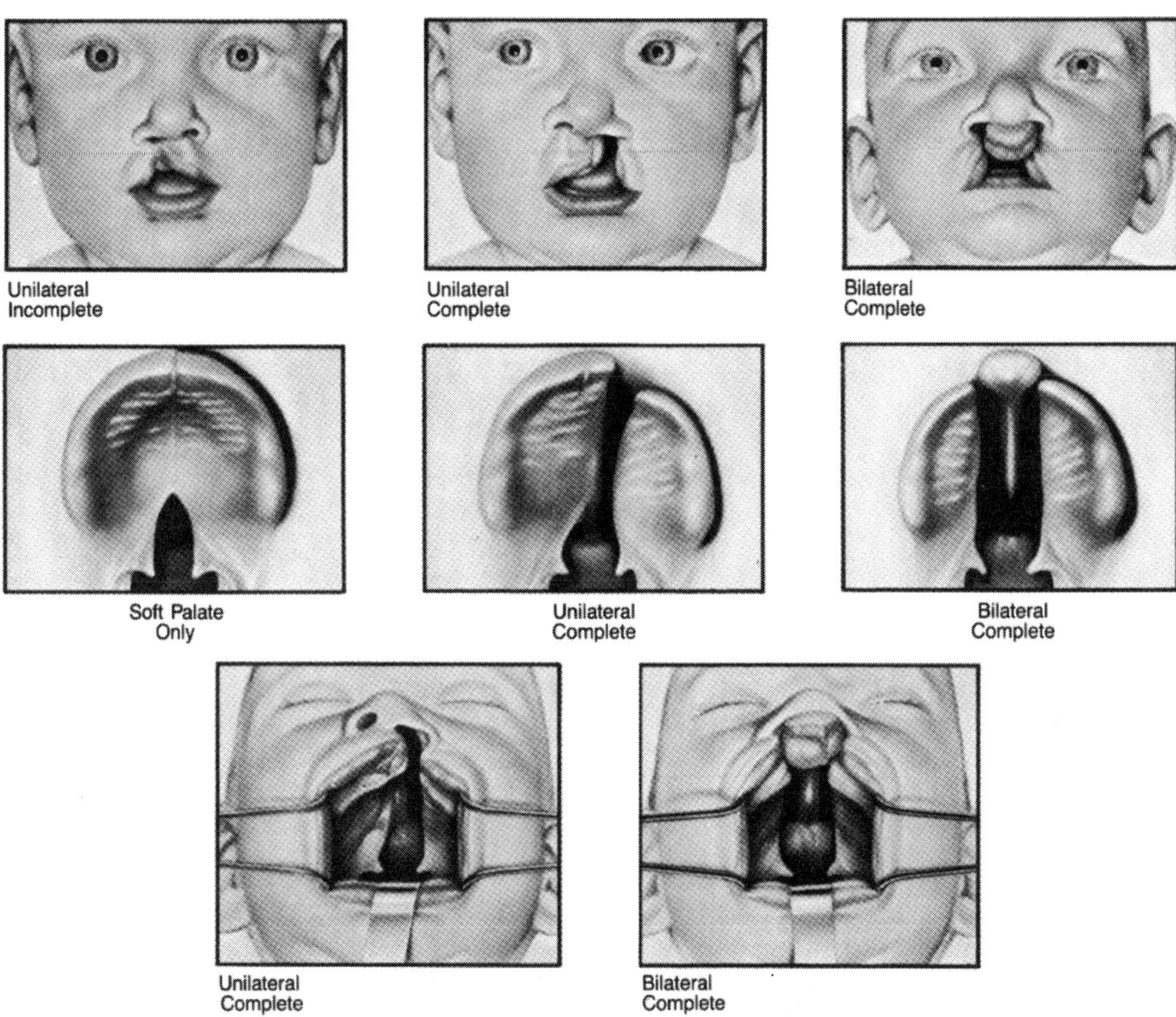

Figure 14-11. Cleft Lip and Cleft Palate (Redrawn from drawings by Ross Laboratories)

From Maternity Nursing: Family Newborn, and Women's Health (17th ed., p. 1178), by S.J. Reeder, L.L. Martin and D. Koniak, 1992, Philadelphia: J.B. Lippincott. Copyright 1992 by J.B. Lippincott.

immature caps of enamel and dentine have poor root formation and are usually loose. These teeth may be aspirated if dislodged, make breast feeding difficult, or cause lacerations on the mucosa, lips, or tongue, they are usually removed during the neonatal period. Fluid-filled cysts found along the alveolar ridge are not associated with an underlying tooth and reabsorb spontaneously (Coen & Koffler, 1987).

Candida albicans (thrush), a common bacterial infection, may be found in the mouth. It is transmitted to the infant during descent through the birth canal, while breast feeding, or from contact with the hands of family members, friends, or other care givers. Thrush can be distinguished from Epstein's pearls because the examiner is able to wipe away the white patches of thrush leaving a reddish area which bleeds easily. Epstein's pearls cannot be removed. Since this bacteria travels throughout the gastrointestinal (GI) tract, the newborn is observed for a characteristic spotty diaper rash. The lesions appear flat, shiny, beefy red, and may bleed. Table 14-6 identifies findings during the physical assessment of the mouth that are abnormal and their related pathology.

TABLE 14-7. Neck

Assessment	Pathology
Multiple skin folds in the lateral, posterior region of the neck (webbing)	Down syndrome Turner syndrome
Soft mass above or lateral to the clavicle, transilluminates well, with or without deviation of the trachea to either side	Cystic hygroma (see Figure 14-12)
Enlarged thyroid	Hyperthyroidism Hypothyroidism
Absence of head control	Prematurity Genetic disorder Asphyxia Neuromuscular disorder

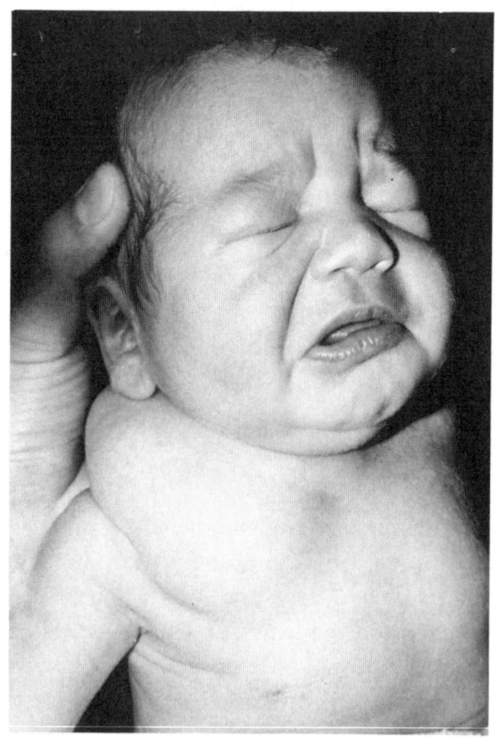

Figure 14-12. Cystic hygroma.

From Principles and Practice of Pediatrics (p. 1749), by F. Oski, 1994, Philadelphia: J.B. Lippincott.

NECK

Inspection and palpation are used to assess the neck. The neck is inspected for symmetry, webbing, and range of motion. Newborns have short, thick necks with multiple skin folds. Full range of motion is present at term. Some newborns are able to raise their head momentarily. Torticollis, an asymmetrical neck deformity due to injury of the sternocleidomastoid muscle, may be present at birth or seen at about 3 weeks of age. The neck is palpated for the trachea along the midline and abnormal masses. The thyroid gland is difficult to palpate unless it is enlarged, an unusual finding during the newborn period. Table 14-7 identifies findings during the physical assessment of the neck that are abnormal and their related pathology.

RESPIRATORY

Auscultation and inspection are used to assess newborn respiratory status. The newborn's chest is cylindrical in shape. Measured at the nipple line, it is approximately 33 cm or 2-3 cm less than the infant's head (Figure 14-1). The xiphoid process is seen as a small protuberant area at the end of the sternum. Respirations are shallow and irregular. Chest movement should be symmetrical and nonlabored. Respiratory rate is counted for 1 full minute, preferably when the newborn is quiet. Newborns are obligatory nose breathers and have an average respiratory rate of 30-60 breaths/minute. With each respiration, abdominal movement is noted.

Increased respiratory rate soon after birth may indicate that fetal lung fluid has not been fully reabsorbed into pulmonary veins and lymphatic system, a condition known as transient tachypnea of the newborn (TTN). This fluid is usually cleared during vaginal birth by compression of the thorax. If tachypnea is present, respiratory rate may reach 120 breaths/minute. The primary healthcare provider is notified, and oral feedings withheld due to risk of aspiration.

Inspection of the newborn's chest includes placement, shape, and amount of palpable breast tissue. Hypertrophy of breast tissue, with or without secretion of milky fluid, may be present the second or third day of life, due to maternal hormones (Figure 14-13). This condition lasts approximately 1 week. Supernumerary nipples (accessory nipples) are considered a benign congenital anomaly. They are often seen below and medial to the normal nipples.

Auscultation of the anterior and posterior chest proceeds in an orderly fashion from top to bottom, comparing from side to side for equality and presence of clear breath sounds. Silverman Index may be used to assess and document newborn respiratory effort and presence of physical symptoms of respiratory distress (Figure 14-14). A score of zero indicates no respiratory distress.

Newborns have a periodic breathing pattern, due to the immaturity of their respiratory and central nervous systems. It is common to observe brief pauses in respiratory effort. Pauses lasting 20 seconds or longer and associated with color change or bradycardia are considered apneic periods and should be reported to the primary healthcare provider (Jackson & Saunders, 1993). Table 14-8 identifies findings during the respiratory assessment that are abnormal and their related pathology.

CARDIOVASCULAR

The cardiovascular system is assessed using inspection, auscultation, and palpation. The examination begins with a visual inspection of the newborn's precordium (anterior chest, where the heart lies). Very little movement should be observed in this area.

Heart rate and rhythm are best auscultated with a small bell stethoscope and diaphragm, while the infant remains quiet. The stethoscope should be warmed prior to placement, so the newborn is not startled. Normal heart rate is 120-160 beats/minute. In deep sleep, the heart rate may be 80-110 beats/minute. Auscultation begins at the point of maximal impulse (PMI), located lateral to the midclavicular line, at the third or fourth intercostal space. A shift in the PMI may indicate a diaphragmatic hernia or pneumothorax. The apical rate is counted for 1 full minute. Heart murmurs in newborns are common during the neonatal period. Ninety percent of all murmurs are related to incomplete closure of the ductus arteriosus or foramen ovale and are transient in nature (Mahlmiester, 1994a). Murmurs are best auscultated at the left lower sternal border in the third or fourth interspace.

Peripheral pulses (brachial, radial, femoral, popliteal, and dorsalis pedis) are evaluated for presence, equality, and strength. Femoral pulses may be difficult to palpate but should be present in all infants. Routine blood pressure screening is not recommended for all newborns (American Adademy of Pediatrics, 1993). Evaluating the blood pressure is usually reserved for newborns showing signs of distress. When the blood pressure is recorded an appropriately sized cuff is necessary. Blood pressure varies depending on birthweight (Figure 14-15). In the lower extremities the blood pressure is usually higher than in the upper extremities (Ziai, Clarke, & Merritt, 1987).

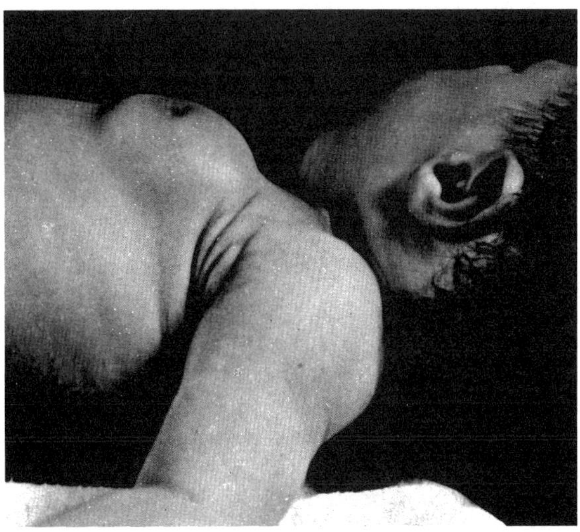

Figure 14-13. Neonatal breast hypertrophy.

From Maternity Nursing: Family Newborn, and Women's Health (17th ed., p. 660), by S.J. Reeder, L.L. Martin and D. Koniak, 1992, Philadelphia: J.B. Lippincott. Copyright 1992 by J.B. Lippincott.

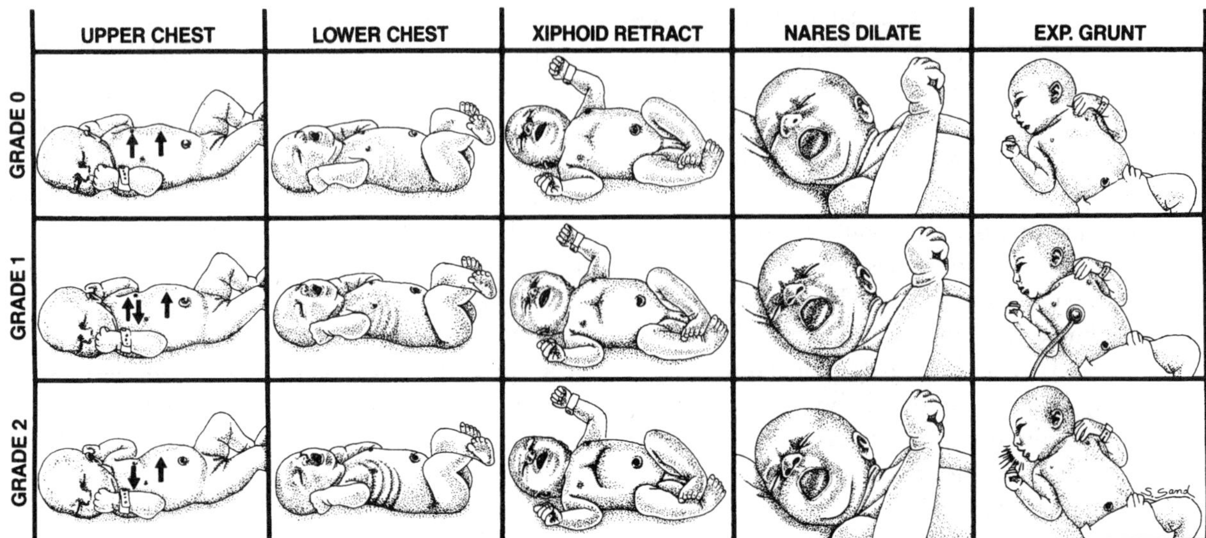

Figure 14-14. Silverman-Anderson Index of Neonatal Respiratory Distress.

From Maternal and Neonatal Nursing: Family-Centered Care (3rd ed., p. 980), by K.A. May and L.R. Mahlmeister, 1994, Philadelphia: J.B. Lippincott. Copyright 1994 by J.B. Lippincott.

TABLE 14-8. Respiratory

Assessment	Pathology
Cessation of breathing for more than 20 seconds	Hypo/hyperthermia
	Sepsis
	Prematurity
	Respiratory disorders
	Cardiovascular disorders
	Neurologic disorders
	Maternal narcotics
Tachypnea—rate greater than 60	Respiratory disorders
	Congestive heart failure
	Sepsis
	Hypothermia
	Hypoglycemia
	Polycythemia
Retractions, grunting, nasal flaring, seesaw respirations	Respiratory distress
Decreased or absent breath sounds	Meconium aspiration
	Atelectasis
	Pneumothorax
Bowel sounds heard in place of breath sounds	Diaphragmatic hernia

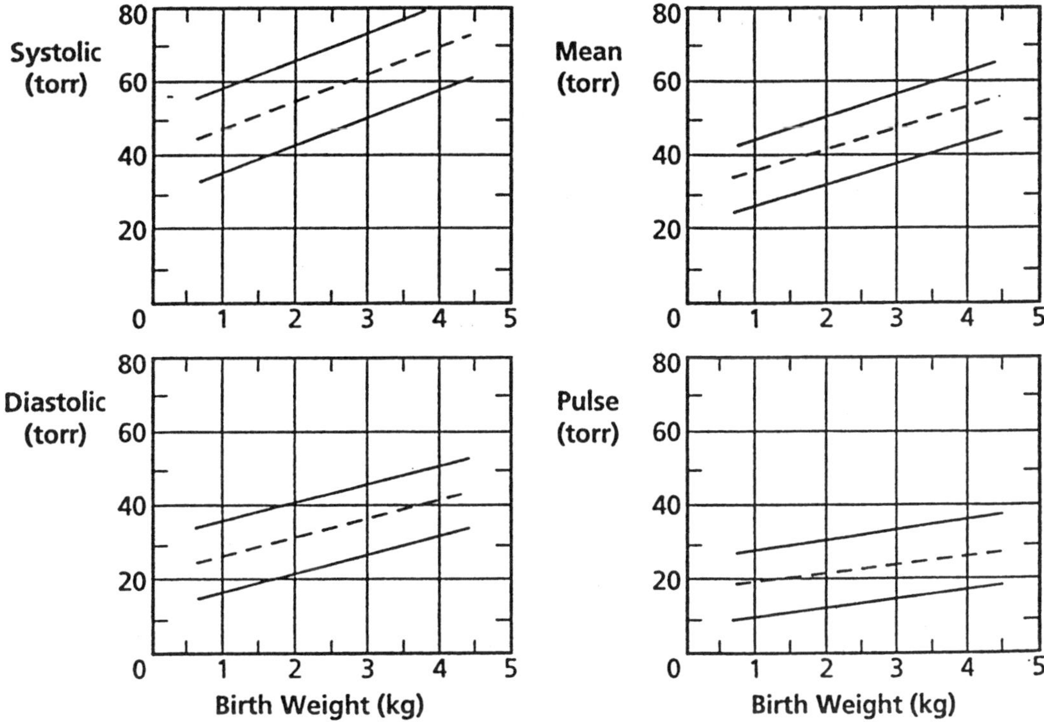

Figure 14-15. Normal Blood Pressure Range. Linear regressions (broken Lines) and 95% confidence limits (solid lines) of systolic (left) and diastolic (right) blood pressure.

From Physical Assessment of the Newborn (p.79), by E. P. Tappero and M.E. Honeyfield, 1993, Petaluma, CA: NICU. Copyright 1993 by NICU; "Aortic Blood Pressure during the First 12 Hours of Life in Infants 610 to 4220 grams," by H.T. Versmold and J.A. Kitterman, 1981, Pediatrics, 76(5), p. 22. Copyright 1981. Adapted with premission.

The blood pressure is assessed in all four extremities if pulses are unequal, a murmur is heard, there is an absence of a femoral pulse, or if it was difficult obtaining a blood pressure (Vargo, 1993). Table 14-9 identifies findings during the cardiovascular assessment that are abnormal and their related pathology.

ABDOMEN

The abdomen is assessed using inspection, auscultation, palpation, and percussion. The abdomen is inspected for size and symmetry, and is normally rounded, symmetrical, protuberant, and soft due to weak abdominal musculature. If abdominal distension is suspected, the circumference of the abdomen is periodically measured at the level of the umbilicus (Figure 14-1). The umbilical cord is examined for number of vessels, color, and condition. The cord should be opaque to whitish blue and contain two arteries and one vein. Variations include a thin, dry cord associated with intrauterine growth restriction or a thick cord seen in LGA newborns. A greenish yellow discoloration of the cord sometimes occurs with relaxation of the anal sphincter and subsequent passage of meconium. The area surrounding the umbilical cord is observed for masses or the herniation of abdominal contents (Figure 14-16). Umbilical hernias are more common in low-birth-weight, and African American newborns. Some hernias are observable only when the newborn is crying.

Abdominal movements correspond with respirations. Separation of abdominorectus muscle (diastasis recti) 1/2 to 2 inches wide may occur along the midline from xiphoid to umbilicus, occasionally extending to the symphysis pubis (Barness, 1991). Separation is due to weak muscles or prematurity.

The perianal region is inspected for the presence of a patent anus. The majority of newborns will pass meconium within the first 24 hours of life. Failure to pass meconium may indicate a GI obstruction and necessitates further evaluation.

TABLE 14-9. Cardiovascular

Assessment	Pathology
Tachycardia greater than 160 beats/minute	Anemia
	Congestive heart failure
	Shock
	Sepsis
	Congenital heart anomalies
	Extremely premature infants
Persistent bradycardia less than 100 beats/minute	Congenital heart block
Persistent murmurs	Persistent fetal circulation
	Congenital heart anomalies
	Fluid overload
Muffled heart sounds	Pneumothorax
	Pneumomediastinum
	Diaphragmatic hernia
	Pneumopericardium
Heart sound muffled on left side, loud on right side	Dextrocardia Pneumothorax with mediastinal shift
Decrease in intensity or absence of femoral pulses	Hip dysplasia
	Shock
Bounding peripheral pulses; active precordium	Patent ductus arteriosus
	Fluid overload
	Ventricular septal defect
	Prematurity
Difference of blood pressure greater than 20 mmHg between upper and lower extremities	Coarctation of aorta

Bowel sounds, normally present within 1 hour of birth, are auscultated in all four quadrants.

Most perinatal nurses conduct a limited assessment of the abdomen using light palpation for consistency and the presence of masses. A more detailed examination is conducted by the primary healthcare provider. The lower border of the liver is palpated in the right upper quadrant 1-2 cm below the costal margin. The spleen, located in the left upper quadrant, may be palpable in preterm newborns but rarely in term newborns (Green, 1992). Kidneys are 4-5 cm in length, and are usually only palpable during the first 6 hours of life (Figure 14-17). After this time, the bowel and stomach become distended with fluid and air, making this assessment difficult. With the newborn's legs flexed against the abdomen, kidneys are located using deep palpations at the level of the umbilicus, lateral to the midclavicular line. The right kidney may be lower then the left kidney (Endo & Nishioka, 1993).

Inspection and palpation of the femoral region is conducted during this portion of the examination or as part of the cardiovascular assessment. Presence of a soft, compressible swelling in the groin may indicate an inguinal hernia or undescended testes (Figure 14-18). Bowel sounds can be auscultated in the testis if swelling is due to herniation of the bowel.

Tympanic sounds are percussed throughout the abdomen except over liver, spleen, and bladder where the percussion note is dull. Table 14-10 identifies findings during the physical assessment of the abdomen that are abnormal and their related pathology.

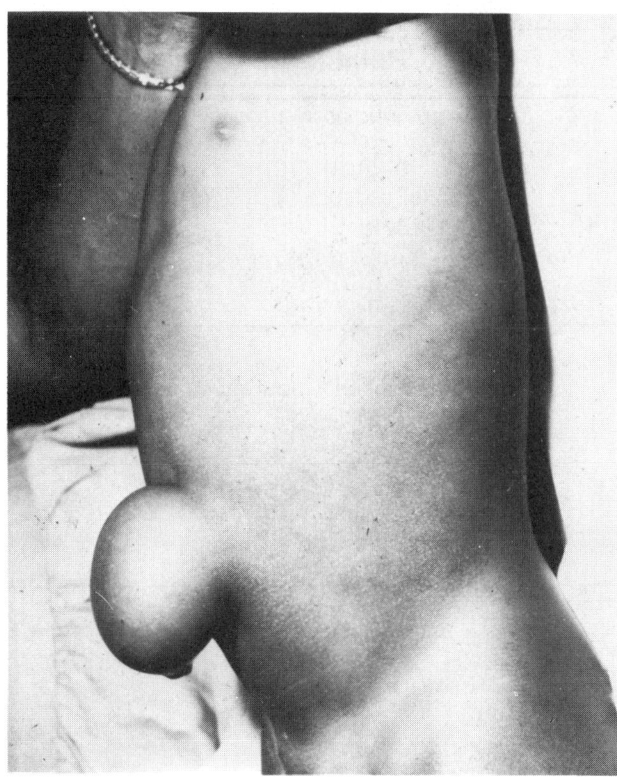

Figure 14-16. Umbilical Hernia (Courtesy of Dr. Mark Ravitch.)

From Nursing Care of Children (9th ed.), by F.G. Waecht, 1976, Philadelphia: J.B. Lippincott.

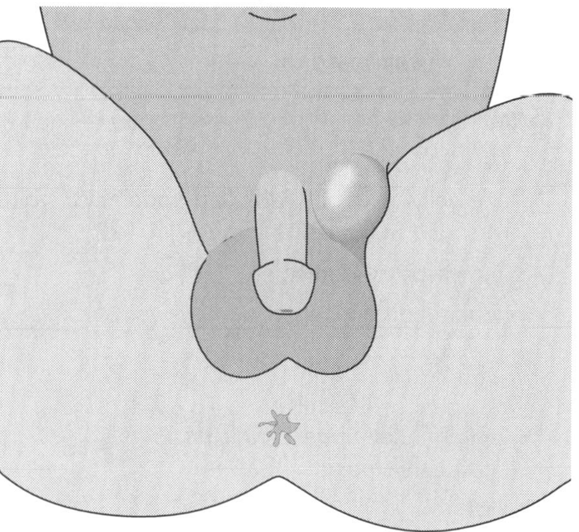

Figure 14-18. Left inguinal hernia producing a bulge in the groin of the affected side.

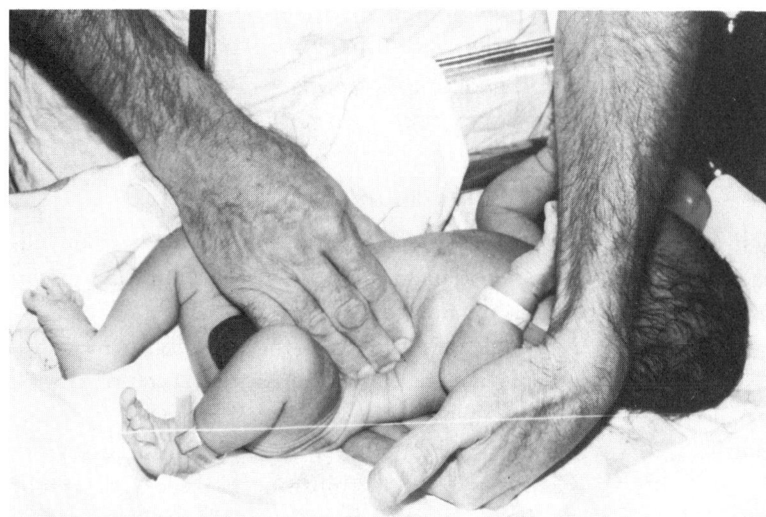

Figure 14-17. Examiner Demonstrating Technique for Palpation of the Left Kidney.

From Principles and Practice of Pediatrics (2nd ed., p. 304), by F. Oski, 1994, Philadelphia:J.B. Lippincott.

TABLE 14-10. Abdomen

Assessment	Pathology
Scaphoid	Diaphragmatic hernia Malnutrition
"Prune belly" – flabby, wrinkled abdominal wall distended in the flanks (Figure 14-19)	Congenital absence of abdominal musculature
Asymmetrical abdomen	Abdominal mass /GI/GU anomalies
Abdominal distention	GI obstruction Renal disease Preterm infant with poor musculature
Distention in left upper quadrant (Endo & Nishioka, 1993)	Pyloric stenosis Duodenal or jejunal obstruction
Ascites	Hydrops fetalis
Umbilical cord with one artery, one vein	Associated with GI/GU anomalies
Thin membrane covering herniation of abdominal contents through a defect in the umbilical ring	Omphalocele
Uncovered protrusion of abdominal contents usually to the right of umbilicus	Gastroschisis
Red, oozing, or foul-smelling cord	Infection
Persistently moist umbilicus; clear discharge from umbilical cord stump (Conner, 1993a)	Alteration in embryologic development- patent urachus omphalomesenteric duct
Failure to pass meconium stool	Imperforate anus Meconium ileus Hirschsprung's disease Meconium plug syndrome
Passage of sticky, thick small plugs of meconium	Meconium ileus Cystic fibrosis
Bruits	Arteriovenous malformations Renal artery stenosis

GENITOURINARY

The genitourinary system is assessed using inspection and palpation. External genitalia is evaluated as part of physical examination and gestational-age assessment. Newborns should void within 24 hours of birth. A rust-colored staining on the diaper, which in some instances can be flaked off, is a normal variation due to the presence of uric acid crystals in the urine.

Female

In full-term newborns, the clitoris and labia minora are covered by the labia majora. The urinary meatus is located beneath the clitoris. The labia majora and clitoris are enlarged due to maternal hormones circulated to the newborn in utero.

In some newborns when the introitus is gently separated, a hymenal tag is seen at the posterior vaginal opening. This tissue, which developed from the hymen and labia minora, will disappear in 1 to 2 weeks (Conner, 1993b). A white mucous discharge from the vagina is not uncommon during the first week of life. Pseudomenstruation, caused by withdrawal of maternal hormones, is a pink-tinged mucous discharge

TABLE 14-11. Genitourinary—Female

Assessment	Pathology
Ambiguous genitalia	Genetic disorder
Urinary meatus near or just inside vagina (hypospadias)	GU anomaly
Urinary meatus above clitoris	
Decrease or no urination within 24 hours	Urinary tract obstruction
	Potter's Syndrome
	Polycystic kidney
	Hydronephrosis
	Renal failure
Fecal discharge from vagina	Fistula between rectum and vagina

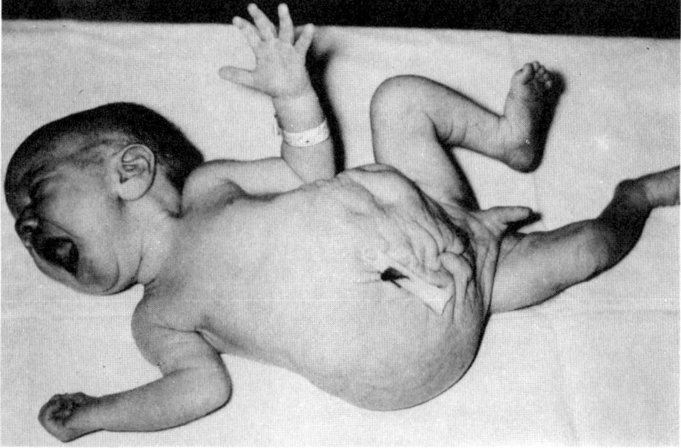

Figure 14-19. Prune-belly syndrome.

From Child Health Nursing (p.1260), by D. Jackson and R. Saunders, 1993, Philadelphia: J.B. Lippincott.

lasting 2 to 4 weeks. The presence of an imperforate hymen causes secretions to pool within the vagina (Figure 14-20). Palpating a suprapubic mass or mass between the labia majora suggests presence of an imperforate hymen. Table 14-11 identifies findings during the physical assessment of the female newborn that are abnormal and their related pathology.

Male

In full-term newborns, external genitalia is observed for a penis (2.8 cm – 4.3 cm in length) with the urethral opening located on the tip of the glans (Endo & Nishioka, 1993). Circumcision should be delayed when an abnormally located urinary meatus is

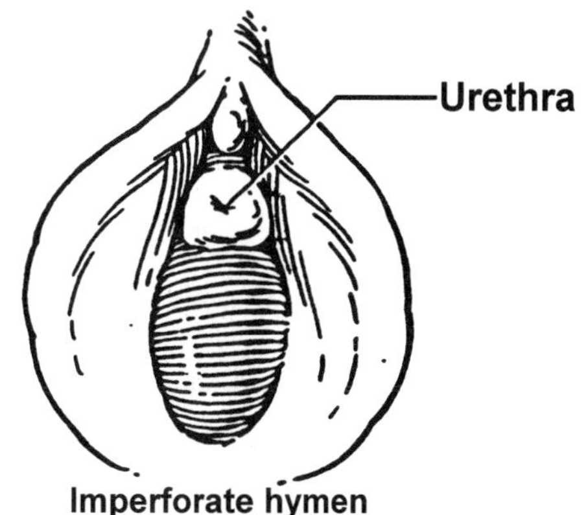

Figure 14-20.

From Child Health Nursing (p.1880), by D. Jackson and R. Saunders, 1993, Philadelphia: J.B. Lippincott.

TABLE 14-12. Genitourinary—Male

Assessment	Pathology
Ambiguous genitalia	Genetic disorder
Epispadias–meatus on dorsal surface of glans Hypospadias–meatus on ventral surface of glans (Figure 4–21)	GU anomaly
Scrotal mass which does not transilluminate	Inguinal hernia (Figure (14-22)
Testes not palpable in scrotum or inguinal canal	Undescended testes
Discoloration or dimpling of scrotal sac (Endo & Nishioka, 1993)	Testicular torsion
Decreased or no urination within 24 hours	Urinary tract obstruction
	Potter's syndrome
	Polycystic kidney
	Hydronephrosis
	Renal failure
Urinary stream not straight	Stenosis of the urethral meatus
	Urinary malformation

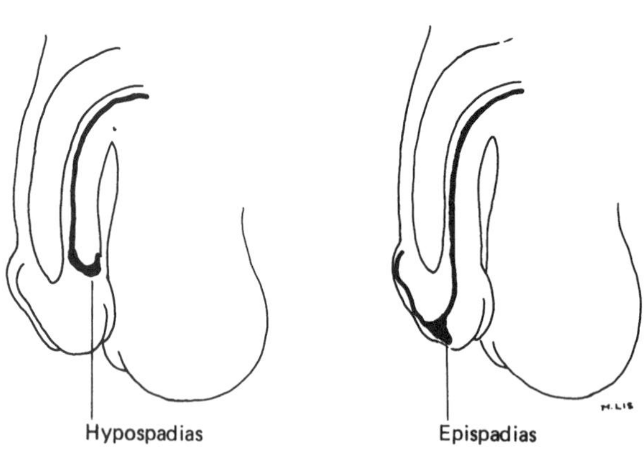

Figure 14-21. Illustration of hypospadias and epispadias.

From Maternity Nursing: Family, Newborn, and Women's Health (17th ed., p. 1180), by S.J. Reeder, L. Martin and D. Koniak, 1992, Philadelphia: J.B. Lippincott.

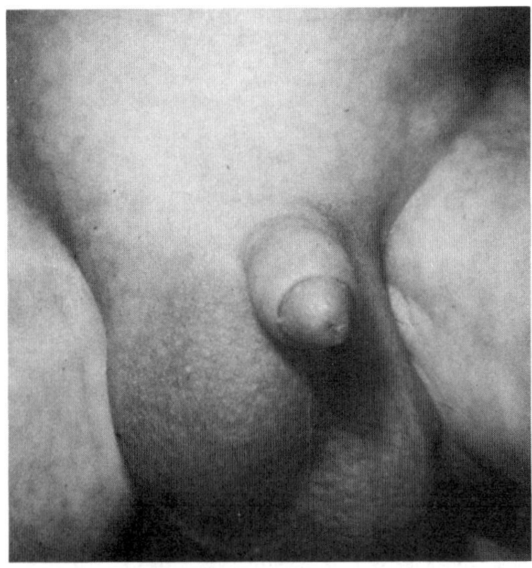

Figure 14-22. Inguinal hernia extending into the scrotum.

From Hernia (4th ed., p. 97), by Nyhus and Cardon, 1995, Philadelphia: J.B. Lippincott.

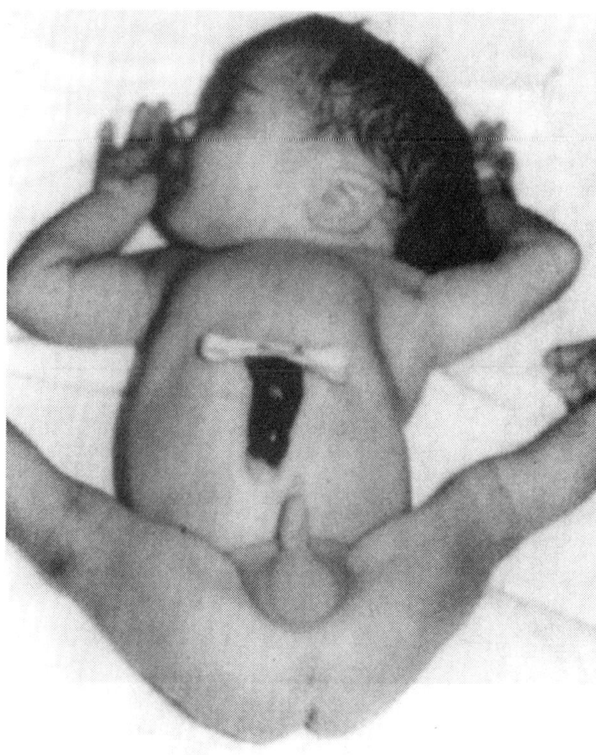

Figure 14-23. Result of a persistent breech position in utero.

Courtesy of Dr. David A. Clark, Louisiana State University Medical Center and Wyeth-Ayerst Laboratories, Philadelphia, PA.

observed. The scrotum is more darkly pigmented than the surrounding skin. It is covered with rugae and is enlarged due to the effects of maternal hormones. Adhesions between the prepuce and glans may prevent the foreskin from being retractable until after the child is 1 to 2 years of age. Small, white cysts filled with epithelial cells may be transiently present on the distal portion of the prepuce (Green, 1992). Smegma, a whitish yellow, cheesy, substance from sebaceous glands, collects between the glans and prepuce.

The scrotum is palpated for presence and size of the testes. Presence of rugae and a pendulous scrotum usually indicates descent of the testes. Before palpating the scrotum, the index finger of the opposite hand is used to apply pressure to the inguinal canal to prevent the testes from slipping out of the scrotum (cremasteric reflex). The ability to palpate either testis high in the inguinal canal suggests prematurity or undescended testes. Undescended testis (cryptorchidism) may be unilateral or bilateral. If undescended at birth, the testes will usually descend by 3 months of age. If undescended at 1 year of age, surgical evaluation and intervention may be necessary.

An enlarged scrotum is evaluated for the presence of a hydrocele, an accumulation of fluid. Fluid accumulates during fetal development, when differentiation of sexes occurs, and usually disappears within 3 months after birth. The ability to transilluminate a hydrocele differentiates it from a solid or blood filled mass.

It is not uncommon for bruising and edema of the genitalia and buttocks to be present in newborns who have been in a breech presentation. Table 14-12 identifies findings during the physical assessment of the male newborn that are abnormal and their related pathology.

MUSCULOSKELETAL

Inspection and palpation are used to assess the musculoskeletal system. The hands and feet are inspected for number of digits and presence of creases. Plantar creases begin to appear between 28 to 30 weeks of gestation and cover the entire sole of the foot at term. The presence and amount of creases on the soles of the feet are noted as part of the gestational age assessment. Nails are soft and cover the entire nail bed. In a postmature newborn, the nail may extend beyond the fingertips. Newborns exposed to meconium in utero have yellow discoloration of their nails.

Arms and legs are inspected for flexion and symmetry. Extremities are well flexed and move symmetrically with full range of motion. Legs appear slightly bowed with everted feet. A persistent breech presentation may result in abducted hips and extended knees (Figure 14-23). Positional deformities seen in the newborn period are often due to intrauterine positioning. Passive range of motion corrects these deformities that may only last several weeks.

Hips are examined using palpation. Presence of congenital hip dislocation is evaluated by Ortolani's maneuver (Figure 14-24). Barlow's maneuver demonstrates how readily the femoral head can be dislocated from the acetabulum (Figure 14-25). Asymmetrical gluteal folds indicate the presence of congenital hip dislocation (Figure 14-26). During this portion of the exam the length of the spinal column is palpated for masses and abnormal curvatures. The sacral area is inspected for the presence of a pilonidal dimple (Figure 14-27), tuft of hair, or skin disruptions that may indicate spina bifida.

Feet are examined for structural and positional deformaties. Talipes equinovarus (clubfoot), usually requires exercises and casting for correction (Figure 14-28). Metatarsus adductus, the inward turning of

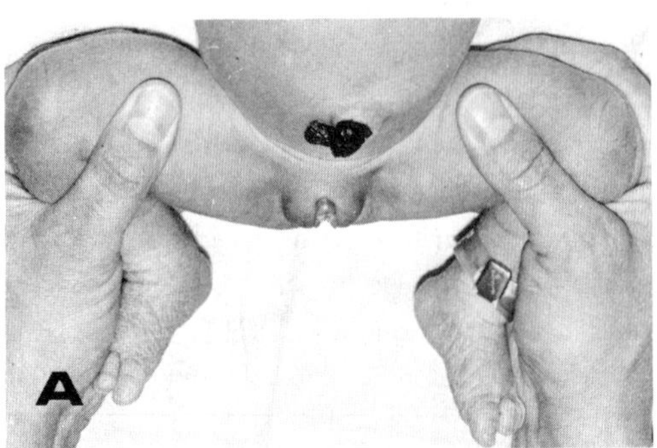

Figure 14-24. Ortalani's Sign. With flexed legs, the thumb on the femur and fingers on the trochanter, the femur is lifted forward as the thighs are abducted toward the bed. If the hip is dislocated a "click" may be heard or felt as the head of the femur moves into the acetabulum.

From Neonatology: Pathophysiology and management of the Newborn (4th ed., p. 1180), by G.B. Avery, 1994, Philadelphia: J.B. Lippincott. Copyright 1994 by J.B. Lippincott.

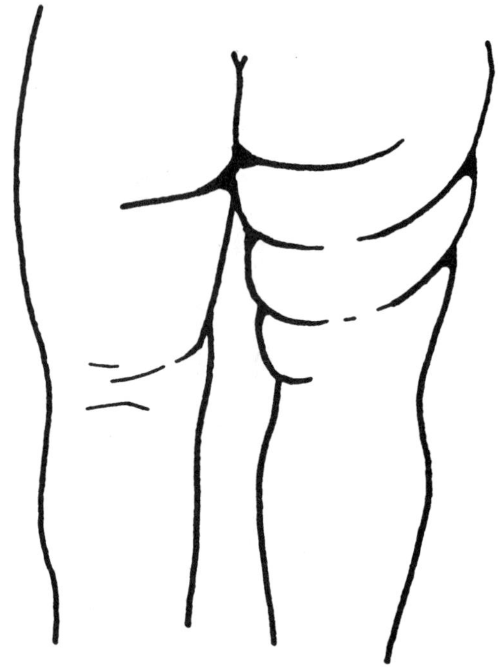

Figure 14-26. Asymmetrical Gluteal Folds.

From Broadribb's Introductory Pediatric Nursing (p.140), by Marks, 1994, Philadelphia: J.B. Lippincott.

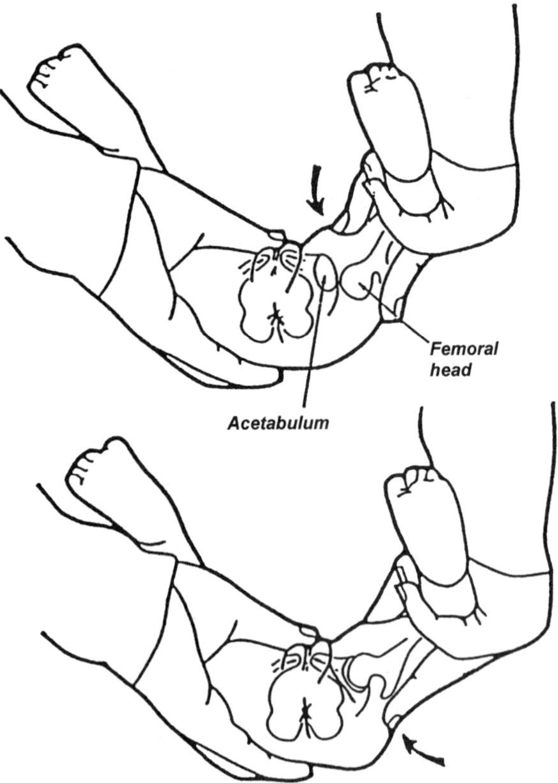

Figure 14-25. Barlow's Sign. With the thumb on the femur and fingers on the trochanter, abducting the thighs causes the head of the femur to be dislocated from the acetabulum.

From Physical Diagnosis: An Introduction to Clinical Medicine (16th ed., p. 246), by J.W. Burnside, 1981, Baltimore: Williams & Wilkins. Copyright 1981 by Williams & Wilkins. Adapted with permission.

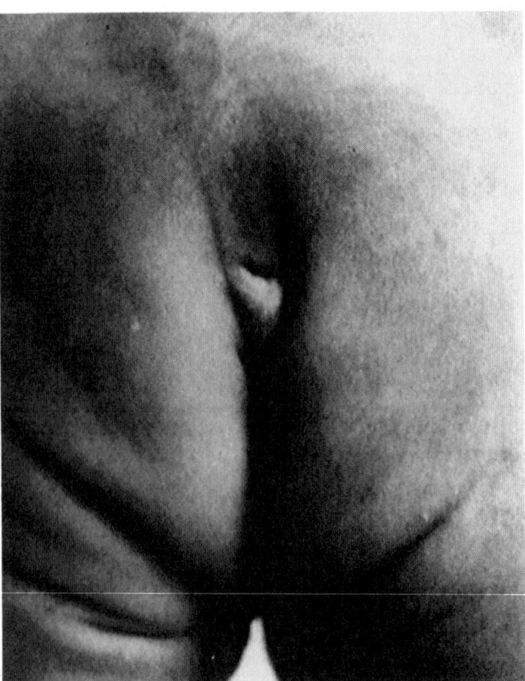

Figure 14-27. Pilonidal dimple.

Courtesy of Dr. David A. Clark, Louisiana State University Medial Center and Wyeth-Ayerst Laboratories, Philadelphia, PA.

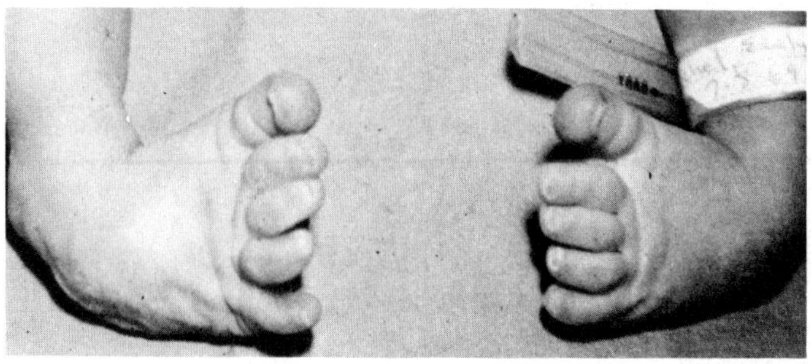

Figure 14-28. Club foot.

From Neonatology (4th ed., p. 1187), by G.B. Avery, M.A. Fletcher and M.G. MacDonald, 1984, Philadelphia: J.B. Lippincott.

the foot, from positioning in utero, can easily be brought to midline and requires no surgical correction. Table 14-13 identifies findings during the musculoskeletal assessment that are abnormal and their related pathology.

NEUROLOGIC

Assessment of the central nervous system is performed throughout the physical examination and includes evaluation of most cranial nerves and all neonatal reflexes. Table 14-14 describes how to illicit a response to determine the integrity of each cranial nerve. The newborn demonstrates two types of reflexes. The first type is protective in nature (i.e., blink, cough, sneeze, and gag). The second type, which disappears during the first year of life, reflects the neurologic immaturity of the newborn. These are sometimes referred to as primitive reflexes. The Chapter Appendix describes how to ellicit these reflexes, normal and abnormal responses and at what age they disappear.

TABLE 14-13. Musculoskeletal

Assessment	Pathology
Weak or absent muscle tone	Neurologic disorder Prematurity Genetic disorder Neuromuscular disease
Extra digit (polydactyly) (Figure 14-29)	Inherited as dominate trait
Partial or complete fusion of digits; more often in feet than hands (syndactyly) (Figure 14-30)	Inherited as dominate trait
Short fingers, incurving of fifth finger, fusion or palmar creases (simian crease), wide space between big toe and second toe	Down syndrome
Jitteriness	Hypoglycemia Hypocalcemia
Arm extended and limp, hand rotated inward, absence of normal movement, absent Moro reflex in effected side	Brachial plexus palsy
Limited movement of arm, crepitus of bone, absent Moro reflex on effected side	Fractured clavicle

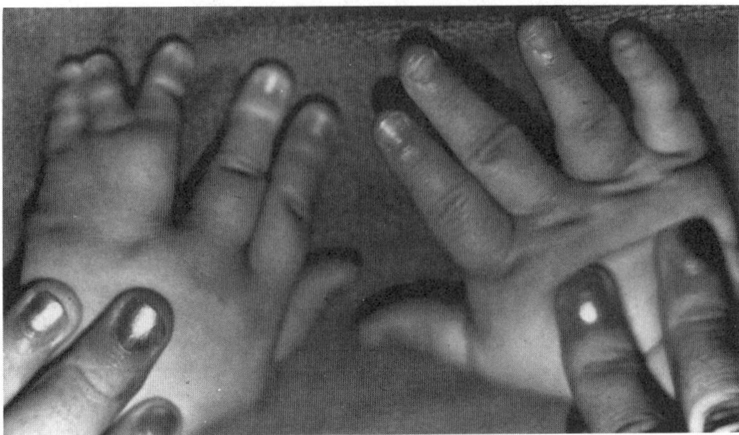

Figure 14-29. Polydactyly.

From Pediatric Orthopedics (3rd ed., Vol. 2, p. 593), by Morrissey, Lovell and Winter, 1990, Philadelphia: J.B. Lippincott.

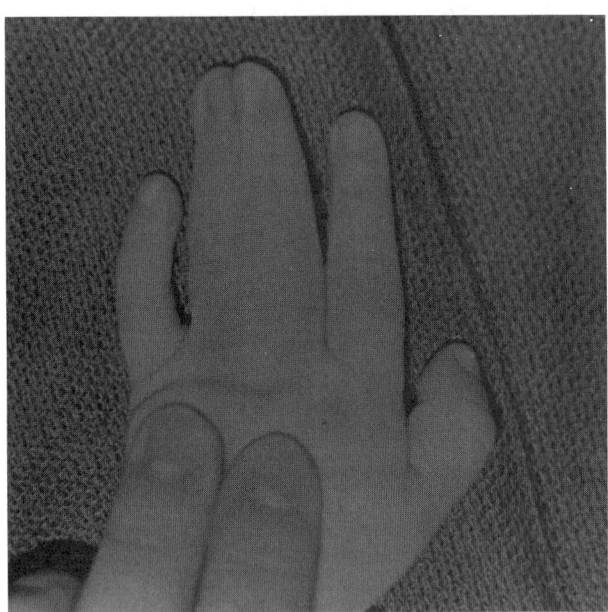

Figure 14-30. Syndactyly

From Pediatric Orthopedics (3rd ed., Vol. 2, p. 578), by Morrissey, Lovell and Winter, 1990, Philadelphia: J.B. Lippincott.

SUMMARY

A formal assessment of all body systems is completed by the perinatal nurse soon after birth and repeated at intervals established by institutional protocol throughout the newborn's hospitalization. Informal assessments occur during caregiving activities. Performing physical assessment provides an ongoing picture of how the newborn is adapting to extrauterine life. The development of keen physical assessment skills allows the perinatal nurse to detect subtle changes in the newborn's condition, identify or anticipate the development of problems, and intervene immediately to prevent or minimize these problems.

TABLE 14-14. Assessing the Integrity of Cranial Nerves

Cranial Nerve	Method of Assessment
CN I Olfactory	Not assessed in the neonate
CN II Optic	Newborn follows brightly colored object or face Blinks in response to light
CN III Oculomotor CN IV Trochlear CN VI Abducens	Constriction of pupils in response to light; normal response to the Doll's Eye maneuver
CN V Trigeminal	Presence of rooting and sucking reflexes
CN VII Facial	Symmetry of facial movement while crying or smiling
CN VIII Acoustic	Positive Moro reflex or movement in the direction of sound
CN IX Glossopharyngeal CN X Vagus	Coordination of suck and swallow; presence of gag reflex
CN XI Accessory	Head turns easily to either side; height of shoulders equal
CN XII Hypoglossal	Tongue remains midline when mouth is open; coordination of suck and swallow

References

American Academy of Pediatrics. (1993). Routine evaluation of blood pressure, hematocrit, and glucose in newborns. Pediatrics, 92(3), 474-476.

Ballard, J.L., Khoury, J.C., Wedig, K., Wang, L., Ellers-Walsman, B.L., & Lipp, R. (1991). New Ballard Score, expanded to include extremely premature infants. Journal of Pediatrics, 119(3), 417-423.

Ballard, J.L., Novak, K.K., & Driver, M. (1979). A simplified score for assessment of fetal maturation of newly born infants. Journal of Pediatrics, 95(5 Pt 1), 769-774.

Barness, L.A. (1991). Manual of pediatric physical diagnosis (6th ed.). St. Louis: C.V. Mosby.

Bates, B. (1990). A guide to physical examination and history taking (5th ed.). Philadelphia: J.B. Lippincott.

Bayne, L.G., & Costas, B.L. (1990). Malformations of the upper limb. In R.T. Morrissy (Ed.), Lovell & Winter's Pediatric Orthopaedics (3rd ed., vol. 2, pp. 563-610). Philadelphia: J.B. Lippincott.

Burnside, J.W. (1981). Physical diagnosis: An introduction to clinical medicine (16th ed.). Baltimore: Williams & Wilkins.

Coen, R.W., & Koffler, H. (1987). Primary care of the newborn. Boston: Little, Brown and company.

Cochran, W.D. (1994). Management of the normal newborn. In F. Oski (Ed.), Principles and Practise of Pediatrics (pp. 302-318). Philadelphia: J.B. Lippincott.

Conner, G.K. (1993a). Abdomen assessment. In E.P. Tappero, & M.E. Honeyfield (Eds.), Physical assessment of the newborn: A comprehensive approach to the art of physical examination (pp. 81-90). Petaluma, CA: NICU INK.

Conner, G.K. (1993b). Genitourinary assessment. In E.P. Tappero, & M.E. Honeyfield (Eds.), Physical assessment of the newborn: A comprehensive approach to the art of physical examination (pp. 91-100). Petaluma, CA: NICU INK.

Endo, A., & Nishioka, E. (1993). Neonatal assessment. In C. Kenner, A. Brueggemeyer, & L.P. Gunderson (Eds.), Comprehensive neonatal nursing (pp. 265-293). Philadelphia: W.B. Saunders.

Frank, C.G., Turner, B.S., & Merenstein, G.B. (1993). Jaundice. In G.B. Merenstein, & S.L. Gardner (Eds.), Handbook of neonatal intensive care (3rd ed., pp. 272-286). St. Louis: Mosby–Year Book.

Fuller, J., & Schaller-Ayers, J. (1994). Health assessment: A nursing approach (2nd ed.). Philadelphia: J.B. Lippincott.

Gerds, R.J. (1992). Assessment of the newborn. In S. J. Reeder, L.L. Martin, & D. Koniak (Eds.), Maternity nursing: Family, newborn, and women's health care (17th ed., pp. 641-680). Philadelphia: J.B. Lippincott.

Green, M. (1992). Pediatric diagnosis: Interpretation of symptoms and signs in infants, children and adolescents. (5th ed.). Philadelphia: W.B. Saunders.

Griffin, P.P. (1994). Orthopedics. In G.B. Avery, M.A. Fletcher, M.G. MacDonald (Eds.), Neonatology: Pathology and management of the newborn (4th ed., pp. 1179-1194). Philadelphia: J.B. Lippincott.

Grosfeld, J.L. (1995). Groin hernia in infants and children. In L.M. Nyhus & R.E. Condon (Eds.), Hernia (4th ed., pp. 93-110). Philadelphia: J.B. Lippincott.

Jackson, D.B., & Saunders, R.B. (1993). Child health nursing: A comprehensive approach to the care of children and their families. Philadelphia: J.B. Lippincott.

Johnson, C.B. (1993). Head, eyes, ears, nose, throat (HEENT) assessment. In E.P. Tappero, & M.E. Honeyfield (Eds.), Physical assessment of the newborn: A comprehensive approach to the art of physical examination (pp. 41-54). Petaluma, CA: NICU INK.

Lepley, C.J., Gardner, S.L., & Lubchenco, L.O. (1993). Initial nursery care. In G.B. Merenstein, & S.L. Gardner (Eds.), Handbook of neonatal intensive care (3rd ed., pp. 76-99). St. Louis: C.V. Mosby.

Mahlmeister, L.R. (1994b). Assessment of the Newborn. In K.A. May, & L.R. Mahlmeister (Eds.), Maternal and neonatal nursing (3rd ed., pp. 877-922). Philadelphia: J.B. Lippincott.

Mahlmeister, L.R. (1994a). Assessment of at-risk neonate. In K.A. May, & L.R. Mahlmeister (Eds.), Maternal and neonatal nursing (3rd ed., pp. 961-985). Philadelphia: J.B. Lippincott.

McAteer, J. (1992). The high-risk infant: Developmental disorders. In S.J. Reeder, L.L. Martin, & D. Koniak (Eds.), Maternity nursing: Family, newborn, and women's health care (17th ed., pp. 1168-1195). Philadelphia: J.B. Lippincott.

McAteer, J. (1992). High Risk Infant: Acquired Disorder. In S.J. Reeder, L.L. Martin, & D. Koniak (Eds.), Maternity Nursing: Family, newborn, and women's health care (17th ed., pp. 1196-1223). Philadelphia: J.B. Lippincott.

Pokorny, W.J. (1994). Congenital malformations of the lymphatic system. In F. Oski (Ed.), Principles and Practice of Pediatrics (pp. 1749-1750). Philadelphia: J.B. Lippincott.

Smith, P.W., & Jones, K.L. (Eds.) (1988). Smith's recognizable patterns of human malformation (4th ed.). Philadelphia: W.B. Saunders.

Tunnessen, W.W. (1994). Pediatric Dermatology. In F. Oski (Ed.), Principles and Practice of Pediatrics (pp. 898-948). Philadelphia: J.B. Lippincott.

Vargo, L. (1993). Cardiovascular assessment of the newborn. In E.P. Tappero, & M.E. Honeyfield (Eds.), Physical assessment of the newborn: A comprehensive approach to the art of physical examination (pp. 67-80). Petaluma, CA: NICU INK.

Versmold, H.T., Kitterman, J.A., Phibbs, R.H., Gregory, G.A., & Tooley, W.H. (1981). Aortic blood pressure during the first 12 hours of life in infants 610 to 4,220 grams. Pediatrics, 67(5), 703-613 .

Whaley, L.F., & Wong, D.L. (1995). Nursing care of infants and children. St. Louis: C.V. Mosby.

Witt, C. (1993). Skin assessment. In E.P. Tappero, & M.E. Honeyfield (Eds.), Physical assessment of the newborn: A comprehensive approach to the art of physical examination (pp. 27-40). Petaluma, CA: NICU INK.

Ziai, M., Clarke, T.A., & Merritt, T.A. (1987). Assessment of the newborn: A guide for the practitioner. Boston: Little, Brown.

APPENDIX 14-A. Neonatal Reflexes

Reflex	How Elicited	Normal Response	Abnormal Response	Duration of Reflex
Rooting and sucking	Touch cheek, lip, or corner of mouth with finger or nipple.	Newborn turns head in direction of stimulus, opens mouth, and begins to suck.	Weak or absent response seen with prematurity, neurologic deficit, or CNS depression secondary to maternal drug ingestion.	Rooting may disappear by 3-4 months but usually disappears by 5-6 months. Rooting is abnormal after 7 months of age. Sucking disappears by 1 year.
Swallowing	Place fluid on back of tongue.	Newborn swallows in coordination with sucking.	Gagging, coughing, or, regurgitation of fluid; possibly associated with cyanosis secondary to prematurity, neurologic deficit, or injury.	Does not disappear
Extrusion	Touch tip of tongue with finger or nipple.	Newborn pushes tongue outward.	Continuous extrusion of tongue or repetitive tongue thrusting seen with CNS anomalies and seizures.	Disappears by about 4 months.
Moro	Change newborn's position suddenly or place on back on flat surface.	Bilateral symmetrical extension and abduction of all extremities, with thumb and forefinger forming characteristic "C." Followed by adduction of extremities and return to relaxed flexion.	Asymmetrical response seen with peripheral nerve injury (brachial plexus) or fracture of clavicle or long bone of arm or leg. No response with severe CNS injury.	Diminished by 4 months; disappears by 6 months.
Stepping	Hold newborn in upright position and touch one foot to flat surface.	Newborn will step with one foot and then the other in walking motion.	Asymmetrical response seen with CNS or peripheral nerve injury or fracture of long bone of leg.	Disappears within 4-7 months.
Prone crawl	Place newborn on abdomen on flat surface.	Newborn will attempt to crawl forward with both arms and legs.	Asymmetrical response seen with CNS or peripheral nerve injury or fracture of long bone.	Disappears within 1-2 months.

APPENDIX 14-A Cont.

Reflex	How Elicited	Normal Response	Abnormal Response	Duration of Reflex
Tonic neck fencing.	Turn newborn's head to one side when infant is resting.	Extremities on side to which head is turned will extend and opposite extremities will flex. Response may be absent or incomplete immediately after birth.	Persistent response after 4 months may indicate neurologic injury.	Diminishes by 4 months.
Startle	Expose newborn to sudden movement or loud noise.	Newborn abducts and flexes all extremities and may begin to cry.	Absence of response may indicate neurologic deficit or deafness. Response may be absent or diminished during sleep.	Diminishes by 4 months.
Crossed extension	Place newborn in supine position and extend one leg while stimulating bottom of foot.	Newborn's opposite leg will flex and extend rapidly as if trying to deflect stimulus to other foot.	Weak or absent response seen with peripheral nerve injury or fracture of long bone.	Disappears by 4-6 months.
Blink	Tap bridge of newborn's nose when eyes are open.	Newborn blinks with first four or five taps.	Persistent blinking and failure to habituate is suggesive of neurologic deficit.	Does not disappear.
Plantar grasp	Place finger against base of toes.	Newborn toes will curl downward.	Diminished response with prematurity. No response with severe neurologic deficit.	Diminishes by 4 months.
Babinski	Stroke one side of foot upward from heel and across ball of foot.	Newborn toes will hyperextend and fan apart	No response with CNS deficit.	Disappears by 1 year.

Newborn Nutrition

Karen Moore
Gwen Chute

The choice of feeding method is made by most women long before they give birth. Many factors, including education, age, previous experience, support from her husband or significant other, the physical condition of mother and newborn, and encouragement from professionals influence the decision. This chapter covers both breastfeeding and formula feeding and includes the physiology of lactation, milk composition, and the mechanics each feeding method. Practical information for management and problem solving related to infant feeding is also provided.

BREASTFEEDING

Advantages of Breastfeeding

The number of women breastfeeding during the immediate postpartum period while still hospitalized has increased steadily over the last 4 years from 51.5% in 1990 to 57.4% in 1994 (Ross Products Division, 1995). These data are slightly less than the peak breastfeeding rate of 59.7% reported in 1984, the highest since 1970 when Ross Laboratories began surveying mothers about feeding methods (Ross Products Division). Women who are college educated, over 30 years of age, with higher incomes, not enrolled in The Special Supplemental Food Program for Women, Infants, and Children (WIC), and who live in the Pacific and Mountain areas of the United States continue to report the highest rates of breastfeeding (Ross Products Division). However, the largest increases in breastfeeding rates since 1970 are among women who are primiparas, have less education, are under 20 years of age, employed full-time, have incomes less than $10,000, are WIC participants, are African American and Hispanic, and live in the South Atlantic and West South Central areas of the United States (Ross Products Division). While the trends in breastfeeding rates are promising, they are still far below the national goal of 75% outlined in *Healthy People 2000: National Health Promotion and Disease Prevention Objectives* from the U.S. Department of Health and Human Services (1991). In 1994, 40.6% of women were breastfeeding at 2 months; 27.1% at 4 months, and 19.7% at 6 months (Ross Products Division). The duration of breastfeeding has not kept pace with the increases reported during postpartum hospitalization. Results of the *Ross Mother's Survey* suggest declines in breastfeeding duration are directly correlated with the new mother's work status outside of the home.

In the United States and Canada, the feeding decision is often viewed as a life-style choice. However, the significant health benefits of breastfeeding far outweigh perceived convenience factors related to formula feeding (Walker, 1993). Some of the advantages of breastfeeding are as follows: (1) it is inexpensive, ecological, readily available, sanitary, warm, and easily digested; (2) it increases maternal-newborn contact; and (3) it reduces the risk of many infant illnesses, such as respiratory infections, otitis media, bacteremia, meningitis, gastrointestinal illness, diabetes mellitus (Cunningham, Jelliffe, & Jelliffe, 1991), SIDS (Mitchell et al., 1991), necrotizing enterocolitis (Lucas & Cole, 1990), and allergies (Bahna, 1987). Research also suggests that breastfeeding confers some protection against adult diseases such as Crohn's disease (Koletzko, Sherman, Corey, Griffiths, & Smith, 1989), and protection against breast cancer for women who breastfeed (United Kingdom National Care Control Study Group, 1993).

Until recently, many components of breast milk were unknown. Sophisticated technology has now made possible the detection of previously unrecognized large, complex proteins in breast milk that are responsible for many of breastfeeding's protective effects. So significant are these discoveries that some argue that breast milk should be considered a medication (Fredrickson, 1994).

Physiology of Human Milk Production

Lactogenesis

Circulating hormones cause changes in breast structure and appearance during pregnancy. Breasts increase in size and superficial veins become more visible. Diameter and pigmentation of the areolae increase. Nipples become more erect and Montgomery glands enlarge. Estrogen causes growth and differentiation of the ductal system, while progesterone influences size of lobes, lobules, and alveoli.

Although prolactin levels rise during pregnancy, lactation is inhibited at this time by high levels of progesterone and estrogen. Following expulsion of the placenta, levels of estrogen and progesterone rapidly decline, initiating the chain of events that leads to the onset of milk production. Prolactin levels fall 2 to 3 hours prior to birth and peak by about 3 hours postpartum (Riordan, 1993). In the breastfeeding woman, the infant's suckling stimulates the release of prolactin and subsequent milk production. The rise and fall in prolactin levels during the early weeks of breastfeeding are directly related to the frequency, intensity, and duration of nipple stimulation.

After the first postpartum weeks, prolactin levels gradually decline, remaining somewhat elevated compared with nonpregnant women as long as breastfeeding continues. Once milk production is established, continuation appears to depend not on hormonal stimulation but instead on removal of milk from the breast. This autocrine control mechanism within the breast itself regulates the amount of milk produced so that it matches the infant's intake. This mechanism is thought to allow for greatly increased milk production in the case of multiples or involution of one breast if milk is not removed from that side (De Coopman, 1993).

While prolactin is essential for initiating milk production, oxytocin is necessary for milk ejection, or "let down." Oxytocin stimulates contraction of myoepithelial cells, which propels milk from the alveoli into the ductal system. Blood levels of oxytocin are related to nipple stimulation, rising quickly during feeding, remaining elevated, and returning to baseline within minutes after the feeding ends. Oxytocin levels continue to rise and fall with each feeding, even during extended lactation (Leake, Waters, Rubin, Buster, & Fisher, 1983). Oxytocin also stimulates uterine contractions that control postpartum bleeding and promote involution. These uterine contractions occur during breastfeeding and continue for a time after the feeding ends.

It is well known that maternal emotional states affect the milk-ejection reflex. Milk ejection may be inhibited in women who are insecure, anxious, fatigued, or in pain. Conversely, it may occur more quickly in women experiencing positive feelings and thoughts about themselves or their newborns.

Stages of Human Milk Development

The composition of human milk changes over the course of pregnancy and postpartum. Stages of milk development are colostrum, transitional milk, and mature milk. Composition at each stage reflects the needs of the newborn.

Colostrum is a thick, yellow fluid. It is present in the mammary glands and ducts at birth and is almost always measurable by 12 hours postpartum, lasting up to 48 hours (Humenick, 1987). Evolution of colostrum to transitional milk is dependent upon the duration and frequency of early feedings (Humenick). Women who have breastfed previously have more colostrum available at birth, and the volume increases more rapidly (Lawrence, 1994). Compared to mature milk, colostrum contains relatively high levels of protein and low levels of fat. It is especially rich in IgA and other immunoglobulins. These antibodies may provide protection against bacteria and viruses. High levels of beta carotene give colostrum its yellow color. The establishment of friendly, bifidus flora in the gut and passage of meconium through the digestive tract are facilitated by the newborn's ingestion of this important first milk.

The production of transitional milk begins on the second to the fifth postpartum day. It is present from 36 to 60 hours postpartum and changes to mature milk by around the ninth day. In some cases, it can take as long as 28 days for milk maturation to occur (Humenick, 1987). The concentration of immunoglobulins and proteins steadily decreases, while lactose, fat, and caloric content increase.

Water is the main constituent of mature milk, while fat provides the largest source of calories. Fat in human milk is highly variable. Concentrations fluctuate with time of day, stage of lactation, and from the beginning to the end of a feeding. The lowest fat content is generally found in the morning and at the beginning of a feeding (foremilk). The highest fat content is found in midafternoon and in the milk produced at the end of a feeding (hindmilk).

Breastfeeding Process

Preparation for Breastfeeding

Physical preparation of the breasts during the prenatal period is of questionable benefit. Prenatal nipple rolling, application of creams, and expression of colostrum does not decrease pain or nipple trauma during the postpartum period (Brown & Hurlock, 1975). Use of methods to improve nipple erectility, such as Hoffman's exercises and breast shells, are not supported by research (Alexander, Grant, & Campbell, 1992). Suggesting that a woman has an inferior nipple in need of correction may decrease her desire and motivation to successfully breastfeed, undermining the entire breastfeeding experience.

Prenatal breastfeeding classes should be recommended to women planning to breastfeed. Current postpartum length of stay has made it nearly impossible to instruct parents on all aspects of breastfeeding in the inpatient setting. Prenatal classes provide

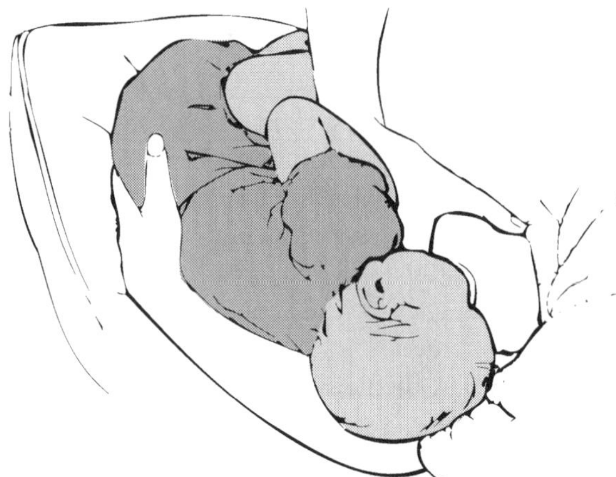

Figure 15-1a. Cradle hold.

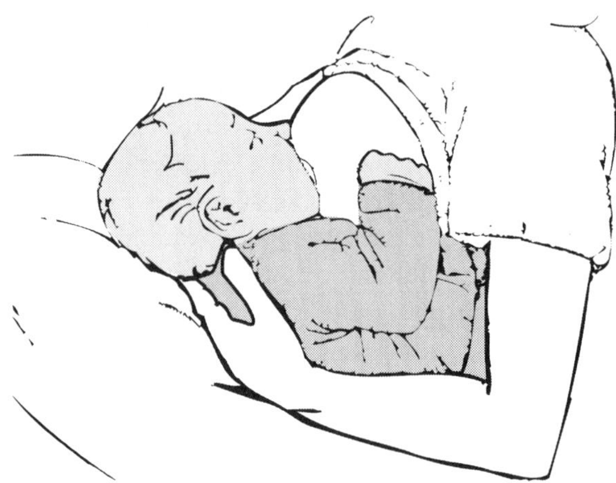

Figure 15-1b. Football hold.

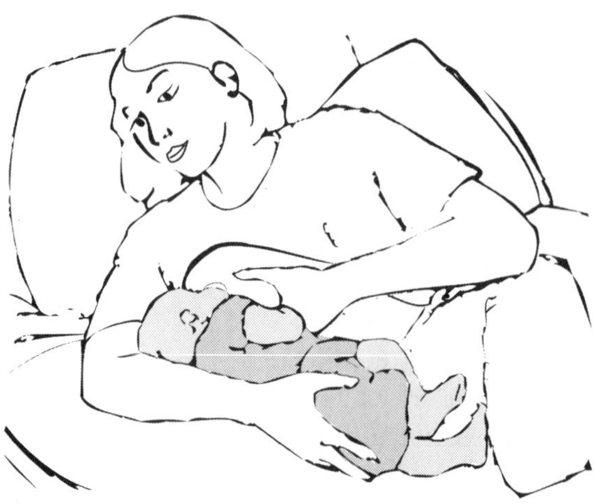

Figure 15-2. Sidelying.

information concerning implications of newborn feeding choice, introduce basic principles such as correct latch-on and positioning, discuss returning to work or school, and identify supportive resources and tips for beginning and maintaining breastfeeding.

Mechanics of Breastfeeding

Positioning. Women breastfeed successfully in many different positions. It is important for the mother to assume a relaxed, comfortable position with her back and arms well supported. Using the cradle or football hold, a pillow provides support for the arm holding the newborn (Figure 15-1A,B). If the mother is sitting in a chair, a foot stool decreases stress on her legs and back. In a side-lying position, the mother may be more comfortable with a pillow behind her back (Figure 15-2).

In most positions, a pillow or blanket can be used to raise the newborn to breast level, eliminating muscle strain caused by either supporting the newborn's entire weight with her arms or as a result of leaning toward the newborn. No matter what position is used, the newborn's body should be turned toward the mother so that the head is facing directly forward. The newborn's back can be supported with a blanket roll or pillow to maintain this position while feeding. The head should be in neutral alignment, not turned to the side, flexed, or extended.

Unwrapping the newborn allows the nurse and mother to clearly see the neonate's body position and helps keep a sleepy newborn awake for feeding. There is no need to be concerned about keeping the newborn warm because both mother and newborn generate body heat during breastfeeding. As the feeding progresses, a light blanket may be placed over the newborn's legs and feet if necessary.

The newborn usually feeds better if the legs are flexed so that the body curves inward in a gentle "C" shape around or beside the mother. The neonate's arms and hands are positioned out of the way around the mother's waist, under her arm, or along the newborn's side, so that they do not interfere with holding the newborn close for latch-on.

Supporting the Breast. Lactation consultants recommend that mothers support the breast in a "C" hold. The mother lifts her breast with her thumb on top and fingers below, against the chest wall. The thumb and fingers are away from the areola. This hold allows the mother to direct her nipple toward the center of the neonate's mouth during latch-on. Mothers are directed to use whichever hand is more comfortable.

In the past, practitioners believed that the breast needed to be compressed under the newborn's nose, permitting the newborn to breathe. Current recommendations are to avoid pressure on the breast. Applying pressure can pull the nipple forward in the infant's mouth and disturb latch-on. The newborn's pug-shaped nose allows breathing through the grooves along the sides of the nares during breastfeeding, even when the nose is touching the breast. In all breastfeeding positions, pulling the newborn's buttocks closer to the mother's body or gently lifting the breast causes the newborn's head to drop back slightly, providing additional room for breathing.

Latch-on. Latch-on is the process of bringing the newborn's mouth to the breast so that the sinuses beneath the areola can be compressed. When positioned as described, the mother lightly and briefly touches the lips with her nipple until the newborn's mouth opens very wide. Once the newborn's mouth is wide open, the mother quickly and in one motion pulls the newborn's entire body and head forward toward the breast so that as much of the areola as possible is drawn into his mouth. Shrago (1992, p. 589) describes the motion as "fitting two puzzle pieces together." The action of the jaws and undulating motion of the tongue during sucking compress sinuses beneath the areola and squeeze milk through the ducts and out of the nipple (Figure 15-3).

The following observations of the newborn indicate correct latch-on:

- lips are rolled outward
- absence of clicking or smacking
- absence of dimpled cheeks
- movement of muscles above and in front of the ear
- both cheeks are equally close to the breast
- chin and nose are touching the breast
- all of the nipple and part of the areola (at least 1 to 1.5") is covered by the newborn's mouth
- more of the areola is covered by the lower lip than the upper lip
- angle at the corner of the mouth is wide
- when the lower lip is gently pulled away from the breast, the tongue is visible over the lower gum line

Management of Breastfeeding

Getting Started. As soon as possible after birth, the mother should be encouraged to put her newborn to breast. Immediately after birth the newborn experiences a state of alertness that lasts for 1 to 2 hours, making this an ideal time for the first feeding (Johnson, 1976). Successful feeding at this time appears to have an imprinting effect on the newborn, and subsequent feedings are positively affected (Righard & Alade, 1990; Widstrom et al., 1987). The mother benefits

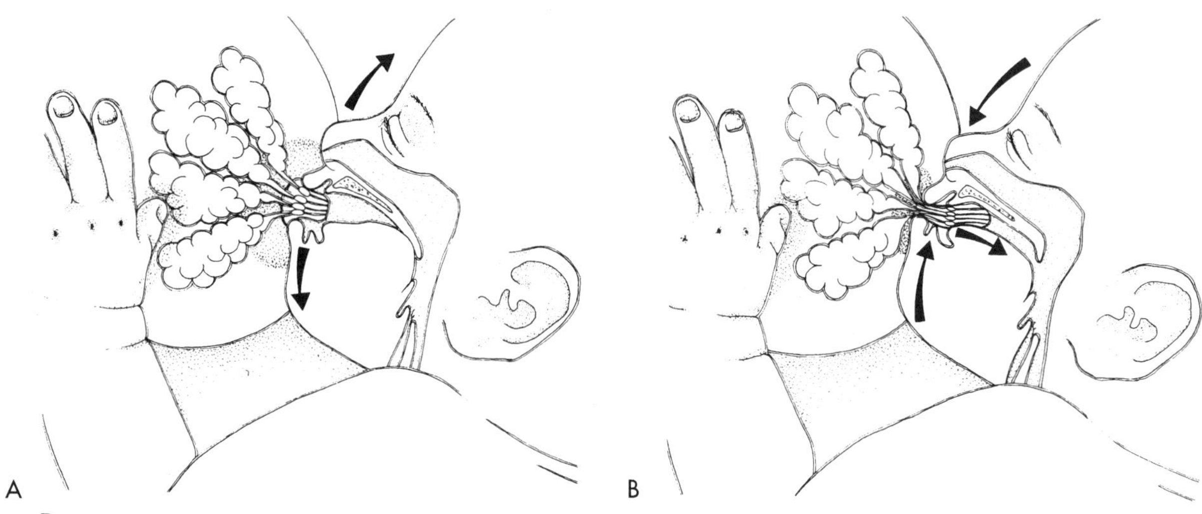

Figure 15-3. A. Newborn opens mouth wide to receive the breast, the tongue comes forward over the lower gum to form a trough under the nipple and areola, and the nipple is pulled far back into the mouth. **B.** Undulations of the tongue from front to back press nipple against hard palate, squeezing milk out of sinuses. Lips form a seal around areola.

From Reeder, S.J., Martin, L.L., & Koniak, D. (Eds). (1993). Maternity nursing: Family, newborn, and women's health care. Philadelphia: J.B. Lippincott.

from increased confidence during and after a successful feeding. The nurse's role in the first feeding is to assist as necessary with positioning and latch-on. Nipple erectility can be unobtrusively observed before and after the feeding. Coordination and vigor of the newborn's suck should also be observed.

Once initial wakefulness has passed, the newborn enters a physiologic sleep cycle lasting from 6 to 12 hours. Depending on length of labor and timing of medications used for analgesia or anesthesia, the newborn may continue to be sleepy and somewhat disorganized during much of the first day or two. A recent study suggests that Stadol (butorphanol) given less than 1 hour prior to birth affects the neonate's ability to suck and delays effective breastfeeding (Crowell, Hill, & Humenick, 1994). Epidural anesthesia has also been implicated in early sucking problems (Sepkoski, Lester, Ostheimer, & Brazelton, 1992). Nurses need to encourage frequent "on cue" breastfeeding during the first 24 hours of life because frequent feedings increase early milk production and newborn weight gain and decrease newborn jaundice and crying (Yamauchi & Yamanouchi, 1990).

Sustained Maternal-Newborn Contact. Twenty-four hour rooming-in provides more opportunities for mothers and family members to learn and understand their newborn's behaviors. Witnessing behavior changes and responding to their newborn's needs prepares new parents for the transition to home. For breastfeeding families, this structure allows more opportunities for identifying hunger cues and responding with a feeding. If the nursing couple are together, when the newborn demonstrates early hunger cues, the breast is offered. If the newborn is in a nursery, a healthcare provider witnesses the hunger cues and transports the newborn to the mother's room. During this delay, the neonate may become increasingly agitated, self-console, and return to sleep or become exhausted from crying and return to sleep. By the time the newborn reaches his mother, he is often sleeping or crying and the optimal feeding opportunity is missed. Sustained maternal-newborn contact should be encouraged during the night. Keefe (1988) found that mothers who kept their newborns at night were able to sleep longer, and that newborns cried less and established a 24-hour circadian sleep pattern more quickly. Lindenberg, Artola, and Jimenez (1990) found that breastfeeding duration was longer in mothers who were kept in contact with their newborns after birth.

Hunger Cues. Recognizing behaviors that indicate hunger is an important step for mothers and other family members. Early feeding cues include the following:

- rooting
- smacking of lips
- sucking on fingers or hands
- flexed arms, clenched fists
- placing hands to mouth
- mouth opening in response to tactile stimulation

Feeding is most successful if initiated while the neonate is in a quiet, alert state. Crying is a late hunger cue, and it is often necessary to console the newborn before he will settle and feed well.

Satiation Cues. Behavioral signs indicating that the newborn is satiated after feeding provide the new parent with positive feedback that increases confidence. In the presence of adequate latch-on, audible swallow, and sufficient time at breast (i.e., at least 10 minutes on each side), behavioral signs that indicate fullness and satisfaction include the following:

- gradual decrease in number of sucks over course of feeding
- pursed lips followed by pulling away from the breast and releasing the nipple
- relaxed body
- legs extended
- absence of hunger cues
- sleep
- small amount of milk drools from mouth
- contented state

Frequency and Duration. Mothers should be instructed to allow their newborns to control both frequency and duration of feedings and not to expect a regular pattern in the early weeks. On average, newborns feed every 2 to 3 hours during the day and when they awake at night for a total of at least eight feedings in 24 hours. Some will feed every 30 to 60 minutes for several times and then sleep for a longer period. This pattern is normal and is called "cluster feeding." If the newborn is feeding more than 14 times in 24 hours and frequently shows signs of hunger after feedings, the mother should consult a healthcare professional for evaluation and guidance.

Time limits should not be imposed on feeding. When the newborn comes off one breast, the mother can try to burp him and, if he is sleepy, check or change his diaper to stimulate him. Generally, mothers are encouraged to offer both breasts at each feeding. In the early days of breastfeeding, a good feeding on one breast may satisfy the newborn's hunger; in this case the next feeding should begin on the opposite breast. Feeding on cue encourages early milk maturation, minimizes engorgement and sore nipples, enhances newborn weight gain, decreases jaundice, and increases breastfeeding duration (Humenick, 1987; Moon & Humenick, 1989).

Assessment

A comprehensive assessment involves more than observation of breastfeeding episodes after birth. An initial assessment includes history of breastfeeding experience, problems with latch-on, sore nipples, engorgement, newborn weight gain, and amount and quality of social support. Knowing how long the mother exclusively breastfed, when or if she introduced pacifiers and/or bottles, how satisfied she was with the feeding experience, and how long she plans to breastfeed this newborn provides insight into the mother's style and potential problem areas.

Women who have had breast surgery require a thorough assessment and counseling about the potential for breastfeeding. Ideally, medical records describing the exact nature of the surgical procedure are available to the primary healthcare provider for review prior to discussion with the woman about potential breastfeeding success. Women who have had breast augmentation can sometimes breastfeed without difficulty, but the nurse should be cautious about false reassurance. Insufficient milk supply following breast augmentation surgery is not uncommon (Neifert, 1992). There is no evidence in the literature to support the perception that this type of surgery is without risk. In addition, the safety of silicone is controversial (Levine & Ilowite, 1994). Breast reduction can interfere with milk transfer if the ducts, nerves, or blood vessels have been severed. All women who have had breast surgery need to be followed closely by a healthcare professional to monitor infant weight gain and intervene for other problems such as severe engorgement or breast pain (Neifert).

Assessing the Breastfeeding Interaction

Assessment of the breastfeeding mother and newborn is ongoing during the hospital stay and encompasses all aspects of the mechanics of feeding as described above. The position of the mother and how she holds the newborn and supports her breast, as well as his response to the mother's attempts to initiate feeding, his ability to successfully latch-on, and his sucking pattern, all are important aspects of the feeding assessment.

Signs of Adequate Intake

Parents, perinatal nurses, and extended family members often express concern about whether the breastfed newborn is receiving adequate fluid and nutrition. Methods to assess intake include noting the presence of audible swallows, elimination patterns, and satiation cues during and following the breastfeeding episode. The mother's breast should also feel noticeably softer after a feeding, once engorgement has subsided.

Described as sounding like a "forceful expiration of air," audible swallow was first labeled by Shrago and Bocar (1990, p. 214). Many lactation consultants and perinatal nurses instruct mothers to recognize audible swallows as a means of ensuring milk intake. The number of audible swallows is related to the abundance of milk supply and rate of milk flow. The ratio of newborn sucks to swallows changes as milk production progresses. On the first day of life, when the intake is small amounts of colostrum, the rate may be five to ten sucks per swallow. Once breast milk is present in larger quantities and the milk ejection reflex becomes conditioned, swallowing occurs with each suck. During milk ejection, the newborn may even stop sucking and swallow two or three times before sucking resumes.

Elimination patterns are a reflection of oral intake. As a general rule, newborns are receiving adequate nourishment if, by the fifth day of life, they produce at least six wet diapers and three bowel movements per day. Many breastfed newborns have a bowel movement with each feed during the first 4 to 6 weeks. Urine is clear or pale yellow and stools look like thin yellow mustard with seeds. Super-absorbent disposable diapers make it difficult to assess wetness. If there is a concern, the lactation consultant or perinatal nurse can suggest switching to cloth diapers for a day. Any signs of decreased elimination should be reported to a physician, nurse practitioner, or lactation consultant so that appropriate interventions may be initiated to increase newborn intake.

Assessment Tools

Common methods of documenting breastfeeding interactions do not always provide adequate information. The primary healthcare provider and healthcare team members need to know detailed data about how

TABLE 15-1. LATCH–Breastfeeding Charting System

	0	1	2
L LATCH	Too Sleepy or Reluctant No latch achieved	Repeated attempts Hold nipple in mouth Stimulate to suck	Grasps breast Tongue down Lips flanged Rhythmical sucking
A AUDIBLE SWALLOWING	None	A few with stimulation	Spontaneous and Intermittent <24 hrs old Spontaneous and Frequent >24 hrs old
T TYPE OF NIPPLE	Inverted	Flat	Everted (After stimulation)
C COMFORT (Breast/Nipple)	Engorged Cracked, bleeding, large blisters or bruises Severe discomfort	Filling Reddened/Small Blisters or Bruises Mild/Moderate Discomfort	Soft Non-tender
H HOLD (Positioning)	Full assist (staff holds infant at breast)	Minimal assist (i.e., place pillows for support, elevate head of bed) Teach one side; mother does other Staff holds and then mother takes over	No assist from staff Mother able to position/hold baby

From Jensen, D., Wallace, S., Kelsey, P. (1994). LATCH: A breastfeeding charting system and documentation tool. Journal of Obstetric, Gynecologic, and Neonatal Nursing 23, 27-32. Copyright 1994 by J.B. Lippincott.

the breastfeeding couple are progressing. The phrase "breastfed well" does not capture information regarding latch-on, audible swallow, time frames, or satiation. Table 15-1 is an example of a breastfeeding assessment tool for use in the hospital or community. Similar to an Apgar score, the tool assists the perinatal nurse to perform and document a thorough assessment and to identify areas where assistance and support are needed. An example of a breastfeeding care path is included in Chapter Appendix.

Potential Problems

Difficult Latch-on and Sucking Problems

When the newborn does not latch-on or latches but does not suck well, breastfeeding can be difficult and frustrating for a new mother. The perinatal nurse should give the newborn time to become organized and awake before intervening. Current length of postpartum hospitalization, however, imposes a time limit on the nurse's ability to wait and watch. It is not advisable to discharge a mother and newborn unless the newborn has demonstrated the ability to breastfeed successfully at least once. The importance of encouraging early breastfeeding after birth cannot be overemphasized. Most latch-on and sucking problems can be avoided by this simple but critical intervention. If the newborn has not latched on at all by 24 hours of age, the mother should begin pumping and the newborn may be fed pumped breastmilk if available or formula by cup, spoon, dropper, feeding tube device, or bottle. If the newborn has demonstrated the ability to latch-on and suck at least once, the nurse may elect to wait a bit longer. These newborns should be followed at home by a lactation consultant or primary healthcare provider. Home visits or follow-up phone calls are essential for on-going assessment and interventions as needed.

Nipple Pain

Contrary to previous assumptions, breastfeeding mothers frequently experience nipple tenderness. In one study, 96% of the mothers experienced nipple pain and 27% of those mothers discontinued breastfeeding by 6 weeks' postbirth (Ziemer, Paone, Schupay, & Cole, 1990). It is difficult to determine accuracy of these data because randomized controlled studies for factors that contribute to sore nipples, such as positioning and maternal skin characteristics, do not exist. Finding solutions to relieve nipple pain is a challenge for perinatal nurses.

In a study comparing warm moist tea bags, warm water compresses, expressed human milk massaged into the nipple and areola, and education only, the most effective treatment for alleviating nipple pain was application of warm water compresses (Buchko et al., 1994). Limiting the duration of feedings or applying ointments and creams does not positively affect pain but may improve healing of the nipple. Moist wound healing techniques such as the application of modified anhydrous, hypoallergenic, pesticide residue-free lanolin to cracked, fissured nipples have been recommended by dermatologists and lactation consultants (Huggins & Billon, 1993). If the nipples are cracked and bleeding, blood may be ingested along with milk during feeding. Seeing the newborn spit up blood-tinged milk after a feeding can be frightening, so when discussing interventions for sore nipples with the new mother, this possibility should be mentioned. The woman can be instructed to call the primary healthcare provider should the newborn spit up blood-tinged milk following a feeding, so she can be reassured this is normal if her nipples are bleeding and other potential newborn complications can be ruled out.

A feeding session must be carefully observed whenever the mother reports pain. Inspect the nipples for any abrasions or cracks. Substantial damage to the nipple can result from a single feeding with poor positioning. Instruct the mother to center her nipple in the newborn's mouth and bring the newborn close to her body during feeding. Assess for signs of correct latch-on during the feeding process, and make sure the mother is breaking the suction before removing the newborn from the breast. Also ask the mother when she experiences the most pain. If the pain begins to subside within a few minutes after latch-on, the mother can be reassured that tenderness is probably transitory and will improve within a few days. If the pain continues through the entire feeding and it feels like the newborn is pinching or biting, the newborn's position and particularly latch-on should be assessed and corrected.

The newborn's mouth and mother's breast are inspected for signs of yeast/candida infection when nipple pain remains unrelieved or the mother complains of sharp pain in her breast or nipple area after the feeding. This infection may occur following antibiotic therapy. Newborns infected with yeast/candida also known as thrush, may have white patches in their mouths which cannot be wiped away or a red, raw diaper rash. Maternal nipples usually have generalized redness, exquisite tenderness, and possibly itching, as well as cracks that do not heal despite other therapies (Johnstone & Marcinak, 1990). Mothers should be referred to their primary healthcare provider for treatment with antifungal medication. The newborn's mouth must also be treated, and objects such as pacifiers that come into contact with it should be meticulously cleaned.

Jaundice

Physiologic jaundice occurs in more than half of all infants (Palmer & Drew, 1993). Bilirubin levels peak on days 3 to 4 and return to normal sometime between days 13 and 21 (Brown, Arnold, Allison, Klein, & Jacobsen, 1993). Breastfeeding should not be terminated or supplemented during this time. Newborns require evaluation for effective breastfeeding and mothers should be encouraged to increase the number of feedings. Lower bilirubin levels are associated with a higher frequency of feedings (De Carvalho, Klaus, & Merkatz, 1982). Pumping excess milk and feeding it to the newborn with a cup or bottle is recommended so that breastmilk intake may be increased. Advice given to mothers can sometimes be conflicting because recommendations for the management of jaundice in the healthy, full-term breastfed newborn have changed over the past few years. The mother should be reassured that in a healthy term newborn this type of jaundice is not harmful (Newman & Maisels, 1992). The importance of frequent feedings should be stressed.

Breastmilk or late-onset jaundice, although rare, occurs on days 4 to 7 when the bilirubin level begins to rise. The bilirubin level peaks at about 14 days and returns to normal by 4 to 16 weeks. The clinical picture is complicated when a newborn with exaggerated physiologic jaundice because of ineffective feeding patterns also experiences breastmilk jaundice. The diagnosis is generally made by eliminating other possible causes of the jaundice. In a healthy, full-term newborn, interrupting breastfeeding is rarely justified, since no harm from this type of jaundice has ever been documented, and even a temporary cessation of breastfeeding can lead to breastfeeding problems and early weaning.

Use of Supplemental Feedings and Pacifiers

Supplemental feedings (in the form of water or formula) and pacifiers should be discouraged for the first 3 to 4 weeks of life. Newborns need to satisfy their sucking needs at the breast during these early weeks to ensure continued adequate milk production. Pacifier use for newborns less than 1 month old is associated with earlier weaning, interference with milk production, and breastfeeding problems (Victora, Tomasi, Olinto, & Barros, 1993; Newman, 1990; Righard and Alade, 1992). Supplemental feedings are strongly discouraged by lactation consultants. When newborns are receiving supplemental feedings, they are not stimulating human milk production, thus potentially jeopardizing the chance for a successful breastfeeding experience. In addition, if they are receiving milk from a rubber nipple, when suckling at the breast they may become "confused" and ineffective.

Engorgement

Engorgement is a condition that occurs when breast tissue becomes distended. Primary engorgement is a result of increased blood and lymph circulation and tissue edema that accompanies lactogenesis on days 3 to 5 after birth. Secondary engorgement is caused by ineffective or lack of milk removal from the breast. Situations that lead to secondary engorgement include infrequent or shortened feedings, a newborn who sleeps through nighttime feeds, separation of mother and newborn without pumping to remove milk, or a sudden decrease in an established feeding or pumping pattern. Secondary engorgement is prevented or minimized by offering unlimited and unscheduled breastfeeds.

If the breast is hard and the nipple has retracted because of breast tissue distention, the newborn will have a difficult time latching on. Instruct the mother to express milk prior to nursing so that the areola softens and the nipple projects, then initiate latch-on and allow the newborn to feed. While nursing, instruct the mother to massage each quadrant of her breast using her thumb or finger tips in small circular motions, moving from the outer portion toward the nipple. Massaging helps to move the milk down the ducts to the nipple. Ice packs may be used before and/or between feedings to reduce edema of the tissue. Ibuprofen is an effective analgesic and is minimally transferred into human milk. Mothers should continue wearing a well-fitted bra if it improves comfort.

Assessment of the breastfeeding couple is necessary whenever a mother experiences engorgement. It is important to determine if engorgement is related to ineffective latch-on or infrequent or shortened feedings. If the newborn is not feeding every 2 to 3 hours and long enough to soften the breast, feedings need to be increased or the mother should pump or express excess milk and feed it to the infant from a cup or bottle.

Insufficient Milk Supply

Insufficient milk supply is the most common reason why women stop breastfeeding before it was planned. The perinatal nurse should be aware of this potential problem and provide appropriate anticipatory guidance about evaluating the newborn's intake, normal breastfeeding behaviors and feeding patterns, and variations such as growth spurts. Growth spurts generally occur at 10 to 14 days, 6 weeks, 3 to 4 months, and 4 to 6 months of age. The mother should be instructed to offer unlimited feedings for 1 to 2 days until her milk supply increases. The mother should be aware that her breasts will not remain heavy and full once engorgement is resolved and her milk supply has adjusted to the newborn's intake at approximately 2 to 4 weeks. She should be instructed in ways to increase her milk production if she perceives that it is faltering. Possible strategies include increasing the number of feedings, lengthening the time at the breast, offering both breasts at each feeding, pumping after each feeding, eliminating supplements and pacifiers, and refraining from use of alcohol and nicotine. Some women notice a reduction in breast size or fullness approximately 4 weeks postpartum. The woman can be reassured this is a normal finding and not an indication of decreasing milk production.

Administration of Medication During Breastfeeding

Interruption of breastfeeding for women who are taking medication is often an unnecessary and potentially damaging recommendation. There are a limited number of medications that can cause actual harm. The degree to which a medication affects a newborn depends upon several factors including the form of the medication, mother's plasma levels, molecular size, and whether it is fat soluble or water soluble. Taking medication after feeding or during a feeding can reduce the medication content in the breastmilk at the next feeding. Unfortunately, even a temporary interruption of breastfeeding can result in development of complications and/or permanent cessation of breastfeeding.

Plugged Duct and Mastitis

Inadequate emptying of a milk duct causes milk stasis which may develop into a plugged duct. Plugged ducts are palpated as a hard mass along the ductal system. Mothers state that they have tenderness and possibly redness or warmth over the plugged duct. Instruct the mother to apply heat to the area before feeding, offer the affected breast first, and firmly massage the plugged area during the feed. Frequent, thorough emptying of the breast is critical for prevention and treatment of plugged ducts and mastitis. If the mother develops a temperature or flu-like symptoms, she should contact her primary healthcare provider for evaluation of mastitis and potential need for antibiotic therapy.

FORMULA FEEDING

Use of a commercially prepared formula is another method of providing neonatal nutrition during the first year of life. Perceived advantages of formula include the possibility for any caregiver to feed the newborn in the mother's absence, increased opportunity for the father or partner to feed the newborn, easily measured intake at each feeding, and avoidance of possible discomfort with breastfeeding in public. Breastfeeding is almost always recommended, but in a few instances it is not appropriate.

Breastfeeding is contraindicated for newborns with galactosemia, a rare lactose intolerance. Mothers receiving chemotherapy are instructed not to breastfeed and mothers infected with HIV (in this country), are discouraged from breastfeeding. In a few other instances, such as a herpetic lesion on the breast or treatment with certain medications, temporary cessation of breastfeeding is advised. Some mothers choose not to breastfeed or find it an undesirable feeding method. Mothers who wean from the breast during the first year of life are advised to feed with formula until the child is 12 months old. Providing support and appropriate instructions to women who choose not to breastfeed is the responsibility of perinatal nurses.

Composition of Formula

Companies promoting the use of formula stress the similarities with breast milk. Actually, formula has been modified or "humanized" by altering protein, vitamins, and minerals. Basic proteins in formula are derived from cow's milk, soy protein, protein hydrolysate, or meat base. The main types of formula are milk based, whey adjusted, and soy isolate.

Mechanics of Formula Feeding

The primary healthcare provider will recommend which formula is appropriate. Formula comes as a ready-to-feed, concentrated preparation to be diluted with water, or as a powder to be mixed with water. Powdered mixes are more economical than ready-to-feed, though it has been suggested that mixing water into the feeding is not always done properly. In one trial, fewer than half of the mothers mixed the feeding correctly, and 26% offered over-strength feedings with the potential for serious consequences to the infants. Infants from this study who received ready-to-feed formula had softer stools and less constipation which are usually reasons parents switch brands (Lockton, Davies, & Lucas, 1992).

Oral water intoxication is a serious consequence of mixing too much water with formula or feeding plain water. It is most common in infants from 3 to 6 months of age; they generally present to the emergency room with seizures and apnea that sometimes are irreversible (McJunkin, Bithoney, & McCormick, 1987; Keating, Schears, & Dodge, 1991; Schaeffer & Ditchek, 1991). Caregivers' explanations for over-feeding with water included running out of formula, mixed more water than suggested so that the formula would last longer, giving water because the baby was fussing, it was a hot day, etc. Formula that is too concentrated can also be a serious problem that is manifested by severe dehydration, further complicated by the infant's immature kidneys' inability to compensate for the water loss (Walker, 1993). Reviewing how to correctly measure powder or concentrate and water is a critical step in teaching parents the preparation process.

Management

Identifying hunger cues is an important part of the feeding process. The mother who responds to hunger cues teaches the newborn that he can elicit a response from his caregiver. Mothers should be encouraged to hold their newborn for feeding and to use this time to communicate with him or her, not to attend to other stimuli such as the television.

The mother or family member should assume a comfortable position for feeding. The newborn is held in a cradle position with the head elevated about 45°. After touching the newborn's lower lip with the bottle nipple, the nipple is inserted well into the newborn's mouth over the tongue. The bottle should be inclined so that the nipple and neck of the bottle remain filled with formula, preventing the newborn from sucking and swallowing air during feeding.

Instruct the parents to begin feeding 0.5 oz of formula at each feeding during the first 24 hours of life. If the newborn exhibits hunger cues after feeding, the feeding may be increased to 1 oz, but that volume should be continued for next 2 to 3 feeds. Remind parents that the newborn's stomach is only the size of a golf ball. During the next 24 hours, the feedings may be increased by 0.5 oz increments, feeding the same volume for 2 to 3 feedings before increasing. Recognizing satiation cues avoids overfeeding which is more likely to happen with formula feeding than breastfeeding. Table 15-2 illustrates typical patterns of formula feedings. The newborn should be burped after every 0.5 oz or half-way through their normal intake. Position the newborn with the head on the caregiver's shoulder, lying across the caregiver's lap, or in a sitting position while supporting the head. Gently rub or pat the newborn's back. Once the newborn burps, feeding can continue.

Safety

Instruct parents on the use of a bulb syringe to suction mucus or regurgitated milk. Propping bottles during feeding should be strongly discouraged since it may cause ear infections, choking, aspiration, caries (bottle-mouth syndrome), and it decreases maternal-infant contact. Formula can be used at room temperature. Heating the formula in a microwave oven should be avoided because of the danger of "hot spots" in the milk (Sando, Gallaher, & Rodgers, 1984). Temperature of the milk is tested by sprinkling a few drops on the wrist. It is important for the nurse to include safety guidelines for the purchase and storage of formula. The expiration date on the can or package should always be checked to ensure freshness. Once a can or bottle has been opened, the contents should be stored in the refrigerator and used within 48 hours (Mead-Johnson Pediatrics, 1994). Any milk remaining in the feeding bottle should be discarded since it is an excellent medium for bacterial growth. Powdered mixes should be kept in a cool, dry place and used before the expiration date.

Lactation Suppression

The most cost-effective and safest methods of suppressing lactation include the following:

- wearing a well-fitting bra or sport bra 24 hours per day until the breasts become soft
- applying ice to the breasts and taking a mild analgesic for discomfort
- avoiding nipple or breast stimulation

TABLE 15-2. Typical Pattern of Infant Feedings with Formula

Age of Infant	Number of Feedings	Volume per Feeding	Total
Birth–2 wk	6–10	1/2–2 oz. (60–90 ml)	3–20 oz. (90–600 ml)
2 wk to 1 month	6–8	3–4 oz. (90–120 ml)	18–32 oz. (540–960 ml)
1–3 month	5–6	5–6 oz. (150–180 ml)	25–36 oz. (750–1080 ml)
3–7 month	4–5	6–7 oz. (180–210 ml)	24–35 oz. (750–1080 ml)
7–12 month	3–4	7–8 oz. (210–240 ml)	21–32 oz. (750–1080 ml)

Adapted from May, K., & Mahlmeister, L. (1994). Maternal and neonatal nursing: Family centered care. Philadelphia: J.B. Lippincott.

TABLE 15-3. Myth and Fact in Breastfeeding Information

Myth	Fact
Limiting the length of feedings prevents or minimizes sore nipples.	Limited feeding duration contributes to engorgement, thereby making latch-on difficult and increasing the likelihood of sore nipples (Moon & Humenick, 1989).
Fair-skinned women are prone to nipple soreness.	No association has been found between hair or skin color and nipple soreness (Hewat & Ellis, 1987).
The breast is emptied during feeding and refills between feedings.	The breast actively produces milk during suckling and therefore is never truly empty (Riordan, 1993).
Breastfeeding is harder work for the infant than bottle feeding.	The infant more actively uses the tongue and jaws to remove milk from the breast than from a bottle. However, sucking and swallowing are more easily coordinated during breastfeeding (Meier, 1988).
Engorgement is a normal part of lactogenesis.	Breast fullness accompanies the onset of lactation. Painful engorgement, however, can be minimized by frequent unrestricted breastfeeding and is not experienced by all breastfeeding women (Auerbach, 1990).
Letdown occurs once in each breast during each feeding.	Letdown occurs several times during a feeding (Auerbach, 1990).
Women with small breasts are at risk for insufficient milk supply.	The size of the breasts is determined mostly by fat deposits, not glandular tissue, and is therefore unrelated to milk-producing ability (Lawrence, 1994a).
Breastfeeding women must drink large amounts of fluid to produce milk.	Drinking large amounts of fluid beyond what is needed to satisfy thirst may decrease milk production (Dusdieker, Booth, Stumbo, & Eichenberger, 1985).
Breastfeeding women must avoid certain foods.	Breastfeeding women can usually eat any food, in moderation (Riordan, 1993).
Women with inverted nipples cannot breastfeed successfully.	Women with inverted nipples can often breastfeed successfully (Riordan & Auerbach, 1993).
Jaundiced newborns require extra water to flush out the bilirubin.	Bilirubin is excreted primarily in the stool. Giving water can interfere with excretion by decreasing the infant's intake of breastmilk (Nicoll, Ginsburg, & Tripp, 1982).
A 24-hour interruption of breastfeeding is a necessary and harmless intervention for breast milk jaundice.	Interruption of breastfeeding is associated with shortened duration of breastfeeding. In the absence of pathology, bilirubin levels will slowly decline with or without interrupting breastfeeding (Riordan & Auerbach, 1993).
Breastfeeding infants feed at regular intervals of 2 to 3 hours.	Breastfeeding infants may cluster several feedings together, then sleep for a longer period of 2 to 5 hours. Feedings are usually quite irregular (Klause, 1987).

TABLE 15-3. Cont.

Myth	Fact
Breastfeeding is never a reliable method of contraception.	Breastfeeding is as effective as an oral contraceptive for the first 6 months postpartum if the woman is amenorrheic and exclusively breastfeeding (Kennedy, 1993).
If a woman becomes pregnant while breastfeeding, she must wean.	Breastfeeding is not contraindicated in a healthy, well-nourished woman. It has not been identified as a risk factor for preterm labor or IUGR (Gromada, 1992).
A child that breastfeeds past the age of 9 to 12 months will be dependent and insecure.	Breastfeeding helps to meet the security needs of the developing child, encouraging independence (Sears & Sears, 1992).

Restricting fluids is not necessary or desirable. The breasts return to normal and tenderness decreases within 48 to 72 hours after swelling (engorgement) occurs.

PROFESSIONAL RESPONSIBILITY RELATED TO INFANT FEEDING

Research studies on every aspect of lactation, formula feeding, and breastfeeding appear in the professional literature every year, providing vastly expanded knowledge and understanding. Nurses need to be open to new recommendations and be willing to question traditional practices that have no scientific basis. Table 15-3 refutes some of the most common breastfeeding fallacies. Hospitals have an obligation to support changes in practice that have been shown to have a positive impact on the breastfeeding experience of mothers and newborns. Clinical nurse specialists, educators, nurse managers, hospital administrators, and physicians must take steps to see that breastfeeding is supported in their institution.

Practices that support breastfeeding include the following:

- educating all nursing and medical staff about benefits, physiology, and management of breastfeeding
- developing policies and protocols that ensure consistent information is given to parents
- offering breastfeeding education to parents
- encouraging mothers to breastfeed their newborns within one half hour of birth
- keeping mothers and newborns together 24 hours per day
- assisting mothers to breastfeed and teaching them how to continue breastfeeding if they must be separated from their newborns
- teaching and encouraging mothers to breastfeed on cue without limits on frequency or duration
- avoiding supplements of formula or water except when medically indicated
- avoiding the use of rubber bottle nipples, pacifiers, and nipple shields
- providing discharge packs with information and items supportive of breastfeeding and that do not contain formula samples or coupons
- following up breastfeeding mothers after discharge with home visits and/or telephone calls
- refering breastfeeding mothers to breastfeeding support groups (WHO/UNICEF Joint Statement, 1989).

SUMMARY

Many health care organizations have endorsed breastfeeding as the infant feeding method of choice. These endorsements recognize that the decision to breastfeed is more than a lifestyle choice. It is a decision with significant health benefits for women and infants and a cost-savings for the healthcare system. Perinatal nurses' interactions with families throughout the perinatal period should reflect recognition of the importance of choice of infant feeding as it relates to development of the parent-infant relationship.

REFERENCES

Alexander, J.M., Grant, A.M., & Campbell, M.J. (1992). Randomized controlled trial of breast shells and Hoffman's exercises for inverted and non-protractile nipples. British Medical Journal, 304 (6833), 1030-1032.

Auerbach, K.G. (1990). Breastfeeding fallacies: Their relationship to understanding lactation. Birth: Issues in Perinatal Care and Education, 17(1), 44-49.

Bahna, S.L. (1987). Milk allergy in infancy. Annals of Allergy, 59(5, Pt. 2), 131-136.

Brown, M., & Hurlock, J. (1975). Preparation of the breast for breastfeeding. Nursing Research, 24(6), 448-451.

Brown, L.P., Arnold, L., Allison, D., Klein, M.E., & Jacobsen, B. (1993). Incidence and pattern of jaundice in healthy breast-fed infants during the first month of life. Nursing Research, 42(2), 106-110.

Buchko, B.L., Pugh, L.C., Bishop, B.A., Cochran, J.F., Smith, L.R., & Lerew, D.J. (1994). Comfort measures in breastfeeding, primiparous women. Journal of Obstetric, Gynecologic, and Neonatal Nursing, 23(1), 46-52.

Crowell, M.K., Hill, P.D., & Humenick, S.S. (1994). Relationship between obstetric analgesia and time of effective breastfeeding. Journal of Nurse-Midwifery, 39(3), 150-156.

Cunningham, A.S., Jelliffe, D.B., & Jelliffe, E.F. (1991). Breastfeeding and health in the 1980s: A global epidemiologic review. Journal of Pediatrics 118(5), 659-666.

De Carvalho, M., Klaus, M.H., & Merkatz, R.B. (1982). Frequency of breast-feeding and serum bilirubin concentration. American Journal of Diseases of Children, 136(8), 737-738.

De Coopman, J. (1993). Breastfeeding after pituitary resection: Support for a theory of autocrine control of milk supply. Journal of Human Lactation, 9(1), 35-40.

Dusdieker, L.B., Booth, B.M., Stumbo P.J., & Eichenberger, J.M. (1985). Effect of supplemental fluids on human milk production. Journal of Pediatrics, 106(2), 207-211.

Fredrickson, D. (1994). Lactation Consultants, Reimbursement and Credibility: Where are we Tomorrow? Paper presented at the meeting of the International Lactation Consultant Association, Atlanta, GA.

Gromada, K.K. (1992). Breastfeeding more than one: Multiples and tandem breastfeeding. NAACOG's Clinical Issues in Perinatal and Women's Health Nursing, 3(4), 656-666.

Hewat, R.J. & Ellis, D.J. (1987). Comparison of the effectiveness of two methods of nipple care. Birth: Issues in Perinatal Care and Education, 14(1), 41-45.

Huggins, K.E. & Billon, S.F. (1993). Twenty cases of persistent sore nipples: Collaboration between lactation consultant and dermatologist. Journal of Human Lactation, 9(3), 155-167.

Humenick, S.S. (1987). The clinical significance of breastmilk maturation rates. Birth: Issues in Perinatal Care and Education, 14(4), 174-181.

Jensen, D., Wallace, S., & Kelsay, P. (1994). LATCH: A breastfeeding charting system and documentation tool. Journal of Obstetric, Gynecologic, and Neonatal Nursing, 23(1), 27-32.

Johnson, N. (1976). Breast-feeding at one hour of age. American Journal of Maternal Child Nursing (1)1, 12-16.

Johnstone, H.A. & Marcinak, J.F. (1990). Candidiasis in the breastfeeding mother and infant. Journal of Obstetric, Gynecologic, and Neonatal Nursing, 19(2), 171-173.

Keating, J.P., Schears, G.J., & Dodge, P.R. (1991). Oral water intoxication in infants. American Journal of Diseases of Children, 145(9), 985-990.

Keefe, M.R. (1988). The impact of infant rooming-in on maternal sleep at night. Journal of Obstetric, Gynecologic, and Neonatal Nursing, 17(2), 122-126.

Kennedy, K. (1993). Sexuality and contraception during lactation. In J. Riordan & K. Auerbach (Eds.), Breastfeeding and human lactation (pp. 429-455). Boston: Jones & Bartlett.

Klaus, M.H. (1987). The frequency of suckling: A neglected but essential ingredient of breast-feeding. Obstetrics and Gynecology Clinics of North America, 14(3), 623-633.

Koletzko, S., Sherman, P., Corey, M., Griffiths, A., & Smith, C. (1989). Role of infant feeding practices in development of Crohn's disease in childhood. British Medical Journal, 298 (6688), 1617-1618.

Lawrence, R. (1994). Anatomy of the human breast. In R. Lawrence (Ed.), Breastfeeding: A guide for the medical profession (4th ed., pp. 37-58). St. Louis, MO: C.V. Mosby.

Leake, R.D., Waters, C.B., Rubin, R.T., Buster, J.E., & Fisher, D.A. (1983). Oxytocin and prolactin responses in long-term breast-feeding. Obstetrics and Gynecology, 62(5), 565-568.

Levine, J.J., & Ilowite, N.T. (1994). Sclerodermalike esophageal disease in children breast-fed by mothers with silicone breast implants. Journal American Medical Association, 271(3), 213-241.

Lindenberg, C.S., Artola, R.C., & Jimenez, V. (1990). The effect of early post-partum mother-infant contact and breastfeeding promotion on the incidence and continuation of breast-feeding. International Journal Nursing Studies, 27(3), 179-186.

Lockton, S., Davies, P., & Lucas, A. (1992). Ready-to-feed baby milks: The way forward? Professional Care of Mother and Child, 2(5), 150-152.

Lucas, A., & Cole, T.J. (1990). Breastmilk and necrotizing enterocolitis. Lancet, 336 (8730), 1519-1523.

May, K., & Mahlmeister, L. (1994). Maternal and neonatal nursing: Family centered care. Philadelphia: J.B. Lippincott.

McJunkin, J.E., Bithoney, W.G., & McCormick, M.C. (1987). Errors in formula concentration in an outpatient population. Journal of Pediatrics, 111(6, Pt. 1), 848-850.

Mead-Johnson Pediatrics. (1994). How to prepare your baby's infant formula. Evansville, IN: Author.

Meier, P. (1988). Bottle and breast feeding: Effect on transcutaneous oxygen pressure and temperature in preterm infants. Nursing Research, 37(1), 36-41.

Mitchell, E.A., Scragg, T., Stewart, A.W., Becroft, D.M., Taylor, B.J., & Ford, R.P. (1991). Results from the first year of the New Zealand cot death study. New Zealand Medical Journal, 104(906), 71-76.

Moon, J.L., & Humenick, S.S. (1989). Breast engorgement: Contributing variables and variables amenable to nursing intervention. Journal of Obstetric, Gynecologic, and Neonatal Nursing, 18(4), 309-315.

Newman, J. (1990). Breastfeeding problems associated with early introduction of bottles and pacifiers. Journal of Human Lactation, 6(2), 59-63.

Newman, J.B., & Maisels, M.J. (1992). Evaluation and treatment of jaundice in the term newborn: A kinder, gentler approach. Pediatrics, 89(5), 809-818.

Nicoll, A., Ginsburg, R., & Tripp, J.H. (1982). Supplementary feeding and jaundice in newborns. Acta Paediatrica Scandinavica, 71(5), 759-61.

Neifert, M. (1992). Breastfeeding after breast surgical procedure or breast cancer. NAACOG's Clinical Issues in Perinatal and Women's Health Nursing, 3(4), 673-682.

Palmer, D., & Drew, J. (1993). Jaundice: A ten year review of 41,000 live born infants. Australian Paediatrics Journal 19(2), 86-89.

Reeder, S.J., Martin, L.L., & Koniak, D. (Eds.). (1993). Maternity nursing: Family, newborn and women's health care. Philadelphia: J.B. Lippincott.

Righard, L., & Alade, M.O. (1990). Effect of delivery room routines on success of first breast-feed. Lancet, 336(8723), 1105-1107.

Righard, L., & Alade, M.O. (1992). Sucking technique and its effect on success of breastfeeding. Birth: Issues in Perinatal Care and Education, 19(4), 185-189.

Riordan, J. (1993). Anatomy and psychophysiology of lactation, In J. Riordan & K. Auerbach (Eds.), Breastfeeding and human lactation, (pp. 81-102). Boston: Jones & Bartlett.

Riordan, J. & Auerbach, K. (1993). Breast-related problems. In J. Riordan & K. Auerbach (Eds.), Breastfeeding and human lactation (pp. 379-398). Boston: Jones & Bartlett.

Ross Products Division. (1995). Ross Mother's Survey. Columbus, OH: Abbott Laboratories.

Sando, W.C., Gallaher, K.J., Rodgers, B.M. (1984). Risk factors for microwave scald injuries in infants. Journal of Pediatrics 105(6), 864-867.

Schaeffer, A.V., & Ditchek, S. (1991). Current social practices leading to water intoxication in infants. American Journal of Diseases in Children, 145(1) 27-28.

Sears, W., & Sears, M. (1992). The Baby Book. Boston: Little, Brown.

Sepkoski, C.M., Lester, B.M., Ostheimer G.W., & Brazelton, T.B. (1992). The effects of maternal epidural anesthesia on neonatal behavior during the first month. Developmental Medicine and Child Neurology, 34(12), 1072-1080.

Shrago, L.C. (1992). The breastfeeding dyad: Early assessment, documentation, and intervention. NAACOG's Clinical Issues in Perinatal and Women's Health Nursing, 3(4), 583-97.

Shrago, L.C., & Bocar, D.L. (1990). The infant's contribution to breastfeeding. Journal of Obstetric, Gynecologic, and Neonatal Nursing, 19(3), 209-215.

United Kingdom National Care Control Study Group. (1993). Breastfeeding and risk of breast cancer in young women. British Medical Journal, 307 (6895), 17-20.

U.S. Department of Health and Human Services. (1991). Healthy People 2000: National health promotion and disease prevention objectives (Public Health Service Publication No. 91-50213). Washington, DC: Author.

Victora, C.G., Tomasi, E., Olinto, M.T., & Barros, F.C. (1993). Use of pacifiers and breastfeeding duration. The Lancet, 341(8842), 404-06.

Walker, M. (1993). A fresh look at the risks of artificial infant feeding. Journal of Human Lactation, 9(2), 97–107.

WHO/UNICEF Joint Statement. (1989). Protecting and Supporting Breastfeeding: The Special Role of Maternity Services. Geneva: World Health Organization.

Widstrom, A.M., Ransjo-Arvidson, A.B., Christensson, K., Matthiesen, A.S., Winberg, J., & Uvnas-Moberg, K. (1987). Gastric suction in healthy newborn infants. Acta Paediatrica Scandinavica, 76(4), 566-572.

Yamauchi, Y., & Yamanouchi, I. (1990). Breast-feeding frequency during the first 24 hours after birth in full-term neonates. Pediatrics, 86(2), 171-175.

Ziemer, M.M., Paone, J.P., Schupay, J., & Cole, E. (1990). Methods to prevent and manage pain in breastfeeding women. Western Journal of Nursing Research, 12(6), 732-44.

APPENDIX 15-1

Breastfeeding Path: Term Infant, Vaginal Delivery 24 Hour Stay

Task	Hours 1–2	Hour 3	Hour 8	Hour 16	Hours 17–24	Discharge At
Positioning	First attempt immediately postdelivery, with the baby on mother's chest uninterrupted for 55–60 minutes First feeding with instruction in the proper positioning, baby at level of the breast, mouth in front of the nipple, four fingers under the breast, thumb on top	Positioning reviewed, alternate positions taught if needed, pillows arranged for comfort, support person taught how to help with positioning; four fingers cup the breast with thumb on top; mother does not lean down; baby is brought up to the breast, breast is not moved to baby	One complete feeding observed, burping, positioning reviewed; Baby in flexed position with no extension in neck or trunk, head and body are at breast level, head is aligned with trunk and is not turned sideways, legs wrapped around mother's waist will draw nose away from breast freeing airway	2nd complete feeding observed; mother demonstrates correct positioning of herself and baby; rolled receiving blanket can be placed under large breasts for extra support	3rd complete feeding observed; instant photograph of proper positioning if needed, for mothers' review at home	Review at-home feeding plan
Latch-on and suckling	Lips touching the nipple, nipple plus 1/4–1/2 of areola drawn into mouth, alternate massage if needed to assist in start of suckling	Latch-on observed at a feeding; if baby's mouth does not open wide enough, use side of index finger to pull down gently on chin, roll nipple erect, express drops of colostrum	Baby's mouth opens wide with upper and lower lips flared out; no smacking or clicking sounds are heard, no dimpling of cheeks; tongue cups nipple; 1–4 sucks per swallow	Baby latches-on with smooth motion; suckling observed as 6–7 sucks per 10 seconds with several swallows	Same	Review latch-on and nutritive suckling patterns
Frequency, Duration, Milk Supply	1–2 feeds during recovery period, no time limits at breast	1–2 feeds during this time, baby left on 1st side until alternate massage no longer causes suck and swallow or baby comes off by himself; other side offered	3–4 feeds or when baby indicates feeding readiness; father or support person is instructed in calming techniques and breastfeeding assistance	3–4 feeds; one or both sides given at each feed; baby fed on cue and at night; no artificial nipples or pacifiers; any supplement needed is given at breast with an alternate feeding device	3–4 feeds	8–12 feedings per 24 hours
Feeding Cues	Baby alert, hand to mouth movements, movements of mouth and tongue	Baby alert or in light sleep state; feeding cues taught to mother include; rapid eye movements, sucking movements of mouth and tongue, increased restlessness	Feeding cues reviewed; support person will be knowledgeable of infant readiness to feed	Mother uses feeding cues to initiate feeds; baby rooms-in with mother; preferable 24 hours	Same	Same
Hydration Caloric Assessment	Diaper check for voiding and meconium	Diaper check for voiding and meconium	Diaper check for voiding and meconium	Diaper check for voiding and meconium	Diaper check for voiding and meconium	8 or more wet diapers per 24 hours, 3 or more bowel movements per 24 hours; stool changes to liquid yellow

Continued

APPENDIX 15-1 Cont.

Task	Hours 1–2	Hour 3	Hour 8	Hour 16	Hours 17–24	Discharge At
Problems: Baby not feeding; sleepy, fussy, sucking incorrectly, sore nipples, engorgement, plugged ducts, hypoglycemia	Place baby at breast, dim lights, express colostrum into his mouth	Offer breast during times of light sleep; alternate massage	Feeding cues used for sleepy baby; alternate massage for slow to start infant, baby put to breast 20 minutes before start of crying; avoid hard crying before feeds; sore nipples need feeding observation with baby's mouth open wide; colostrum or D5 with feeding tube device—no artificial nipples if sugar needed	Lactation specialist called if baby is still not feeding; reduce stimulation at feedings (dim lights, quiet room, avoid stroking, talking to, or jiggling baby, no visitors). Feeding tube device to encourage latch-on; avoid nipple shields	Lactation specialist if baby still not established at breast; pumping started if baby not suckling correctly or at all; written feeding plan developed for at home; return demo of feeding tube device; engorgement explained; pump if baby cannot keep up or breasts become over full; hot soaks and massage for plugged ducts	Referral made for any unresolved problems to community lactation consultant or other expert; pediatrician's office notified of feeding problems
Maternal self care; nipple and breast care; nutrution; rest	Express colostrum onto nipples and air dry following feedings	Avoid using creams, oils, etc., on nipples; rest and reduce visitors	Drink to thirst, no special foods to avoid; discourage visitors and telephone	No soap or creams on nipples at home; sleep when baby does; eat same as when pregnant, no food restrictions; drink to thirst; fluid does not increase milk supply	Help at home reviewed; decrease visitors and obligations; review breastfeeding and paid employment if needed; sexuality and relationships reviewed; father's role reviewed with no bottles	No discharge packs with formula; names and phone numbers of community support sources
Teaching		Positioning, duration and frequency; latch-on, feeding cues, alternate massage have been taught	8–12 feeds per 24 hours; 8 or more wet diapers and 3 or more stools per 24 hours by day 5; breast-feeding class and in-house videos discussed, breast-feeding literature given (not from formula companies)	Babies do not need bottles of water or formula; ask for patient's concerns and questions	Frequency and duration of feedings at home; sleeping not an indication of baby getting enough; diaper counts reviewed; siblings; normal weight gain ranges; engorgement and importance of frequent feeds for abundant milk supply; pumps and pumping	Reminder of pediatric appointment for 2 week weight check
Charting	Note position taught, the response of infant, latch and swallowing	Note teaching of the above, chart response of infant after observing a feeding; document swallowing	Note nutritive sucking pattern with swallowing; elongated nipple when baby comes off the breast; condition of nipples; number of times baby fed; number of diapers; subjective feeling of mother regarding how feedings are progressing	Same; noting any concerns voiced by mother	Same; noting any problems still not resolved	Concerns regarding feeds; referrals made
Consults		Interpreter if needed		Lactation specialist for continued problems; dietary if mother has special nutritional needs; social services alerted if outside referrals are needed (VNA, WIC, etc.)	Same as needed	Same as needed

Source: Walker, M. (1992). Breastfeeding Care Path: Term Infant, Vaginal Delivery, 24 hour stay. Unpublished manuscript.

Common Neonatal Complications

Patricia Nash

The majority of newborns with complications are identified and cared for in community hospitals or level II perinatal centers. Perinatal nurses must have a thorough understanding of the pathophysiology and clinical signs of alterations from the normal course during the immediate newborn period. Decreasing length of stay limits time to identify behavioral cues or subtle changes that could potentially compromise newborn well-being.

Common complications discussed in this chapter include respiratory distress, hyperbilirubinemia, hypoglycemia, and sepsis. Neonatal abstinence syndrome is also included, due to emerging data about chemical dependency among women during the childbearing years. The chapter concludes with a discussion of neonatal transport since in some cases the severity of the disease process necessitates transfer to a tertiary-care center.

RESPIRATORY DISTRESS

Respiratory distress is a major cause of neonatal morbidity and mortality despite significant technologic and pharmacologic advances during the past 30 years (Obladen & Maier, 1993). Respiratory distress is likely the most common neonatal complication seen by the perinatal nurse and is a principle indication for neonatal transfer to tertiary-care units. Perinatal events and the respiratory diseases associated with them are described in Table 16-1. The pathophysiology or causative factor of respiratory distress varies; however, the result is decreased ability to exchange the oxygen and carbon dioxide necessary to ensure perfusion of well-oxygenated blood to vital organs and to remove metabolic waste products. Respiratory distress occurs in the presence of obstruction or malformation, develops as a consequence of acute lung injury, reflects prolonged transition to extrauterine life, or occurs in the presence of other medical or systemic problems.

Five of the most common respiratory diseases occurring during the neonatal period are presented and include respiratory distress syndrome (RDS), meconium aspiration syndrome (MAS), pneumonia, transient tachypnea of the newborn (TTN), and persistent pulmonary hypertension of the newborn (PPHN).

TABLE 16-1. Clinical Correlates of Perinatal History

History	Associated Respiratory Disease
Premature Birth Maternal diabetes Maternal hemorrhage Perinatal asphyxia	RDS
Multiple gestation	RDS more common in second twin
Postmature Birth Nonreassuring fetal heart rate pattern Meconium-stained amniotic fluid Perinatal asphyxia	MAS Persistent pulmonary hypertension
Oligohydramnios	Pulmonary hypoplasia
Polyhydramnios Choking on feedings Drooling	Tracheoesophageal fistula with esophageal atresia
Cesarean birth	Transient tachypnea
Prolonged rupture of fetal membranes Maternal fever	Pneumonia/sepsis
Traumatic delivery	Poor respiratory effort
Narcotics in labor	Poor respiratory effort

Adapted from Kenner, C., Brueggemeyer, A., & Gunderson, L.P. (1993). Comprehensive Neonatal Nursing. Philadelphia: W.B. Saunders.

Pathophysiology

Respiratory Distress Syndrome

RDS classically occurs in preterm infants; the incidence varies inversely with advancing gestational age. In the United States, 20,000 to 30,000 infants are born each year with RDS (Whitsett, Pryhuber, Rice, Warner, & Wert, 1994). Development of RDS is due to insufficient amounts of surfactant or delayed/impaired surfactant synthesis. Surfactant decreases surface tension in the alveoli and functions as a stabilizer to prevent deflation during expiration. Without surfactant, atelectasis (alveoli collapse) occurs, resulting in a series of events that progressively increases disease severity. These events include hypoxemia, hypercapnia, acidosis, pulmonary vasoconstriction, alveolar endothelial and epithelial damage, and subsequent protein-rich interstitial and alveolar edema. This cascade of events results in a further decrease in surfactant synthesis, storage and release, and worsening respiratory distress.

Meconium Aspiration Syndrome

Chronic or acute hypoxia may result in meconium passage in utero. Under normal intrauterine conditions, amniotic fluid does not enter the fetal lung. However, when the fetus experiences hypoxemia, gasping may occur which can result in aspiration of meconium-stained amniotic fluid. MAS occurs in approximately 4% of all live births. Approximately 35% of births complicated with thick meconium-stained amniotic fluid result in a newborn who develops MAS (Whitsett, Pryhuber, Rice, Warner, & Wert, 1994). Amount and thickness of the meconium appears to directly affect the severity of respiratory distress. Once aspirated, meconium can obstruct large and small airways. Obstruction of the large or upper airways results in an acute hypoxic event postnatally. This may be prevented by suctioning the mouth and pharynx once the head is delivered and by suctioning the trachea via a laryngoscope immediately after birth. Meconium present in the small or lower airways may result in obstruction of these airways or in an inflammatory response in the lung tissue. This may or may not be preventable by suctioning at birth. An inflammatory response, pneumonitis, results in acute lung injury with protein-rich interstitial and alveolar edema. When meconium only partially obstructs the airway, a ball-valve effect results where air enters the lower airways on inspiration but cannot escape on expiration. This causes overdistention of alveoli and terminal air sacs, leading to alveolar rupture and pulmonary

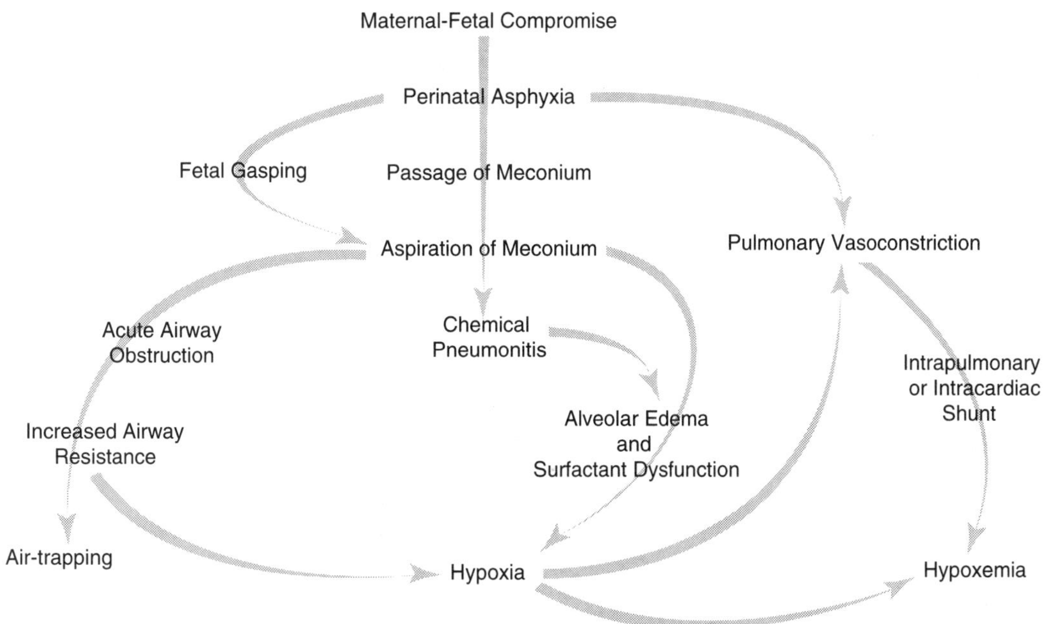

Figure 16-1. Pathogenesis of meconium aspiration syndrome

From Avery, G.B., Fletchar, M.A., MacDonald, M.G., (Eds.), Neonatology, pathophysiology and management of the newborn (4th ed., p. 439). Philadelphia: J.B. Lippincott. Copyright 1994 by J.B. Lippincott.

air leaks. Pneumonitis and airway obstruction result in hypoxemia and acidosis, which cause increased pulmonary vascular resistance and subsequent PPHN (Eichenwald, 1991; Obladen & Maier, 1993). Figure 16-1 illustrates the pathogenesis of MAS.

Pneumonia

Pneumonia may be acquired as an ascending infection following rupture of membranes. Table 16-2 identifies common organisms responsible for pneumonia in the newborn. Pneumonia, like MAS, causes an inflammatory process, disrupting the normal barrier function of the pulmonary endothelium and epithelium, leading to abnormal protein permeability and edema of lung tissue. Hypoxemia and acidosis result, causing increased pulmonary vascular resistance and PPHN (Bland, 1991).

Transient Tachypnea of the Newborn

Fetal lungs contain a fluid volume of approximately 25-30 cc/kg at term, which is maintained by continuous secretion of lung fluid at a rate of about 5 cc/kg per hour. At birth, fluid secretion ceases and with the onset of breathing, this fluid is absorbed from the airspaces via blood vessels, lymphatics, and upper airways. TTN occurs in approximately 11 per 1,000 live births (Whitsett et al., 1994). Generally, TTN is a mild self-limiting disorder lasting 2-5 days. TTN was historically thought to be related to delayed resorption of fetal lung fluid. Some authors suggest that TTN could result from mild immaturity of the surfactant system, supported by lack of phosphatidyglycerol in amniotic fluid samples from infants with TTN (Whitsett et al., 1994). Newborns who develop TTN are usually born at or near term and frequently are delivered by cesarean section with or without labor (Jobe, 1991, 1992; Stark & North, 1991).

Persistent Pulmonary Hypertension of the Newborn

In fetal circulation, pulmonary blood vessels are relatively constricted, causing the majority of the blood flow to bypass the lungs. This is appropriate for the fetus since the placenta rather than the fetal lung acts as the organ of gas exchange. PPHN of the newborn is the result of a sustained elevation of the pulmonary vascular resistance (PVR) after birth, preventing transition to the normal extrauterine pattern of circulation. When

TABLE 16-2. Organisms that may Cause Pneumonia in the Neonate

Bacterial	Viral	Other
Group B streptococcus	Cytomegalovirus	Candida
Escherichia coli	Adenovirus	Pneumocystitic carinii
Klebsiella	Rhinovirus	Tuberculosis
Staphylococcus aureus	Respiratory syncytial virus	
S. epidermidis	Parainfluenza	
Listeria	Enterovirus	
Enterobacter	Rubella	
Haemophilus influenzae	Herpes simplex	
Pneumococcus	Varicella	
Pseudomonas		
Bacteroides		
Ureaplasma		
Mycoplasma		
Chlamydia		
Syphilis		

From Kenner, C., Brueggemeyer, A., & Gunderson, L.P. (1993). Comprehensive Neonatal Nursing. Philadelphia: W.B. Saunders.

PVR remains elevated, blood bypasses the lungs by flowing through the foramen ovale and/or ductus arteriosus. This pattern of circulation is referred to as right-to-left shunting because blood is diverted from the venous circulation on the right side of the heart to the arterial circulation on the left side of the heart without going through the pulmonary vascular system. See Chapter 14 for comparison of fetal and adult circulation. Severe prolonged hypoxemia progresses to hypoxia and results in metabolic acidosis and worsening pulmonary vasoconstriction. A vicious cycle ensues. PPHN may be idiopathic, due to abnormal development of pulmonary vessels or secondary to pathophysiologic events such as asphyxia, MAS, pneumonia, and RDS (Van Marter, 1991).

Assessment

Symptoms of respiratory distress may be present at birth, or occur at any time in the early neonatal period (Carter, 1989). These symptoms include tachypnea, grunting, retractions, nasal flaring, and cyanosis. Tachypnea is defined as a respiratory rate greater than 60 breaths per minute (Lapido, 1989). Tachypnea develops when the newborn attempts to improve ventilation by increasing rate or depth of inspiration. Due to the very compliant chest wall, especially in the preterm infant, it is more energy efficient for the newborn to increase respiratory rate, breathing at rates greater than 100 breaths per minute for sustained periods of time, rather than increase depth of respiration.

On expiration, a grunting sound is heard in neonates with respiratory distress. Grunting is the result of expired air passing through a partially closed glottis. The glottis closes in an effort to increase intrapulmonary pressure by keeping alveoli open during expiration and is a compensatory response to decreased PO_2. Grunting develops in an attempt to prevent atelectasis and improve oxygenation and ventilation abnormalities (Lapido, 1989; Mahlmeister, 1994).

Retractions are depressions noted between the ribs, above the sternum, or below the zyphoid process when an infant in respiratory distress inhales. Retractions are the result of a very compliant chest wall and noncompliant lung. Compliance refers to the stiffness or distensibility of the chest wall and lung parenchyma. As the amount of negative intrathoracic pressure increases on inspiration, the rib cage expands until the soft tissue of the thorax and weak intercostal muscles are pulled inward toward the spine. The result is worsening atelectasis with marked oxygenation and ventilation abnormalities (Lapido, 1989).

Nasal flaring occurs in neonates with respiratory distress, as they attempt to decrease airway resistance and increase the inflow of air (Lapido, 1989). Nasal flaring may be seen immediately after birth; if noted beyond this period, it is considered abnormal (Askin, 1993).

Cyanosis results from inadequate oxygenation due to atelectasis, poor lung compliance, and right-to-left shunting (Liley & Stark, 1991). Although the newborn's color is an indication of oxygenation, it is more appropriately monitored by using pulse oximetry and/or intermittently by arterial/capillary blood gases.

Interventions

Care for newborns with respiratory distress focuses on oxygenation and ventilation, warmth, nourishment, and protection from harm (Peters, 1992).

Oxygenation

Adequate oxygenation and ventilation requires supportive mechanisms ranging from supplemental oxygen only to supplemental oxygen with mechanical ventilation. Pulse oximetry, arterial catheterization, and blood gas monitoring are the current methods of ensuring adequate gas exchange. In a preterm infant, delivery of oxygen should be sufficient to maintain arterial oxygen tension at 50-80 mmHg, which corresponds to a pulse oximeter reading of approximately 90%. Since oxygen may be toxic to some tissue, care is taken to avoid hyperoxia which increases the risk of developing chronic lung disease and retinopathy of prematurity (ROP) (Liley & Stark, 1991; Peters, 1992). In a full-term newborn at risk for PPHN, oxygen delivery should be sufficient to maintain an arterial oxygen tension of more than 100 mmHg, an oxygen saturation of 99-100%. In these infants, hypoxemia must be avoided because it is one of the most powerful stimuli for pulmonary vasoconstriction and subsequent cycle of PPHN. The full-term or near-term newborn is at a low risk for the development of ROP (Van Marter, 1991).

Thermoregulation

A neutral thermal environment is crucial in the care of newborn with respiratory distress. Hypothermia or hyperthermia increase metabolic demands, leading to decreased oxygenation, metabolic acidosis, and potentially to respiratory distress (Dodman, 1987).

Newborns with respiratory distress are cared for under a radiant warmer or in an isolette. Chapter 13 presents a thorough discussion of thermoregulation.

Nutrition

Adequate nutrition frequently requires the administration of intravenous fluids during the early neonatal period. Care is taken to prevent hypoglycemia that may occur secondary to respiratory distress and increased metabolic demands, since hypoglycemia can worsen respiratory distress and cyanosis (Downey & Cloherty, 1991).

HYPOGLYCEMIA

Establishing incidence of symptomatic and asymptomatic neonatal hypoglycemia is difficult due to lack of agreement on the definition. One of the major difficulties associated with defining hypoglycemia is the lack of correlation between a given blood glucose level and adverse central nervous system (CNS) and neurodevelopmental outcomes. Hypoglycemia may be a life-threatening event (Zinn, 1992), and although the vast majority of neonates recover completely, there remains the possibility of neurologic sequelae such as brain injury, learning disabilities, and cerebral palsy (Cole, 1991).

Hypoglycemia is defined as blood levels ranging from 18 mg/dl to as high as 72 mg/dl (American Academy of Pediatrics [AAP], 1993; Cole, 1991; Cornblath, Schwartz, Aynsley-Green, & Lloyd 1990; Cowett, 1992; Downey & Cloherty, 1991). Some authors designate different hypoglycemic levels for preterm and full-term neonates (Cornblath et al., 1990; Cowett). Reported incidence of transient symptomatic hypoglycemia varies from 0.1-28.6% (AAP; Cole; Pildes & Lilien, 1992). For purposes of this discussion, hypoglycemia is defined as a blood glucose level less than 40 mg/dl (Cole).

TABLE 16-3. Etiology of Neonatal Hypoglycemia

Increased utilization of glucose hyperinsulinemia	Infant of a diabetic mother
	Islet cell hyperplasia
	Beckwith-Weidemann syndrome
	Insulin-producing tumors
	Maternal tocolytic therapy
	Hypothermia
	Malpositioned umbilical artery catheter
	Exchange transfusion
	Excessive maternal fluid administration in labor
	Rapid tapering of high glucose infusion
	Macrosomic infant
Decreased production or stores of glucose	Prematurity
	Small for gestational age
	Maternal starvation
Increased utilization and/or decreased production of glucose	Asphyxia
	Sepsis
	Shock
	Defects in carbohydrate or amino acid metabolism
	Endocrine deficiency
	Polycythemia

Pathophysiology

During fetal life, insulin is secreted by the fetal pancreas in response to glucose that readily crosses the placenta. At birth, the newborn's blood glucose level is approximately 70-80% that of the mother's. Following removal of placental circulation, the newborn must maintain glucose homeostasis. This requires initiation of various metabolic processes, including gluconeogenesis (forming glucose from noncarbohydrate sources such as protein and fat) and glycogenolysis (conversion of glycogen stores to glucose), as well as an intact regulatory mechanism and an adequate supply of substrate (Cole, 1991). The etiology of hypoglycemia is overutilization of glucose, underproduction of glucose, or a combination of both. Table 16-3 identifies clinical situations associated with overutilization and/or underproduction of glucose.

Hypoglycemia develops at various hours of life depending on etiology. Transient symptomatic hypoglycemia usually occurs within the first 24 hours after birth, but may not present until 72 hours or later in some infants (Pildes & Lilien, 1992). Symptomatic hypoglycemia, secondary to maternal or intrapartum causes, generally occurs during the first 2 hours after birth. Iatrogenic symptomatic hypoglycemia occurs at anytime, depending on the associated process. Hypoglycemia associated with hyperinsulinism, such as in the infant of a diabetic mother, occurs between 1 and 3 hours of age and is followed by spontaneous recovery in most infants (Pildes & Lilien).

Assessment

Identification of infants at risk for developing neonatal hypoglycemia facilitates planning and implementation of appropriate nursing care. This process begins with a review of maternal prenatal and intrapartum history, for risk factors associated with neonatal hypoglycemia, and a careful physical examination. Symptoms of hypoglycemia are nonspecific and not easily differentiated from many other common neonatal conditions (Display 16-1). Glucose values in normal full-term newborns fall after birth. Lowest levels are reached at 1 to 1.5 hours of age, after which they begin to rise.

Universal blood glucose screening of all infants before symptoms develop, is not currently recommended by the AAP (1993). Selective screening of at-risk infants is more appropriate and does not appear to decrease quality of care or result in adverse outcomes. Each perinatal unit should develop a protocol for identifying and treating newborns with hypoglycemia. Display 16-2 identifies newborns at high risk for hypoglycemia, who may benefit from routine screening.

Interventions

Newborns who are at risk for hypoglycemia or demonstrate symptoms of hypoglycemia should have routine blood glucose screening soon after birth. Testing is performed using a bedside glucose oxidase stick method such as the Chemstrip or a glucometer approved by the United States Food and Drug Administration for use with neonates. Although glucose oxidase sticks are widely used, results are dependent on the hematocrit. They have been shown to have considerable variance from actual blood glucose levels (AAP, 1993) and to lack reproductibility, especially with blood glucose levels < 50 mg/dl (Cornblath, Schwartz, Aynsley-Green, & Lloyd, 1990). One possible reason for variance and lack of reproducibility is improper storage or outdated shelf-life of test strips, which may result in inaccurate results. Another potential problem is contamination with isopropyl alcohol falsely elevating the results (Cornblath et al., 1990; Downey & Cloherty, 1991). To increase accuracy of blood glucose determination, isopropyl alcohol should be allowed to dry thoroughly, before the skin is punctured, and the first drop of blood wiped away, before a blood drop is placed on the test strip.

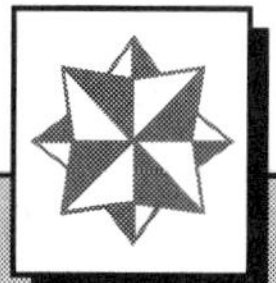

DISPLAY 16-1

Symptoms of Hypoglycemia

- Jitteriness/tremors
- Tachypnea/grunting
- Diaphoresis
- Cyanosis
- Lethargy
- Hypotonia
- Irritability
- Temperature instability
- Apnea
- Seizures/coma

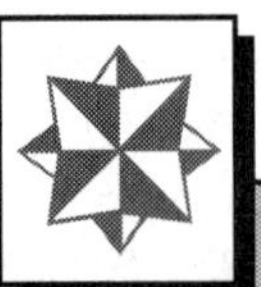

DISPLAY 16-2

Criteria for Routine Screening for Hypoglycemia

Weight < 2,500 g or > 4,082 g
Small for gestational age
Large for gestational age
<37 weeks gestation
Infants of diabetic mothers

Newborns with asymptomatic hypoglycemia should be fed immediately and then retested. If results continue to be low (< 40 mg/dl), they should be corroborated by laboratory determination and intravenous therapy started. It is important to note that laboratory measurements may also result in inaccurate values since failure to determine the glucose level promptly after blood sampling results in red blood cell oxidation of glucose and produces falsely low values (Cowett, 1992). Newborns who have had a glucose level less than 40 mg/dl are at risk for subsequent episodes of hypoglycemia and should have bedside screening performed prior to feedings and anytime symptoms occur (AAP, 1993; Pildes & Lilien, 1992).

Newborns with symptomatic hypoglycemia and a low bedside blood glucose determination should be treated immediately and a blood sample drawn and sent to the laboratory for glucose evaluation. Treatment consists of an oral feeding of 5% glucose water or formula if the newborn's condition is stable. Newborns who are unable to nipple or those whose blood glucose does not respond to oral feedings are given a 200 mg/kg (2 cc/kg) bolus of 10% dextrose water intravenous (IV) over 1 minute, followed by a continuous infusion, until the blood glucose level is stabilized (Cowett, 1992; Downey & Cloherty, 1991). Correction of hypoglycemia should result in resolution of the symptoms. IV administration is tapered off slowly and blood glucose level monitored every 1 to 4 hours initially, then intermittently before feedings, until stable (Downey & Cloherty, 1991).

The focus of nursing care in the perinatal unit is to prevent hypoglycemia when possible. Newborns should be put to breast, or receive formula (if the woman has chosen not to breastfeed) within the first 2 hours of life. Care is taken to avoid cold stress and to recognize symptoms of respiratory distress and sepsis that, if present, increase the newborn's risk for developing hypoglycemia.

HYPERBILIRUBINEMIA

Hyperbilirubinemia resulting in clinical jaundice is noted in almost 50% of full-term and more than 75% of preterm newborns (McFadden, 1991). Unconjugated hyperbilirubinemia results from physiologic (Display 16-3) or pathologic causes (Display 16-4).

Pathologic hyperbilirubinemia is most commonly associated with isoimmune hemolytic disease, due to blood group incompatibility that results in an increased bilirubin load. Other causes include extravascular blood, polycythemia, intestinal obstruction, various metabolic conditions, prematurity, infection, and RDS (Cloherty, 1991).

Pathophysiology

Bilirubin is produced from the catabolism or breakdown of heme-containing proteins (Cloherty, 1991; Wilkerson, 1988). The major heme-containing protein is hemoglobin, which is the source of approximately 75% of the bilirubin produced. The degradation of every 1 gm of hemoglobin produces 34 mg of bilirubin (Cloherty). Bilirubin, which is water insoluble, binds with albumin, a carrier protein, for transport to the liver. Bilirubin, but not albumin, diffuses into the liver cell plasm, where it is transported to the endoplasmic reticulum for conjugation. Bilirubin combines with glucuronate, with the help of glucuronyl transferase, the conjugating enzyme. Conjugated bilirubin is water soluble and excreted into bile and subsequently into the small intestine via the common bile duct. Once in the gut, conjugated bilirubin is excreted from the body or converted to unconjugated bilirubin by a gut enzyme (beta-glucuronidase). If conversion to unconjugated bilirubin occurs, it is resorbed into the enterohepatic circulation.

Excretion of conjugated bilirubin is facilitated by bacteria in the gut. Excretion is inhibited in the normal newborn due to sterility of the gut. Normal colonization of bacteria occurs over time. Lack of bacterial flora promotes conversion of conjugated bilirubin back to an unconjugated form. The newborn gut contains meconium which contains large amounts of

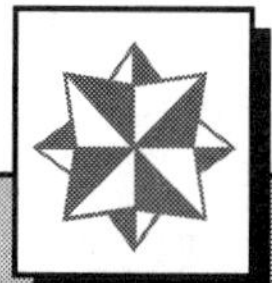

DISPLAY 16-3

Mechanisms Attributed to Physiologic Unconjugated Hyperbilirubinemia

- Increased bilirubin related to relative polycythemia and short (80-90 day) life span of fetal red blood cells (RBCs)
- Decreased uptake of bilirubin by the liver
- Decreased enzyme activity and ability to conjugate bilirubin
- Decreased ability to excrete bilirubin
- Breastfeeding

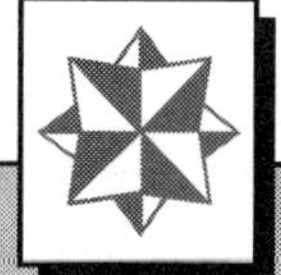

DISPLAY 16-4

Causes of Pathologic Unconjugated Hyperbilirubinemia

- Hemolytic disease of the newborn
- Bruising/hemorrhage
- Polycythemia
- Intestinal obstruction
- Metabolic conditions
- Prematurity
- Infection
- Respiratory distress

bilirubin; approximately 100-200 mg/dl in a full-term newborn (Ennever, 1992). This, along with greater red cell mass per kilogram in the newborn compared to the adult and shorted red cell life span, sets the stage for development of physiologic hyperbilirubinemia.

Assessment

In a full-term newborn, physiologic unconjugated hyperbilirubinemia is characterized by a progressive increase in serum bilirubin to a peak of 5-8 mg/dl at 72 hours of age. In a preterm newborn, bilirubin continues to rise until the fifth postnatal day, reaching a peak of 10-15 mg/dl (Gartner & Lee, 1992). A normal adult bilirubin level of less than 2 mg/dl may not be reached until 1 month of age in both full-term and preterm newborns.

Pathologic, unconjugated hyperbilirubinemia occurs in full-term and preterm newborns. Criteria used to identify pathologic hyperbilirubinemia includes clinical jaundice within the first 24 hours after birth, a rise in serum bilirubin of more than 5 mg/dl per 24 hours, total bilirubin greater than 15 mg/dl in a formula fed newborn, total bilirubin more than 17 mg/dl in a breastfed newborn, and clinical jaundice persisting beyond 7 days in a full-term newborn and 14 days in a preterm newborn (Cloherty, 1991).

As bilirubin levels rise, there is concern that bilirubin encephalopathy (kernicterus) will develop. Permanent damage to the CNS results from deposition of unconjugated bilirubin in the brain; specifically the basal ganglia, hippocampal cortex, subthalamic nuclei, and cerebellum (Gartner & Lee, 1992; McFadden, 1991). Kernicterus can be conclusively diagnosed only at autopsy by a characteristic yellow staining of the brain. Clinical characteristics associated with kernicterus include poor Moro reflex, decreased tone, lethargy, poor feeding, high-pitched cry, opisthotonos, seizures, rigidity, and paralysis of upward gaze. There is currently no absolute level at which kernicterus occurs in all newborns. Gestational age, postnatal age, clinical condition, and the pathophysiologic process involved all play a part in determining what level of unconjugated bilirubin causes encephalopathy in a particular newborn.

Clinical jaundice is apparent at serum bilirubin levels of 5-7 mg/dl (Gartner & Lee, 1992; Wilkerson, 1988) and progresses in a caudal direction from head to the lower extremities. A careful physical examination of any newborn presenting with jaundice aids in determining the cause of pathologic hyperbilirubinemia. The newborn should be examined for signs of prematurity, small size for gestational age, microcephaly, extravascular blood such as bruising and cephalhematoma, petechiae, and hepatosplenomegaly. In conjunction with the clinical examination, a number of laboratory tests may be done in the event of clinical jaundice (Display 16-5). See Appendix D for an algorithm for management of hyperbilirubinemia in the healthy term newborn.

Interventions

In the late 1940s, exchange transfusion was the only available treatment for newborns with hyperbilirubinemia (Funato, Tamai, Shimada, & Nakamura, 1994; Wilkerson, 1989). Then, in the mid-1950s an observant nurse noted that newborns exposed to sunlight had less clinical jaundice over exposed areas as well as decreased serum bilirubin levels (Polin, 1990; Wilkerson, 1989). This observation led to the use of phototherapy, which has become the treatment of choice for newborns with hyperbilirubinemia. During the past 30 years, no real improvement has occurred in the delivery of phototherapy despite multiple research studies (Ennever, 1992).

In nearly all newborns, phototherapy decreases or blunts the rise in serum unconjugated bilirubin regardless of gestational age, race, or presence or absence of hemolysis (Gartner & Lee, 1992). Phototherapy is used both for treatment and prophylaxis of hyperbilirubinemia. To date, no serious long-term side effects have been reported. Consensus does not exist in the literature or clinical practice about criteria for phototherapy initiation or discontinuation.

The goal of phototherapy is to decrease the level of unconjugated bilirubin in a jaundiced infant (Ennever, 1992). To attain this goal, three separate steps must occur: (1) absorption of the light by bilirubin; (2) photoconversion of bilirubin by photochemical reaction, restructuring the molecule; and (3) excretion via the urine and the bile (Ennever, 1992; Polin, 1990; Wilkerson, 1989).

The optimal light source is still under investigation; however, to be effective there must be illumination of an adequate area of exposed skin at a sufficiently short distance. There are currently several types of phototherapy lamps available: daylight white fluorescent, fluorescent green, special blue fluorescent, and quartz halogen (Wilkerson, 1989). Since bilirubin absorbs visible light in the 400-500 nm range, any light source with irradiance in this range is effective (Cloherty, 1991). There is a known dose-response relationship between the light intensity and the rate of bilirubin decline. The standard recommended irradiance is 6-12 micro Watts/cm^{2}per nanometer (Ennever, 1992; Polin, 1990). Irradiance should also be monitored using an irradiance meter; an ideal radiance is 8-9 micro Watts/cm^2 per nanometer. Bank lights, with a plexiglass shield placed closer than 36 cm from the newborn, should deliver adequate doses. Phototherapy can also be provided using a fiberoptic blanket that delivers irradiance of 15-20 micro Watts/cm^2 per nanometer. The newborn is placed naked under the phototherapy light and repositioned at least every 2 hours to ensure adequate light exposure to all areas. If a fiberoptic blanket is used, the blanket is wrapped around the newborn's trunk, then clothing is placed over the blanket. It is possible to provide "double" phototherapy by using either two phototherapy lamps placed above and at an angle to the newborn, or by placing the newborn on the fiberoptic blanket while a phototherapy lamp is above.

Although phototherapy has not been associated with any serious long-term effects, short-term side effects exist. The focus of nursing care is to prevent or minimize side effects if they occur. Newborns receiving phototherapy from phototherapy lamps are placed in an isolette or under a radiant heat source, and axillary temperature is monitored at least every 2 hours to assess for hyperthermia. Hyperthermia can result in tachycardia and increased insensible water loss and dehydration. Loose stools are an unavoidable effect of phototherapy and can also result in increased insensible water loss and dehydration. Therefore accurate intake and output and urine-specific gravity are measured and documented (McFadden, 1991; Wilkerson, 1989). Meticulous skin care is necessary to prevent skin breakdown resulting from loose stools. Use of creams and lotions on skin is avoided during

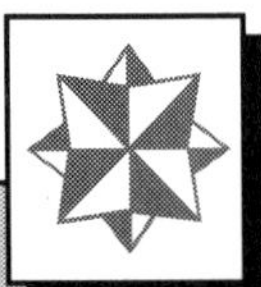

DISPLAY 16-5

Laboratory Tests to Evaluate Etiology of Jaundice

Total and direct bilirubin
Blood type
Coombs
Hematocrit
Peripheral smear for RBC morphology
Liver enzymes
Viral and/or bacterial cultures
pH
Serum albumin

phototherapy, since these may increase the risk of burns (McAteer, 1992). A generalized macular rash frequently develops and resolves spontaneously when phototherapy is discontinued.

The newborn's eyes are covered at all times while under phototherapy lamps to prevent retinal damage. An advantage of the fiberoptic blanket is that eye protection is not necessary. Eye patches should be removed during feedings or at least every 4 hours to observe for drainage and to promote social stimulation and visual development. Corneal abrasions can result from eye patches that apply excessive pressure to the eyes (Slater & Brewer, 1984).

Although human studies have not shown irradiance effects on the developing gonads, animal studies have shown DNA strand breaks and chromatid exchanges and mutations. Therefore small diaper-like devices are used as a shield for the testicles or ovaries (Wilkerson, 1989). Finally, bilirubin levels should be followed as ordered, until they decrease to normal physiologic levels.

NEONATAL ABSTINENCE SYNDROME

The types of illegal drugs used in this country have changed since the drug epidemic began in the 1960s. Heroine, methadone, and cocaine use is now more prevalent than marijuana, sedatives, and amphetamines. Commonly abused drugs can be divided into three groups: potent opioids, less-potent opioids and opioid-like agents, and non-opioid CNS depressants (Display 16-6).

Incidence of in utero exposure to illicit drugs is currently unknown. Despite multiple research studies, methodology issues such as design flaws and sample errors have resulted in underestimation of intrauterine exposure (Adams, Eyler & Behnke, 1990; Hansen, Evans, Gillogley, Hughes and Krener, 1992; Hite & Shannon, 1992; Robins & Mills, 1993; vonWindeguth & Urbano, 1989; Weiss & Hansell, 1992). Rates reported in various studies have been based on individual hospitals or communities. These rates vary considerably across populations. Differences

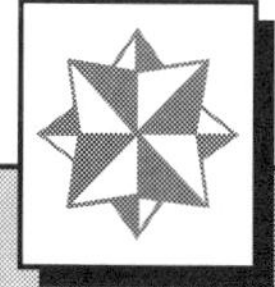

DISPLAY 16-6

Drugs Associated with Neonatal Abstinence Syndrome

Opioids	Heroin
	Methadone
	Morphine
	Meperidine (Demerol)
Less-potent opioids	Propoxyphene hydrochloride
	Codeine
	Pentazocine (Talwin)
Non-opioid CNS depressants	Bromides
	Chlordiazepoxide (Librium)
	Desipramine (Pentofrane; Norpramin)
	Diazepam (Valium)
	Ethylchlorvynot (Placidyl)
	Glutethimide (Doriden)
	Hydroxine HCL (Atarax)
	Oxazepam (Serax)

From Merenstein, G.B., & Gardner, S.L. (1993). Handbook of neonatal intensive care. St. Louis, MO: Mosby-Year Book.

in hospital practice as well as sample studied may account for this variation (Amaro, Zuckerman & Cabral, 1989; Chasnoff, Landress, & Barrett, 1990; Frank et al., 1988). The National Institute on Drug Abuse (NIDA) is currently investigating incidence of in utero exposure, using a cohort of hospitals representative of hospitals currently delivering 95% of the nation's newborns. Routine urine specimens obtained from women, on admission to the hospital, will be tested anonymously for commonly abused drugs (Robins & Mills, 1993).

Pathophysiology

Maternal drug use in pregnancy has been associated with pregnancy complications, abnormal fetal development, and neonatal complications. It is difficult to know whether substance abuse alone is responsible or (more likely) the multifactorial influence of drug abuse and social problems. Drug abuse in pregnancy is frequently associated with poverty and family disruption, increasing the risk that women will place less value on seeking early and consistent prenatal care. General health of these women may be poor, predisposing them to less-than-optimal weight gain and anemia (Robins & Mills, 1993).

Complete information on transmission of illicit drugs to the fetus is unavailable, but most appear to pass easily through the placenta. Based on animal studies, it is known that rates of transmission and metabolism vary from drug to drug and depend on fetal age. Increased maternal blood flow in later gestation appears to improve transport of substances to the fetus (Robins & Mills, 1993).

Vasoconstricting effects cause abruptio placentae (Handler, Kistin, Davis, & Ferre, 1991; Meeker & Reynolds, 1990), elevated blood pressure (Robins & Mills, 1993), precipitous labor (Tabor, Smith-Wallace, & Yonekura, 1990), inadequate contraction pattern, and decreased fetal oxygenation (Robins & Mills, 1993). While researchers note that lifestyle as a variable should be examined independently in future studies, Fried (1985) suggests that chemical dependency during pregnancy increases risk of preterm birth. All maternal complications increase risk to the fetus and newborn.

Urogenital malformations are strongly associated with cocaine use in the first trimester (Centers for Disease Control and Prevention, 1989). Cocaine is also thought to increase fetal vasoconstricting hormones leading to increased blood pressure and elevated heart rate (Woods, Plessinger, & Clark, 1987). These physiologic responses increase risk of cerebral ischemia and hemorrhagic lesions (Dixon & Bejar, 1989). Use of cocaine and heroin (Robins & Mills, 1993), amphetamine (Little, Snell, & Gilstrap, 1988), and marijuana and PCP (Tabor, Smith-Wallace, & Yonekura, 1990) is associated with intrauterine growth restriction.

Assessment

Neonatal abstinence syndrome describes a range of symptoms the newborn experiences during withdrawal (Table 16-4). While the most severe withdrawal symptoms are seen in the newborn exposed to opioids, symptoms can also occur following exposure to other drugs. Depending on the chemical agent the mother used, after several weeks or months, symptoms no longer represent withdrawal but instead represent the long-term effects of in utero drug exposure.

Symptoms of opioid withdrawal usually begin 24 to 48 hours after birth, but may not appear for as long as 10 days. Symptoms generally last for less than 2 weeks, but some infants show mild signs for up to

TABLE 16-4. Symptoms of Neonatal Abstinence Syndrome

Central nervous system	irritability shrill cry tremors hyperreflexia altered sleep patterns occasional seizures
Gastrointestinal dysfunction	vomiting diarrhea excessive sucking poor feeding
Respiratory distress	tachypnea stuffy nose flaring retractions apnea
Other	yawning sneezing mottled color fever cyanosis

6 months (Robins & Mills, 1993). The severity of the syndrome is dependent upon the drug or drugs used (Vinci, Parker, Bauchner, Zuckerman, & Cabral, 1989). Withdrawal from narcotics plus cocaine is more severe than withdrawal from narcotics alone. Methadone withdrawal is more severe than any other narcotic alone or cocaine alone (Flanagan-Everett, 1991).

Heroin withdrawal begins anytime within the first 2 weeks after birth, with an average onset at 72 hours. The duration of symptoms lasts 8 to 16 weeks or longer. There has been no correlation between maternal heroine abuse and the severity of neonatal withdrawal (Flandermeyer, 1987). It is impossible to predict which newborns will develop severe symptoms of neonatal abstinence.

Methadone withdrawal begins later and lasts longer than heroin withdrawal. Approximately 75% of infants with prenatal exposure to methadone develop withdrawal symptoms (Robins & Mills, 1993). Time of onset is variable. The newborn may have early withdrawal beginning at 24 to 48 hours or one or two types of late withdrawal: (1) symptoms may appear shortly after birth, improve, then reappear in 2 to 4 weeks or (2) there may be no symptoms until 2 to 3 weeks of age.

Cocaine addiction differs from opioid addiction because there is no predictable sequence of withdrawal symptoms (Flandermeyer, 1987). Whether or not withdrawal indeed occurs is still under investigation. If cocaine withdrawal does exist symptoms include hypertonia, hyperactive startle reflex, irritability, tremulousness, tachypnea, loose stools, state disorganization, and poor feeds. These symptoms may actually be a direct effect of cocaine itself rather than withdrawal (vonWindeguth & Urbano, 1989).

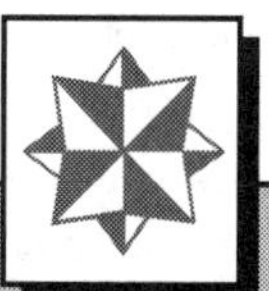

DISPLAY 16-7

Interventions to Support the Newborn Experiencing Withdrawal

Swaddling
Rocking
Decrease tactile stimulation
Dark room
Decrease environmental noise and stimulation
Water bed
Small frequent feedings
Use of a pacifier

Interventions

Since neonatal abstinence syndrome is one complication for which treatment exists, the perinatal nurse should be familiar with symptoms of drug withdrawal in the newborn and potential complications.

Appropriate care of drug-exposed newborns begins with early identification and recognition of maternal drug abuse. Careful prenatal and postnatal maternal screening for substance abuse is essential. All women, regardless of racial or social background and perceived risk status, should be asked directly in a nonjudgemental manner about drug and alcohol use during pregnancy. Illicit drug use should be considered in women who (1) received no prenatal care, (2) have a history of sexually transmitted diseases, (3) insist on leaving the hospital shortly after birth, (4) demonstrate signs of drug use such as needle marks and malnutrition, or (5) demand medication frequently and in large doses (Robins & Mills, 1993; vonWindeguth & Urbano, 1989).

When indicated, a maternal urine toxicology screen can be included as part of laboratory tests routinely ordered during the hospital admission process. If results are positive, or not obtained, a urine toxicology screen or meconium assay is collected from the newborn's first void or stool (Hansen, Evans, Gillogley, Hughes, & Krener, 1992; Jessup, 1990; Rosengren et al., 1993). All newborns should be observed for symptoms of neonatal abstinence syndrome. Many withdrawal symptoms can be successfully treated with basic nursing interventions (Display 16-7). These interventions increase the newborn's ability to regulate behavioral state, improve neuromotor control, and promote maternal newborn attachment.

Newborns who do not respond to symptomatic treatment alone may need medication. Ideally, the decision to begin medication is based on an objective assessment of symptoms such as the Neonatal Abstinence Scoring System (Figure 16-2). The newborn is assessed and scored every 2 hours for the first 48 hours and then every 8 hours while symptoms of withdrawal persist. Points are given for all behaviors or symptoms noted during the scoring interval. The newborn must be awake and calm to assess muscle tone, respirations and, Moro reflex. Observations should be made after feeding whenever possible, since hunger can mimic withdrawal. Temperature recorded on the scoring sheet should be obtained rectally, although an axillary temperature 2° cooler may also indicate withdrawal. If the average of any three successive scores exceed eight and is not reduced by nursing interventions, medications are initiated (Flanagan-Everett, 1991).

A variety of medications are used to treat neonatal abstinence syndrome. The three most commonly used are diluted tincture of opium (DTO), paregoric, and phenobarbital. A protocol for administration tapering and discontinuing these drugs was proposed by Flanagan-Everett (1991). DTO controls all withdrawal symptoms, causes little impairment of the suck reflex, and contains few additives. Dosage is 0.05 ml/kg or 2 gtts/kg every 4 to 6 hours; the dose may be increased by 2 gtts every 4 hours until the desired effect is achieved. Side effects of DTO are sedation and constipation. Paregoric also contains opium 0.4% and numerous additives. Dosage, tapering, and side effects are similar to DTO. Phenobarbital eases irritability, although it has little effect on relieving the gastrointestinal symptoms of withdrawal. Phenobarbital is given at a dose of 5-8 mg/kg per day in three divided doses, although some infants may require higher doses. Side effects of phenobarbital include sedation, poor suck reflex, and heightened sensitivity to pain.

Tapering and discontinuation of medications is best achieved using the Neonatal Abstinence Scoring sheet. Once medication has been initiated, the newborn should be scored every 8 hours and reevaluated on a daily basis. If all scores are eight or less or the mean of any three successive scores is seven or less, the dose should be maintained for 72 hours. If, after 72 hours, the scores are consistently eight or less or the mean of three successive scores is seven or less, the dose should be decreased by 10%. This dose is maintained for 24 hours. If the mean score remains less than eight, the dose is decreased by 10% every 24 hours. When the dose of DTO is 0.03 mg/kg per day or less or phenobarbital is 5 mg/kg per day or less, the medication is discontinued. After the medication has been discontinued, scoring continues until scores are eight or less for 72 hours.

Symptoms of neonatal abstinence may not be completely resolved at the time of discharge, so parents need education to successfully care for the newborn. Parents should spend extended periods of time observing and interacting with their newborn in the presence of the nurse. These opportunities can be used by the nurse to observe parental interaction. Since drug-exposed newborns are discharged into an environment where drug use may still be a factor, families are followed after discharge to ensure that growth and development is adequate and that parents are aware of and receive available community resources.

NEONATAL SEPSIS

Incidence of neonatal sepsis is 1 to 10 per 1,000 live births (Freij & McCracken, 1994). Variations in reported morbidity and mortality rates are related to methodologic factors such as healthcare institution practice, risk status of population or community investigated, and clinical factors such as gestational age and birth weight (Table 16-5). Diagnosis of neonatal sepsis is made based on clinical symptoms and evidence of a positive blood culture (Freij & McCracken, 1994). As technologic advances allow for the survival of progressively smaller preterm newborns, neonatal sepsis can potentially develop beyond the first month of life to 4 to 6 months of age (Witek-Janusek & Cusack, 1994).

Pathophysiology

Many microorganisms are responsible for infection during the neonatal period (Display 16-8). Life-threatening neonatal sepsis is usually polymicrobial in nature. The most common causative bacterial agents are group B beta hemolytic streptococcus (GBS), Escherichia coli (E. coli), and Hemophilus influenza (O'Donnell & Merenstein, 1993). Infection occurs as a result of (1) intrauterine exposure via ascending infection from one or more of the endogenous flora of the cervix or vagina or (less commonly) transplacentally from microorganisms in the maternal circulation, (2) cutaneous transmission as the fetus passes through the birth canal, and (3) environment contamination following birth.

Two patterns of development, early onset, and late onset, are observed in neonatal sepsis. Early onset sepsis occurs within 7 days of life. Frequently inoculation occurred in utero. If symptoms are not present immediately after birth, most newborns become symptomatic within 12 hours. Development of symptoms in early onset sepsis is generally very sudden and may rapidly progress to septic shock (Witek-Janusek & Cusack, 1994). Late-onset infection may occur as early as 1 week of age but more commonly after the first week of life. Late-onset infection usually results from

Figure 16-2. Neonatal Abstinence Scoring System

CENTRAL NERVOUS SYSTEM DISTURBANCES													
SIGNS AND SYMPTOMS	SCORE	AM							PM				
Excessive High-pitched Cry	2												
Continuous High-Pitched Cry	3												
Sleeps <1 Hour After Feeding	3												
Sleeps <2 Hours After Feeding	2												
Sleeps <3 Hours After Feeding	1												
Hyperactive Moro Reflex	2												
Markedly Hyperactive Moro Reflex	3												
Mild Tremors Disturbed	1												
Moderate–Severe Tremors Disturbed	2												
Mild Tremors Undisturbed	1												
Moderate–Severe Tremors Undisturbed	4												
Increased Muscle Tone	2												
Excoloration (Specify Area):	1												
Myoclonic Jerks	3												
Generalized Convulsions	5												
METABOLIC/VASOMOTOR /RESPIRATORY DISTURBANCES													
Sweating													
Fever <101(99–100.8°F./37.2–38.2°C)	1												
Fever >101(38.2°C. and Higher)	2												
Frequent Yawning (>3–4 times/interval)	1												
Mottling	1												
Nasal Stuffiness	1												
Sneezing (>3–4 times/interval)	1												
Nasal Flaring	2												
Respiratory Rate >60/Min.	1												
Respiratory Rate >50/Min. with Retractions	2												
GASTROINTESTINAL DISTURBANCES													
Excessive Sucking	1												
Poor Feeding	2												
Regurgitation	2												
Projectile Vomiting	3												
Loose Stools	2												
Watery Stools	3												
TOTAL SCORE													

From Cloherty, J.P., & Stark, A.R. (1993). Manual of neonatal care (3rd ed., pp. 26-27). Boston: Little, Brown.

TABLE 16-5. Neonatal Sepsis—Incidence and Mortality Rate

Birth Weight	Incidence	Mortality Rate
>2,500 g	1 per 1,000	3%
1,000–2,500 g	4–9 per 10,000	30%
<1,000	26 per 1,000	90%

From Remington, J.S., & Klein, J.O. (Eds.), (1995). Infectious diseases of the fetus and newborn (4th ed., pp. 835-890). Philadelphia: W.B. Saunders.

exposure during the birth process or is the result of nosocomial transmission after birth from caregivers or invasive procedures. Table 16-6 describes bacterial pathogens responsible for early- and late-onset sepsis. Due to immaturity of the newborn immune system and inability to localize infection, the most common clinical manifestations of sepsis are septicemia, pneumonia, and meningitis. Approximately 30% of septic newborns develop meningitis (Korones, 1986).

GBS acquired from the mother is the most common gram-positive organism causing sepsis in the newborn. Controversy exists as to timing of antibiotic therapy in the treatment of intraamniotic infection. In the past, treatment delay was advocated in order to obtain antibiotic-free cultures in the newborn; however, recent research has shown significant advantage for the newborn if antibiotics are initiated during the newborn period. Current recommendations are to treat the mother with broad-spectrum antibiotic therapy as soon as clinical signs of intraamniotic infection are apparent. Prophylactic antibiotic therapy, during the intrapartum period for asymptomatic women who have cultured positive for GBS, has been shown to be beneficial in preventing early-onset sepsis (Allen, Navas, & King, 1993).

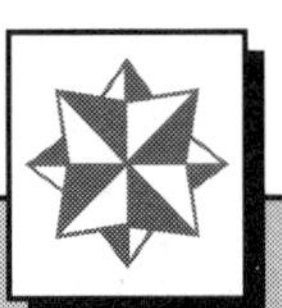

DISPLAY 16-8

Organisms Responsible for Neonatal Infection

Toxoplasmosis
Rubella
Cytomegalovirus
Herpes
Acquired immunodeficiency syndrome
Syphilis
Chlamydia trachomatis
Enterovirus
Bacterial infections
Hepatitis B
Human papillomavirus

Assessment

As with all neonatal complications, early identification of newborns at risk and prompt recognition of developing symptoms decreases morbidity and mortality and increases the chances of survival. Recognizing multiple risk factors for infection is the first step in identifying newborns whose early days may be complicated by their illness. Risk factors can be categorized as maternal, neonatal, and environmental.

Maternal factors are frequently apparent in the antepartum and intrapartum period (Display 16-9). A thorough review of antepartum and intrapartum history, specifically looking for conditions that increase risk of early onset sepsis, is important. If the mother and newborn are cared for by different nurses, communication between team members is essential to ensure that maternal complications with potential impact on the newborn are not overlooked. The nurse caring for the woman during the postpartum period should notify the neonatal care provider if fever or other symptoms of infection develop.

The primary neonatal factors influencing development of sepsis are gestational age and birth weight. Gestational age and birth weight vary inversely to morbidity and mortality from sepsis. Preterm infants may be exposed to the same organisms as term infants; however, the ability of preterm infants to fight

TABLE 16-6. Common Causative Bacterial Pathogens for Neonatal Sepsis

Early Onset	Late Onset
Common organisms	Coagulase-negative Staphylococcus
Group B streptococcus	*Escherichia coli*
Escherichia coli	Klebsiella species
Haemophilus influenzae	Enterobacter species
Unusual organisms	Candida species
Staphylococcus aureus	*Malassezzia furfur*
Staphylococcus epidermidis	Other enteric organisms
Neisseria meningitidis	*Group B streptococcus*
Streptococcus pneumoniae	Methicillin-resistant Staphylococcus aureus
Listeria monocytogenes	
Rare organisms	
Klebsiella pneumoniae	
Pseudomonas aeruginosa	
Enterobacter species	
Serratia marcescens	
Group A streptococcus	
Group B streptococcus	
Anaerobic species	

From Remington, J.S., & Klein, J.O. (Eds.), (1995). Infectious diseases of the fetus and newborn (4th ed., pp. 835-890). Philadelphia: W.B. Saunders.

infection is lessened. Several other factors are associated with increased risk of sepsis including resuscitation at birth or low Apgar scores. Presence of congenital anomalies, especially where skin or mucus membrane is not intact, increases risk due to a cutaneous port of entry for microorganisms. History of a nonreassuring fetal heart rate pattern during labor, with or without meconium in the amniotic fluid, may identify fetuses at risk for infection. More male than female newborns develop sepsis, suggesting that the susceptibility may be sex linked (Witek-Janusek & Cusack, 1994).

The most obvious environmental risk for developing sepsis is admission to a newborn intensive care unit (NICU). Newborns in the NICU are compromised due to the reason for admission along with being subjected to manipulation and invasive procedures which frequently puncture skin, the first line of defense against infection. Environmental risk of nosocomial infection includes use of equipment, indwelling catheters and chest tubes, inadequate handwashing or cleaning procedures, breaks in skin integrity, oxygen therapy and mechanical ventilation, and surgical procedures. Overcrowding in the nursery or inadequate attention to isolation precautions increases the risk of cross-contamination.

In addition to reviewing antepartum and intrapartum history, identifying the newborn with neonatal sepsis requires a thorough physical examination, evaluation of vital signs and laboratory data, and recognition of symptoms consistent with the diagnosis of sepsis. Like many conditions complicating the newborn period, the early symptoms of neonatal sepsis are vague and frequently nonspecific. Symptoms such as apnea, tachypnea, temperature instability, tachycardia, lethargy, and poor feeding may be early symptoms of sepsis, while petechiae, seizures, enlarged liver and spleen, and conjugated hyperbilirubinemia are symptoms which develop later in the disease process. Figure 16-3 identifies clinical signs of neonatal sepsis.

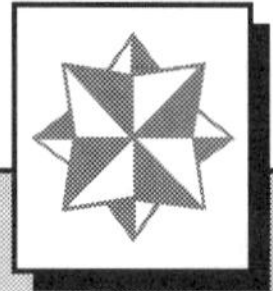

DISPLAY 16-9

Maternal Factors Predisposing Newborns to Sepsis

Preterm labor
Premature rupture of the membranes
Prolonged rupture of membranes
Maternal sepsis
Chorioamnionitis
Intraamniotic infection
Vaginal colonization with *GBS*
Perineal colonization with *E. coli*
Prior birth of an infant with *GBS*
Chemical dependency/substance abuse
Urinary tract infection
Foul-smelling amniotic fluid

Anaerobic and aerobic blood cultures should be obtained prior to the initiation of antibiotic therapy from any newborn suspected of being septic. A positive blood culture is the only way to make a definitive diagnosis of bacterial sepsis. Superficial cultures from sites such as nares, ear, throat, axillary, and umbilicus and cultures of gastric aspirate are rarely performed because they document colonization with a particular organism rather than bacteremia or sepsis. Lumbar puncture for culture and Gram's stain of cerebral spinal fluid is indicated when meningitis is suspected, especially in newborns who are symptomatic, have GBS sepsis, or late-onset disease (O'Donnell & Merenstein, 1993). In addition, a complete blood count with differential is obtained.

Interventions

Many institutions have developed protocols for evaluations to rule out sepsis including laboratory data and frequency of vital signs and clinical assessment. (See Appendix E for algorithm to rule out neonatal sepsis). Caring for the newborn with sepsis involves supporting all physiologic systems. Respiratory

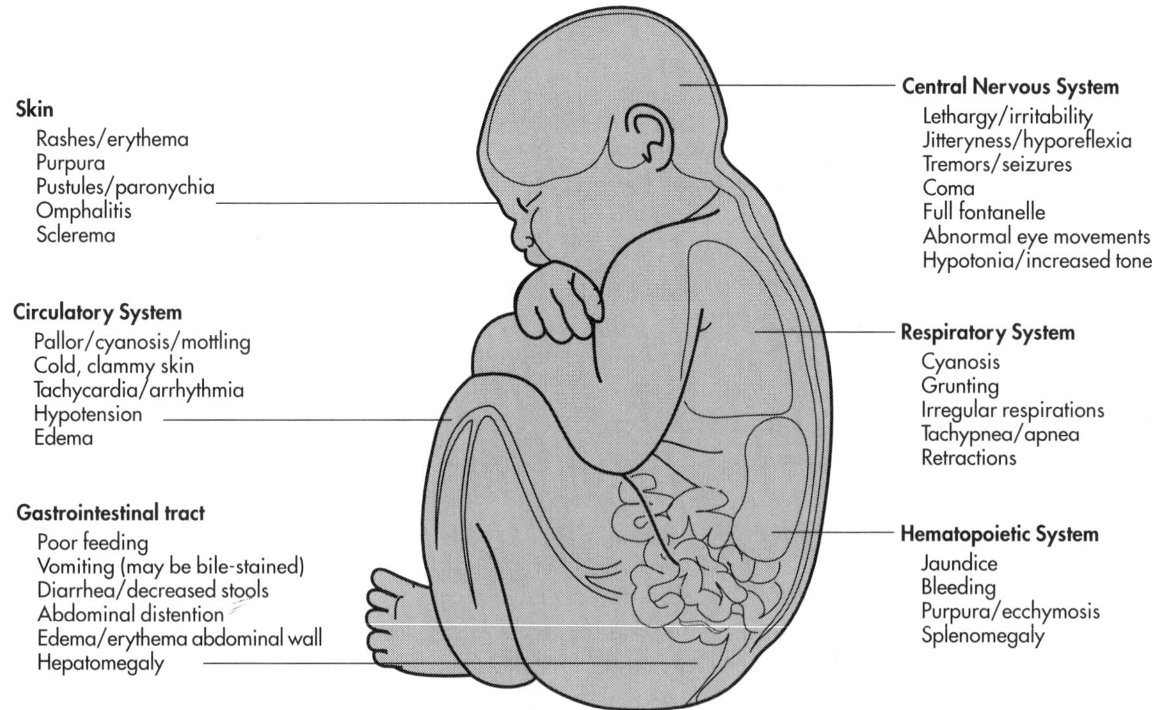

Figure 16-3. Clinical signs of neonatal sepsis

From Wasserman, R. L. (1982). Neonatal sepsis: The potential of granulocyte transfusion. Hospital Practice, 17(5), p. 98.

symptomatology may require initiation of oxygen therapy. Metabolic and nutritional management is dependent on physical condition. Intravenous therapy may be initiated via an umbilical line with progression to breastfeeding or formula feeding as the newborn's condition improves.

After blood cultures are obtained, antibiotics are initiated. For early onset sepsis, Ampicillin, a broad-spectrum antibiotic that is bactericidal for both gram-positive and gram-negative bacteria, is used in combination with an aminoglycoside such as gentamicin. Usual dose of Ampicillin is 50-100 mg/kg every 8 to 12 hours. When sepsis is complicated by meningitis, the dose is increased to 100-200 mg/kg. The dose of gentamicin, effective against Pseudomonas, Klebsiella, and E. coli, is 2.5 mg/kg every 12 to 24 hours. Treatment for sepsis continues for 7 to 10 days. If a diagnosis of meningitis is made, treatment may continue for 14 days. A spinal tap is usually done by day 10; if results remain positive, antibiotics are continued for 21 days and/or until two sterile spinal fluid specimens are obtained. Antibiotics are changed if results of blood cultures indicate a different medication would be more effective against the involved organism and/or less toxic to the newborn. After 48 to 72 hours, if culture result is negative, antibiotics may be discontinued.

SUMMARY

Many conditions complicating the neonatal period do not begin with dramatic clinical symptoms. Experience and well-developed assessment skills allow perinatal nurses to recognize subtle changes and intervene before the newborn's condition worsens. Occasionally, condition of the newborn and services available at a particular perinatal center necessitate transport to a level III NICU. The goal of neonatal transport is to bring a sick newborn to a tertiary-care center in stable condition. Stabilization is ongoing, beginning with the referring hospital, through consultation with the tertiary center as needed, until the arrival and eventual departure of the transport team. Stabilization of the neonate may take many forms, due to the diversity in disease process and gestational age. Basic care needs of newborns requiring transport to a tertiary center include adequate oxygenation, prevention of hypothermia, prevention of hypoglycemia and conservation of energy, and maintenance of physiologic integrity. In order to provide newborns with the best care possible, healthcare professionals within the referring hospital and between the referring hospital and tertiary center must communicate and work together as a team. See Appendix S for an example of a care path designed to facilitate transfer to a level III NICU and a care path for return to the transferring hospital after the newborn's condition is stable.

REFERENCES

Adams, C., Eyler, F.D., & Behnke, M. (1990). Nursing intervention with mothers who are substance abusers. Journal of Perinatal and Neonatal Nursing, 3(4), 43-52.

Allen, U.D., Navas, L., & King, S.M. (1993). Effectiveness of intrapartum penicillin prophylaxis in preventing early-onset group B streptococcal infection: Results of a meta-analysis. Canadian Medical Association Journal, 149(11), 1659-1665.

Amaro, H., Zuckerman, B., & Cabral, H. (1989). Drug use among adolescent mothers: Profile of risk. Pediatrics, 84(1), 144-151.

American Academy of Pediatrics. (1993). Routine evaluation of blood pressure, hematocrit and glucose in newborns. Pediatrics, 92(3), 474-476.

Askin, D.F. (1993). Chest and lung assessment. In E.P. Toppero & M.E. Honeyfield (Eds.), Physical assessment of the newborn: A comprehensive approach to the art of physical examination (pp. 55-66). Petaluma, CA: NICU INK.

Bland, R.D. (1991). Pathophysiology of neonatal lung injury. International Journal of Technology Assessment in Health Care, 7 (Suppl. 1), 56-60.

Carter, M.B. (1989). Problems and nursing management strategies related to respiratory distress syndrome in the very preterm baby. International Care Nursing, 5(2), 55-64.

Centers for Disease Control and Prevention. (1989). Urogenital anomalies in the offspring of women using cocaine during early pregnancy. Morbidity and Mortality Weekly Report, 38(31), 536, 541-542.

Chasnoff, I.J., Landress, H.J., & Barrett, M.E. (1990). The prevalence of illicit drug or alcohol use during pregnancy and discrepancies in mandatory reporting in Pinellas County, Florida. The New England Journal of Medicine, 322(17), 1202-1206.

Cloherty, J.P. (1991). Neonatal hyperbilirubinemia. In J.P. Cloherty & A.R. Stark (Eds.), Manual of neonatal care (3rd ed., pp. 298-334). Boston: Little, Brown.

Cole, M.D. (1991). New factors associated with the incidence of hypoglycemia: A research study. Neonatal Network, 10(4), 47-50.

Cornblath, M., Schwartz, R., Aynsley-Green, A., & Lloyd, J.K. (1990). Hypoglycemia in infancy: The need for a rational definition. A CIBA Foundation discussion meeting. Pediatrics, 85(5), 834-837.

Cowett, R.M. (1992). Hypoglycemia and hyperglycemia in the newborn. In R.A. Polin & W.W. Fox (Eds.), Fetal and neonatal physiology (Vol. 1, pp. 406-418). Philadelphia: W.B. Saunders.

Dixon, S.D., & Bejar, R. (1989). Echoencephalographic findings in neonates associated with maternal cocaine and methamphetamine use: Incidence and clinical correlates. Journal of Pediatrics, 115, (5, Pt. 1), pp. 770-778.

Dodman, N. (1987). Newborn temperature control. Neonatal Network, 5(6), 19-23.

Downey, J.C., & Cloherty, J.P. (1991). Metabolic problems. In J.P. Cloherty & A.R. Stark (Eds.), Manual of neonatal care (3rd ed., pp. 431-437). Boston: Little, Brown.

Eichenwald, E.C. (1991). Meconium aspiration. In J.P. Cloherty & A.R. Stark (Eds.), Manual of neonatal care (3rd ed., pp. 246-250). Boston: Little, Brown.

Ennever, J.F. (1992). Phototherapy for neonatal jaundice. In R.A. Polin & W.W. Fox (Eds.), Fetal and neonatal physiology (Vol. 2, pp. 1165-1173). Philadelphia: W.B. Saunders.

Finnegan, L.P., & Weiner, S.M. (1993). Drug withdrawal in the neonate. In G.B. Merenstein & S.L. Gardner (Eds.), Handbook of neonatal intensive care (3rd ed., pp. 40-54). St. Louis, MO: Mosby-Year Book.

Flanagan-Everett, M. (1991). Drug abuse and withdrawal. In J.P. Cloherty & A.R. Stark (Eds.), Manual of neonatal care (3rd ed., pp. 22-33). Boston: Little, Brown.

Flandermeyer, A.A. (1987). A comparison of the effects of heroin and cocaine abuse upon the neonate. Neonatal Network, 6(3), 42-48.

Frank, D.A., Zuckerman, B.S., Amaro, H., Aboagye, K., Bauchner, H., Cabral, H., Fried, L., Hingson, R., Kayne, H., Levenson, S.M., Parker, S., Reece, H., & Vinci, R. (1988). Cocaine use during pregnancy: Prevalence and correlates. Pediatrics, 82(6), 888-895.

Frank, C.G., Turner, B.S., & Merenstein, G.B. (1993). Jaundice. In G.B. Merenstein & S.L. Gardner (Eds.), Handbook of neonatal intensive care (3rd ed., pp. 272-286). St. Louis, MO: Mosby-Year Book.

Freij, B.J., & McCracken, G.H. (1994). Acute infections. In G.B. Avery, M.A. Fletcher, & M.G. MacDonald (Eds.), Neonatology: Pathophysiology and management of the newborn (4th ed., pp. 1082-1116). Philadelphia: J.B. Lippincott.

Fried, P.A. (1985). Postnatal consequences of maternal marijuana use. NIDA Research Monograph, 59, 61-72.

Funato, M., Tamai, H., Shimada, S., & Nakamura, H. (1994). Vigintiphobia, unbound bilirubin, and auditory brainstem responses. Pediatrics, 93(1), 50-53.

Gartner, L.M., & Lee, K.S. (1992). Jaundice and liver disease. In A.A. Fanaroff & R.J. Martin (Eds.), Neonatal-perinatal medicine diseases of the fetus and infant (5th ed., pp. 1075-1117). St. Louis, MO: Mosby-Year Book.

Handler, A., Kistin, N., Davis, F., & Ferre, C. (1991). Cocaine use during pregnancy: Perinatal outcomes. American Journal of Epidemiology, 133(8), 818-825.

Hansen, R.L., Evans, A.T., Gillogley, K.M., Hughes, C.S., & Krener, P.G. (1992). Perinatal toxicology screening. Journal of Perinatology, 12(3), 220-224.

Haywood, J.L., Coghill, C.H., Carlo, W.A., & Ross, M. (1993). Assessment and management of respiratory dysfunction. In C. Kenner, A. Brueggemeyer, & L.P. Gunderson, Comprehensive neonatal nursing (pp. 294-354). Philadelphia: W.B. Saunders.

Hite, C., & Shannon, M. (1992). Clinical profile of apparently healthy neonates with in utero drug exposure. Journal of Obstetric, Gynecologic, and Neonatal Nursing, 21(4), 305-309.

Jessup, M. (1990). The treatment of perinatal addiction. Identification, intervention, and advocacy. The Western Journal of Medicine, 152(5), 553-558.

Jobe, A.H. (1991). Pathogenesis of respiratory failure in the preterm infant. Annals of Medicine, 23(6), 687-691.

Jobe, A.H. (1992). Pathogenesis of respiratory distress syndrome. In R.A. Polin & W.W. Fox (Eds.), Fetal and Neonatal Physiology (Vol. 2, 995-1001). Philadelphia: W.B. Saunders.

Klein, J.O., & Marcy, S.M. (1995). Bacterial sepsis and meningitis. In J.S. Remington & J.O. Klein (Eds.), Infectious diseases of the fetus and newborn (4th ed., pp. 835-890). Philadelphia: W.B. Saunders.

Korones, S.B. (1986). High risk newborn infants (4th ed., pp. 214-235). St. Louis, MO: C.V. Mosby.

Lapido, M. (1989). Respiratory distress revisited. Neonatal Network, 8(3), 9-14.

Liley, H.G., & Stark, A.R. (1991). Respiratory distress syndrome/hyaline membrane disease. In J.P. Cloherty & A.R. Stark (Eds)., Manual of neonatal care (3rd ed., pp. 189-195). Boston: Little, Brown.

Little, B.B., Snell, L.M., & Gilstrap, L.C. (1988). Methamphetamine abuse during pregnancy: Outcome and fetal effects. Obstetrics and Gynecology, 72(4), 541-544.

Mahlmeister, L.R. (1994). Assessment of the at-risk neonate. In K.A. May, & L.R. Mahlmeister (Eds.), Maternal and neonatal nursing: Family-centered care (3rd ed., pp. 961-985). Philadelphia: J.B. Lippincott.

McAteer, J. (1992). The high risk infant: Acquired disorders. In S.J. Reeder, L.L. Martin, & D. Koniak (Eds.), Maternity nursing: Family, newborn and women's health care (17th ed., pp. 1196-1220). Philadelphia: J.B. Lippincott.

McFadden, E.A. (1991). The Wallaby Phototherapy System: A new approach to phototherapy. Journal of Pediatric Nursing, 6(3), 206-208.

Meeker, J.E., & Reynolds, P.C. (1990). Fetal and newborn death associated with maternal cocaine use, Journal of Analytical Toxicology, 14(6), 379-382.

Obladen, M., & Maier, R.F. (1993). Respiratory disorders of the neonate. Current Opinions in Pediatrics, 5(2), 156-161.

O'Donnell, J.P., & Merenstein, G.B. (1993). Infection in the neonate. In G.B. Merenstein & S.L. Gardner, Handbook of Neonatal Intensive Care (3rd ed., pp. 287-310). St. Louis, MO: Mosby-Year Book.

Peters, K.L. (1992). Does routine nursing care complicate the physiologic status of the premature neonate with respiratory distress syndrome? Journal of Perinatal and Neonatal Nursing, 6(2), 67-84.

Pildes, R.S., & Lilien, D. (1992). Symptomatic transient idiopathic neonatal hypoglycemia. In A.A. Fanaroff & R. J. Martin (Eds.), Neonatal-perinatal medicine: Diseases of the fetus and infant (5th ed., pp. 1158-1180). St. Louis, MO: Mosby-Year Book.

Polin, R.A. (1990). Management of neonatal hyperbilirubinemia: Rational use of phototherapy. Biology of the Neonate, 58 (Suppl. 1), 32-43.

Robins, L.N. & Mills, J.L. (1993). Effects in utero exposure to street drugs. American Journal of Public Health, 83 (Suppl.), 1-32.

Rosengren, S.S., Longobucco, D.B., Bernstein, B.A., Fishman, S., Cooke, E., Boctor, F., & Lewis, S.L. (1993). Meconium testing for cocaine metabolite: Prevalence, perceptions, and pitfalls. American Journal of Obstetrics and Gynecology, 168(5), 1449-1456.

Slater, L., & Brewer, F. (1984). Home versus hospital phototherapy for term infants with hyperbilirubinemia: A comparative study. Pediatrics, 73(4), 515-519.

Srinivasan, G., Pildes, R.S., Cattamanchi, G., Voora, S., Lilien, L.D. (1986). Plasma glucose values in normal neonates: A new look. Journal of Pediatrics, 109(1), 114-117.

Stark, A.R., & North, J.M. (1991). Transient tachypnea of the newborn. In J.P. Cloherty & A.R. Stark (Eds.), Manual of neonatal care (3rd ed., pp. 235). Boston: Little, Brown.

Tabor, B.L., Smith-Wallace, T., & Yonekura, M.L. (1990). Perinatal outcome associated with PCP versus cocaine use. American Journal of Drug and Alcohol Abuse, 16(3-4), 337-348.

Van Marter, L.J. (1991). Persistent pulmonary hypertension of the newborn. In J.P. Cloherty & A.R. Stark (Eds.), Manual of neonatal care (3rd ed., pp. 227-235). Boston: Little, Brown.

Vinci, R., Parker, S., Bauchner, H., Zuckerman, B., & Cabral, H. (1989). Maternal cocaine use and impaired fetal oxygenation. Pediatric Research, 25, 231.

vonWindeguth, B.J., & Urbano, M.T. (1989). Cocaine-abusing mothers and their infants: A new morbidity brings challenges for nursing care. Journal of Community Health Nursing, 6(3), 147-153.

Wasserman, R.L. (1982). Neonatal sepsis: The potential of granulocyte transfusion. Hospital Practice, 17(5), 95-104.

Weiss, J., & Hansell, M.J. (1992). Substance abuse during pregnancy; Legal and health policy issues. Nursing and Health Care, 13(9), 472-479.

Whitsett, J.A., Pryhuber, G.S., Rice, W.R., Warner, B.B., & Wert, S.E. (1994). Acute respiratory disorders. In G.B. Avery, M.A. Fletcher & M.G. MacDonald (Eds.), Neonatology, pathophysiology and management of the newborn (4th ed., pp. 429-451). Philadelphia: J.B. Lippincott.

Wilkerson, N.N. (1988). A comprehensive look at hyperbilirubinemia. Part 1. American Journal of Maternal Child Nursing, 13(5), 360-364.

Wilkerson, N.N. (1989). Treating hyperbilirubinemia. American Journal of Maternal Child Nursing, 14(1), 32-36.

Witek-Janusek, L., & Cusack, C. (1994). Neonatal sepsis: Confronting the challenge. Critical Care Nursing Clinics of North America, 6(2), 405-419.

Woods, J.R., Plessinger, M.A., & Clark, K.E. (1987). Effect of cocaine on uterine blood flow and fetal oxygenation. Journal of the American Medical Association, 257(7), 957-961.

Zinn, A.B. (1992). Inborn errors of metabolism. In A.A. Fanaroff & R.J. Martin (Eds.), Neonatal-perinatal medicine: Diseases of the fetus and infant, (5th ed., pp. 1118-1151). St. Louis, MO: Mosby-Year Book.

PART 6

Perinatal Home Care

Discharge Planning

Marilyn Lowe
Diane Millea
Kathleen Rice Simpson

- Prenatal Patient Data Base
- Prenatal Classes
- Educational Methods and Materials
- Family Preference Plan
- Learning-Needs Assessment
- Case Management
- The Role of the Staff Nurse
- Clinical Pathways
- Home Follow-Up Telephone Calls
- Evaluation

Current length of stay (LOS) in the United States varies from 8 to 24 hours postpartum. Therefore, discharge planning can no longer be delayed until admission for childbirth. Clearly, the woman in active labor is not a candidate for assessing maternal-newborn learning needs and implementing a teaching plan. The woman's focus during the intrapartum period is on safe passage through labor and on a healthy childbirth experience. Rubin's (1961) classic research suggests that during the immediate postpartum period the new mother is not physically or emotionally ready to listen to extensive presentations of how to care for herself and newborn. Priorities for many women in the first 24 hours postpartum are rest and a desire to discuss their labor and birth. The childbearing experience is very different today than it was from the 1950s through the 1970s, when most of Rubin's research was conducted. Major changes include availability of prenatal classes, women as active participants in all aspects of childbirth, fathers and other support persons present for labor and birth, epidural anesthesia, analgesia, open visiting, and couplet care models. Despite progression toward a healthcare environment where childbearing women have more control, much of Rubin's work about the taking-in and taking-hold phases of the postpartum period is still valid today.

Rather than waiting for the inpatient stay, perinatal nurses can take advantage of other opportunities for teaching maternal-newborn care to childbearing women and families. The prenatal period provides a window of opportunity to prepare families, not only for the birth process but also for the postpartum period after discharge (Menke, 1993). Prenatal visits to the primary healthcare provider are an ideal time for the perinatal nurse to assess family learning needs and provide information on a one-on-one basis. Because length of postpartum hospitalization has decreased, the focus of prenatal classes must expand from strictly labor and birth content to maternal-newborn care content. Critical concepts can then be reviewed and reinforced during the postpartum stay. Home visits and follow-up telephone calls allow for clarification and answering of any additional questions. Prenatal assessment and educational programs complement postpartum instruction provided by the inpatient perinatal nurse.

Many perinatal nurses and physicians have expressed concern about quality and safety issues related to current and decreasing postpartum LOS. Insurance companies and government programs are frequently blamed for sending women and newborns home too soon. However, third-party payors are only partially responsible for the emergence of shorter hospital stays. Both healthcare provider and consumer attitudes about childbirth have shifted from an illness to a wellness orientation. More women are desiring a childbirth experience in which they have meaningful input into key decisions. When provided with information about caring for themselves and their newborns, women discharged within 24 hours feel more in control and express greater feelings of maternal confidence and competence (Hall & Carty, 1993). Women discharged within 24 hours after childbirth without complications have outcomes similar to women with traditional LOS (Beck, 1991; Carty & Bradley, 1990; Grubbs, 1990; Harrison, 1990).

This chapter describes strategies for developing a comprehensive approach to discharge planning. Through the use of prenatal data bases, prenatal classes, case-management models, clinical pathways, individualized assessment tools, follow-up telephone calls, and a variety of innovative teaching methods, perinatal nurses can ease the transition from hospital to home so that childbearing families have enough information to safely care for the mother and newborn.

PRENATAL PATIENT DATA BASE

Prenatal preparation for hospitalization and postpartum discharge can be facilitated by early identification and entry into the system. Successful programs require communication between primary healthcare providers, prenatal educators, and the perinatal center. A simple, user-friendly system that incorporates demographic data, estimated date of birth, significant clinical history, family assessment and learning needs, participation in prenatal education programs, and a mechanism to communicate all pertinent information to the inpatient unit is critical. A computerized data base is ideal, but traditional file systems also work well. Individual institutions can develop a prenatal patient data base to meet specific needs. For example, early in pregnancy when a woman registers intent to give birth at the institution, demographic and insurance coverage data can be entered into the system. Primary healthcare providers and community prenatal clinics that refer women for inpatient care can be encouraged to send notification regarding women who have selected the institution for childbirth. Increasingly, managed-care contracts involve geographic exclusivity clauses so that all pregnant women enrolled in the healthcare plan are required to use a particular institution. These third-party payors are excellent sources of data about future patients. A system can be designed that involves notification of the institution when a member of the health plan becomes pregnant.

Periodically, material appropriate to the pregnancy trimester such as fetal growth and development information, health promotion advice, parenthood preparation tips, and sibling issues can be mailed to the family. Also, the family can be encouraged to participate in prenatal classes and tours. Brochures listing all perinatal services available at the institution, together with appropriate telephone numbers, are especially helpful. By the thirty-sixth week of pregnancy, a record of prenatal care should be received from the primary healthcare provider and added to the data base. When the woman is admitted for childbirth, the perinatal nurse has valuable information about the current maternal-fetal health status and family learning needs. The increase in quality and quantity of prenatal data about the childbearing family enhances individualized care and teaching.

PRENATAL CLASSES

The traditional prepared childbirth education model is a series of six classes, focusing on pregnancy, labor, birth, breathing and relaxation techniques, and to a lesser extent, maternal-newborn care during the postpartum period. For many working couples, making the time commitment necessary to attend a series of six classes is often difficult. Multiple factors such as transportation issues, work schedules, childcare availability, and previous birth and newborn care experiences influence the decision to attend prenatal classes. Many institutions and perinatal educators have responded to consumers needs by streamlining content to decrease program length, and offering alternatives such as weekend programs, flexible hours, and antepartum home visits.

Perinatal education classes should be designed based on needs of the population served. A comprehensive program offering a variety of options is ideal. In addition to the traditional prepared childbirth classes, other class series can be developed that incorporate content on maternal-newborn care. (Display 17-1 is a sample curriculum for a combined Lamaze/Infant Care class in the traditional 6-week format.) For couples unable to make the 6-week time commitment, classes that meet less frequently can be designed. Options can include a 1-, 2-, or 3-week series covering critical content that is prioritized based on class time limitations. (Display 17-2 lists sample curricula for prenatal classes based on a 1-, 2,- and 3-class series.) Classes focusing on preparation for breastfeeding, vaginal birth after a cesarean birth, cesarean birth for women with a medical indication for cesarean birth, or multiple pregnancy can be offered as an additional option for women with special needs. Classes designed for health promotion in early pregnancy complement a comprehensive perinatal education program. Subjects covered in these

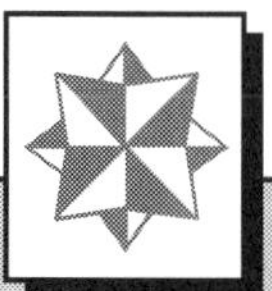

Display 17-1

Lamaze/Infant Care Class Curriculum Overview

Lamaze	Infant Care
Class I	
Introduction	Selecting a Pediatrician
Discomforts of Pregnancy	Immunizations
Preterm Labor	Childcare
Exercises	Babytime
Relaxation and Breathing Patterns	
Slow-Paced Breathing and Progressive Relaxation	
Class II	
Preview of Labor	Bathing Video or
Relaxation and Breathing Patterns	Bathing Baby Demonstration
Favorite Place, Slow-Paced, and Bridged Breathing	Changing/Diapering
Position Changes for Labor	Holding Baby
Class III	
Birth Video	Breastfeeding versus Bottlefeeding Video
Goodybag	Burping
Relaxation and Breathing Patterns	Sleeping patterns
Transition	Pacifiers
Class IV	
Labor, Birth, and Nursery Tour	Newborn Characteristics
Medical Interventions	
Class V	
Labor Rehearsal	Infant CPR
Review Breathing and Relaxation	Choking Demonstration
Emergency Childbirth	Illness/When to call pediatrician
Cesarean Birth Video	Parents as Teachers Video
Medication/Analgesia/Anesthesia	
Class VI	
Postpartum Discussion	Safety Video
Postpartum Video	
Party	

From Harper, J. (1995) Prenatal Class Content Outline. St. John's Mercy Medical Center, St. Louis, MO. Used with permission.

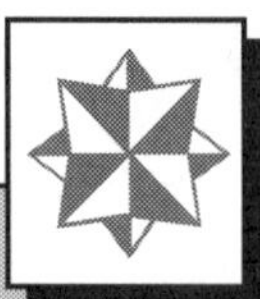

DISPLAY 17-2

Class Content: One 3-Hour Prenatal Class

Essentials to bring to the hospital
Early signs of labor/When to come to the hospital
What to expect during labor and birth
Formulating a birth plan
Anesthesia/analgesia options
Visiting policies
How to anticipate LOS, third-party payor issues, precertification, deductibles and copayments
Choosing a pediatrician
Warning signs of pregnancy complications, including preterm labor and preeclampsia

Maternal Care Issues:
Episiotomy care, normal lochia, afterpains, incision care, breast care, nutrition, rest, "baby blues"

Newborn Care Issues:
Umbilical cord care, circumcision care, breastfeeding, formula feeding, diapering, bathing, behavioral and satiation cues, crying, comforting, car seats, sleeping positioning, and other safety issues

Videotapes and booklets to reinforce class content
Parent hotline number for additional questions
Community and institutional resources

Class Content: Two 3-Hour Prenatal Classes

Class I
Essentials to bring to the hospital
Formulating a birth plan
Early signs of labor, relaxation, and breathing techniques
When to come to the hospital
The admission process
Ambulation in early labor
Electronic fetal monitoring/intermittent auscultation
Labor induction/augmentation
Amniotomy
Active labor
Transition
Second stage of labor
Anesthesia/analgesia options, review of pain relief and comfort measures, nonpharmacologic and pharmacologic
The unanticipated cesarean birth
Visiting policies
How to anticipate LOS, third-party payor issues, precertification, deductibles, and copayments
Warning signs of pregnancy complications, including preterm labor and preeclampsia

Class II
Choosing a pediatrician
Maternal Care Issues:
Episiotomy care, normal lochia, afterpains, incision care, breast care, nutrition, rest, baby blues, sexuality issues, contraception/family planning

DISPLAY 17-2 cont.

Newborn Care Issues:

Umbilical cord care, circumcision care, breastfeeding, formula feeding, diapering, bathing, behavioral and satiation cues, sleep-awake state, crying, comforting, car seats, sleeping positioning, other safety issues

Videotapes and booklets to reinforce class content
Parent hotline number for additional questions
Community and institutional resources

Class Content: Three 3–Hour Prenatal Classes

Class I

Brief overview of fetal development
Changes during pregnancy
Nutrition and lifestyle modification
Sexuality during pregnancy
Formulating a birth plan
Relaxation and breathing techniques
Childbirth options
Visiting policies
How to anticipate LOS, third-party payor issues, precertification, deductibles, and copayments
Choosing a pediatrician
Tour of perinatal unit
Warning signs of pregnancy complications, including preterm labor and preeclampsia

Class II

Essentials to bring to the hospital
Early signs of labor/When to come to the hospital
The admission process
Ambulation in early labor
Electronic fetal monitoring/intermittent auscultation
Labor induction/augmentation
Amniotomy
Active labor
Transition
Second stage of labor
Anesthesia/analgesia options, review of pain relief and comfort measures, nonpharmacologic and pharmacologic
Reinforcement of relaxation and breathing techniques
The unanticipated cesarean birth

Class III

Maternal Care Issues:

Episiotomy care, normal lochia, afterpains, incision care, breast care, nutrition, rest, baby blues, sexuality issues, contraception/family planning

Newborn Care Issues:

Umbilical cord care, circumcision care, breastfeeding, formula feeding, diapering, bathing, behavioral and satiation cues, sleep-awake state, crying/comforting, car seat, sleeping positioning, other safety issues

Videotapes and booklets to reinforce class content
Parent hotline number for additional questions
Community and institutional resources

classes include fetal growth and development; nutrition; the effects of smoking, alcohol, and tobacco; expected changes of pregnancy; lifestyle modifications, activity and exercise; discomforts of pregnancy; and warning signs of pregnancy complications, including symptoms of preterm labor.

EDUCATIONAL METHODS AND MATERIALS

When developing teaching methods and materials, consideration should be given to language and basic level of understanding of family members as well as to work schedules and ability to attend classes. Various education approaches can be individualized for specific needs. Group demonstrations are very effective for some learners while others prefer one-on-one demonstrations. Support group formats sponsored by the institution, such as a New Mom's Network or Breastfeeding Mother's Club, have been successful in providing additional teaching opportunities during the postpartum period.

In-hospital television channels with programs on newborn bath, cord, and circumcision care, and breast or formula feeding are effective. Videos that are either purchased or developed in-house are another means of instruction. They can be loaned to families, given as gifts, or available for purchase in the hospital gift shop.

Standardized written material, in the form of specific texts or handouts, can be a time-saving and cost-effective strategy. This approach increases the likelihood of the patient receiving consistent information, provides a ready resource for parents at a later date, and potentially decreases unnecessary calls to the primary healthcare provider and/or perinatal center. The perinatal staff can develop educational booklets or purchase and distribute existing parenting texts. There are a number of excellent resources in print. Selection is based on education level of populations served and financial resources available. Before adopting an existing text, collaboration with primary healthcare providers is essential.

FAMILY PREFERENCE PLAN

Involving women and families in childbearing decision making increases satisfaction and promotes a collaborative relationship between healthcare providers and patients. Advantages of tools that encourage women to develop a birth plan or list of family preferences include family knowledge of available birthing options and perinatal center policies, as well as healthcare provider awareness of the family's special needs and requests (Display 17-3). Women who are asked about care preferences feel their unique needs will be met by nurses and other healthcare providers who value patient input. A family preference or birth plan can be sent to all pregnant women registered for birth or can be given to couples during prenatal classes. The plan can then be completed and mailed back to the institution or collected by the perinatal educator. A copy is included in the woman's prenatal file on the inpatient unit so that it is available to the nurse when the woman is admitted in labor.

LEARNING-NEEDS ASSESSMENT

Needs-assessment tools assist nurses and families in identification of maternal-newborn learning needs and in documentation of type and time of prenatal education (Memke, 1993). The needs-assessment tool can be initiated at various times during pregnancy, depending on when a woman first enters the hospital system. Opportunities include prenatal classes, prenatal visits, hospital tours, telephone contact with a case manager, or on admission to the hospital. Many couples attending prenatal classes are first-time parents. A detailed needs assessment introduced during the first prenatal class alerts prospective parents to information they need prior to discharge. As the information is reviewed in class, the perinatal educator documents initial instructions given. At the conclusion of a class series, tools are forwarded to the perinatal unit to be stored in the woman's prenatal data file. They are immediately available when a woman is admitted to the hospital. Display 17-4 is an example of a learning-needs assessment tool that follows the woman through the prenatal period and then becomes the discharge teaching record. Content with an asterisk is reviewed with all women prior to discharge. Referencing specific content to written educational materials provides reinforcement and promotes use of materials as a reference.

For women who have not attended prenatal class or completed a learning-needs assessment during a prenatal visit or meeting with the case manager, the process begins on admission to the hospital. With the help of the labor nurse, families select topics they want covered during the inpatient stay. Whether the needs assessment is completed prior to admission, during

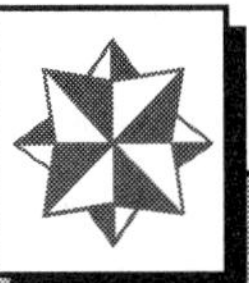

DISPLAY 17-3

Family Preference Plan

My name: ______________________________ My doctor's name: ______________________________

1. I would like to have these persons visit during labor:

   ______________________________ ______________________________

   ______________________________ ______________________________

2. My main support person is: ______________________________

   Relationship: ______________________________

3. For pain control/positioning during labor and birth, I would like to:

   ______ walk in room/halls ______ listen to special music

   ______ sit in recliner ______ use special focal point

   ______ use shower ______ use my own pillows

   ______ use jacuzzi ______ use squat bar

   ______ use heat/cold/massage ______ use foot pads on bed

4. I would like to have these persons present during birth:

   ______________________________ ______________________________

5. I have these religious requests:

   ______ birth blessing by chaplain

   ______ eucharist or communion

   ______ have visit by my own clergy

   ______ other: ______________________________

   ______ none

6. After birth: I would like to:

   ______ place baby skin to skin

   ______ wrap baby in blanket before holding

   ______ breastfeed my baby

   ______ bathe my baby

   ______ have doctor circumcise my son

   ______ have pictures taken of my baby

   ______ keep baby in my room as long as he/she is stable

7. During my hospital stay, I would like to have my support person:

   put baby skin to skin to him or her

   ______ assist with baby care

   ______ give the baby's first bath

   ______ spend the night in my room

   ______ take pictures of birth experience

8. I plan to attend, or have already attended, these classes/services during this pregnancy:

   ______ prenatal class

   ______ hospital OB tour

   ______ sibling class

DISPLAY 17-3 cont.

______ exercise sessions
______ lamaze

9. Child care has been arranged for other dependent children:
   ______ during the hospital stay
   ______ after mom and baby go home
   ______ not applicable
   ______ other:
10. I plan to have my other child(ren) come to visit:
   ______ during labor
   ______ during birth
   ______ in the first 2-hour recovery time
   ______ after I arrive in my postpartum room
   ______ not at all
   ______ not applicable
11. After going home, these persons will help out for the first 2 days:

   ______________________ ______________________

   ____

12. Additional ideas:

   ____

   ____

   ____

   ____

From Methodist Perinatal Center, Omaha, NE (1994).

early labor, or after birth, the educational process begins as soon as possible.

Primary responsibility for patient and family teaching varies with institution. Postpartum education may be coordinated by a case manager or perinatal educator; however, in any practice model, the staff nurse plays a key role. Several areas have been identified as critical concepts, that is, essential information for all women regardless of past experience or self-assessment. Critical concepts include the following:

- Maternal care
  - Activity/rest
  - Care of the perineum and episiotomy
  - Postoperative cesarean birth instructions
  - Signs of postpartum complications
- Newborn care
  - What to do if the newborn is choking
  - Use of bulb syringe
  - Umbilical cord care
  - Circumcision care
  - Position after feeding and for sleep
  - Signs of newborn complications
  - Breastfeeding basics
  - Formula feeding basics
  - Use of car seat
- When to call the primary healthcare provider
- Suggestions for when to schedule the first mother and newborn office visits

Before discharge, maternal-newborn knowledge and skills are validated. Validation can be accomplished by discussion with the new mother during which understanding is verbalized or by demonstration of critical skills such as positioning, feeding, or umbilical cord care. Written validation tools can also be used (Stevens, 1993). (See Display 17-5 for a sample written self-assessment.) No one method of validation

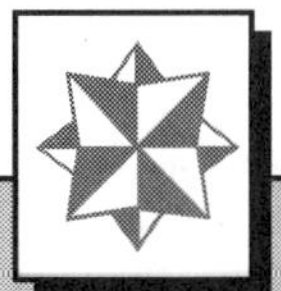

DISPLAY 17-4

Please go through the following list and check whether you understand each topic or need to know more.

Please read ...*For Moms and Babies* booklet given to you **after** the birth of your baby.

NURSES MUST INITIAL

I know this already	Doesn't apply to me	I need to know more	Topic	Booklet page #	Mother & family reviewed/ demonstrated
			POSTPARTUM		
			Activity — how much is OK	11	*
			Care of perineum and episiotomy	7,8	*
			Postoperative C-section instructions	9	*
			Signs of postpartum complications	11	*
			Changes in vaginal bleeding, return of my period	7	
			Comfort measures for afterpains, constipation and hemorrhoids	7,9	
			Postpartum "baby blues," depression, hormonal changes	10	
			Postpartum exercises for the first weeks	11	
			How to minimize milk production if I'm not nursing	8	
			BABY CARE		
			What to do if baby is choking or gagging	14	*
			How to do skin care/cord care	14	*
			How to take care of the circumcision or genital area Type: Bell/Gomco	13	*
			How to know if my baby is sick and what to do	21	
			What is jaundice and how to detect it	15	
			Use and cleaning of bulb syringe	14,15	*
			How and when to burp baby	17	
			How to position baby after feeding	17	*
			How to complete and obtain a birth certificate	20,21	
			BREASTFEEDING		
			I attended Breastfeeding class/watched Breastfeeding video ☐YES ☐NO		
			How to position baby for feeding	23	*
			How to get baby to latch onto my nipple properly	23	*
			Removal of baby from my nipple	24	*
			What is the supply and demand concept	23,24	*
			When does breast milk come in	25	
			Implications of supplementing for breastfeeding mothers	24	
			Prevention and comfort measures for sore nipples	24	
			Prevention and comfort measures for engorgement	25	
			How to express milk by hand/breast pump	25	
			BOTTLE FEEDING		
			How and when to feed my baby a bottle	16	*
			Reasons for NOT propping bottles	17	
			What formula should my baby drink	16	
			State Law requires use of infant car seat. I have a baby/infant car seat and know how to use it. ☐YES ☐NO		

Discharge weight_____lb _____oz

Medications:

Mother: None_____ Prescriptions: ____________________

Baby: None_____ Prescriptions: ____________________

Discharge Instructions: ____________________

Follow-up doctor's appointment:

Mother: Date: ____________________

Baby: Date: ____________________

Please call your doctor if you have any questions or concerns.

My discharge instructions have been explained to me and I have received a copy.

Signature: ____________________

Person receiving infant: ____________________

Postpartum Discharge Nurse: ____________ Date:______ Time:______

Nursery Nurse:____________________ Date:__________

White—Mother's Record; **Canary**—Baby's Record; **Pink**—Mother

MOTHER-BABY DISCHARGE RECORD

St. John's Mercy Medical Center/St. Louis, MO

Form 583 (11/93)

PKU (Repeat) Instructions (if needed): By state law your baby must be tested for these metabolic diseases. Bring your baby to the admitting lab on 2L (next to the escalators) within 3-5 days after discharge. No appointment is necessary. You may come Monday through Friday and Saturday morning. There will be no additional charge. Call 569-6814 for specific hours.

Metabolic Screen (PKU/Thyroid/Galactosemia)

Date:__________Time: __________ Repeat needed: ☐YES ☐NO (If yes - see instructions above.)

Nurses Signature(s) and Initials	

PATIENT IDENTIFICATION

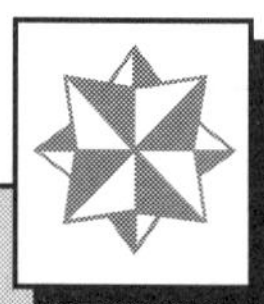

Display 17-5

New Mother Self-Assessment

Mother Care

1. Call the doctor if any of the following occur:
   a. Fever, chills, flu-like symptoms.
   b. Foul odor, a heavy bleeding—heavier than the heaviest day of period.
   c. Reddened area or extreme pain in the breasts, or a lump which does not vanish after breastfeeding.
   d. All of the above.
2. Which of the following is not a reliable form of birth control?
   a. Condoms (rubbers)
   b. Contraceptive sponges
   c. Breastfeeding
3. Which of the following is true regarding emotional changes?
   a. Will be lessened by rest.
   b. Can be caused by hormonal changes.
   c. Emotional changes include sudden feelings of sadness, feelings of inadequacy, crying or having trouble sleeping.
   d. All of the above.

Baby Care

4. Which of the following is true about giving your baby a bath?
   a. Bathing baby 2–3 times per week is adequate.
   b. Wash baby from clean to dirty (face to bottom).
   c. Stimulate scalp with hairbrush during bath to avoid cradle cap.
   d. All of the above.
5. Call the baby's doctor for which of the following:
   a. Yellow coloring of the skin or the whites of the eyes.
   b. Less than 6 wet diapers in 24 hours.
   c. Temperature of 100 degrees or above.
   d. All of the above.
6. Which of the following statements is true?
   a. Children must be in a safety-approved restraint by Nebraska State Law until they are 4 years of age or over 40 pounds.
   b. Car accidents are one of the leading causes of injury and death to young children.
   c. Be certain that the car seat is used according to the manufacturer's instructions.
   d. All of the above.

DISPLAY 17-5 cont.

7. How often should baby be burped?
   a. Only after baby has finished feeding.
   b. During and after feeding.
   c. Every five minutes.
8. How often should baby be fed?
   a. Every time he/she cries.
   b. Wake up baby every 3–4 hours.
   c. As often as every 2 hours but no longer than 5 hours during the day.
9. How much formula should baby get at each feeding?
   a. 8 ounces.
   b. As much as the baby tolerates.
   c. Until he/she burps or spits up.

Breastfeeding: Answer these questions if you are breastfeeding:

10. The MOST important factor in preventing sore nipples is:
    a. Positioning the baby.
    b. Length of the feeding.
    c. Applying ointment.
11. Which of the following will help prevent engorgement:
    a. Delayed feedings.
    b. Giving water after feedings.
    c. Frequent feedings.

Comments/Concerns

____

____

____

Key Answers eg: 1(d), 2(c), 3(d), 4(d), 5(d), 6(d), 7(b), 8(c), 9(b), 10(a), 11(c)

From Methodist Perinatal Center, Omaha, NE (1994)

is superior; rather, each perinatal center can develop a system with enough flexibility to meet individual needs. Validation ensures that women who indicate no information is needed are, in reality, prepared and knowledgeable. The goal is for all women to verbalize understanding or demonstrate skills related to critical concepts. Women with special needs are referred for follow-up care as indicated. Referrals are made to the clinical nurse specialist, lactation consultant, dietician, social worker, and/or homehealth agency. Follow-up care can include telephone calls, postpartum home visits, enrollment in support groups, community programs, or healthcare provider office visits.

CASE MANAGEMENT

Case management is an excellent method to enhance the quality of perinatal services. In a case-management model, the case manager interacts with expectant women and families over the continuum of care from entry into the system and through the postpartum period, including follow-up home care. The case man-

coordinates a case load of families in collaboration with nursing staff, physicians, and other healthcare professionals. An obvious advantage of this approach is that there is one person with comprehensive knowledge of each family and responsibility for ensuring all needs are met. Coordination and collaboration enhances continuity of care, promotes cost-effective use of resources, ensures expected maternal-newborn outcomes occur in a timely manner, and improves family and healthcare provider satisfaction. As the case manager follows the woman and her family during pregnancy, potential risk factors are identified, and educational needs and availability of support systems are assessed. Thus appropriate referrals can be initiated as needed (Display 17-6).

The case manager uses a variety of opportunities to access pregnant women during the prenatal period. Ideally, women are initially contacted by the care manager after referral from the healthcare provider's office or from lists of pregnant members provided by third-party payors. Contact is usually made by telephone; however, some institutions report success by sending newly pregnant women information about prenatal classes and inviting tours of the perinatal center. The woman then initiates contact with the case manager at her convenience. Method and type of initial contact is based on the population served.

Women are encouraged to attend prenatal classes during which learning needs and risks are identified. For women who are unable to attend prenatal classes, assessment can be accomplished by alternative methods. For example, a prenatal visit with the case manager can be arranged to coincide with a prenatal office appointment. Women who present to the hospital without prenatal care or who are emergently transferred from another facility are managed from the time they arrive or when contact is made for tertiary care referral.

During the inpatient stay, the case manager and primary nurse work in close collaboration. The learning-needs assessment completed during the prenatal period is reviewed by the primary nurse. Discussion with the woman will determine if the data are still accurate and if there are new needs or areas of concern. A new mother or father may not have confidence in their ability to care for the newborn despite participation in prenatal classes, presentation of maternal-newborn care content, and satisfactory demonstration of expected skills such as umbilical cord care, diapering, feeding, and holding the newborn. Maternal confidence affects family discharge needs. It is also important to identify and address those concerns the mother and family feel are important, even though data may not have been identified by the primary nurse or case manager as significant. Common issues that can inhibit confidence are perceived feeding difficulties, inability to soothe the crying newborn, prior parenting experience, limited financial resources, and past physical or emotional problems.

The medical record is reviewed for indications of preexisting physical and psychosocial conditions. If complicating factors with potential for affecting the discharge needs of the mother and/or newborn are identified, the case manager is notified. The family's knowledge and current use of institutional and community resources are evaluated. Possession of supplies/equipment in the home that are necessary to provide safe care for the newborn is determined.

Based on the needs assessment form, the case manager or primary nurse initiates or reinforces maternal-newborn teaching. As the case manager completes the teaching process, or makes referrals, there is communication with the primary staff nurse. Referrals to institution and community resources are made as appropriate. Examples of inpatient referrals are to the clinical nurse specialist, lactation consultant, nutritionist, nurse-midwife, nurse practitioner, physician, and/or social worker. Outpatient referral can be made to community services such as home healthcare agencies, parent support groups, WIC services, breastfeeding support groups, and community health clinics. The case manager may also coordinate services that include follow-up telephone calls and/or postpartum home visits.

THE ROLE OF THE STAFF NURSE

Not all perinatal centers have developed case manager positions. Staff nurses coordinate and participate in successful discharge planning programs. Prenatal classes are taught by perinatal staff nurses in many institutions. Benefits of this approach include presentation of realistic expectations of what will happen during hospitalization by someone providing direct patient care, and a heightened awareness of consumer desires and concerns related to the childbearing experience. Staff nurse committees develop clinical pathways, care plans, individualized maternal-newborn learning-needs assessment tools, and prepare patient educational materials. The staff nurse has the most interaction with the woman and family during

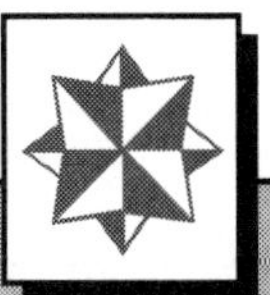

Display 17-6

Care Management Discharge Planning Form

Assessments

Anticipated LOS Date ______ Time ______ Payment Source ______

Insurance # ______ Contact Person ______

Newborn physician ______ Mother physician ______

Admission Date ______ Time ______ Delivery Date ______ Time ______

Marital Status S ______ D ______ M ______

Lives with Self ______ Significant Other ______ Spouse ______ Parent ______

Other dependent children ______ Ages ______

Temporary residence (specify) ______ Length of time ______

Identifies most supportive person(s) as ______

Available for assistance during Day ______ Evening ______ Night ______

Community Resource Utilization

WIC ______ Visiting nurse ______ MaMa and Me ______ Caseworker ______ Other

Available Equipment/Supplies

Clothing ______ Crib ______ Diapers ______ Car seat ______

Equipment/Supplies needed ______

Teaching

Completed ______ In process ______ Needs (specify) ______

Complicating Factors

Antepartum ______

Intrapartum ______

Postpartum ______

Family Crisis ______

Patient Concerns

Ability to care for newborn ______ or self ______

(specify) ______

Feeding: Breast ______ Bottle ______

Lack of support or assistance ______

Financial (specify) ______

Newborn Sex ______ Newborn Health Status ______

Physical or Emotional Status of Self:

Physical (specify) ______

Emotional (specify) ______

HX of Depression ______ Postpartum Depression ______

Limited or no experience with newborn care ______

Interventions

Teaching Initiate ______ Reinforce ______

Communicate Needs with Assigned Staff ______

Referrals (specify date & time if appropriate)

Social Service ______ CNS ______

Physician ______ WIC ______

Pastoral Care ______

Postpartum Support Group ______

Lactation Support Group ______

Childbirth Education Classes (specify) ______

Health Touch One ______ Other ______

Homeward Health ______ VNA ______

Home Followup Phone Call ______

From Methodist Perinatal Center, Omaha, NE (1994)

postpartum hospitalization. Ultimately, responsibility for ensuring that the woman and family have an adequate grasp of necessary information related to maternal-newborn care usually rests with the staff nurse.

Opportunities for teaching occur during most aspects of clinical care. Assessment of the episiotomy site can include instructions for perineal care after discharge, review of characteristics of normal lochia, suggestions to minimize discomfort, and sexuality issues. Fundal assessment can include a discussion of normal involution processes. The initial newborn bath can occur at the bedside with a presentation of newborn physical traits, crying cues, behavioral states, and sleeping and waking patterns. The discussion of normal newborn sleeping and awake states can lead to suggestions for ensuring adequate maternal rest after discharge. If family members are present, involving them in discussions promotes family-newborn attachment and may encourage help with newborn care at home. Assisting the new mother with breastfeeding is an excellent opportunity to discuss proper positioning, latch-on, demand feeding schedules, and satiation cues.

Ideally, the staff nurse has sufficient time prior to discharge to review the critical areas of maternal-newborn education content and answer questions or concerns. Use of a maternal-newborn teaching checklist is one method to ensure all new mothers are provided similar key information that can serve as a documentation tool as well. Staff nurses also play an important role in answering patient questions by telephone after discharge. Some units have "warm lines" with designated staff nurses to triage these calls and refer them to other appropriate healthcare providers as necessary. The inpatient postpartum nurse can influence successful transition from hospital to home by assessing each woman's individual learning needs, giving appropriate information, encouraging self and newborn care independence, and promoting confidence in the mothering role. A positive experience during childbirth and the immediate postpartum period sets the stage for continued adaptation to parenthood at home.

CLINICAL PATHWAYS

The clinical pathway is used to ensure that assessments, interventions, and appropriate outcomes are accomplished within a limited time span (Display 17-7). Ability to look at care in distinctive time frames prevents, or at least decreases, the incidence of delaying teaching until immediately prior to discharge.

The clinical pathway is used as a prospective overview of the entire childbearing process beginning during the prenatal period through postpartum follow-up, including evaluation of program effectiveness and patient satisfaction. The clinical pathway provides a timeline for assessments, interventions, teaching, and evaluation for further follow-up.

Critical maternal-newborn content that must be discussed with all families prior to discharge is listed. Teaching may be completed before the scheduled time frame but ideally should occur no later than the scheduled time. The same format is used for a cesarean birth clinical pathway with time frame adjustments to account for a 2- or 3-day stay.

A corresponding family clinical pathway is given at the first prenatal class or whenever entry into the system occurs (Display 17-8), (See also appendix P). Providing the woman and family with a clinical pathway written in lay terms about what to expect is invaluable in promoting collaboration between the childbearing woman and the perinatal healthcare team. Women and families have a concise resource related to their anticipated childbirth experience and they can be reassured that their clinical, education, and emotional needs will be met over the course of their care. (See Chapter 3 for a detailed discussion of clinical pathway development.)

Clinical pathway models provide an organized approach to meeting clinical care and teaching goals in specific time frames; however, other methods can be equally successful in streamlining perinatal services and accomplishing desired patient care and educational outcomes. Use of routine intrapartum and postpartum order sets and maternal-newborn teaching checklists can ensure that all women are provided similar clinical care and educational opportunities in the inpatient setting.

HOME FOLLOW-UP TELEPHONE CALLS

Results of an informal survey of perinatal centers indicate that follow-up telephone calls are handled in a variety of ways. In some perinatal centers, primary staff nurses call their own patients so that all women receive at least one follow-up call after they go home. Other perinatal centers have designated nurses whose sole responsibility is follow-up postpartum telephone calls. The decision to include follow-up telephone calls as part of a comprehensive discharge planning pro-

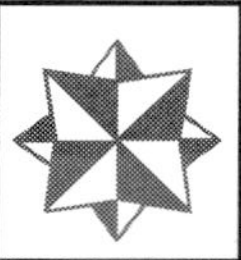

DISPLAY 17-7. Vaginal Birth

Aspect of Care:	Prenatal	Admit L&D	Early Labor	Active Labor	Recovery Period 1º	1–8 Hours P.P.	8–16 Hours P.P.	16–24 Hours P.P.	Follow up
HOME CARE NEEDS/ EDUCATIONAL NEEDS **Outcome Goal:** Patient/Support person will be able to manage self & newborn care at home (24 hours post-delivery) -Demonstrates and/or verbalizes understanding of information in regard to identified needs -Post test score 100% -Verbalizes awareness of appropriate resources & phone numbers for assistance after discharge	Encourage attendance in 1 or more of the classes/clinic **PRENATAL CLASSES** -Needs Assessment initiated -Course content includes information needed for hospital & discharge to home: -Maternal care -Newborn care -Breastfeeding -Analgesia/anes. -Pain scale -Comfort measures -Lamaze -Siblings **PREADMISSION CLINIC VISIT** -Obtain prenatals from Dr's offices (about 5-6 months) -Contact client for preadmission clinic visit -Initiate needs assessment tool (if not already initiated) -Review payment plan: -LOS -Insurance/HMO benefits -Self pay status -Review birth plan -Hospitals plan of care -Patients plan of care -Identification of support system -Assess need for prenatal classes	Complete home care needs assessment section of L&D admit history within 30 min Assess need for referral Assess support system on admission	Teach patient about: (if appropriate) 1X & prn -Phases & stages of labor -Proper positioning -NPO status -Comfort measures -Ext/Int fetal monitoring -IUPC -Oxytocin -Epidural Assess support system Initiate needs assessments (if not already completed)	Reinforce teaching	Teach patient about: 1X & prn -Self fundal massage -Peri care/ episiotomy -Pain control (pain scale, medication schedule) -Comfort measures Teaching/Assist with breastfeeding (if appropriate) 1X & prn -Latch on -Positioning Assess nipple condition 1X & prn Initiate needs assessment (if not already completed)	Review needs assessment 1X Teach/demonstrate based on needs assessment: 1X & prn -Vaginal flow -Breastfeeding -Supply & demand -Frequency of feedings -Formula feeding -Use of bulb syringe -Handwashing Assess support person Assess availability &/or need for car seat at discharge X1 Assess need for further follow up: -Home visit -WIC -Lactation Consultant -Social Services	Teach/Demonstrate based on needs assessment 1X & prn -Baby bath -Cord care -Circumcision care -Stooling & wetting patterns -Baby's sleep/ wake cycles -Breastfeeding: -Breast milk expression -Storage of breast milk -Care of sore/ cracked nipples -Measures to reduce engorgement Assess support system at home Referrals made (if appropriate)	Teach based on needs assessment 1X & prn: -Contraception -Emotional changes Instruct *all* patient about: -When to call Dr. -Maternal & newborn s/s -Detection of NB jaundice -Safety measures (positioning, car seats) Administer post test: 1X -Evaluate score -Reinforce information missed on test -Readminister if test score not 100% Advise of follow up appointments -Maternal & newborn Inform of support groups: -Breastfeeding support group -Post–partum support group	Follow up phone call within 48 hours after delivery Complete follow up phone form Home visit within 72 hours (if ordered & as needed) **EVALUATION** Compare follow up data to needs assessment to evaluate teaching effectiveness Evaluate expected outcomes based on outcome criteria for quarterly QI.

From Methodist Perinatal Center, Omaha, NE (1994)

DISPLAY 17-8. Family Clinical Pathway

Prenatal	Admit L & D	Early Labor	Active Labor	Recovery Period 2°	3–8 Hrs P.P.	9–24 Hrs P.P.	Follow-up
Attendance at 1 or more of learning sessions **Prenatal Classes** -Needs assessment completed -Course content to include information needed for hospital & discharge to home -Maternal care -Newborn care -Breastfeedings -Analgesia/anesthesia -Comfort measures -Relaxation techniques -Sibling information Develop family preference plan Obtain a car seat and learn to use Do you need information on: -Financial assistance -Length of stay (LOS) -Insurance -WIC -Social Services -Parenting -Child care needs	Bring car seat to hospital Bring education books given to you in classes	Receive information on: (if appropriate) -Phases & stages of labor -Proper positioning/activity -Pain control options -Fetal monitoring -Pitocin Initiate needs assessment (if not already completed)	Information reinforced as needed	Receive information/review: -Self fundal massage -Pericare/episiotomy -Pain control Receive information/assistance with breastfeeding (if appropriate) -Latch on -Positioning -Nipple condition Initiate needs assessment (if not already completed) Let your nurse know if you need information on: -Home visits by a nurse -WIC -Lactation consultants -Social Services	Review needs assessment identify areas you need more information on: -Vaginal flow -Breastfeeding -Supply & demand -Frequency of feedings -Formula feeding -Use of bulb syringe -Handwashing -Baby bath -Cord care -Temperature taking -Stooling & wetting patterns -Baby sleep/wake	Identify areas you need more information on: -Breastfeeding & breast milk expression -Storage of breast milk & care of sore/cracked nipples -Measures to reduce engorgement -Contraception -Emotional changes All families are instructed: -When to call the Dr. -Mother & newborn signs of illness -How to detect jaundice -Safety measures (positioning car seat, etc.) Make a follow-up appointment -Mother & newborn	-Breastfeeding support group available -Call your Dr. or Health Touch One nurse for mother or newborn questions 331-1111

Display 17-8. Family Clinical Pathway cont.

Prenatal	Admit L&D	Early Labor	Active Labor	Recovery Period 2°	3–8 Hrs P.P.	9–24 Hrs P.P.	Follow-up
	Admission history interview Fetal monitor applied Vaginal Exam for dilation & efface-ment No fluids other than ice chips (NPO) Sibling screening completed	Periodic check of: -Baby's heart beat (FHT's) -Contractions -Mother's BP, P, R (vital signs) NPO Walk in halls, shower, take a whirlpool, sit in chair REMEMBER: change your positions and activity frequently	Occasional &/or continuous monitoring of: -FHT's -Contractions -Mother's vital signs Vaginal exams for dilation and effacement NPO Urinate frequently to keep bladder empty IV started Use pain control as needed Continue to change position/activities frequently	Checks every 15 min x 4 then 30 min x 2 -Top of uterus for firmness (fundus) -Massage fundus if needed -Mother's vital signs -Vaginal flow (lochia) Change peri pad as needed Ice to perineum Pain control as needed Empty bladder Start breastfeeding (if appropriate) Newborn (NB) will receive: -Aqua Mephyton shot (Vit. K) -Erythromycin ointment to eyes -Monitoring for: -Temperature -Vital signs -Blood sugar Teaching started to prepare you for discharge (see discharge activity list)	Check every 1 hour x 2, then every 4 hours x 2: -Fundus -Lochia -Vital signs -Episiotomy (if appropriate) Up and about in room or halls Ice to perineum Change peri pads with each bathroom use -About every 2 hours Pain pills (Ibuprofen) every 8 hours Keep bladder empty - use your peri bottle after urination NB activities: -First bath -Vital signs -First physical exam -Temperature -First formula feed (if appropriate) -Feed baby when hungry Handwashing: -After each bathroom use -Before handling the baby -For all visitors & siblings	Check every 8 hours until discharge -Fundus -Lochia -Vital signs -Episiotomy (if appropriate) Check legs and calves for tenderness (Homan sign) Change pads with each bathroom use Pain pills every 8 hours Keep bladder empty Enjoy baby Feed baby when hungry	

From Methodist Perinatal Center, Omaha, NE (1994)

Display 17-9

Early Discharge Follow–Up Telephone Call Report

Mother: Age ________ G/P ________ Vag Birth ________ C/Birth ________

Marital status: S M W Discharge date: ________

Baby: Sex: M F Gestational age: ________

Newborn birth weight ________ ________ Discharge weight

Breast ________ Formula ________ Person making call: ________

BABY CARE	NO CONCERNS	PROBLEM IDENTIFIED	SUGGESTION MADE
Circumcision assessment			
Cord assessment			
Jaundice			
Changes in Newborn:			
Behavior			
Feeding			
Temperature			
Breastfeeding:			
# wet diapers			
# & character of stools			
latch on/positioning			
Frequency of feeding/24 hours			
Breast & nipple assessment:			
sore nipples			
cracked nipples			
breast fullness			
Suck/swallow assessment			
Other concerns			
Formula Feeding:			
# wet diapers			
# & characteristics of stools			
Ounces/feedings			
Frequency of feedings			
Skin appearance			
Sleep patterns			
Ability to care for newborn			

DISPLAY 17-9 cont.

MATERNAL CARES	NO CONCERNS	PROBLEM IDENTIFED	SUGGESTION MADE
Lochia			
Episiotomy			
Incision			
Discomforts:			
Breast			
Perineal			
Incisional			
Cramping			
Calf/leg tenderness			
Hemorrhoids			
Voiding			
Frequency			
Dysuria			
Bowel Movement			
Emotional			
Weepy			
Fatigue			
Sadness			
Onset of feelings			
Duration of feelings			
Adequate rest			
Taking naps			
Sleeps well when baby sleeps			
Other			
Ability to care for self			
REFERRALS	**DATE**	**PROBLEM IDENTIFIED**	**SUGGESTION MADE**
Lactation Consultant			
Social Services			
Physician			
Clinical Specialist			
Home Heath Care			
WIC			
Other			

From Methodist Perinatal Center, Omaha, NE (1994)

gram is based on multiple factors such as personnel and financial resources available and risk status of populations served. Suggested criteria for women who may benefit from follow-up telephone calls include the following:

- LOS less than 24 hours after a vaginal birth
- LOS less than 48 hours after a cesarean birth
- Limited or no prenatal care
- No prenatal class attendance
- Lack of adequate support systems
- Women who seem overwhelmed, anxious, or depressed
- Discharge evaluation indicates need for further teaching

Ideally, the initial call is made within the first 24 hours after discharge. The use of a Follow-up Phone Call Report (Display 17-9) ensures comprehensive assessment. Results of phone conversations should be documented and maintained as a permanent part of the medical record, including referrals to appropriate institutional and community resources. If referral for postpartum homecare is indicated, visits can be made by the institution's home healthcare services or by other community homecare agencies (see Chapter 18).

EVALUATION

While much has been written about prenatal education curricula and inpatient discharge teaching, limited data exist about prenatal program evaluation (Biasella, 1993; Gennaro, 1993; Stevens, 1993). Perinatal healthcare resources will be allocated to programs with proven success records. An essential first step in program evaluation is identification of goals and expected outcomes. Primary outcome criteria are family knowledge about maternal-newborn care, ability to identify support persons and community resources, and familiarity with signs and symptoms of complications that warrant a call to the primary healthcare provider. Criteria met both at discharge and in the immediate postpartum period at home should be included in the evaluation process. Both quantitative and qualitative approaches are useful.

Quantitative evaluation may be concurrent or retrospective review of medical record data, tracking readmissions, and/or keeping a log of parent phone calls to the nursery or postpartum unit (Gennaro, 1993). Clinical pathway variance data provides information about maternal-newborn teaching completed within suggested time frames during the inpatient stay. Primary healthcare providers can also participate in data collection by tracking phone calls, commonly asked questions, and other than routine office visits. Results of individual follow-up phone calls and home visits assessments can be compared with learning-needs assessments completed prior to discharge. If data analysis suggest specific topics should be covered in more depth in the inpatient setting, staff nurses can make appropriate revisions in patient teaching strategies.

Qualitative methods of evaluation such as patient interviews, focus groups, and letters or phone calls from parents who have used programs and services are additional valuable sources of data. Women and families frequently identify important issues not addressed on surveys or evaluation tools. Tracking data trends and adjusting discharge plans accordingly leads to improvements in the system. For example, if analysis of the parents' phone call log indicates many calls about a particular issue, parent teaching plans can be redesigned to include comprehensive coverage of that topic (Gennaro, 1993). Childbearing family surveys may suggest a need to offer more flexibility in class schedules. Prenatal class evaluations provide information about class content and teaching methods that parents found useful (Stevens, 1993). Prenatal classes can be revised based on consistent themes in participant feedback.

An additional benefit of soliciting patient feedback about services provided is the ability to share with perinatal educators and staff nurses positive remarks about their individual contributions. Often women will take the time to write lengthy comments about their prenatal class instructor and the nurses who cared from them during the inpatient stay and/or visited them at home during the postpartum period. The role of the perinatal nurse in contributing to a positive childbirth experience can not be overemphasized. While perinatal nurses many times feel rushed to accomplish all there is to do in the limited time available, it is gratifying to know we can still make a difference. Conversely, comments about individuals who could use some improvement in clinical and/or interpersonal skills, are also valuable because they allow those individuals to see how they are perceived by patients and family members, and thus can lead to appropriate behavior changes.

A well-designed postpartum discharge planning program can be cost effective if unnecessary calls or return visits to the institution or primary healthcare provider are decreased. However, in order to note a decrease in readmissions or unnecessary phone calls, a systematic method of data collection and analysis must be in place. As healthcare dollars become more scarce, increased sophistication in linking positive outcomes (both clinical and financial) to prenatal education and discharge planning programs will be critical.

SUMMARY

Current and decreasing postpartum LOS continue to provide challenges for perinatal nurses. Traditional approaches to prenatal education and discharge planning are obsolete. Opportunities for teaching in the inpatient setting are limited. Innovative educational programs that begin during the prenatal period and continue after discharge are essential to meet the needs of today's childbearing families. Evaluative data about program effectiveness is a critical component of discharge planning.

References

Beck, C.T. (1991). Early postpartum discharge programs in the United States: A literature review and critique. Women and Health, 17(1), 125-138.

Biasella, S. (1993). A comprehensive perinatal education program. AWHONN's Clinical Issues in Perinatal and Women's Health Nursing, 4(1), 5-19.

Carty, E.M., & Bradley, C.F. (1990). A randomized controlled evaluation of early postpartum hospital discharge. Birth: Issues in Perinatal Care and Education, 17(4), 199-204.

Gennaro, S. (1993). Perinatal education for parents of high-risk infants. AWHONN's Clinical Issues in Perinatal and Women's Health Nursing, 4(1), 147-157.

Grubbs, L.M. (1990). Early postpartum discharge: Implications for HMOs. HMO Practice, 4(3), 94-99.

Hall, W.A., & Carty, E.M. (1993). Managing the early discharge experience: Taking control. Journal of Advanced Nursing, 18(4), 574-582.

Harrison, L.L. (1990). Patient education in early postpartum discharge programs. American Journal of Maternal-Child Nursing, 15(1), 39.

Memke, K.L. (1993). Linking patient education with discharge planning. In B.E. Giloth (Ed.), Managing hospital-based patient education (pp. 153-164). Chicago: American Hospital Publishing.

Rubin, R. (1961). Puerpural change. Nursing Outlook, 11, 828-831.

Stevens, K.A. (1993). Developing a perinatal education program. AWHONN's Clinical Issues in Perinatal and Women's Health Nursing, 4(1), 44-54.

CHAPTER

18

Perinatal Homecare Services

Kathleen Rice Simpson
Linda Seibold
Kim Stremsterfer

Critical to the success of quality perinatal nursing care delivery during the postpartum period is a well-designed, universally accessible homecare follow-up program for childbearing women and their families. Today, length of stay (LOS) for most uncomplicated vaginal births is 8 to 24 hours after childbirth. Therefore, what was once referred to in the literature as an "early" postpartum discharge program has become the current practice in much of the United States. Fundamental changes in reimbursement for perinatal services, a continued emphasis on cost reduction, consumer demands for more natural childbirth experiences and increased care participation, and favorable outcomes for women and infants discharged within 24 hours after birth are factors that have influenced this trend.

SUPPORTIVE DATA

Decreasing LOS for childbirth is not a new phenomenon. As early as 1943 there were reports in the literature related to efforts to discharge women 2 to 5 days postpartum with homecare follow-up services, instead of the then traditional 10-day stay (Guerriero, 1943; Beck, 1991). During the 1960s, early discharge programs were instituted in response to maternity hospital bed shortages (Hellman, Kohl, & Palmer, 1962). During the 1970s and 1980s similar programs were developed; however, not until the 1990s did the practice become widespread. Norr and Nacion (1987) reviewed all postpartum early discharge programs published between 1960 and 1985 and concluded that discharge under 48 hours after birth has generally been safe for mothers and infants. Beck's (1991) review of early discharge programs in the United States provided similar results concerning the favorable statistics on maternal and infant morbidity. Infant hyperbilirubinemia was the main reason for readmission in both reviews.

Several randomized studies comparing early postpartum discharge and follow-up home visits have been published (Carty & Bradley, 1990; Waldenstrom, 1987; Yanover, Jones, & Miller, 1976). Yanover et al. found that discharge as early as 12 hours after birth, when combined with home visits by a perinatal nurse practitioner, was safe, economically feasible, and well accepted by childbearing women. No differences in morbidity or readmissions were noted between women who went home early and those with traditional LOS. Women's choice in staying in the hospital or going home early had an influence on patient satisfaction with the postpartum experience in Waldenstrom's qualitative study. However, in those families randomized to the early discharge group, 92% of women and 83% of men reported positive experiences. Men were also more involved in changing, bathing, and holding the newborn in the early discharge group (Waldenstrom, 1988). In the most recent study (Carty & Bradley, 1990), postpartum women were randomly assigned to three discharge times; 12 to 24 hours, 25 to 48 hours, and 4 days. Based on LOS, women received from one to five home visits by a perinatal nurse during the first 10 days postpartum. Results indicated low maternal and neonatal morbidity for all groups. Breastfeeding success at 1 month and satisfaction with nursing care was significantly higher for early discharge groups. Women with 4-day LOSs scored higher on measures of depression and lower on scores of confidence in the mothering role than did the early discharge groups (Carty & Bradley, 1990).

Previously published studies have limited generalizability due to differences in criteria for discharge and inconsistencies in definition of the term "early", type of care providers, and number of visits. Few authors describe programs with LOSs similar to current practice of less than 24 hours (Carty & Bradley, 1990; Drummond, Boucher, Chisholm, Geraci, & Kay, 1984; Scupholme, 1981; Yanover et al., 1976). Most postpartum homecare services do not provide nurse practitioners for all patients. Rarely do number of postpartum home visits exceed one or two. While limitations of available published studies exist, all authors cite the need for comprehensive follow-up perinatal care for women and infants after discharge. More data is needed on what constitutes a quality homecare follow-up program, including types of service most beneficial for selected populations. Only one group studied the impact of early discharge with home follow-up visits for low-income women and infants (Norr, Nacion, & Abramson, 1989). In this study, women who were discharged less than 48 hours after birth with their newborns reported higher maternal satisfaction and less maternal concerns than the control group. No differences in maternal-newborn morbidity was noted for traditional versus shorter LOS (Norr, Nacion, & Abramson).

While consensus in the literature and in practice does not exist concerning number of visits and type of service provided, there is enough evidence to support the benefits of postpartum homecare follow-up for childbearing women and newborns. The perinatal nurse can ease the transition from hospital to home by providing thorough physical, psychosocial and learning needs assessments, appropriate nursing interventions and teaching, and coordination of referrals to other healthcare resources as necessary.

MODELS OF SERVICES

Different strategies for providing perinatal homecare follow-up services have developed in each market area. Financial incentives, nursing resources, institutional goals, third-party payor influence, and homecare agency availability are variables that have influenced these models in various geographic regions. Although there are differences in who pays for the service and in who employs the perinatal nurses providing the service, generally phone contact and one to two home visits are included. Ideally, the same nurse who cares for the woman during childbirth and the postpartum period during hospitalization visits the woman and family in the home after discharge, but this practice model is not feasible in many perinatal settings. Some institutions have reported success with programs using their own postpartum nurses who see the woman initially during hospitalization and then provide homecare follow-up nursing care. Others contract with local homecare agencies to provide care. In an effort to decrease LOS, third-party payor groups in some market areas need to offer incentives for women to choose early discharge. As a result, homecare services are provided by agencies contracted for and paid by these insurance plans. Each perinatal center must develop strategies based on financial and nursing resources available. The goal of perinatal discharge programs and homecare services is (1) to bridge the interests of families, providers, payors, and community resources; (2) coordinate efforts; (3) minimize duplication; and (4) fill gaps in the healthcare system (Stern, 1991).

ESSENTIAL COMPONENTS OF QUALITY PERINATAL HOMECARE SERVICES

Discharge Criteria

Successful outcomes are dependent on a commitment from healthcare providers to comprehensive discharge planning, thorough patient and family assessment, education, and support, with coordination of institutional and community resources. Expected LOS for uncomplicated vaginal births should be discussed with women and support persons during prenatal visits. The childbearing family can then make appropriate plans. Increasingly, third-party payors mandate LOS based on condition of mother and newborn so options for longer LOS are limited, unless the patient has financial resources to pay for additional hospitalization. It is essential that home visits remain a covered source of both private and government insurance as 24-hour LOS (or less) becomes the standard (Welt, Cole, Myers, Sholes, & Jelovsek, 1993).

The American Academy of Pediatrics (AAP) and the American College of Obstetricians and Gynecologists (ACOG) have established guidelines and suggested criteria for discharging childbearing women within 24 hours after birth (AAP & ACOG, 1992; ACOG, 1989). The Association of Women's Health, Obstetric, and Neonatal Nurses (AWHONN) has developed guidelines for nursing practice, health education and counseling, and policies, procedures, and protocols for postpartum homecare (NAACOG, 1991; AWHONN, 1994). These criteria and guidelines are helpful in designing a comprehensive perinatal homecare follow-up service. Careful screening is essential to avoid sending women and newborns who are at risk for complications home too soon. Plans that include patient and family education and assessment of support persons' availability are also important (Display 18-1).

Perinatal centers may find it helpful to use checklists or similar evaluation tools to assess mothers' readiness for discharge. Chapter 17 includes a sample checklist. Teaching needs assessment and physical assessment can be combined on a single form or documented separately. Some institutions use a single documentation tool for both mother and baby while others have maintained two medical records. Preference of nursing staff and ease of documentation must be considered when designing medical record forms. As practice changes related to decreased LOS occur, a task force representing staff nurses who use the form, physicians, and nurse managers can be organized to periodically review existing forms and propose modifications and revision. Examples of medical record forms are included in Book Appendices. Clinical pathways are also excellent tools for determining patient and family status at discharge because expected goals and outcomes are evaluated and appropriate nursing interventions can be initiated prior to sending the mother and infant home (see Chapters 4 and 17).

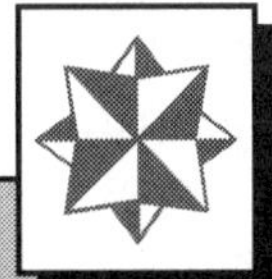

DISPLAY 18-1

Suggested Criteria for Discharge Within 24 Hours After Birth

- The mother had an uncomplicated vaginal birth following a normal term antepartum course and immediate postpartum course.
- Pertinent laboratory data, as selected by the practitioner, are within normal limits for both mother and newborn.
- The newborn is stable and able to maintain thermal homeostasis as well as demonstrate feeding abilities.
- Family members or other support persons are available to the mother for the first few days following discharge.
- The mother is aware of possible complications and has been instructed to notify the appropriate practitioner, as necessary.
- The institution has in place mechanisms to address patient questions that arise after discharge.

From American Academy of Pediatrics and American College of Obstetricians & Gynecologists. (1992). Guidelines for perinatal care. Elk Grove Village, IL: Author.

Selected Programs

Although number of nursing visits, follow-up telephone calls, and additional services offered vary with each perinatal homecare agency, a basic program is presented based on review of national practice (Display 18-2).

Ideally, the perinatal homecare nurse initially visits the woman during hospitalization. However, if this approach is not possible, a practical alternative is phone contact on the day of discharge. A mutually agreeable time can then be set for the first home visit. Opportunity for questions and answers is also provided during this conversation. It is important to attempt to schedule the first visit within 24 hours after discharge to meet the immediate care needs of both mother and newborn and to identify complications that may require timely interventions. Because nutritional stability may not be established prior to discharge, newborns are especially at risk for dehydration and jaundice. The AAP & ACOG (1992) guidelines for early newborn discharge include the recommendation for follow-up home visits at least within 48 hours after birth. Evidence of adequate nutrition, normal stool pattern, degree of jaundice, quality of mother-infant interaction, and details of newborn behavior are critical assessments in the first 48 hours (AAP & ACOG, 1992). Maternal ability for self-care, understanding of normal lochia characteristics, presence of discomfort, voiding and elimination pattern, nutritional status, adaptation to the parenting role, and social support systems are also assessed (NAACOG, 1991).

The first home visit is of sufficient duration for the perinatal nurse to complete a thorough physical examination of both the mother and newborn as well as to reinforce teaching and answer questions that may arise. The second and subsequent visits may be shorter, with additional physical assessment and follow-up of earlier questions and concerns. Home visits are an opportunity for return demonstration of feeding and newborn care techniques. The goal is for the woman to be able to adequately and safely care for herself and her newborn. If the newborn appears jaundiced, a heel stick for bilirubin may also be done at this time. Some agencies work with protocols or standing orders for newborns with jaundice, while others require nurses to contact the pediatrician for an order to obtain a blood specimen to be tested for bilirubin. Depending on state law, laboratory specimens [e.g., phenylketonuria (PKU)] are usually obtained during the second home visit, after feeding has been established.

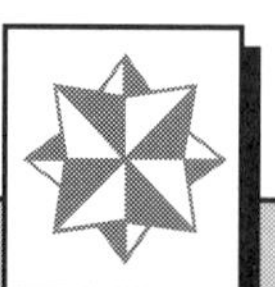

DISPLAY 18-2

Suggested Perinatal Homecare Services

Vaginal Births
- 1 to 2 home nursing visits*
- 2 follow-up phone calls
- 24 hours phone availability of a perinatal nurse for 2 weeks

Cesarean Births
- 1 to 3 home nursing visits*
- 3 follow-up phone calls
- 24 hours phone availability of a perinatal nurse for 2 weeks

*If possible, the first visit is made within 24 hours postdischarge.

PLAN OF CARE

The first few days at home can be challenging and stressful, even when the childbirth experience has been wonderful and the newborn eagerly anticipated. The process of integrating a new baby into the household coincides with major changes and adjustments in the lives of parents. If adequate social support systems, (i.e., grandparents, family members, friends, doulas, childcare, or housekeeping services) are not available or financially feasible, new parents may be overwhelmed by a greatly increased workload related to diapers, feeding, and newborn care. In addition, the new mother must cope with fatigue, discomfort, changes in body image, and possible frustration as she tries to learn her newborn's patterns and ways of communicating (Reeder, Martin, & Koniak, 1992). Fatigue is frequently reported by new mothers in the first few days at home with their newborn and can have a cumulative effect on physical discomforts, mood swings, and changes in relationships inherent in the physical and emotional transition to motherhood (Ruchala & Halstead, 1994).

Adaptation to the parenting role and successful transition from hospital to home can be facilitated by the perinatal nurse during home visits. While increased maternal confidence and satisfaction have been described (Carty & Bradley, 1990), not all women are eager to leave the hospital within hours of giving birth (Patterson, 1987; Waldenstrom, 1989). Some women feel they need more time to rest and recuperate before taking on the challenge of caring for a very needy newborn. Since LOS is generally predetermined by insurance coverage, most women do not have the choice to select additional inpatient days. The postpartum nurse has an important role in promoting the positive aspects of the current LOS. Women's perceptions of adequacy of postpartum LOS are significantly influenced by caregiver attitudes (Patterson). Even women who plan for a brief postpartum LOS may be more fatigued and overwhelmed than anticipated and wish they had extra recovery time in the hospital. The perinatal nurse can listen to the fatigue-related concerns of new mothers and together they can strategize approaches to ensure that adequate rest is obtained. Simple suggestions, such as enlisting assistance from family members and friends and sleeping when the baby sleeps, can help the woman get through the first few weeks.

Adjustment and coping with the stress of a newborn varies with each family. During the first few days postpartum, women have a need to describe the labor and birth process (Rubin, 1961). Asking the woman about her childbirth experience assists in fulfilling a developmental task in the transition to motherhood and can be the first opening to successful nurse/patient communication. Really listening as she relates her unique experience gives the woman the sense that the nurse is interested in her concerns and feelings, as well as her physical status. This discussion is also an excellent starting point for the perinatal nurse to pick up cues about the physical and emotional experience the woman brings to these early days. A thorough physical, psychosocial, and environmental assessment is essential to determine individual needs and to formulate a plan of care. Nursing assessments and interventions occur concurrently. During the assessment of physical status, learning needs, and psychological adaptation to parenting, the nurse has the opportunity to reinforce earlier teaching, answers questions and concerns, and refer to appropriate community resources as needed. It is especially important for the nurse to act as a helpful resource rather than telling the woman what to do. A collaborative approach is more successful in promoting maternal confidence in parenting skills (Hall & Carty, 1993). Each new mother has unique abilities and learning needs. The following maternal/newborn assessments may be included in the care provided during home visits.

NURSING ASSESSMENTS

Physical Assessment

Maternal

- Review of antepartum, intrapartum, and immediate postpartum events
- Vital signs
- Fundal location
- Episiotomy
- Abdominal incision
- Pain/discomfort level
- Homan's sign
- Color, consistency, and amount of lochia
- Breasts and nipples
- Elimination patterns: voiding and bowel movements
- Nutritional status
- Sleeping patterns
- General physical condition
- Self-care ability

Newborn

- Vital signs
- Color
- Evaluation for newborn jaundice
- Activity
- Reflexes: suck, grasp, Moro
- Skin condition
- Fontanels
- Cord
- Circumcision
- Abdomen
- Elimination patterns: voiding and stooling
- Nutritional status: feeding patterns
- Sleeping patterns

Learning-Needs Assessment

Maternal

- Pericare
- Incision/episiotomy care
- Breastfeeding/Breast care:
  - Support bra
  - Nipple care
  - Engorgement
  - Strategies to cope with sore nipples
  - Strategies to cope with well-meaning, non-supportive family and friends
  - Importance of rest and increased diet/fluid intake

    - 24-hour availability of perinatal nurse to answer breastfeeding questions and provide support
    - Availability of certified lactation nurse consultant for phone consultation and/or visit
- Diet/fluid intake
- Sexuality
- Contraception
- Body image changes
- Activity level
- Rest requirements
- Normal baby blues versus postpartum depression/psychosis
- Potential complications
- When to call perinatal nurse, nurse midwife, or obstetrician
- When to return for postpartum office visit

Newborn Care

- Bathing
- Cord care
- Circumcision care
- Vaginal discharge/hormonal influence/normals
- Diapering/rash treatment
- Newborn positioning: side and back versus prone
- Use of bulb syringe for suctioning secretions
- Temperature assessment
- Comforting techniques
- Normal growth and development
- Maternal-newborn attachment process
- Sibling rivalry
- Safety issues, including car seats
- Infant CPR
- Potential complications
- When to call perinatal nurse, pediatric nurse practitioner or pediatrician
- When to return for first newborn office visit

Newborn Feeding

- Bottle feeding:
    - Amount, type, and frequency
    - Positioning
    - Burping

Breastfeeding

- Demand, frequency
- Positioning
- Latching on
- Let down
- Burping
- Strategies to assess breastfeeding adequacy
- Strategies for successful breastfeeding experience

Newborn behaviors and cues

- Crying
- Sleeping and waking pattern
- Individual temperaments
- Response to parenting and reciprocal cues

Psychosocial Assessment

- Maternal/newborn attachment process
- Emotional response
- Perceptions of childbirth experience
- Family interactions
- Coping and adaptation abilities
- Maternal role assumption
- Body image adjustment
- Identification of support persons
- Social, economic, and cultural factors
- Knowledge of community resources

Environmental Assessment

- Obvious safety issues
- Adequate heat and temperature control
- Telephone availability
- Infant crib

Adapted from: Standards for the Nursing Care of Women and Infants (NAACOG, 1991) and Protocols and Practice Guidelines for Perinatal Homecare Services (Healthy Homecomings, Inc., 1994)

NURSING INTERVENTIONS

Nursing interventions are based on the needs of the childbearing woman and family that are identified by nursing assessments of physical, psychosocial, learning needs, and environmental factors. Previous chapters have covered in depth interventions for postpartum and newborn care, as well as educational strategies. Generally, perinatal nursing interventions during home visits are directed toward reinforcing earlier instructions, providing assistance with self-care, promoting health education, providing emotional support, validating childbirth experiences, and emphasizing support and referral resources available in the community (NAACOG, 1991). Additional services that may be provided on an as-needed basis are staple removal for abdominal incisions, obtaining samples for laboratory testing (e.g., newborn PKU and bilirubin or maternal hemoglobin and hematocrit), and initiating and monitoring newborn phototherapy.

OUTCOME MONITORING AND QUALITY CARE

Documentation of nursing assessments, interventions, evaluations, and discharge summary must be as meticulous and complete during perinatal home visits as during inpatient care. It is also important to record nurse-patient phone consultations. Examples of documentation tools (Pregnancy Assessment, Maternal Assessment, Infant Assessment, and Discharge Summary) are presented here in Chapter Appendix 18-1. If complications arise, nursing interventions, physician orders, and follow-through are included. Most physicians and nurse midwives request that copies of homecare medical records be sent to the office so they can be maintained as a permanent part of the record.

For appropriately screened childbearing women and newborns, morbidity is low in the postpartum period. The most common complication is neonatal jaundice. Statistics from one program reported here are consistent with morbidity statistics found in the literature (Avery, Fournier, Jones, & Sipovic, 1982; Carty & Bradley, 1990; Gibbs, Rodgers, Casteneda, & Ramzy, 1980; Jansson, 1985; Mehl, Peterson, Sokolosky, & Whitt, 1976; Welt, Cole, Myers, Sholes, & Jelovsek, 1993; Yanover, Jones, & Miller, 1976). The 1991 through 1994 maternal and neonatal statistics are as follows: newborns with neonatal jaundice requiring in-home phototherapy—15%; newborn infections either in the cord stump or circumcision site—2%; mothers with complications such as infection at incision site, mastitis, hypertension, postpartum hemorrhage, or clinical depression—2–5% (Healthy Homecomings, Inc., Morbidity Data, 1995). Display 18-3 provides suggested categories for a Morbidity Statistics Data Base.

Ability to track readmissions related to perinatal complications is essential in the evaluation of nursing care provided and in planning future care strategies. Some complications that would have required readmission in the past, such as neonatal jaundice, can be successfully managed in the homecare setting. Additional nursing visits are arranged on a daily basis to initiate home phototherapy and monitor newborn improvement. Neonatal readmissions have been greatly reduced since the availability of home phototherapy. Maternal infections can be identified by the perinatal nurse and antibiotics may be taken by the mother after consultation with a physician and the appropriate prescription is obtained. Other complications may necessitate a return visit to the healthcare provider's office. Obtaining blood samples in the home for PKU testing avoids an outpatient visit for this purpose. Any interventions performed at home instead of the hospital are cost effective and can be more convenient for the childbearing woman and family.

PATIENT AND FAMILY SATISFACTION

In addition to morbidity and cost data, maternal satisfaction with perinatal homecare services is also important in the evaluation of the services provided and for future planning. Literature reports of high levels

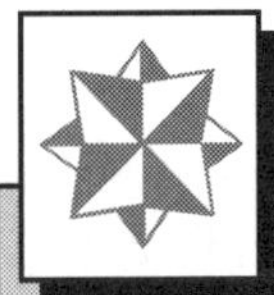

DISPLAY 18-3

Suggested Categories for Morbidity Statistics Database

- All Readmissions
- Maternal Complications
  - Infections: Incision, episiotomy, breast, urinary tract, endometrium
  - Vaginal Bleeding
  - Anemia
  - Fever
  - Gastrointestinal
  - Inadequate maternal-newborn attachment
  - Clinical depression
  - Social support deficit
  - Abuse/battering
  - Unsafe/inadequate environment
- Newborn Complications
  - Jaundice
  - Dehydration
  - Feeding instabilities
  - Failure to thrive/inadequate weight gain
  - Infections: cord stump, circumcision, eyes, thrush
  - Unsafe/inadequate environment
  - Abuse

of maternal satisfaction (Avery, Fournier, & Jones, 1982; Carty & Bradley, 1990; Drummond, Boucher, Chisholm, Geraci, & Kay, 1994; Yanover, Jones, & Miller, 1976) are consistent with data collected from one agency; 98% of those surveyed (see Chapter Appendix 18-2 for a Quality Assurance Survey) were satisfied with their early discharge experience and the perinatal nursing care provided in the home (Healthy Homecomings, Inc., Quality Assurance Data, 1995). The only validated maternal satisfaction tool related to early discharge and perinatal homecare services identified in the literature is Satisfaction With Nursing Care (Bradley, Carty, & Hall, 1989) (Book Appendix Q). Researchers using this tool found women who were discharged early were significantly more satisfied with their experience than women with traditional LOS (Carty & Bradley, 1990). Similar results of high levels of maternal satisfaction and confidence in the mothering role were found in a study of 100 postpartum women when the Satisfaction with Nursing Care Tool and the Maternal Confidence Scale (see Book Appendix R) were used (LaMartina, 1994).

NURSE PROVIDERS OF PERINATAL HOMECARE

Orientation/Education

AWHONN (1994) has published guidelines for didactic content and clinical skills verification for professional nurse providers of perinatal homecare services that are useful in planning a comprehensive orientation program. A thorough knowledge base in normal postpartum and newborn care, as well as in potential complications and appropriate nursing interventions, is essential for the perinatal nurse providing care in the home. Experience in nursing care of childbearing women and infants in the inpatient setting is an ideal way to gain this level of expertise. Practice in the home setting requires a high degree of autonomy and independence. It is important to remember that the perinatal nurse is a guest in the home and is there to facilitate the family's ability to cope using their own resources.

A didactic course covering the content outline suggested in the AWHONN (1994) guidelines will provide basic knowledge needed for homecare practice. A clinical practicum with an experienced preceptor is an essential part of a comprehensive orientation to perinatal homecare nursing. Evaluation and documentation of core competencies through clinical skills verification and knowledge base assessment should be as thorough as those in the inpatient setting. Requirements for continuing education are also desirable to maintain excellence in practice. Suggested criteria for employment is as follows:

- Registered professional nurse
- 3 years' perinatal nursing experience
- Successful completion of orientation
- Attend at least one agency meeting annually
- Attend at least one agency inservice annually
- 7 contact hours of continuing education in perinatal nursing per year

Annual performance evaluations are based on patient satisfaction data; accurate, complete and timely documentation; and consistent, appropriate nursing interventions and follow-up. A perinatal center manager spends time with each perinatal nurse during home visits in preparation for individual annual performance evaluations. This effort has proven to be an effective method of assessing the nurse in the practice setting (Healthy Homecomings, Inc., 1990).

Personal Safety

A final issue unique to nursing practice in the home setting is that of personal safety. Each agency should have in place policies to address various situations that could potentially compromise the safety of the nurse in the community. There should be a system to locate the nurse if necessary and a reliable method for communication between agency and the nurse. Beepers and cellular telephones are ideal ways to ensure rapid communication and the ability to call for help in unanticipated dangerous situations. Orientation should include directions regarding the immediate actions the nurse will take when encountering potentially unsafe situations such as abusive others in the home, weapons, illegal drugs, and hazardous pets. Self-defense techniques should be addressed as well as situations to avoid, such as groups of people in doorways or corners leading to the home. If travelling by car, preventive maintenance and adequate fuel are important in order to avoid being stranded. A heightened awareness of personal safety and common sense are the best approaches to decrease the likelihood of involvement in a potentially dangerous situation. Conditions that necessitate community resources follow-up such as obvious health hazards (poor sanitation or infestation) and/or physical hazards (broken windows, lack of heat, poor lighting, other unsafe housing conditions) should also be covered during employee orientation. Nursing knowledge of community resources and referral options is invaluable in assisting the new mother to provide the best possible home setting for herself and newborn.

SUMMARY

Research to date has suggested that discharge within 24 hours after childbirth is safe and effective for appropriately screened women and newborns. There appears to be a high level of satisfaction with early discharge when followed with perinatal homecare nursing services. Data related to the financial benefits are also encouraging. As healthcare services are increasingly scrutinized for both quality and cost impact, programs such as perinatal homecare, with positive clinical outcomes, high levels of patient satisfaction, and cost reduction potential, will continue. The role of the traditional postpartum nurse has evolved over the last decade to include more than routine or custodial care (Lukacs, 1991). Clinical assessment, supportive care, and teaching provided over a several-day period in past practice, must now be accomplished in a few hours. Postpartum nursing has moved to the home where our patients now spend the first few days after birth. We are challenged to expand our practice to the community to meet the needs of childbearing women and families. Perinatal nurses have the opportunity to improve outcomes and enhance the childbirth experience by providing quality nursing care in the home setting.

REFERENCES

American Academy of Pediatrics & American College of Obstetricians and Gynecologists. (1992). Guidelines for Perinatal Care. Elk Grove Village, IL: Author.

American College of Obstetricians and Gynecologists. (1989). ACOG: Standards for obstetric-gynecologic services (7th ed.). Washington, DC: Author.

Association of Women's Health, Obstetric, and Neonatal Nurses. (1994). Didactic content and clinical skills verification for professional nurse providers of perinatal home care. Washington, DC: Author.

Avery, M.D., Fournier, L.C., & Jones, P.L. (1989). An early postpartum hospital discharge program: Implementation and evaluation. Journal of Obstetric, Gynecologic & Neonatal Nursing, 11, 233-235.

Beck, C.T. (1991). Early postpartum discharge programs in the United States: A literature review and critique. Women and Health, 17(1), 125-138.

Bradley, C.F. (1983). Psychological consequences of intervention in the birth process. Canadian Journal of Behavior Science, 15(4), 422-438.

Bradley, C.F., Carty, E.M., & Hall, W.A. (1989). An evaluation of early postpartum discharge from a tertiary maternity hospital (Final Report). Vancouver, British Columbia: Canada. University of British Columbia, School of Nursing.

Carty, E.M., & Bradley, C.F. (1990). A randomized, controlled evaluation of early postpartum hospital discharge. Birth: Issues in Perinatal Care and Education, 17(4), 199-204.

Drummond, R.C., Boucher, J.D., Chisholm, D., Geraci, R.C., & Kay, S. (1984). Mother care: Cost effective program in maternal-infant care: mother and newborn to return home within twenty-four hours. Home Healthcare Nurse, 2(5), 41-43.

Gibbs, R.S., Rogers, P.J., Castenada, Y.S., & Ramzy, I. (1980). Endometritis following vaginal delivery. Obstetrics and Gynecology, 56(5), 555-558.

Guerriero, W. (1943). A maternal welfare program for New Orleans. American Journal of Obstetrics and Gynecology, 46, 312-313.

Hall, W.A., & Carty, E.M. (1993). Managing the early discharge experience: Taking control. Journal of Advanced Nursing, 18(4), 574-582.

Healthy Homecomings, Inc. (1990). Personnel Policies. St. Louis, MO: Author.

Healthy Homecomings, Inc. (1994). Protocols and practice guidelines for perinatal homecare services. St. Louis, MO: Author.

Healthy Homecomings, Inc. (1995). Morbidity data. St. Louis, MO: Author.

Healthy Homecomings, Inc. (1995). Quality Assurance Data. St. Louis, MO: Author.

Hellman, L., Kohl, S., & Palmer, J. (1962). Early hospital discharge in obstetrics. Lancet, 1 (Jan 27), 227-232.

Jansson, P. (1985). Early postpartum discharge: Home visiting an integral part. American Journal of Nursing, 85(5), 547-550.

LaMartina, M.B. (1994). Client satisfaction with home nursing care and perception of maternal role confidence in early postpartum discharge. Unpublished master's thesis, University of Missouri, St. Louis.

Lukacs, A. (1991). Issues surrounding early postpartum discharge: Effects on the caregiver. Journal of Perinatal and Neonatal Nursing, 5(1), 33-42.

Martin, L.L., & Reeder, S.J. (1991). Clinical manual for essentials of maternity nursing. Philadelphia: J.B. Lippincott.

Mehl, L., Peterson, G., Sokolosky, W., & Whitt, M. (1976). Outcomes of early discharge after normal birth. Birth and the Family Journal, 3, 101-107.

Nurses Association of the American College of Obstetricians and Gynecologists. (1991). Standards for the nursing care of women and newborns (4th ed.). Washington, DC: Author.

Norr, K.F., & Nacion, K. (1987). Outcomes of postpartum early discharge, 1960-1986: A comparative review. Birth Issues in Perinatal Care and Education, 14(3), 135-141.

Norr, K.F., Nacion, K.W., & Abramson, R. (1989). Early discharge with home follow-up: Impact on low-income mothers and infants. Journal of Obstetric, Gynecologic and Neonatal Nursing, 18(2), 133-141.

Patterson, P.K. (1987). A comparison of postpartum early and traditional discharge groups. Quarterly Review Bulletin, 13(11), 365-371.

Reeder, S.J., Martin, L.L., & Koniak, D.G. (1992). Maternity nursing: Family, newborn, and women's health care (17 ed.). Philadelphia: J.B. Lippincott.

Rubin, R. (1961). Puerperal change. Nursing Outlook, 9, 753-755.

Ruchala, P., & Halstead, L. (1994). The postpartum experience of low-risk women: A time of adjustment and change. Maternal-Child Nursing Journal, 22(3), 83-89.

Scupholme, A. (1981). Postpartum early discharge: An inner city experience. Journal of Nurse-Midwifery, 26, 19-23.

Stern, T.E. (1991). An early discharge program: An entrepreneurial nursing practice becomes a hospital affiliated agency. Journal of Perinatal and Neonatal Nursing, 5(1), 1-8.

Waldenstrom, U. (1987). Early discharge with domiciliary visits and hospital care: Parents' experiences of two modes of postpartum care. Scandinavian Journal of Caring Sciences, 1(2), 51-58.

Waldenstrom, U. (1988). Early and late discharge after hospital birth: Father's involvement in infant care. Early Human Development, 17(1), 19-28.

Waldenstrom, U. (1989). Early discharge as voluntary and involuntary alternatives to a longer postpartum stay in hospital: Effects on mothers' experiences and breast feeding. Midwifery, 5, 189-196.

Welt, S.I., Cole, J.S., Myers, M.S., Sholes, D.M., & Jelovsek, F.R. (1993). Feasibility of postpartum rapid discharge: A study from a community hospital population. American Journal of Perinatology, 10(5), 384-387.

Yanover, M.J., Jones, D., & Miller, M.D. (1976). Perinatal care of low-risk mothers and infants: Early discharge with home care. New England Journal of Medicine, 294(13), 702-705.

APPENDIX 18-1

HEALTHY HOMECOMINGS® PREGNANCY ASSESSMENT

Patient Name:________________ Social Security No.__________ OB/GYN:__________

RN Signature:________________ Date:_______ ☐ High Risk/At Risk Initial Visit ☐ Pre-Delivery Visit

EDC:___/___/___ Gestational Age:__________ Height:__________ Weight:__________ Age:__________

Occupation:________________ Cervical Status:__________ Date:___/___/___ Findings:________

Gravida:__________ No. Term Deliveries:______ No. Preterm Deliveries:________ No. AB:_________ No. Living:______

Risk Factors/Diagnosis:______________________________

____

Allergies:______________________________

Medications (Dose/Route/Frequency/Contraindications):______________________________

____

____

Past Medical/Surgical History:______________________________

____

Significant Obstetrical History:______________________________

____

Support Systems:______________________________

Educational Information/Booklets Given: ☐ Yes ☐ No Able to Activate EMS in an Emergency: ☐ Yes ☐ No

PHYSICAL ASSESSMENT

Vital Signs	Heart Sounds	Extremities	Elimination	Nutrition
T:_______ P:_______ R:_______ BP:_______ ☐ RA ☐ LA Position:______	☐ Normal **Breath Sounds** ☐ Clear to Auscultation **Respirations** ☐ Non-Labored	☐ No Edema ☐ Neg Homan's **Reflexes** ☐ Normal Right Patellar ☐ Normal Left Patellar	☐ Voiding without difficulty ☐ Regular Bowel Movements ☐ Hemmorrhoids **Functional Limitations** ☐ None	☐ Three Balanced Meals a day ☐ 2 Snacks/Day ☐ 8 glasses of water daily ☐ Increase Fiber **Activity** ☐ Up Ad Lib

Psycho-Social Evaluation	Hospital Information	DOCUMENTATION
☐ Appropriate Affect ☐ Intact Support System ☐ Drug Use__________ ☐ Alcohol Use__________ ☐ Caffeine__________ ☐ Smoking__________ Other Significant Findings:______ __________ __________ __________	Delivering Hospital: __________ Planned: ☐ Vag Del ☐ C-Section Plans to: ☐ Breast-Feed ☐ Bottle Feed Planned length of hospital stay:________ __________ Pediatrician:________ __________	Document all Abnormal Findings, Needs and/or Interventions (***include any home safety concerns***):______ __________ __________ __________ __________ __________ __________ __________ __________ __________ __________

Baby Assessment	Current Complaints
FHTs__________ ☐ Baby Active ☐ Fetal Kick Counts__________	__________ __________ __________

FORM3.DOC

Infant Name:________	Physician:________	Mother's Name________
Infant's DOB:____/___/____	Metabolic Screen Drawn:____/___/____	Educational Booklets Given: ☐ Yes ☐ No

HEALTHY HOMECOMINGS® INFANT TEACHING GUIDE

Key: ① 1st Visit ② 2nd Visit	Verbal Instructions Given	Reinforced	Demonstration Given	Verbalizes Understanding	Return Demonstration
1. Signs & Symptoms of Infection/Complications					
2. Feeding Instructions (Lactation Physiology/ Formula Preparation)					
3. Hygiene (cord care, circumcision care, bathing, diapering, etc.)					
4. Jaundice					
5. Temperature Taking					
6. Positioning of Baby					
7. Use of Suction Bulb					
8. Safety (car seats, cribs, home conditions, bottle propping)					
9. Comfort Techniques					
10. Normal Elimination Pattern					
11. Normal Sleep/Awake Cycles					
12. Infection Control (good handwashing, visitors)					

Additional Instructions:

NOTIFY YOUR BABY'S PHYSICIAN FOR:

- Temperature Less Than 97.2°F or Greater Than 99.4°F.
- Excessive Spitting Up.
- Vomiting or Watery Stools.
- Feeding Difficulties.
- Inconsolable Crying.
- Fewer Than 6-8 Wet Diapers in 24 Hours.
- No Bowel Movement After 48 Hours.
- Difficulty Waking Baby.
- Breathing Difficulty.
- Increasing Jaundice.
- Foul Odor or Red Ring Around Cord.
- Redness or drainage from circumcision.

Signature indicates teaching has been given, is understood by the mother, and a copy of this guide has been received:

Mother's Signature________ Date________ RN Signature________

INFANT ASSESSMENT

1st Visit Date:________ 2nd Visit Date:________ Circle One:
RN Signature:________ RN Signature:________ Male/Female

Vital Signs	Respirations	Head	Color	Activity	Heart Sounds	Muscle Tone	Cord
① ②	Non-Labored ①___②___	Symmetrical: ①___②___	Pink ①___②___	Alert ①___②___	Normal ①___②___	Strong ①___②___	Clean & Dry ①___②___
T: ___ ___	Breath Sounds	Fontanels	Skin	Nose	Pulses	Reflexes	Circumcision
P: ___ ___	Clear to Auscultation ①___②___	Flat ②___②___	Good Turgor ①___②___	Normal ①___②___	Strong ①___②___	Intact ①___②___	Clean & Healing ①___②___
R: ___ ___							

Eyes	Extremeties	Neck	Ears	Abdomen	Jaundice	
Normal ①___②___	Symmetrical ①___②___	Normal ①___②___	Normal ①___②___	Soft ①___②___	① Yes No	② Yes No
Face	Capillary Refill	Ears	Genitalia	Bowel Sounds	☐ Head	☐ Head
Normal ①___②___	Normal ①___②___	Normal ①___②___	Normal ①___②___	Active ①___②___	☐ Head & Chest	☐ Head & Chest
					☐ Head & Abdomen	☐ Head & Abdomen
					☐ Head to Feet	☐ Head to Feet

Elimination	Bottle Feeding	Breast Feeding	Appropriate Mother/Infant Attachment ①________②________
No. of Stools in last 24 hours. ①____②____	Type:________	Minutes/Breast ①___②___	Allergies:________
Consistency ①________ ②________	Oz./Feeding ①____②____	Frequency: ①___②___	Medications: Dose/Frequency/Route/Contraindications:________
No. of Wet Diapers in last 24 hours ①____②____	Frequency: ①____②____	Proper latch-on①___②___	Document all Abnormal Findings, Needs and/or Interventions (*include any home safety concerns*):________
	Suck & Swallow	Assistance needed: ①____②____	
	Normal ①____②____	Supplementation: ①____②____	
	Spitting Amount ①____②____	Type:________ Amt:________ Frequency:________	

FORM2.DOC

APPENDIX 18-1 cont.

Patient Name:	Social Security Number:	Delivery Date: / /
OB/GYN Physician:	Breast Feeding ☐ Bottle Feeding ☐	Educational Booklets Given: Yes ☐ No ☐

HEALTHY HOMECOMINGS® MATERNAL TEACHING GUIDE

Key: ① 1st Visit ② 2nd Visit	Verbal Instructions Given	Reinforced	Demonstration Given	Verbalizes Understanding	Return Demonstration
1. Signs & Symptoms of Infection/Complications					
2. Medications Reviewed					
3. Pericare (Kegal Exercises, Cleansing, Sitz Bath)					
4. Breast/Nipple Care					
5. Postpartum Emotional Adjustments					
6. Activity/Exercise					
7. Diet/Fluid Intake					
8. Incision Care					
9. Vaginal Discharge					
10. Sexual Activity					
11. Contraception					
12. Self Breast Exams					
13. Community Resources					

Additional Instructions:

Notify Your Physician For:

- Fever above 100.4°F for over 24 hours
- Breast Pain-tender reddened area or the entire breast.
- Leg Pain-area is hot, red and swollen.
- Headache, nausea, vomitting, chills or visual changes.
- Urinary Difficulty
- Intense vaginal, pelvic, episiotomy or incisional pain.
- Vaginal Discharge - itchy or foul odor or bright red bleeding.
- Prolonged feelings of sadness, depression.

Signature indicates teaching has been given, is understood by patient, and a copy of this guide has been received:

Patient Signature________________ Date__________ RN Signature________________

MATERNAL ASSESSMENT

1st Visit Date:_________ 2nd Visit Date:__________ Circle One:

RN Signature:__________ RN Signature:__________ Vag Del / C-section

Vital Signs	Fundus	Lochia	Incision	Perineum	Gastrointestinal	Bladder
① ② T: ____ ____ P: ____ ____ R: ____ ____ B/P: ____ ____	Firm ①____②____ Position: ①________ ②________ **Extremeties** No Edema ①____②____ Negative Homan's ①____②____	Type: ①________ ②________ Amount ①________ ②________ **Activity** Up Ad Lib ①____②____	Type:________ Clean, dry & well approximated ①____②____ **Functional Limitations** None ①____②____	☐ No Epis ☐ Episiotomy Type:________ Clean, dry & well approximated ①____②____ Hemorrhoids ①____②____	Bowel Sounds Present ①____②____ Bowel Movement ①____②____	Voiding without difficulty ①____②____ **Breast** Nipples intact ①____②____ Soft ①____②____ Milk Present ①____②____

PsychoSocial	
Appropriate Affect ①____②____ Intact Support System ①____②____ Appropriate Mother/ Infant Attachment ①____②____ Appropriate Family/ Infant Attachment ①____②____	Allergies:________ Medications: Dose/Frequency/Route/Contraindications________ Document all Abnormal Findings, Needs and/or Interventions (***include any home safety concerns***):________

FORM1.DOC

APPENDIX 18-1 cont.

HEALTHY HOMECOMINGS, INC.

Discharge Summary

Patient's	**Mother/Infant**	Date of Birth: __________
Name: ________________________	Cesarean: ______________	Vaginal: __________
Address: ________________________		
Telephone number: __________________	Physician: ____________________	

Date

Nurse's Signature: ____________________ Date of discharge from home care: ____________

Adapted from Healthy Homecomings, Inc. 1994.

APPENDIX 18-2 cont.

HEALTHY HOMECOMINGS, INC.

QUALITY ASSURANCE SURVEY
MATERNAL-NEWBORN HOME VISIT/S

To maintain or improve the quality of our service, your evaluation of **Healthy Homecomings, Inc.** is very important to us. We appreciate your time and effort...your comments are welcome.

Nursing Care Evaluation:

1. Were the postpartum visits and assessments thorough and complete? ☐ Yes ☐ No
2. Were the assessments and evaluations of your baby thorough and complete? ☐ Yes ☐ No
3. Did you enjoy having a professional nurse assist you with the care of your infant? ☐ Yes ☐ No
4. Did you experience problems with breast/bottle feeding during the first week at home? ☐ Yes ☐ No
5. Did the nurse assist you with feeding your baby (breast/bottle)? ☐ Yes ☐ No
6. Did we do, or not do, something which caused you to make an extra visit to your physician or hospital emergency room?
7. Was this a pleasant, satisfying, and learning experience? ☐ Yes ☐ No
8. Did you read our booklets for yourself and your baby? ☐ Yes ☐ No
9. Were the booklets helpful and enable you to apply the information? ☐ Yes ☐ No

Nurse Evaluation:

1. Was your nurse friendly and courteous? ☐ Yes ☐ No
2. Was your nurse professional and responsive to your needs? ☐ Yes ☐ No

Phone Service

1. Were you made aware of our 24 hour phone service? ☐ Yes ☐ No
2. Was the 24 hour phone service a comfort to you? ☐ Yes ☐ No
3. Did you place any calls? ☐ Yes ☐ No
4. Was your call(s) answered promptly (within a half hour)? ☐ Yes ☐ No

Did we meet your emotional and psychological needs? ☐ Yes ☐ No

Would you recommend **Healthy Homecomings, Inc.** to your friends and family? ☐ Yes ☐ No

Comments:

____

Your Nurse's Name: ____________________

Your Signature: ____________________ Month of Service: ____________________

Insurance Carrier: ____________________

Adapted from Healthy Homecomings, Inc. 1990

Appendices

APPENDIX A. Maternal Services Assessment Questionnaire (MSAQ)*

Please circle the best response to each item. If an item does not apply to you, leave the item blank. This informations will be used for the purpose of meeting our goal to provide better patient care on this unit.

The following items 1 thru 8 refer to your meals.

		STRONGLY AGREE	AGREE	UNSURE	DISAGREE	STRONGLY DISAGREE
1.	My meals were served warm.	5	4	3	2	1
2.	The food was good to eat.	5	4	3	2	1
3.	I received a morning snack when I requested one.	5	4	3	2	1
4.	I received an afternoon snack when I requested one.	5	4	3	2	1
5.	I received a bedtime snack when I requested one.	5	4	3	2	1
6.	I was given a menu each day for selection of my food.	5	4	3	2	1
7.	I received the food I ordered.	5	4	3	2	1
8.	My tray was picked up promptly after each meal.	5	4	3	2	1

The following items 9 and 10 refer to your room.

		STRONGLY AGREE	AGREE	UNSURE	DISAGREE	STRONGLY DISAGREE
9.	My room was kept neat and clean at all times.	5	4	3	2	1
10.	My bathroom was kept neat and clean at all times.	5	4	3	2	1

* J. Sandridge, RN, MSN; L. Alexander, RN, MSN; L. Moore, RN, EdD (1987). The University of Texas Medical Branch Hospitals, Galveston, TX 77550.

APPENDIX A. Maternal Services Assessment Questionnaire (MSAQ)* cont.

The following items 11 thru 21 refer to your experiences with the nurses who cared for you on this unit.

	STRONGLY AGREE	AGREE	UNSURE	DISAGREE	STRONGLY DISAGREE
11. My call light was answered promptly.	5	4	3	2	1
12. I knew the names of the nurses caring for me.	5	4	3	2	1
13. The nurses were available to answer questions about myself.	5	4	3	2	1
14. The nurses were available to answer questions about my baby.	5	4	3	2	1
15. After requesting pain medications, I received it promptly.	5	4	3	2	1
16. The nurses were kind and pleasant.	5	4	3	2	1
17. The nurses gave me the attention and care that I needed.	5	4	3	2	1
18. I understand the reason certain treatments, procedures and/or medications were ordered for me.	5	4	3	2	1
19. My privacy was maintained during treatments, interviews and exams.	5	4	3	2	1
20. I was given adequate assistance in the care of my baby.	5	4	3	2	1
21. The nurses were understanding regarding my feelings (happiness, sadness, anxiety).	5	4	3	2	1

APPENDIX A. Maternal Services Assessment Questionnaire (MSAQ)* cont.

The following items 22 thru 34 refer to the information given to you by the nurses.

	STRONGLY AGREE	AGREE	UNSURE	DISAGREE	STRONGLY DISAGREE
The nurses gave me enough information about:					
22. how to use the call light	5	4	3	2	1
23. how to rent the TV	5	4	3	2	1
24. how to use the telephone	5	4	3	2	1
25. how to use the bed controls	5	4	3	2	1
26. visiting hours	5	4	3	2	1
27. rooming–in options	5	4	3	2	1
28. when to call a nurse for assistance.	5	4	3	2	1
29. how to use the peri–light (for episiotomy/stitches)	5	4	3	2	1
30. how to use the heat lamp (for episiotomy/stitches)	5	4	3	2	1
31. how to use the spray (for episiotomy/stitches)	5	4	3	2	1
32. how to use nipple cream (for breastfeeding)	5	4	3	2	1
33. how to use the peribottle	5	4	3	2	1
34. how to use the emergency button in the bathroom	5	4	3	2	1

The following items 35 thru 37 refer to the first time you fed your baby.

	STRONGLY AGREE	AGREE	UNSURE	DISAGREE	STRONGLY DISAGREE
35. The nurse explained the use of the bulb syringe.	5	4	3	2	1
36. The nurse explained how much to feed my baby (if bottlefeeding).	5	4	3	2	1
37. The nurse told me how long to breastfeed my baby (if breasfeeding).	5	4	3	2	1

APPENDIX A. Maternal Services Assessment Questionnaire (MSAQ)* cont.

The following items 38 thru 42 refer to your experiences with the nurses caring for your baby in the nursery.

	STRONGLY AGREE	AGREE	UNSURE	DISAGREE	STRONGLY DISAGREE
38. The nurses identified themselves when talking to me about my baby.	5	4	3	2	1
39. The nurses were available to answer questions about my baby.	5	4	3	2	1
40. The nurses were kind and pleasant.	5	4	3	2	1
41. I understand the reasons certain treatments, and/or procedures, were done on my baby.	5	4	3	2	1
42. I was given adequate assistance in the care of my baby.	5	4	3	2	1

The following items 43 thru 47 refer to your understanding of self care and infant care after you go home.

	STRONGLY AGREE	AGREE	UNSURE	DISAGREE	STRONGLY DISAGREE
43. I feel I was given enough information on how to feed my baby.	5	4	3	2	1
44. I feel I was given enough information about baby care to feel comfortable taking care of my baby at home.	5	4	3	2	1
45. The nurses gave me enough information about caring for myself when I get home.	5	4	3	2	1
46. I feel I was given enough information about the Infant Car Safety Seat Law to buy or rent one before discharge.	5	4	3	2	1
47. I feel I was given enough information about the signs and symptoms of infant illness to know when to call my baby's doctor or clinic.	5	4	3	2	1

The following items 48 thru 50 refer to hospital policies and routines.

	STRONGLY AGREE	AGREE	UNSURE	DISAGREE	STRONGLY DISAGREE
48. The hospital allows enough visiting time for my friends and family.	5	4	3	2	1
49. Hospital personnel entering my room were wearing name badges.	5	4	3	2	1
50. I was able to get the rest and sleep I felt I needed.	5	4	3	2	1

Comments:

APPENDIX B. Perinatal Unit Core Competencies

PERINATAL UNIT CORE COMPETENCIES

KEY: METHOD OF EVALUATION AND FOLLOW-UP

Preceptor Observation	PO	Peer Review	PR	Patient Feedback	PFB
Return Demonstration	RD	Written Self-Assessment	WSE	Computer Assisted Instruction	CAI
Skills Checklist	SC	Medical Record Audit	MRA	None Needed	NN
Video Tape Viewing	VTV	Learning Module Completion	LMC		

Competency	Advanced Beginner	Competent	Proficient	Expert	Method of Evaluation	Follow-up	Initials
ANTEPARTUM							
Able to complete a comprehensive assessment of women during the antepartum period experiencing complications of pregnancy including preterm labor, premature rupture of membranes, pregnancy-induced hypertension, preeclampsia, diabetes, bleeding, and infection.							
Plans and delivers care to women with pregnancy complications appropriate to the specific clinical situation.							
Has a thorough understanding of the warning signs of preterm labor and is able to discuss this information with women at risk in a manner that facilitates their understanding.							
Has a thorough understanding of the psychosocial aspects of a high-risk pregnancy and uses that knowledge to provide care sensitive to those special needs.							
Has knowledge of both institutional and community resources available to women with complications of pregnancy and makes referrals as appropriate.							
Able to provide information to women with pregnancy complications needed prior to discharge such as signs and symptoms of specific clinical situation, and when to call the obstetrician/primary healthcare provider, or come to the hospital.							
INTRAPARTUM							
Able to complete a comprehensive perinatal nursing assessment on pregnant women admitted to labor-delivery-recovery unit.							
Able to identify pregnant women at high risk for pregnancy and/or medical complications.							

St. John's Mercy Medical Center, St. Louis, MO.

PERINATAL UNIT CORE COMPETENCIES cont'd

KEY: METHOD OF EVALUATION AND FOLLOW-UP

Preceptor Observation	PO	Peer Review	PR	Patient Feedback	PFB
Return Demonstration	RD	Written Self-Assessment	WSE	Computer Assisted Instruction	CAI
Skills Checklist	SC	Medical Record Audit	MRA	None Needed	NN
Video Tape Viewing	VTV	Learning Module Completion	LMC		

Competency	Advanced Beginner	Competent	Proficient	Expert	Method of Evaluation	Follow-up	Initials
INTRAPARTUM cont'd							
Plans and delivers care to normal laboring women.							
Plans and delivers care to women with perinatal and/or medical complications including pregnancy-induced hypertension, preterm labor, bleeding in pregnancy, and multiple gestations.							
Has a thorough understanding of the physiology of electronic fetal heart rate monitoring.							
Able to interpret electronic fetal heart rate monitor tracings, identify reassuring and nonreassuring FHR patterns, and initiate appropriate nursing interventions.							
Has a thorough understanding of the normal labor and birth process.							
Plans and delivers care to women who labor without anesthesia.							
Has a thorough understanding of the nursing care for laboring women with epidural anesthesia.							
Has a thorough understanding of the pharmacokinetics of oxytocin.							
Acts as labor coach and circulating nurse for both vaginal and cesarean births.							
Able to complete a systematic assessment of the newborn, including evaluating the need for resuscitation and assigning Apgar scores.							

St. John's Mercy Medical Center, St. Louis, MO.

APPENDIX B. Perinatal Unit Core Competencies cont.

PERINATAL UNIT CORE COMPETENCIES cont'd

KEY: METHOD OF EVALUATION AND FOLLOW-UP

Preceptor Observation	PO	Peer Review	PR	Patient Feedback	PFB
Return Demonstration	RD	Written Self-Assessment	WSE	Computer Assisted Instruction	CAI
Skills Checklist	SC	Medical Record Audit	MRA	None Needed	NN
Video Tape Viewing	VTV	Learning Module Completion	LMC		

Competency	Advanced Beginner	Competent	Proficient	Expert	Method of Evaluation	Follow-up	Initials
INTRAPARTUM cont'd							
Provides supportive care to the woman and her family in situations involving fetal loss or fetal abnormalities.							
Assesses the woman's educational needs during the intrapartum period and provides appropriate information to the woman and her family.							
POSTPARTUM							
Able to perform a comprehensive assessment of the woman in the immediate postpartum period.							
Has a thorough understanding of normal physiologic processes occurring during the postpartum period.							
Plans and delivers care to women without complications during the postpartum period.							
Able to identify women at risk for complications during the postpartum period, including hemorrhage, infection, pregnancy-induced hypertension and preeclampsia.							
Plans and delivers care to women with complications during the postpartum period.							
Has a thorough knowledge of breastfeeding and supports the woman who wants to initiate breastfeeding in the immediate postpartum period.							
Has a thorough understanding of the physiology of human lactation.							
Facilitates the breastfeeding process including supporting the women during initial breasting as soon as possible after birth, positioning, latch on, satiation cues, breast care, measures to manage engorgement, and use of manual or electric breast pumps.							

St. John's Mercy Medical Center, St. Louis, MO.

APPENDIX B. Perinatal Unit Core Competencies cont.

PERINATAL UNIT CORE COMPETENCIES cont'd

KEY: METHOD OF EVALUATION AND FOLLOW-UP

Preceptor Observation	PO	Peer Review	PR	Patient Feedback	PFB
Return Demonstration	RD	Written Self-Assessment	WSE	Computer Assisted Instruction	CAI
Skills Checklist	SC	Medical Record Audit	MRA	None Needed	NN
Video Tape Viewing	VTV	Learning Module Completion	LMC		

Competency	Advanced Beginner	Competent	Proficient	Expert	Method of Evaluation	Follow-up	Initials
POSTPARTUM cont'd							
Facilitates the formula feeding process including providing information about amount of feeding, satiation cues, demand feeding, positioning, burping, formula preparation and measures to prevent or decrease breast engorgement.							
Promotes maternal-newborn attachment including encouraging examining, touching, talking to newborn, keeping couplet together as much as possible, providing information about newborn behavior states, sleeping and waking patterns, and comforting strategies.							
Provides information about maternal self-care and newborn care prior to discharge including safety issues, feeding techniques, and signs and symptoms indicating need to call the pediatrician, obstetrician, or other primary healthcare provider.							
NEWBORN							
Able to perform a comprehensive assessment of the newborn.							
Has a thorough understanding of normal newborn transitional care including thermoregulation, glucose monitoring, respiratory status.							
Plans and delivers care to the healthy full term newborn.							
Able to identify newborns at risk for complications during the first hours of life including temperature, glucose, and respiratory instabilities.							
Plans and delivers care to the newborn with complications.							

St. John's Mercy Medical Center, St. Louis, MO.

APPENDIX C. Daily Postpartum Assessments & Interventions

DAILY POSTPARTUM ASSESSMENTS & INTERVENTIONS

* Indicates further documentation in Integrated Progress Notes.																
	DATE															
	TIME															
SKIN	COLOR Normal, Pale, Cyanotic, Flushed															
	TEMPERATURE Warm, Hot, Cool															
	HUMIDITY Dry, Moist, Clammy, DIA =Diaphoretic															
	IV/CONDITION OF SITE Patent, Occluded, △=Changed, D/C=Discontinued (indicate time) ✓ = No signs of infection * = Refer to Progress Notes (may have signs of infection or infiltration)															
BREASTS	CONDITION Soft, FIlling, Full, Engorged, Red, Pain,															
	NIPPLES Normal, Red, Pain, Cracked, Inverted															
UTERUS	HEIGHT U/U = At Umbilicus (measure in finger breaths) FB/U — Above U/FB — Below															
	POSITION Midline, Right of Umbilicus, Left of Umbilicus															
	CONSISTENCY Firm, Boggy, FM = Firm with Massage															
LOCHIA	COLOR Rubra, Serosa, Alba															
	AMOUNT 0 = no flow, Scant, Small, Moderate, Heavy, Clots (larger than quarters)															
	ODOR + = Present 0 = Absent/Normal															
PERINEUM	CONDITION Intact, Ecchymosis, Hematoma, Puffy, Edema, Clean															
	EPISIOTOMY N = Clean, dry, intact, Separated, Edema, Red															
	HEMORRHOIDS + = Present, Edematous, Thrombosed, Soft, Painful															
CESAREAN SECTION	ABDOMEN Soft, Distended															
	BOWEL SOUNDS Normal, ↑ = Hyperactive, ↓ = Hypoactive, O = Absent, Flatus															
	INCISION Normal (clean, dry, intact), Edema, Red, Drainage, Separated, Unseen															
	DRESSING Dry & Intact, △ = Changed, No Dressing															
	SUTURES/STAPLES REMOVED = ✓															
	BREATH SOUNDS Equal, Unequal, Clear, Congested WI = Wheezing on Inspiration WE = Wheezing on Expiration Rales, Rhonchi															
	POSITIONING Left, Right, Supine, Prone, Self, Fowlers															

Palos Community Hospital, Palos Heights, IL.

APPENDIX C. Daily Postpartum Assessments & Interventions cont.

	DATE															
	TIME															
CARDIO-VASCULAR	EDEMA 1+ Minimal edema of the pedal & pretibial areas 2+ Marked edema of the lower extremities and hands 3+ Edema of the face and hands, lower abdominal wall & sacrum. 4+ Anasarca (Generalized massive edema) & ascites															
	CALF TENDERNESS + = Present (indicate R or L), 0 = Absent															
	HOMAN'S SIGN 0 = Negative + = Positive (indicate R or L)															
LOC/ SEDATION	Alert, Confused, Lethargic, Oriented, Sleeping, Nonresponsive, Arousable															
EMOTIONAL STATUS	Calm, Apprehensive, Anxious, Hostile, Depressed, Labile, Flat Affect															
TREATMENTS	K-PAD Back, Incision, Legs, Other															
	Abdominal binder = ✓															
	Supportive Bra, Breast Binder															
	Breast Pump (hand) (electric) ✓ each time pumping occurs.															
	Breast Shells															
	Ice to Perineum = ✓															
	Sitz = ✓ (check each time used)															
	Inflatable Cushion = ✓															
ACTIVITY	Bed, Chair, Dangle, Ambulatory, BR = Bathroom BRA = Bathroom w/assistance															
HYGIENE	Complete, Partial, Shower Foley Care, Pericare															
DIET	APPETITE NPO, Good, Fair, Poor															
	TYPE General, Clear Liquids, Full Liquids, Soft, Other															
ELIMINATION	STOOLS Formed, Semisolid, Liquid															
	URINATION Void, Straight Cath															
	FOLEY Patent, Irrigated, Changed, D/C = Discontinued (indicate time)															
	SS Enema, Fleets, Suppository															
SAFETY	SIDERAILS ↕ = Up, ↕ = Down (indicate #)															
	CALL LIGHT + = ✓															
	I.D. BAND + = ✓															
INITIALS																

Palos Community Hospital, Palos Heights, IL.

APPENDIX C. Initial Assessment

INITIAL ASSESSMENT

DOB ______________________ Initial Bath: ______________ (Time/Initials) Length: ________ cm. ________ in.

TIME ______________________ Triple Dye to Cord ______________ (Time/Initials) Head: ________ cm. ________ in.

TRANSITIONAL CARE ADMINISTERED IN: Infant Removed from Radiant Warmer: Chest: ________ cm. ________ in.

☐ LDRP ☐ Special Care Nursery Date: ____________ Time: __________ Abdomen: ________ cm. ________ in.

Weight: _____ gms. lbs. _____ oz. _____

										SILVERMAN							
Time	Radiant Warmer Temp	Temp	Pulse	Resp.	Breath Sounds	B/P	Color	Activity	Muscle Tone	Upper Chest	Lower Chest	Xiphoid	Flare	Grunt	Total	Chest PT	Initials

COLOR
Pink, Pale, Dusky, Jaundiced, Plethoric, Mottled, Cyanosis, Acrocyanosis

✓ = chest PT

MUSCLE TONE
Normal flexion, Flaccidity, Spasticity

ACTIVITY
Active, Active With Stimulation, Quiet, alert, Irritable, Lethargic, Hyperactive, Tremors, Sleeping

BREATH SOUNDS
Equal, Rales, Clear, Diminished, Rhonchi

SKIN
_____ Pink _____ Acrocyanosis
_____ Central cyanosis _____ Dusky
_____ Pale _____ Plethoric
_____ Mottled _____ Jaundice
_____ Abrasions ______________
_____ Birthmarks ______________
_____ Dry _____ Meconium stained
_____ Ecchymosis ______________
_____ Lacerations ______________
_____ Milia _____ Peeling
_____ Mongolian spots ______________
_____ Petechiae _____ Pustules
_____ Rash ______________
_____ Skin tags ______________
_____ Vesicles

CHEST
_____ Symmetrical _____ Asymmetrical
_____ Barrel chest
_____ Breast engorgement
_____ Supranummary nipples
_____ Breast discharge

RESPIRATIONS
_____ Normal _____ Labored
_____ Apnea _____ Grunting
Length ______________

BREATH SOUNDS
_____ Equal _____ Clear
_____ Rales _____ Rhonchi

CLAVICLES
_____ Straight _____ Smooth
_____ Crepitus ____ Rt ____ Lt

REFLEXES
_____ Moro _____ Suck _____ Grasp

CRY
_____ Normal _____ Weak _____ Shrill
_____ No cry, quiet, alert

HEAD
_____ Symmetrical _____ Molding
_____ Caput ______________
_____ Cephalohematoma ____ Lt ____ Rt
_____ Forcep marks ______________
_____ Fontanels normal

FACE
_____ Symmetrical _____ Asymmetrical

EYES
_____ Clear _____ Discharge
_____ Lid edema
_____ Subconjunctival hemmorhage

NECK
_____ Full ROM _____ Limited ROM

HEART
_____ Regular _____ Irregular
_____ Murmur _____ Abnormal PMI
Location: ______________

FEMORAL PULSES
_____ Equal _____ Unequal

EXTREMITIES
_____ Symmetrical _____ Asymmetrical
_____ Normal ROM _____ Limited ROM
_____ Hipclicks ____ Rt ____ Lt
_____ Polydactylism _____ Syndactylism
_____ Abnormal foot position

FEMALE GENITALIA
_____ Normal _____ Discharge
_____ Vaginal skin tag

MALE GENITALIA
_____ Normal
_____ Epispadias
_____ Hypospadias
_____ Undecended testicle
____ Rt ____ Lt
_____ Hydrocele

EARS
_____ Normal _____ Low set
_____ Sinus _____ Skin tags

NOSE
_____ Normal _____ Discharge

MOUTH
_____ Clear

MUCUS MEMBRANE
_____ Pink _____ Cyanosis _____ Thrush
_____ Cleft palate _____ Cleft lip
_____ Hard _____ Soft

CORD
_____ 3 vessels _____ 2 vessels
_____ Meconium stained

ABDOMEN
_____ Symmetrical _____ Asymmetrical
_____ Flat _____ Scaphoid
_____ Rounded _____ Distended
_____ Soft _____ Hard

BOWEL SOUNDS
_____ Present _____ Absent

RECTUM
_____ Patent

SPINE
_____ Closed vertebral column
_____ Asymmetry _____ Mass
_____ Dimple _____ Tuft of hair

Initials __________ **Date/Time** ______________

PALOS COMMUNITY HOSPITAL
PALOS HEIGHTS, ILLINOIS

P-768
91480
Rev. 6/94

NEWBORN CARE RECORD

APPENDIX C. Initial Assessment cont.

	DATE																		
	TIME																		
	TEMPERATURE																		
	ROUTE																		
	HEART RATE																		
	RESPIRATIONS																		
	WEIGHT																		
HEAD	FONTANELS Normal-flat, Sunken, Full, Bulging, Tense																		
	SHAPE Normal, Molding, Caput, Cephalohematoma, Symmetrical, Asymmetrical																		
EYES	Clear, Jaundiced, Conjunctivitis, Puffy, Hemorrhage, Discharge																		
MOUTH	Clear, Pink, PL = Pale, Cyanotic																		
SKIN	COLOR Pink, Pale, Dusky, Jaundiced, Acrocyanosis, Mottled, Cyanotic, L = Plethoric																		
	CONDITION Clear, Peeling, Dry, Erythema Toxicum, Rash, Ecchymosis, Forcep Mark, Petechiae, Milia, Stork Bites																		
	TURGOR Good, Fair, Poor																		
	BATH = ✓																		
ABDOMEN	Normal, Distended, Flat, Soft, SC = Scaphoid																		
CORD	CONDITION Dry, Clamped, Moist, Clamp, Off																		
	CARE = ✓ (each time care given)																		
EXTERNAL GENITALIA	Discharge = * (Describe in progress notes anything other than mucous in girls)																		
DIAPER AREA	CONDITION Clear, Chafed, Rash																		
	CARE __________ (type) = ✓ (each time care given)																		
	Double Diaper = ✓																		
CIRCUMCISION	CONDITION Healing, Bell Intact, Bleeding, Oozing, Redness, Swelling																		
	CARE = ✓																		
ACTIVITY	LEVEL Active, Active With Stimulation, Quiet, Irritable, Lethargic, Tremors, Sleeping																		
	CRY Normal, Weak, Shrill, No Cry, Hoarse																		
	REFLEXES PRESENT = ✓ for Moro, Grasp, Suck																		
	TONE Normal flexion, Flaccidity, Spasticity																		
	ROM Normal, Restricted																		
	I.D. Band = X1 or X2																		
	Initial Exam = ✓																		
	INITIALS																		

DATE

Time	INTAKE						OUTPUT				INITIALS
	BREAST			BOTTLE			Urine = ✓	STOOL			
	Time	Position	Behavior	Formula Type	Amount	Behavior		Amount	Color	Consis-tency	
11											
12											
1											
2											
3											
4											
5											
6											
7											
8											
9											
10											
11											
12											
1											
2											
3											
4											
5											
6											
7											
8											
9											
10											

DATE

Time	INTAKE						OUTPUT				INITIALS
	BREAST			BOTTLE			Urine = ✓	STOOL			
	Time	Position	Behavior	Formula Type	Amount	Behavior		Amount	Color	Consis-tency	
11											
12											
1											
2											
3											
4											
5											
6											
7											
8											
9											
10											
11											
12											
1											
2											
3											
4											
5											
6											
7											
8											
9											
10											

BREAST FEEDING

TIME	POSITION	BEHAVIOR
# of minutes Right side / Left side	C = Cradle F = Football L = Lying	G = Good F = Fair P = Poor R = Regurgitation L = Large M = Medium S = Small J = Projectile

STOOL

AMOUNT	COLOR	CONSISTENCY
Large Medium Small	Meconium Transitional Yellow Green Brown Clay	Soft Curdy Loose Pasty Formed

BOTTLE FEEDING

FORMULA TYPE

SW = Sterile water
GW = Glucose water
SIM = Similac ↓ iron
↑SIM = Similac ↑ iron
ENF = Enfamil ↓ iron
↑ENF = Enfamil ↑ iron
SMA = ↓ iron
↑SMA = SMA ↑ iron
NT = Nutramigen

ISO = Isomil
PRO = Prosobee
NU = Nursoy
PED = Pediolyte
Other = ______ type

AMOUNT

Indicate amount in oz.
S = Sips (◄ ½ oz.)

SPECIMEN COLLECTED

DATE/TIME	TYPE

Palos Community Hospital, Palos Heights, IL.

APPENDIX D. Algorithm Part 1

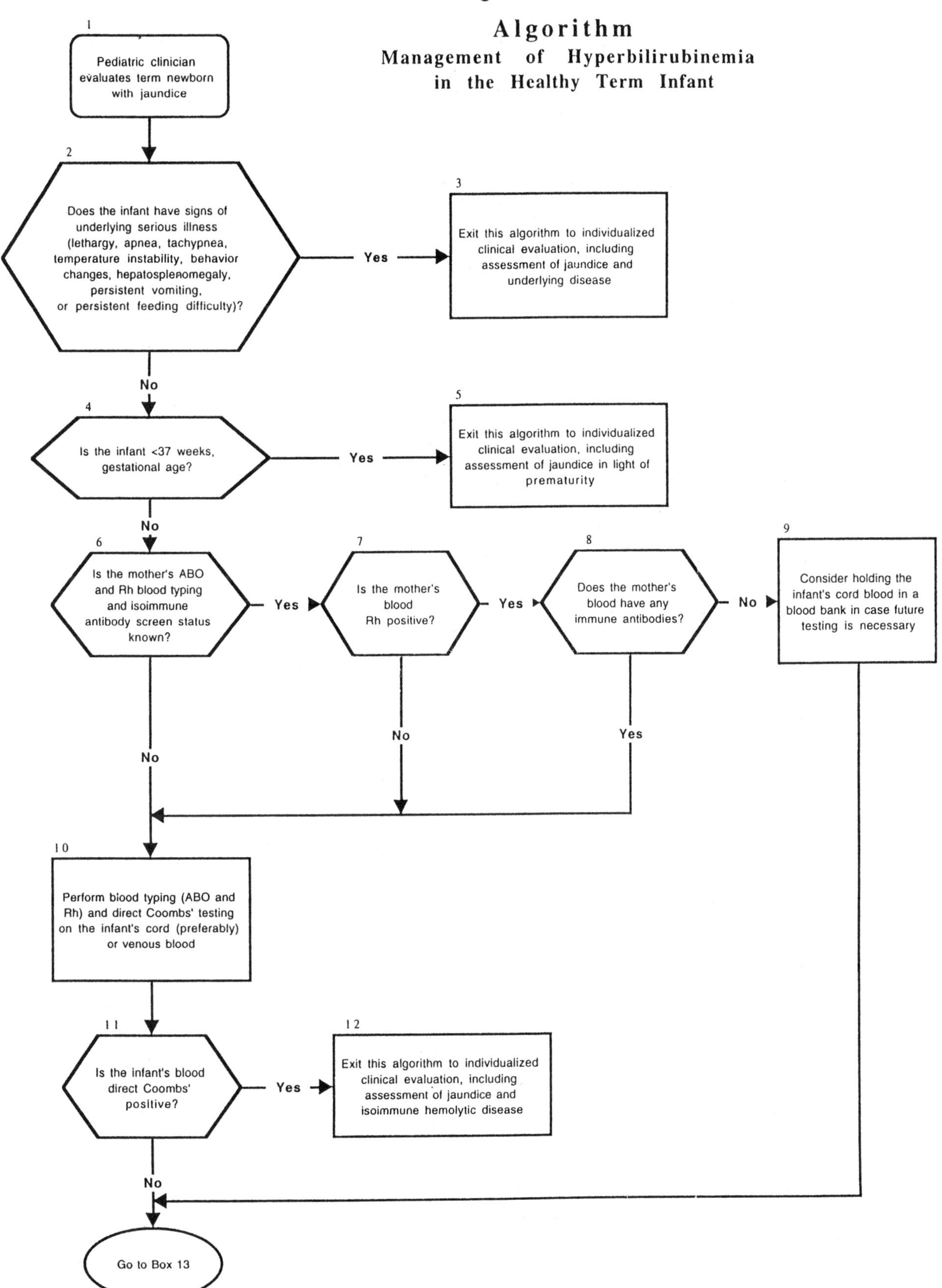

APPENDIX D. Algorithm Part 2

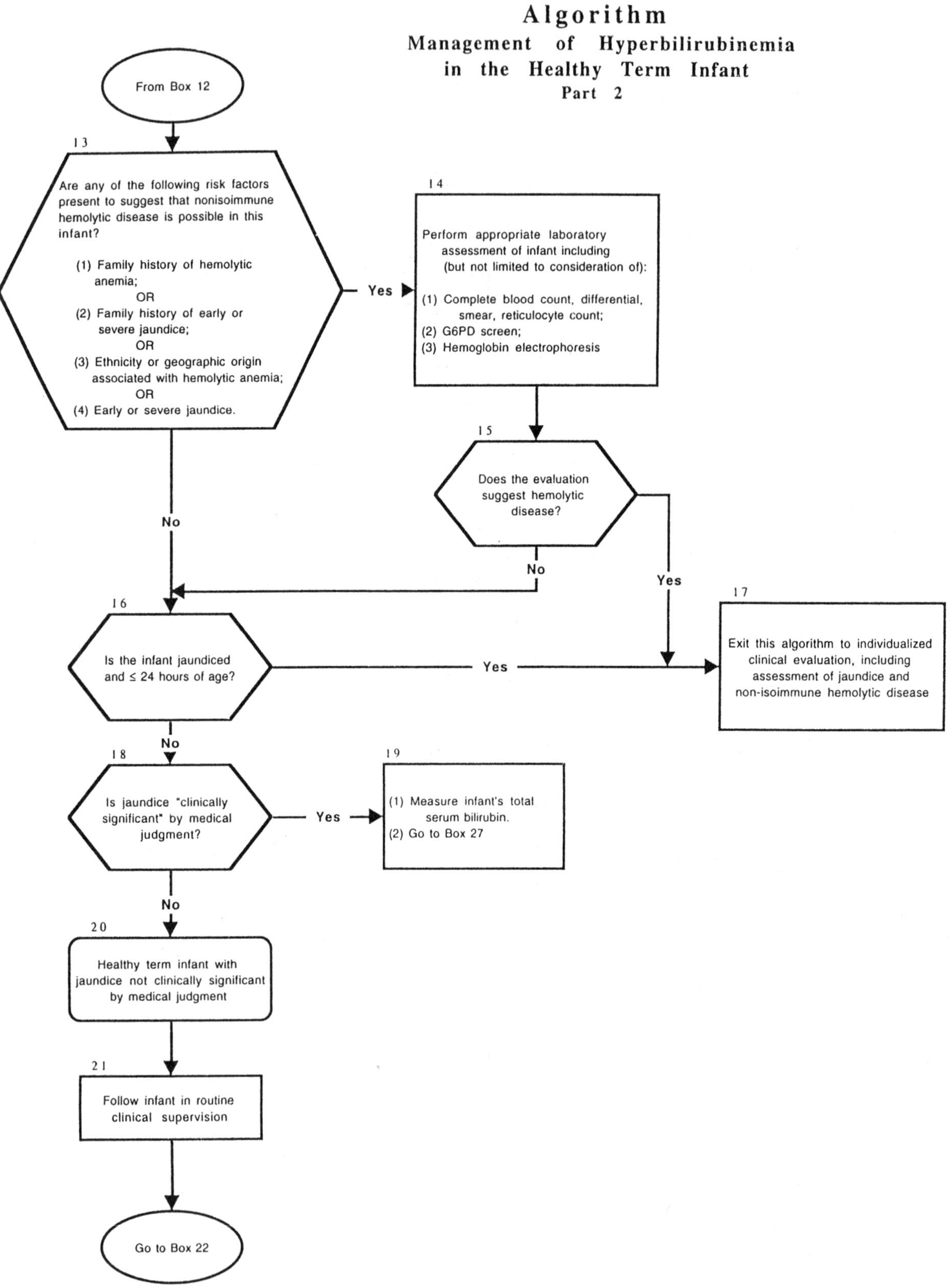

APPENDIX D. Algorithm Part 3

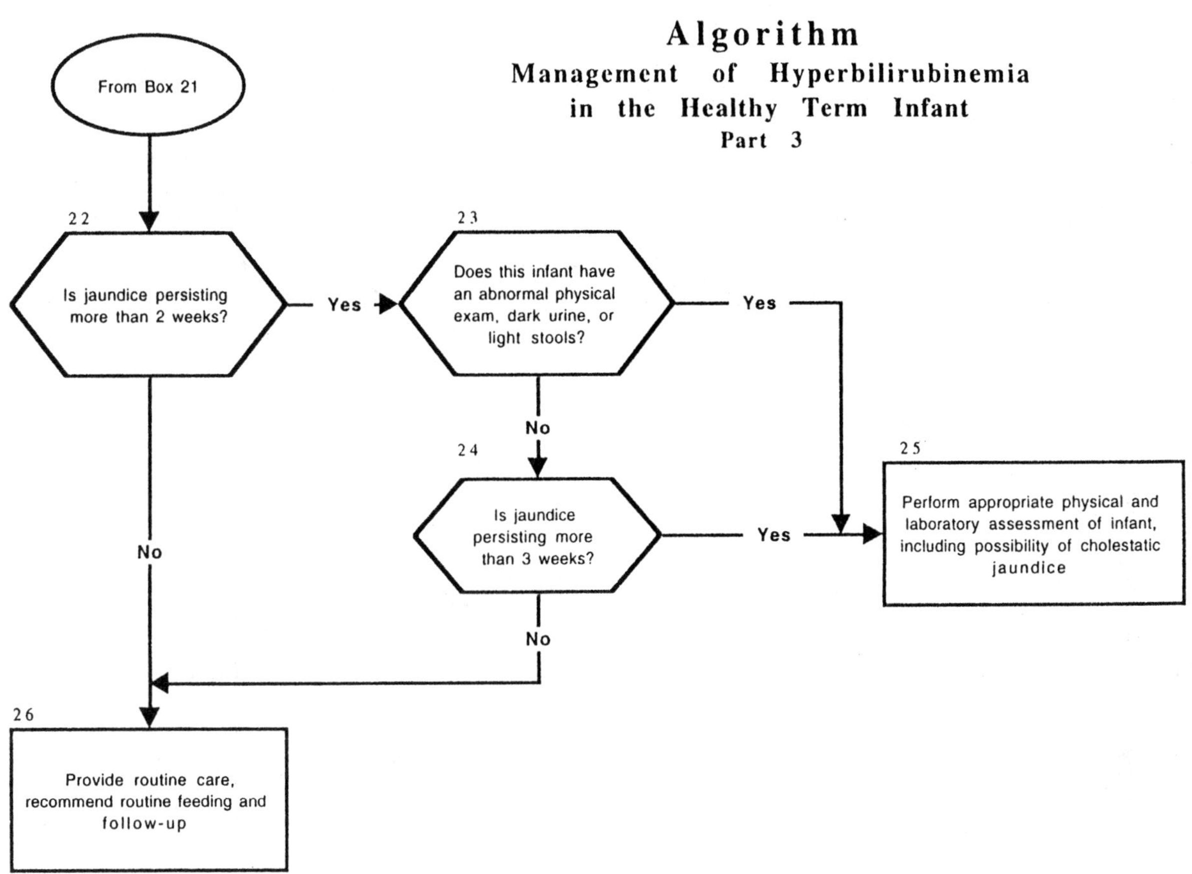

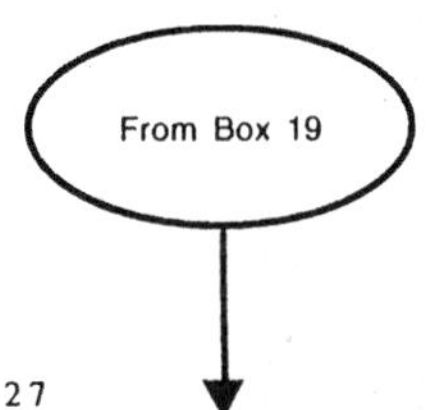

27

TABLE 2. Management of Hyperbilirubinemia in the Healthy Term Newborn*

TSB Level, mg/dL (µmol/L)

Age, hours	Consider phototherapy†	Phototherapy	Exchange Transfusion if Intensive Phototherapy Fails‡	Exchange Transfusion and Intensive Phototherapy
≤ 24	...	...	...	...
25-48	≥ 12(170)	≥ 15(260)	≥ 20(340)	≥ 25(430)
49-72	≥ 15(260)	≥ 18(310)	≥ 25(430)	≥ 30(510)
> 72	≥ 17(290)	≥ 20(340)	≥ 25(430)	≥ 30(510)

TSB LEVEL (mg/dL)[c]

* TSB indicates total serum bilirubin

† Phototherapy at these TSB levels is a clinical option, meaning that the intervention is available and may be used ***on the basis of individual clinical judgment.*** For a more detailed description of phototherapy see the Appendix.

‡ Intensive phototherapy (Appendix) should produce a decline of TSB of 1 to 2 mg/dL within 4 to 6 hours and the TSB level should continue to fall and remain below the threshold level for exchange transfusion. If this does not occur, it is considered a failure of phototherapy.

§ Term infants who are clinically jaundiced at ≤24 hours old are not considered healthy and require further evaluation (see text).

APPENDIX E. Newborn Sepsis
Diagnosis and Mangement of Symtomatic Neonates

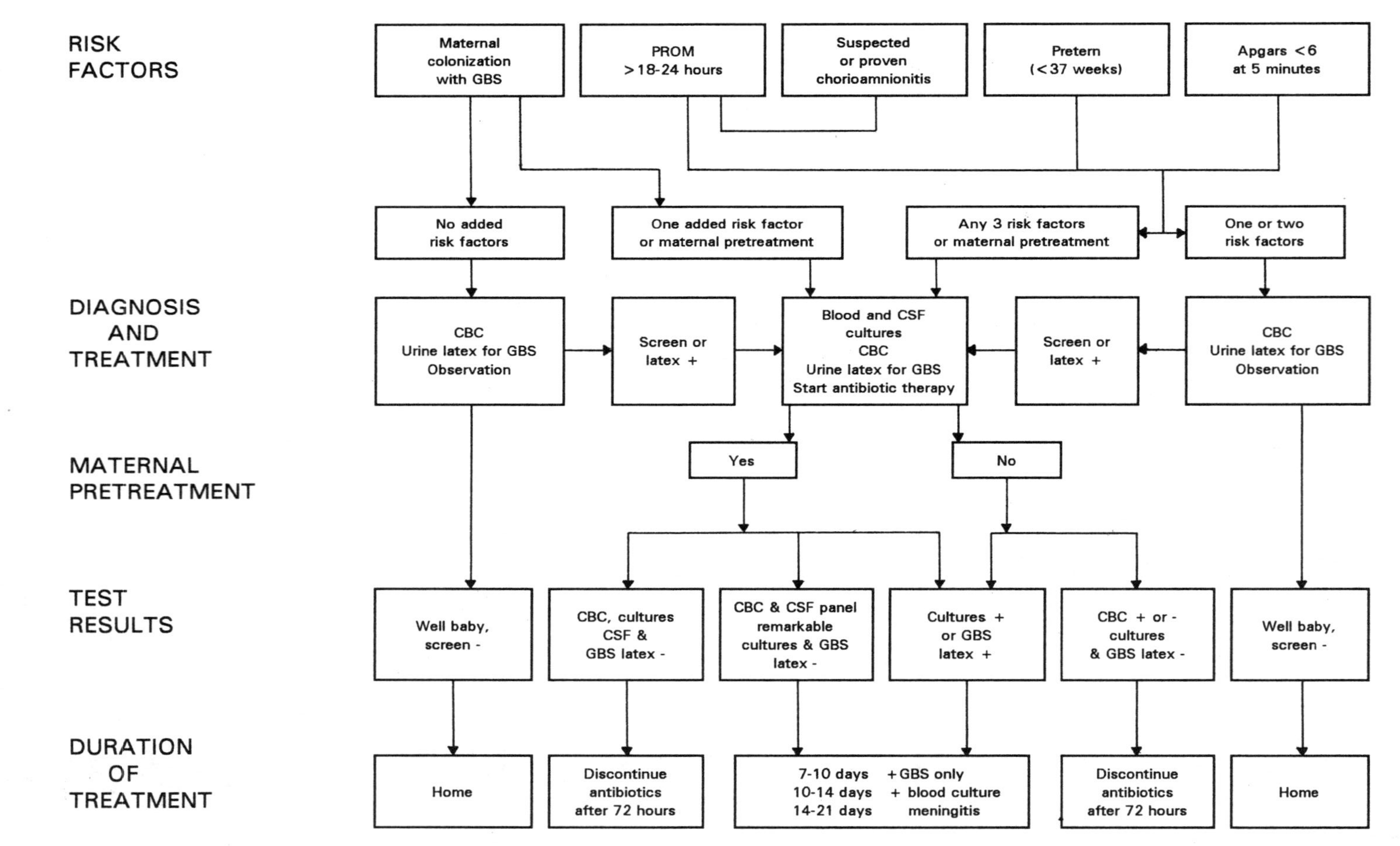

Adapted by Jeanne Fischesser, RNC, NNP
St. John's Mercy Medical Center, St. Louis, MO

APPENDIX E. Newborn Sepsis Diagnosis and Mangement of Symtomatic Neonates

Newborn Sepsis

Diagnosis and Management of Symtomatic Neonates

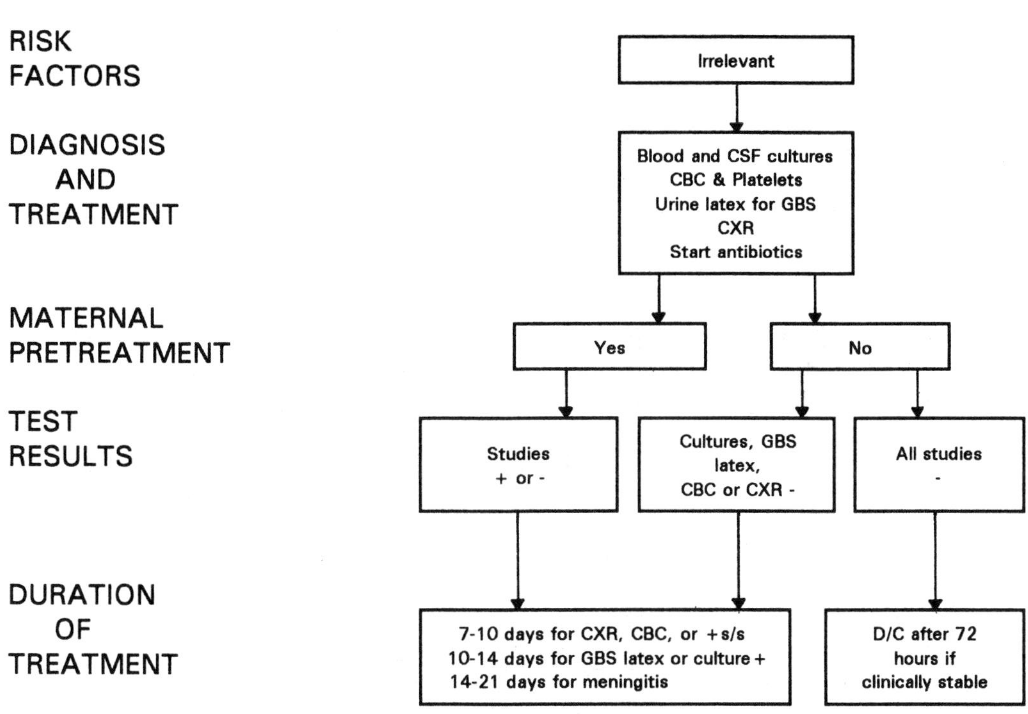

Adapted by Jeanne Fischesser, RNC, NNP
St. John's Mercy Medical Center, St. Louis, MO

APPENDIX F. Nonreassuring Fetal Heart Rate Pattern Clinical Algorithm

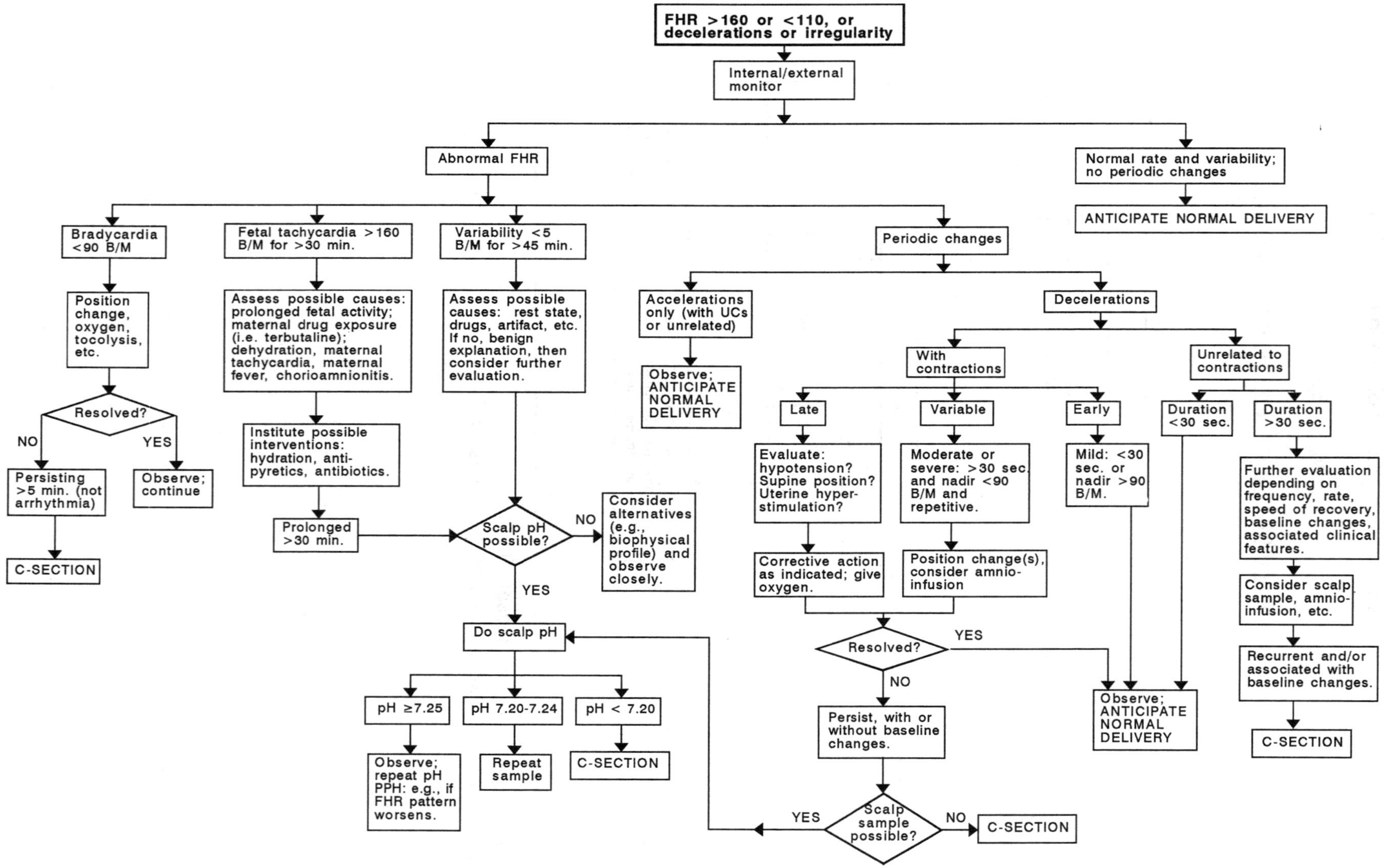

FHR >160 or <110, or decelerations or irregularity

Internal/external monitor

Abnormal FHR

Normal rate and variability; no periodic changes

ANTICIPATE NORMAL DELIVERY

Bradycardia <90 B/M

Position change, oxygen, tocolysis, etc.

Resolved?

NO

Persisting >5 min. (not arrhythmia)

C-SECTION

YES

Observe; continue

Fetal tachycardia >160 B/M for >30 min.

Assess possible causes: prolonged fetal activity; maternal drug exposure (i.e. terbutaline); dehydration, maternal tachycardia, maternal fever, chorioamnionitis.

Institute possible interventions: hydration, anti-pyretics, antibiotics.

Prolonged >30 min.

Variability <5 B/M for >45 min.

Assess possible causes: rest state, drugs, artifact, etc. If no, benign explanation, then consider further evaluation.

Scalp pH possible?

NO

Consider alternatives (e.g., biophysical profile) and observe closely.

YES

Do scalp pH

pH ≥7.25

Observe; repeat pH PPH: e.g., if FHR pattern worsens.

pH 7.20-7.24

Repeat sample

pH < 7.20

C-SECTION

Periodic changes

Accelerations only (with UCs or unrelated)

Observe; ANTICIPATE NORMAL DELIVERY

Decelerations

With contractions

Late

Evaluate: hypotension? Supine position? Uterine hyper-stimulation?

Corrective action as indicated; give oxygen.

Variable

Moderate or severe: >30 sec and nadir <90 B/M and repetitive.

Position change(s), consider amnio-infusion

Early

Mild: <30 sec. or nadir >90 B/M.

Resolved?

YES

NO

Persist, with or without baseline changes.

Scalp sample possible?

YES

NO

C-SECTION

Unrelated to contractions

Duration <30 sec.

Observe; ANTICIPATE NORMAL DELIVERY

Duration >30 sec.

Further evaluation depending on frequency, rate, speed of recovery, baseline changes, associated clinical features.

Consider scalp sample, amnio-infusion, etc.

Recurrent and/or associated with baseline changes.

C-SECTION

Meriter Health Services

LABOR DYSTOCIA CLINICAL ALGORITHM

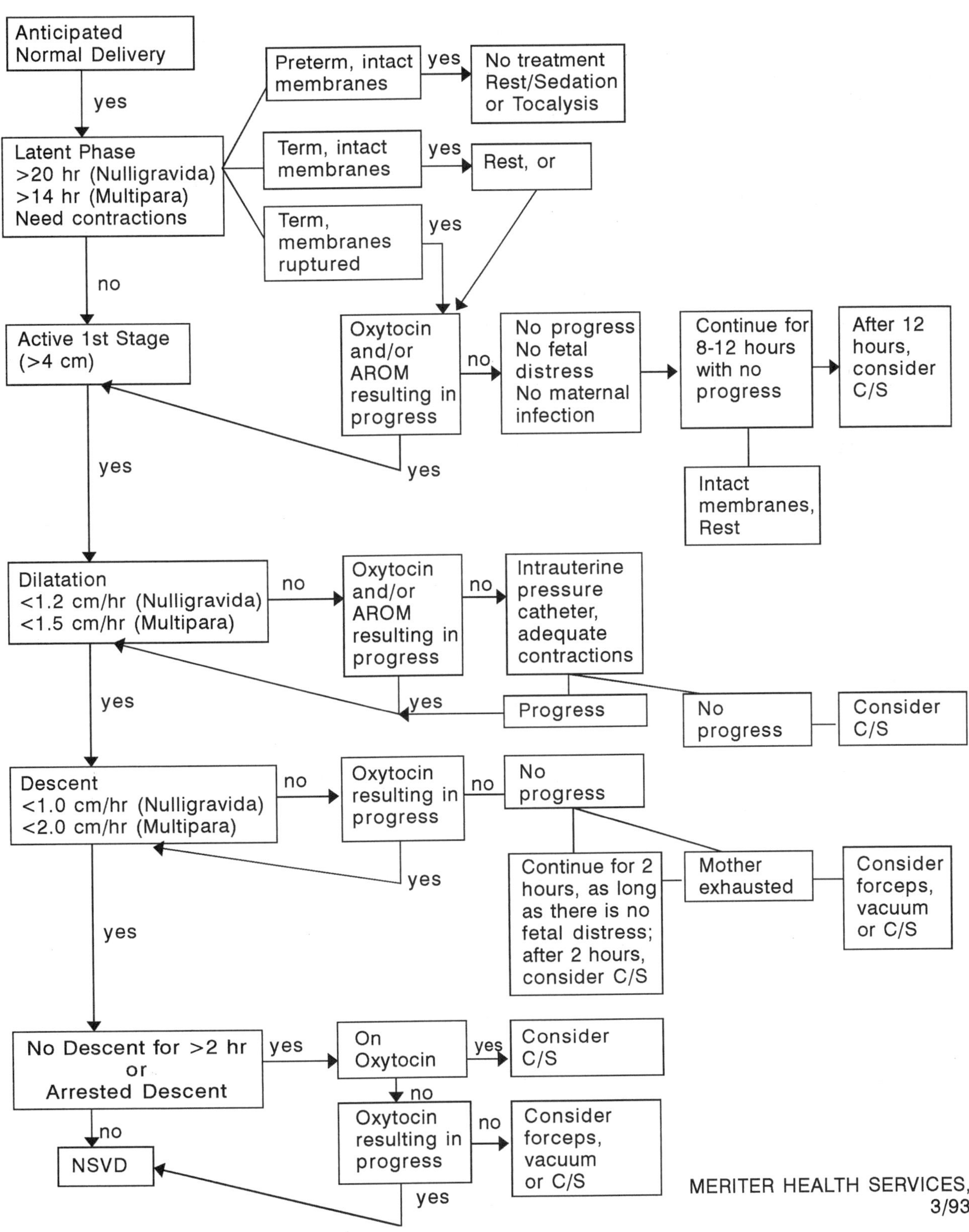

APPENDIX H. Care Path: Obstetric Prenatal

Name: ____

This care path is a guideline and is not intended to create a standard of care. This guideline may be modified based on individual patient's needs.

	Consults Date	Proced/Tests Date	Pt/Family Ed Date	Routine visits	Meds Date	Other Date	Initials
Pre-conception	MD RD, prn RN, prn MSW, prn	PAP, breast exam Hx/family hx screen for Sickle cell, TaySach prn	Wellness ed. Nutrition Self br. exam Abstain from Tob, ETOH, etc	Yearly and prn	PNV FeSO-4 Folic acid		
Week 1-8	MD RD RN MSW	Preg test, prn Initial labs HIV, prn Sickle cell, prn	Given prenatal handbook Additional info:	1/Mo. First 32 Weeks, and prn ↓	PNV, FeSO-4 ↓		
Week 8-12	MD RD, prn RN, prn MSW, prn	PAP, breast exam DNA probe Urine tox.					
Week 12-16	MD RD, prn RN, prn MSW, prn	Order MSAFP to be done in weeks 15-17					
Week 16-20	MD RD, prn RN, prn MSW, prn	Order U/S to be done in weeks 18-22	Refer to childbirth/ VBAC class				
Week 20-24	MD RD, prn RN, prn MSW, prn	Order 1 hr GTT, H&H ~ 24 weeks	Epidural class Breastfeed or bottle				
Week 24-28	MD RD, prn RN, prn MSW, prn	GBS 28 weeks, prn	Additional info.		(Rhogam 28 wks prn)		
Weeks 28-32	MD RD, prn RN, prn MSW, prn		S/Sx PTL				
Weeks 32-36	MD RD, prn RN, prn MSW, prn	Vag exam at 36 wks if ctx	S/Sx labor	Bi-monthly		NST, prn Fetal/pelvic index, prn	
Weeks 36-40	MD RD, prn RN, prn MSW, prn			Weekly til del.			
Week 40-del.	MD RD, prn RN, prn MSW, prn						
Postpartum	MD RD, prn RN, prn MSW, prn	PAP, breast exam	Care of self PP (care of infant) Family planning Wellness	(2 wks for C/S) 6 weeks	(Rhogam prn) (Rubella prn)		

Patient Problems Identified:

____

____

____

____

PATIENT IDENTIFICATION

CARE PATH: Obstetric Prenatal
Care Path Code: 080

ST. JOHN'S MERCY MEDICAL CENTER, ST. LOUIS, MO

Rev. 9/95

APPENDIX H. Care Path: Antepartum Complications

Name: ______________________________

This care path is a guideline and is not intended to create a standard of care. This guideline may be modified based on individual patient's needs.

Prob. #		Day 1/Day of Admission Date:	LOS Day____ Date:	LOS Day____ Date:	LOS Day____ Date:
	ADL	☐ Bedrest ☐ BR/BRP ☐ Wheelchair ☐ Bedside commode ☐ Shower ☐ Up ad lib	☐ Bedrest ☐ BR/BRP ☐ Wheelchair ☐ Bedside commode ☐ Shower ☐ Up ad lib	☐ Bedrest ☐ BR/BRP ☐ Wheelchair ☐ Bedside commode ☐ Shower ☐ Up ad lib	☐ Bedrest ☐ BR/BRP ☐ Wheelchair ☐ Bedside commode ☐ Shower ☐ Up ad lib
	Assessment/ Monitor	Maternal assessments: ☐ VS q 4 hours ☐ VS q 4 hours while awake ☐ VS q shift ☐ VS BID Vaginal bleeding Uterine activity Membrane status Vaginal discharge Fetal assessments: ☐ FHR q 4 hours ☐ FHR q shift ☐ Fetal kick counts (DFMR)	Maternal assessments: ☐ VS q 4 hours ☐ VS q 4 hours while awake ☐ VS q shift ☐ VS BID Vaginal bleeding Uterine activity Membrane status Vaginal discharge Fetal assessments: ☐ FHR q 4 hours ☐ FHR q shift ☐ Fetal kick counts (DFMR)	Maternal assessments: ☐ VS q 4 hours ☐ VS q 4 hours while awake ☐ VS q shift ☐ VS BID Vaginal bleeding Uterine activity Membrane status Vaginal discharge Fetal assessments: ☐ FHR q 4 hours ☐ FHR q shift ☐ Fetal kick counts (DFMR)	Maternal assessments: ☐ VS q 4 hours ☐ VS q 4 hours while awake ☐ VS q shift ☐ VS BID Vaginal bleeding Uterine activity Membrane status Vaginal discharge Fetal assessments: ☐ FHR q 4 hours ☐ FHR q shift ☐ Fetal kick counts (DFMR)
	Consults	☐ Perinatal CNS ☐ House officers ☐ NICU staff ☐ Social Services ☐ Pastoral Services	☐ Perinatal CNS ☐ House officers ☐ NICU staff ☐ Social Services ☐ Pastoral Services	☐ Perinatal CNS ☐ House officers ☐ NICU staff ☐ Social Services ☐ Pastoral Services	☐ Perinatal CNS ☐ House officers ☐ NICU staff ☐ Social Services ☐ Pastoral Services
	Procedures/ Tests	Laboratory tests: ☐ CBC ☐ CRP ☐ 24 hour urine ☐ UA for proteinuria Perinatal Center ☐ NST ☐ Modified BPP	Laboratory tests: ☐ CBC ☐ CRP ☐ 24 hour urine ☐ UA for proteinuria Perinatal Center ☐ NST ☐ Modified BPP	Laboratory tests: ☐ CBC ☐ CRP ☐ 24 hour urine ☐ UA for proteinuria Perinatal Center ☐ NST ☐ Modified BPP	Laboratory tests: ☐ CBC ☐ CRP ☐ 24 hours urine ☐ UA for proteinuria Perinatal Center ☐ NST ☐ Modified BPP
	Treatments				
	Meds/IVs	☐ Prenatal vitamins ☐ Refer to Medication Administration Record	☐ Prenatal vitamins ☐ Refer to Medication Administration Record	☐ Prenatal vitamins ☐ Refer to Medication Administration Record	☐ Prenatal vitamins ☐ Refer to Medication Administration Record
	Nutrition	Regular Diet	Regular Diet	Regular Diet	Regular Diet
	Pt./Family Education	Purpose and course of tx S&S PTL	Purpose and course of tx S&S PTL	Purpose and course of tx S&S PTL	Purpose and course of tx S&S PTL
	Discharge Planning	Appropriate to clinical and social situation Ongoing reinforcement	Appropriate to clinical and social situation Ongoing reinforcement	Appropriate to clinical and social situation Ongoing reinforcement	Appropriate to clinical and social situation Ongoing reinforcement
	Spiritual/ Psycho/Social/ Emotional Needs	Assess support system Assess family separation anxiety Assist in dealing with high-risk pregnancy Assist in developing coping skills Make available information on Pastoral Services Evaluate spiritual needs and respond as appropriate PRN Provide significant sacraments and rituals as requested	Assess support system Assess family separation anxiety Assist in dealing with high-risk pregnancy Assist in developing coping skills Evaluate spiritual needs and respond as appropriate PRN	Assess support system Assess family separation anxiety Assist in dealing with high-risk pregnancy Assist in developing coping skills Evaluate spiritual needs and respond as appropriate PRN	Assess support system Assess family separation anxiety Assist in dealing with high-risk pregnancy Assist in developing coping skills Evaluate spiritual needs and respond as appropriate PRN
Multidisciplinary Team Signatures					

Patient Problems

1. Potential preterm birth
2. Vaginal bleeding
3. Stress related to high-risk pregnancy
4. Stress related to family separation

PATIENT IDENTIFICATION

CARE PATH: Antepartum Complications
Code 089

Rev. 7/95

St. John's Mercy Medical Center, St. Louis, MO.

APPENDIX H. Care Path: Vaginal Birth

Name: ______________________________

This care path is a guideline and is not intended to create a standard of care. This guideline may be modified based on individual patient's needs.

Prob. #		Intrapartum	0-4 Hours Date:	4-8 Hours Date:	8-12 Hours Date:	12-24 Hours Date:
3	ADL	Bedrest or ambulation as tolerated	Bedrest or ambulation as tolerated	Up ad lib (assist PRN)	Up ad lib (assist PRN)	**Up ad lib (assist PRN)**
3	Assessment Monitor	Perinatal Unit admission assessment Ongoing assessments PRN	Immediate postpartum assessments VS Q 15″ until stable, then Q 4 h VS are WNL	VS Q 4h, VS are WNL Postpartum checks Q 4h - are WNL Assess mother/infant attachment	**VS Q 4h, VS are WNL** **Postpartum checks Q 4h - are WNL** **Assess mother/infant attachment**	**VS Q 4h, VS are WNL** **Postpartum checks Q 4h - are WNL** **Assess mother/infant attachment**
1,2,4	Consults	Perinatal CNS Anesthesia PRN House officer PRN Resolve PRN NICU staff PRN	——► ——► ——► ——► ——►	Lactation consultant PRN Social Service PRN/ WIC PRN	Lactation consultant PRN Social Service PRN/ WIC	Lactation consultant PRN Social Service PRN/ WIC
3	Procedures/ Tests	Hct PRN	Assess Rubella Titer status Assess need for Rhogam		Rhogam screen PRN	
1	Treatments	External EFM Internal EFM PRN	Ice to perineum Cath PRN	Ice to perineum Cath PRN Supportive bra PRN	Ice to perineum Cath PRN Supportive bra PRN Sitz bath PRN	Ice to perineum Supportive bra PRN Sitz bath PRN
1,2	Meds/IVs	Pain medication IV or IM PRN Alternative D_5LR/LR when in active labor PRN Epidural/ Pudendal/ Pericervical Pitocin augmentation PRN	Pain medication PRN Tucks PRN Anusol PRN Pitocin 20u IV then D/C	Pain medication PRN Tucks PRN Anusol PRN Stool softener PRN	Pain medication PRN Tucks PRN Anusol PRN Stool softener PRN	Pain medication PRN Tucks PRN Anusol PRN Stool softener PRN Rhogam PRN Rubella vaccine PRN
1	Nutrition	Ice chips PRN	Tolerate PO fluids Regular diet	Adequate fluids Regular diet	Adequate fluids Regular diet	Adequate fluids Regular diet
2	Pt./Family Education	EFM Labor support coaching - encourage support person in role	Self peri care/safety issues Perineum care - comfort measures Mother/baby booklet Initiate bottle or breastfeeding Initiate infant care	Bath/cord care and baby care demo Self care reinforcement and demos Discuss normal involution, lochia, fatigue, activity levels, and nutritional needs	——► ——► ——►	Breast pump if indicated
2	Discharge Planning	Mother/baby teaching form	Determine LOS Begin discharge instructions	Continue discharge instructions	——►	Assess parent/infant interaction Assess need for home health follow-up Discharge instructions reviewed with mother and S.O.
2,4	Spiritual/ Psycho/ Social/ Emotional Needs	Support patient/S.O. Facilitate a positive childbirth experience	Assess maternal role strengths	Assist mother's transition through tasks of taking on maternal role	——►	——►
	Multi-disciplinary Team Signatures	____ ____ ____ ____	____ ____ ____ ____	____ ____ ____ ____	____ ____ ____ ____	____ ____ ____ ____

Patient Problems

1. Discomfort/pain
2. Learning needs
3. Potential for instability - postpartum
4. Potential alteration in coping related to childbirth

PATIENT IDENTIFICATION

CARE PATH: VAGINAL BIRTH — DRG# 373

Rev. 12/94

St. John's Mercy Medical Center, St. Louis, MO.

APPENDIX H. Care Path: Cesarean Birth

Name: ____________________

This care path is a guideline and is not intended to create a standard of care. This guideline may be modified based on individual patient's needs.

Prob. #		Intrapartum	0-4 Hours Date:	4-8 Hours Date:	8-12 Hours Date:	12-24 Hours Date:
3	ADL	Bedrest or ambulation as tolerated	Bedrest PRN	Dangle x 1 Ambulate with assist PRN Chair/rocker PRN	→ →	→
1,3	Assessment Monitor	Perinatal Unit admission assessment Ongoing assessments PRN	Immediate postpartum assessments VS q 15 min x4, q 30 min, then q 4 hr VS are WNL	Immediate postpartum assessments - are WNL Assess mother/infant interaction VS q 4 hr while awake VS are WNL	Listen for bowel sounds → → **VS are WNL**	→ → → **VS are WNL**
1,2,4	Consults	Perinatal CNS Anesthesia PRN House officer PRN Resolve PRN NICU staff PRN	→ → → → →	→ → → → →	Lactation consultant PRN Social Service PRN WIC PRN	Lactation consultant Social Service, WIC PRN
3	Procedures/ Tests	CBC Type and screen	Assess Rubella Titer status Assess need for Rhogam	→ →	Rhogam screen PRN	
1,3	Treatments	EFM IV Foley catheter Abdominal shave prep	Ice to incision Foley cath TCDB q 2 hr Peri care q 4 hr I&O q shift x 48 hr	→ → → → →	→ → → → → Dressing removed PRN	→ Foley cath PRN → Peri care q 4 hr PRN → →
1,3,5	Meds/IVs	Epidural IVF - LR/D5LR	PCA/Epidural IV fluids Pitocin to IV Antiemetic PRN Antibiotics PRN Benadryl PRN	→ → → → → →	→ → → → → →	→ IV fluids PRN Pitocin PRN → → →
1,2	Nutrition	NPO (as ordered for scheduled sections)	Ice chips PRN (sips and chips)	→	Clear liquids	Advance as tolerated
2,4	Pt./Family Education	EFM Explain procedures	Mother/Baby booklet Safety issues Pharmacologic and non-pharmacologic pain control and comfort measures Initiate breast feeding/ bottle feeding	Initiate infant care Normal involution, lochia, perineal care	Initiate self care	Reinforce self care with demos Baby/cord care demo Breast pump if indicated
2,4	Discharge Planning	Mother/baby teaching form	Determine LOS	Begin discharge instructions	→	→ Assess parent interaction
2,4	Spiritual/ Psycho/ Social/ Emotional Needs	Support patient/significant other Facilitate positive childbirth experience	Assess maternal role strengths	Assist mother's transition through tasks of taking on maternal role	→	→
	Multi-disciplinary Team Signatures					

Patient Problems

1. Discomfort/pain
2. Learning needs
3. Potential for instability - postpartum involution
4. Potential alteration in coping related to childbirth
5. Potential for infection

PATIENT IDENTIFICATION

CARE PATH: CESAREAN BIRTH — DRG# 371

Rev. 12/94

St. John's Mercy Medical Center, St. Louis, MO.

APPENDIX H. Care Path:Cesarean Birth Cont.

Care Path: Cesarean Birth - DRG # 371

Prob. #		24-48 Hours Date:	48-72 Hours Date:
3	ADL	**Encourage ambulation**	Up ad lib
1,3	Assessment Monitor	**Bowel sounds present** **Assessments BID are WNL** Assess mother/infant interaction VS q 4 hr while awake **VS are WNL**	VS QID
1,2,4	Consults	Lactation consultant Social Service, WIC PRN	Lactation consultant Social Service, WIC PRN
3	Procedures/ Tests		H&H
1,3	Treatments	Cath PRN I&O q shift x 48 hr Dressing removed PRN Supportive bra PRN	Staple removal PRN
1,3,5	Meds/IVs	PO analgesics PRN Pitocin PRN Antiemetic PRN Antibiotics PRN Benadryl PRN IV fluids PRN Rhogam PRN Rubella vaccine PRN Mylicon PRN Stool softeners PRN	Mylicon PRN Stool softeners PRN PO analgesics PRN Suppositories/laxative PRN
1,2	Nutrition	Advance as tolerated	Regular diet
2,4	Pt./Family Education	Breast pump if indicated	Self care and infant care return demos
2,4	Discharge Planning	Discharge instructions Assess parent interaction Assess need for home health follow-up	Reinforce discharge instructions Assess parent interaction Assess need for home health follow-up
2,4	Spiritual/ Psycho/ Social/ Emotional Needs	Assist mother's transition through tasks of taking on maternal role Encourage family and other support systems	Assist mother's transition through tasks of taking on maternal role
	Multi-disciplinary Team Signatures	____________ ____________ ____________ ____________	____________ ____________ ____________ ____________

APPENDIX H. Care Path: Normal Newborn

Name: ______________________________

This care path is a guideline and is not intended to create a standard of care. This guideline may be modified based on individual patient's needs.

Prob. #		Birth	0-4 Hours Date:	4-8 Hours Date:	8-12 Hours Date:	12-24 Hours Date:
1	ADL	Bedrest and position for holding	————►	————►	————►	————►
1,3	Assessment Monitor	Apgars Newborn assessment	Newborn assessment on admission and Q 8h **VS, Respiratory status, skin color, and temp WNL** Observation: check for maternal hepatitis surface antigen	Temp PRN and Q shift	————► Newborn assessment Q 8h VS WNL	————► ————►
1,2,3	Consults	**NICU Team in attendance PRN**	**Orthopedics PRN** **Genetics PRN** **Infectious disease PRN**	**Orthopedics PRN** **Genetics PRN** **Infectious disease PRN**	**Orthopedics PRN** **Genetics PRN** **Infectious disease PRN**	**Orthopedics PRN** **Genetics PRN** **Infectious disease PRN**
1,2,3	Procedures/ Tests	Cord blood PRN	Chemstrips PRN BP PRN **O_2 sat PRN · O_2 sat WNL** Attach security sensor Assess hepatitis titer	Chemstrips PRN		Metabolic screen
1-4	Treatments	Gastric lavage PRN	————► Initial Newborn bath Cord care	Cord care Cath PRN Ultrasounds PRN Circumcision PRN and circ care	Cord care Cath PRN Ultrasounds PRN Circumcision PRN and circ care	Cord care Ultrasounds PRN Circumcision PRN and circ care Discharge weight
3	Meds/IVs	Ilotycin ointment	Vitamin K IM		Hepatitis vaccine PRN	
2	Nutrition	Initiate breastfeeding	Continue breastfeeding Initiate formula feeding	————► Continue formula feeding	————► ————►	————► ————►
1-4	Pt./Family Education	See Maternal Care Path				
1-4	Discharge Planning	See Maternal Care Path				Assess need for home health follow-up
1-4	Spiritual/ Psycho/ Social/ Emotional Needs	See Maternal Care Path				
	Multi-disciplinary Team Signatures	________ ________ ________ ________	________ ________ ________ ________	________ ________ ________ ________	________ ________ ________ ________	________ ________ ________ ________

Patient Problems

1. Alteration in body temperature
2. Alteration in nutritional requirements
3. Potential for infection
4. Alteration in skin integrity

PATIENT IDENTIFICATION

CARE PATH: NORMAL NEWBORN — DRG# 391

Rev. 12/94

St. John's Mercy Medical Center, St. Louis, MO.

APPENDIX H. Care Path: Normal Newborn cont.

Care Path: Normal Newborn — DRG # 391

Prob.		Day 2 Date:				
1	ADL	Bedrest and position for holding				
1,3	Assessment Monitor	Temp PRN and Q shift VS WNL				
1,2,3	Consults	**Orthopedics PRN** **Genetics PRN** **Infectious disease PRN**				
1,2,3	Procedures/ Tests					
1-4	Treatments	Cord care Ultrasounds PRN Circumcision PRN and circ care Discharge weight				
3	Meds/IVs					
2	Nutrition	Continue breastfeeding Continue formula feeding				
1-4	Pt./Family Education					
1-4	Discharge Planning	Assess need for home health follow-up				
1-4	Spiritual/ Psycho/ Social/ Emotional Needs					
	Multi-disciplinary Team Signatures	____________ ____________ ____________ ____________				

St. John's Mercy Medical Center

CARE PATH EXCEPTION LOG

PATH______________

This is a confidential and privileged Quality Record for Peer Review only.

Patient/Family		Community	
CODE	**DESCRIPTION**	**CODE**	**DESCRIPTION**
1	Patient too ill/pain/unable	201	Placement not available
2	Patient/Family refused/non-compliant	202	Home care not available
3	Patient cognition	**299**	***Community Other****
99	***Patient/Family Other****		
Health Caregiver HCTM Required		**System** Dept Code Required	
CODE	**DESCRIPTION** After HCTM Code, identify discipline.	**DEPT CODE**	**DESCRIPTION** After Dept Code, identify Dept.
301	**HCTM** Action/Decision	402	Equip./Supply not available
302	**HCTM** Inaction	403	Dept. overbooked
305	**HCTM** Overbooked	404	Department closed
399	***HCTM Other****	**409**	***System Other****

** All "Other" codes must have an explanation*

Date	Hosp Day	Exception / Event	Code	Action Taken

APPENDIX I. Vaginal Delivery Clinical Path

PATIENT PROBLEM LIST		PHYSICIAN CONSULTS
A. Potential lack of knowledge re: Labor, Self Care, newborn care	Delivery Date__________ Delivery Time________	
B. Potential alteration fetal tissue perfusion re: Labor	Mother Blood Type_______ Baby Blood Type_______	
C. Pain re; Labor, P.P. uterine involution, Episiotomy	RPR ____ Rubella ____ Hep. Sag. ____	
	Breast______ Bottle______ Sex________	
	Pediatrician Notified Y N	

LEGEND

Breast WNL = Soft to Firm	Reflexes WNL = 2(+) <	Episiotomy/Perineum WNL = Intact & (-) Edema
Nipples WNL = Evert & Intact	Lochia WNL = Scant to moderate flow	
Edema WNL = Absent	Fundus Location WNL = U/U to U/2	

	Path Suspended/Resumed Intrapartum Time	Path Suspended/Resumed 2 Hours Post Delivery	Path Suspended/Resumed 8 Hours Post Delivery
NURSING ASSESS-MENT	Problem list prioritized Pain level: Coping Mental Status WNL Skin intact, pink, warm & dry Lungs clear Bowel sounds (+) Edema WNL Reflexes WNL ***Assess FHT & contractions:*** ***Latent Phase Q60min,*** ***Active Phase Q30min,*** ***2nd stage Q15min*** *Maternal VS Q1h or Q15-30min with epidural* *Temp Q4h until ROM, then Q1-2hrs* Assumed Care Initials Assumed Care Time	Problem list re-prioritized Pain level: Coping Breast/Nipples WNL Fundus firm, Location WNL Q4h Lochia WNL Q4h Episiotomy/Perineum WNL Hemmorhoids/Varicosities (-) Voids QS Homans negative Skin intact, pink, warm & dry Lungs clear Bowel sounds (+) Edema WNL Reflexes WNL ***V.S.. Q4h*** ***Notify Dr. temp > 101*** Assumed Care Initials Assumed Care Time	Pain level: Coping Breast/Nipples WNL Fundus firm, Location WNL Q4h Lochia WNL Q4h Episiotomy/Perineum WNL Hemmorhoids/Varicosities (-) Voids QS Homans negative Skin intact, pink, warm & dry Lungs clear Bowel sounds (+) Edema WNL Reflexes WNL ***V.S.. Q4h*** ***Notify Dr. temp > 101*** Assumed Care Initials Assumed Care Time
SAFETY	Oriented to room Call light in reach Bed in low position Side rail position________ Nursing rounds Q2h Consents on chart Advanced Directives/pamphlet received & no ?s Bill of Rights received Fall Risk Score ________ If >= to 50 fall prevention path implemented Isolation (other than BSI)	Oriented to room Call light in reach,bed low Side rail position________ Nursing rounds Q2h Infant Safety Sheet Signed Fall Risk Score ________ If >= to 50 fall prevention path implemented Isolation (other than BSI) ________ Pt./Visitors instructed on precautions	Call light in reach Bed in low position Side rail position________ Nursing rounds Q2h Isolation (other than BSI) ________ Pt./Visitors instructed on precautions
ACTIVITY	***Encourage ambulation until active labor or epidural*** Position change Q1h	***Bathroom with assistance***	***Up ad lib*** ***Bathroom with assistance PRN***
DIET	***NPO active labor with ice chips*** ***Obtain order for clears early labor***	***Regular***	***Regular***
TEST	***CBC*** ***RPR if not done in last trimester*** ***Urine dip on admission, contact Dr. if abnormal*** ***Protein/Ketones dip PRN*** ***T&S if VBAC or >Para 5***		
	Date:	Date:	Date:

Key: Users Initials = Met U = Unmet ☐ **= N/A**

***Any unmet must have a reason documented in progress note**

*** Circled initial = Change in assessment requiring documentation**

*** A Physician's order is required for anything bolded & italicized**

ADDRESSOGRAPH

VAGINAL DELIVERY CLINICAL PATH
UNIVERSITY COMMUNITY HOSPITAL TAMPA, FLORIDA
Rev. 10/09/95 Page 1 of 4

APPENDIX I. Vaginal Delivery Clinical Path cont.

	Intrapartum	2 Hours Post Delivery	8 Hours Post Delivery
TREAT-MENT	***IV access 18G@125/hr assess Q2h*** ***Initiate IV fluids when active labor & NPO or for Epidural*** ***1000cc LR bolus prior to Epidural*** FSE placement PRN per protocol V.E. on admission, prior to pain med, q2H after 4cm (Epidural or IV analgesia) & PRN I&O (if has IV) ***Straight cath PRN X2*** ***Obtain order for foley prn***	***D/C IV if stable*** Ice packs to perineum ***Tucks PRN*** ***Sitz bath PRN*** Assess 1st 2 voids ***Cath PRN unable to void*** Assist with peri care Epidural cath removed and intact ***Hemorrhage protocol PRN***	***Sitz bath PRN*** Ice packs to perineum ***Tucks PRN*** Massage Therapist (10-15 min chair massage to relieve stress in muscles. Back, glutes, arms hands, & neck are massaged)
RESPIR-ATORY THERAPY	See MAR for Respiratory medication tratments ordered & R.T. log for treatments performed.	See MAR for Respiratory medication tratments ordered & R.T. log for treatments performed.	See MAR for Respiratory medication tratments ordered & R.T. log for treatments performed.
MEDI-CATIONS	***May use 1% Lidocaine SQ for IV start per protocol PRN*** Obtain order for pain med PRN ***Pitocin induction/augmentation protocol: 10U/1000cc D5LR IVPB, initial .5-1.0mu/min then up by 1-2mu Q30-60 min until adequate pattern***	***Initiate SAM meds*** ***PRN narcotics as*** prescribed	SAM packet @ bedside Pt achieved pain relief with SAM Pt achieved pain relief PRN with narcotics
CLINICAL CONSULT	Perinatal CNS for birth plans	Consult Lactation Specialist if breast feeding PRN	
PSYCHO-SOCIAL	Encourage support person involvement	Support system Bonding WNL	Support system Bonding WNL
SOCIAL WORK SERVICES	Consult PRN	Consult PRN	Consult PRN
TEACHING	Family support/coaching Phases/stages of labor Position changes Childbirth prep NPO status Comfort measures Ext/Int EFM Oxytocin (PRN) Epidural (PRN) Bladder emptying Q1h Breast feeding Comprehension level WNL	Discharge pamphlets at bedside Newborn Care: Infant feeding Self Care: Peri Care Fundal Massage Breast Feeding Bonding Normal newborn behavior Comprehension level WNL	Discharge pamphlets reviewed Newborn Care: Infant Feeding Diaper change Cord care Temp. taking Circumcision Care Self Care: Postpartum Care Breast Feeding Give Dietary Food/Drug Interaction Sheet Comprehension level WNL
DIS-CHARGE PLANNING	Assess home support Transfer to MBU per criteria M/B couplet via W/C or Stretcher Time transfered______Report to ____________RN Infant only transferred by ________ @ ____	Support systems at home intact	Support systems at home intact
	Date:	Date:	Date:

Key: Users Initials = Met U = Unmet ☐ **= N/A**

***Any unmet must have a reason documented in progress note**

*** Circled initial = Change in assessment requiring documentation**

*** A Physician's order is required for anything bolded & italicized**

ADDRESSOGRAPH

VAGINAL DELIVERY CLINICAL PATH
UNIVERSITY COMMUNITY HOSPITAL TAMPA, FLORIDA
Rev. 10/09/95 Page 2 of 4

APPENDIX I. Vaginal Delivery Clinical Path cont.

	Path Suspended/Resumed 12-24 hours Postpartum			Path Suspended/Resumed 24-36 hours Postpartum			Path Suspended/Resumed 36-48 hours Postpartum		
NURSING ASSESS-MENT				Problem list reprioritized______					
	Breast/Nipples WNL			Breast/Nipples WNL			Breast/Nipples WNL		
	Fundus Firm Location WNL Q4h			Fundus Firm Location WNL Q4h			Fundus Firm Location WNL Q4h		
	Lochia WNL Q4h			Lochia WNL Q4h			Lochia WNL Q4h		
	Episiotomy/Perineum WNL			Episiotomy/Perineum WNL			Episiotomy/Perineum WNL		
	Hemmorhoids/Varicosities (-)			Hemmorhoids/Varicosities (-)			Hemmorhoids/Varicosities (-)		
	Voiding QS			Voiding QS			Voiding QS		
	Homans negative			Homans negative			Homans negative		
	Skin intact. pink, warm & dry			Skin intact. pink, warm & dry			Skin intact. pink, warm & dry		
	Lungs clear			Lungs clear			Lungs clear		
	Bowel sounds (+)			Bowel sounds (+)			Bowel sounds (+)		
	Edema WNL			Edema WNL			Edema WNL		
	Reflexes WNL			Reflexes WNL			Reflexes WNL		
	V.S. Q4h			V.S. Q12h			V.S. Q12h		
	Assumed Care Initials			Assumed Care Initials			Assumed Care Initials		
	Assumed Care Time			Assumed Care Time			Assumed Care Time		
SAFETY	Call light in reach,bed low			Call light in reach,bed low			Call light in reach,bed low		
	Side rail position__________			Side rail position__________			Side rail position__________		
	Fall Risk Score ________			Fall Risk Score ________			Fall Risk Score ________		
	If >= to 50 fall prevention path implemented			If >= to 50 fall prevention path implemented			If >= to 50 fall prevention path implemented		
	Nursing rounds Q2h			Nursing rounds Q2h			Nursing rounds Q2h		
	Car seat prepared			Car seat prepared			Car seat prepared		
ACTIVITY	***Up ad lib***			***Up ad lib***			***Up ad lib***		
DIET	***Regular***			***Regular***			***Regular***		
TEST	***CBC or Hgb/Hct in AM after delivery if meets criteria***								
TREAT-MENT	***Sitz bath PRN***			***Sitz bath PRN***			***Sitz bath PRN***		
	Massage Therapist								
RESPIR-ATORY THERAPY	See MAR for Respiratory medication tratments ordered & R.T. log for treatments performed.			See MAR for Respiratory medication tratments ordered & R.T. log for treatments performed.			See MAR for Respiratory medication tratments ordered & R.T. log for treatments performed.		
MED-ICATIONS	SAM packet @ bedside			SAM packet @ bedside			SAM packet @ bedside		
	Pt achieved pain relief with SAM			Pt achieved pain relief with SAM			Pt achieved pain relief with SAM		
	Pt achieved pain relief PRN with narcotics			Pt achieved pain relief PRN with narcotics			Pt achieved pain relief PRN with narcotics		
	RhoGAM if indicated			***RhoGAM if indicated***			***RhoGAM if indicated***		
	Rubella as indicated			***Rubella as indicated***			***Rubella as indicated***		
	Date:			Date:			Date:		

Key: Users Initials = Met U = Unmet
***Any unmet must have a reason documented in progress note**
*** Circled initial = Change in assessment requiring documentation**
*** A Physician's order is required for anything bolded & italicized**

ADDRESSOGRAPH

VAGINAL DELIVERY CLINICAL PATH
UNIVERSITY COMMUNITY HOSPITAL TAMPA, FLORIDA
Rev. 10/09/95 Page 3 of 4

	12-24 hours Postpartum	24-36 hours Postpartum	36-48 hours Postpartum
CLINICAL CONSULTS			
PSYCHO-SOCIAL	Support system present Bonding with newborn	Support system present Bonding with newborn	Support system present Bonding with newborn
SOCIAL WORK SERVICES			
TEACHING	Discharge pamphlets reinforced Newborn care: Infant feeding Diaper change Cord care Self care: Postpartum care Videos: Breast feeding Diapers/Delerium CPR Pt./S.O. verbalizes understanding of D/C instructions, Dr. follow-up date Verbalizes understanding of teaching	Discharge pamphlets reinforced Newborn care: Infant feeding Diaper change Cord care Self care: Postpartum care Videos: Breast feeding Diapers/Delerium CPR Pt./S.O. verbalizes understanding of D/C instructions, Dr. follow-up date Verbalizes understanding of teaching	Discharge pamphlets reinforced Newborn care: Infant feeding Diaper change Cord care Self care: Postpartum care Videos: Breast feeding Diapers/Delerium CPR Pt./S.O. verbalizes understanding of D/C instructions, Dr. follow-up date Verbalizes understanding of teaching
DIS-CHARGE PLANNING	***Discharge:*** ***When meets discharge criteria*** Birth Certificate	***Discharge:*** ***When meets discharge criteria*** Birth Certificate	***Discharge:*** ***When meets discharge criteria*** Birth Certificate
	Date:	Date:	Date:

Key: Users Initials = Met U = Unmet

***Any unmet must have a reason documented in progress note**

*** Circled initial = Change in assessment requiring documentation**

*** A Physician's order is required for anything bolded & italicized**

VAGINAL DELIVERY CLINICAL PATH
UNIVERSITY COMMUNITY HOSPITAL TAMPA, FLORIDA
Rev. 10/09/95 Page 4 of 4

ADDRESSOGRAPH

APPENDIX I. Cesarean Birth Clinical Path

PATIENT PROBLEM LIST		Delivery Date________ Delivery Time________	PHYSICIAN CONSULTS
*A. Potential lack of knowledge re: cesarean birth, self care, newborn care	*C. Hemmorhage, potential for	Mother Blood Type_______ Baby Blood Type______	
*B. Pain, potential for	*D. Infection, potential for	Rubella____ RPR_____ Hepatitis______	
		Breast_______ Bottle________ Sex_______	
		Pediatrician Time notified	

NURSING ASSESS MENT

Pre-op	Post-op	Post-op Day 1
Path Suspended/Resumed	Path Suspended/Resumed	Path Suspended/Resumed
Pre-op	Post-op	Post-op Day 1
Hospital day:	Hospital day:	Hospital day:
Preoperative	Problem list reprioritized	Problem list reprioritized
Problem list prioritized	*(most important first)_________	*(most important first)_________
*(most important first)_________	Alert & Oriented X 3	Alert & Oriented X 3
Alert & Oriented X 3	Bil. breath sounds clear	Bil. breath sounds clear
Skin turgor & color WNL	Breasts & Nipples WNL	Breasts & Nipples WNL
Bil. breath sounds clear	Skin turgor & color WNL	Skin turgor & color WNL
Bowel sounds present	Edema minimal	Edema minimal
Edema minimal	Homan's negative	Homan's negative
Reflexes WNL	Abdomen soft	Abdomen soft
Refer to vaginal path for preop assessment	Bowel sounds present	Bowel sounds present
Fetal heart tones WNL (rate 110-160)	Fundus firm, location WNL Q4h	Fundus firm, location WNL Q4h
Vital signs X 1	Lochia WNL Q4h	Lochia WNL Q4h
Pre-op checklist done*	Hemor./Varicosities(-)	Hemor./Varicosities(-)
*see page 2	Urine clear, yellow	Urine clear, yellow
Intraoperative	Foley output >30cc/hr	Voiding Q.S.
Problem list reprioritized	Intake sufficient	Intake sufficient
FHT Q5min after placement of anesthesia until abdominal prep	Pain level:coping	Pain level:coping
Uterine displacement	Abdominal drsg. D & I	Incision clean & dry
Complete perioperative record	Reflexes WNL	Staples intact
Perioperative Safety Management record completed	***VS Q1h X 4 then Q4h***	Reflexes WNL
Support person present		***VS Q4h***
PACU		***Call Physician if temp > 101 X 2*** '*(2 hours apart)
Support person present		Reassessed Q4h
Urine output >30cc/hr		
Epidural cath removed intact per protocol		
Location of Pain:__________		
Acceptable Level of Pain(0-10)		
Level of Pain(0-10)		
Pain Controlled		
Discharged per protocol	Assumed Care Initials	Assumed Care Initials
Transfered to PP per stretcher	Time assumed care	Time assumed care
Date::	Date::	Date::

LEGEND

Breast WNL = Soft to firm	Lochia WNL = Scant to moderate flo
Nipple WNL = Evert and inta	Fundus Location WNL = U/U to U/2
Reflexes WNL = 2(+) <	

Key : Users Initials = Met, U = Unmet, [ ] = N/A

*Any unmet must have a reason documented in progress note

*Circled initials = Change in assessment requiring documentation

* A Physician's order is required for anything bolded & in italics

ADDRESSOGRAPH

CESAREAN BIRTH CLINICAL PATH

UNIVERSITY COMMUNITY HOSPITAL TAMPA, FLORIDA

10/09/95 Rev Average Length of Stay 3 Days Page 1 of 7

	Path Suspended/Resumed	
	Pre-op	
	Hospital day:	

Preoperative

NURSING ASSESS MENT

Pre-op Checklist Completed
Signed Operative Consent
Blood consent signed
Physicians orders noted
Consultation done
Anesthesia record completed & on chart
History & Physical on chart
Pre-op teaching completed (See Pg. 4)
Test Results reviewed and on chart
Abnormal Test results reported to Dr.
Addressograph plate on chart
Identification bracelet on
T&S bracelet on arm
Patient in hospital gown
Removed Dentures, Prosthesis, Contact Lenses,
Glasses, Wig,Hairpins, Makeup,gum & Jewelry
Wedding band taped
Preop medication given
Siderails up after medicated

Most recent vital signs
Temp________ B/P________
Pulse________ Resp.__________
Weight _________________
List Allergies:______________________

Allergy bracelet on

Disposition of valuables to ____________________

To OR via stretcher @ :____________

Old record to OR

Antibiotic to OR
Preop variances noted Y________ N________
Reported to_________________________________

Date:: | Date:: | Date::

Key : Users Initials = Met, U = Unmet, ☐ = N/A
*Any unmet must have a reason documented in progress note
*Circled initials = Change in assessment requiring documentation
* A Physician's order is required for anything bolded & in italics

ADDRESSOGRAPH

CESAREAN BIRTH CLINICAL PATH
UNIVERSITY COMMUNITY HOSPITAL TAMPA, FLORIDA
10/09/95 Rev Average Length of Stay 3 Days Page 2 of 7

APPENDIX I. Cesarean Birth Clinical Path cont.

	Pre-op Hospital day:	Post-op Hospital day:	Post-op Day 1 Hospital day:
SAFETY	Oriented to unit Call light in reach Advanced Directive pamphlet received Bill of Rights received Fall risk score______ If >or=to 50 Fall protocol initiated Reassessed for fall risk Isolation(other than BSI)______ Pt./visitors instructed on precautions	Oriented to unit Call light in reach Side rail position______ Bed in low position Fall risk score______ If >or=to 50 Fall protocol initiated Reassessed for fall risk Nursing Rounds Q2h Isolation(other than BSI)______ Pt./visitors instructed on precautions Infant Safety Sheet signed	Call light in reach Side rail position______ Bed in low position Fall risk score______ If >or=to 50 Fall protocol initiated Reassessed for fall risk Nursing Rounds Q2h Isolation(other than BSI)______ Pt./visitors instructed on precautions
ACTIVITY	***BRP with assist***	***OOB in 6-8 hours with assistance***	***OOB ad lib minimum tid***
DIET	***NPO***	***Clear Liquids***	***Full Liquids*** ***Progress to Soft when passing flatus***
TESTS	***CBC*** Preop H&H results______ ***Type & Screen*** ***RPR if none in last 4 weeks*** ***UA***		***CBC*** ***Hgb/Hct*** ***UA prior to foley D/C***
TREAT-MENT	***IV access with 18G & assess Q2h*** ***May use local per protocol*** ***IV 1000cc LR bolus prior to Epidural*** ***Foley to straight drainage after epidural / spinal*** ***Abdomen shave in OR***	***Epidural catheter removed & intact per protocol*** Peri Care ***T, C, DB Q2h X 24hrs*** ***I&O balance assessed***	***Foley D/C'd*** ***Cath PRN X 2 if unable to void*** ***T, C, DB Q2h X 24hrs*** ***I & O maintained until IV D/C'd and voids X 2***
RESPIR-ATORY	See MAR for Respiratory medication treatment ordered & R.T. log for treatments performed.	See MAR for Respiratory medication treatment ordered & R.T. log for treatments performed.	See MAR for Respiratory medication treatment ordered & R.T. log for treatments performed.
	Date:	Date:	Date:

Key : Users Initials = Met, U = Unmet, ☐ = N/A
***Any unmet must have a reason documented in progress note**
***Circled initials = Change in assessment requiring documentation**
*** A Physician's order is required for anything bolded & in italics**

ADDRESSOGRAPH

CESAREAN BIRTH CLINICAL PATH
UNIVERSITY COMMUNITY HOSPITAL TAMPA, FLORIDA
10/09/95 Rev Average Length of Stay 3 Days Page 3 of 7

APPENDIX I. Cesarean Birth Clinical Path cont.

	Pre-op Hospital day:	Post-op Hospital day:	Post-op Day 1 Hospital day:
MEDI-CATIONS	***30cc BiCitra approximately 30 min prior to surgery***	***IV D5.45NS with 20u Pitocin 1st liter PP @ 125cc/hr*** ***Medications as per Duramorph protocol***	***IV D5.45NS@125cc/hr*** ***SAM packet @ bedside*** Patient achieved pain relief with SAM Patient achieved pain relief with narcotics PRN
CLINICAL CONSULTS	Birth plan:Perinatal CNS Anesthesiologist notified	Lactation Specialist if breast feeding PRN	examined baby Lactation Specialist if Breast feeding PRN
PSYCHO-SOCIAL	Encouraged support person involvement	Support systems present Bonding with newborn	Support systems present Bonding with newborn
SOCIAL WORK SERVICES			
TEACHING	Verbalizes understandin after instructed about: (P.A.T. / FLOOR) Cesarean Birth NPO IV Foley Catheter Other possible equipment Abdominal Prep Support person in OR Breast Feeding Technique Fundus/Bleeding check Post anesthesia recovery procedure, including pain relief meds Proper T, C, & DB Food & drug interaction pamphlet given to Pt./SO Support Person involved in teaching	Discharge Pamphlets at bedside Newborn Care:Infant feeding Self Care:Postpartum care Breast feeding Teaching reinforced on pain managment: PCA Duramorph Pt../Support Person verbalizes understanding of instruction	Discharge Pamphlets at bedside Newborn Care: Infant feeding Diaper change Cord care Self care: Postpartum care Breast feeding Aware signs/symptoms to report to D @ d/c for self or baby Videos: Infant CPR Breast Feeding Diaper Delirium Pt../Support Person verbalizes understanding of instruction
DIS-CHARGE PLANNING	Assess home & family support system	Assess home & family support system	Assess home & family for post-hospital care needs Birth Certificate complete
	Date:	Date:	Date:

Key : Users Initials = Met, U = Unmet, [ ] = N/A

*Any unmet must have a reason documented in progress note

*Circled initials = Change in assessment requiring documentation

* A Physician's order is required for anything bolded & in italics

ADDRESSOGRAPH

CESAREAN BIRTH CLINICAL PATH

UNIVERSITY COMMUNITY HOSPITAL TAMPA, FLORIDA

10/09/95 Rev Average Length of Stay 3 Days Page 4 of 7

	Post-op Day 2	Post-op Day 3	Post-op Day 4
	Path Suspended/Resumed	Path Suspended/Resumed	Path Suspended/Resumed
	Post-op Day 2	Post-op Day 3	Post-op Day 4
	Hospital day:	Hospital day:	Hospital day:
	Problem list reprioritized ______	Problem list reprioritiz ______	Problem list reprioritiz ______
NURSING ASSESS MENT	Alert & Oriented	Alert & Oriented	Alert & Oriented
	Bil. breath sounds clear	Bil. breath sounds clear	Bil. breath sounds clear
	Breasts & Nipples WNL	Breasts & Nipples WNL	Breasts & Nipples WNL
	Skin turgor & color WNL	Skin turgor & color WNL	Skin turgor & color WNL
	Edema minimal	Edema minimal	Edema minimal
	Homan's negative	Homan's negative	Homan's negative
	Abdomen soft	Abdomen soft	Abdomen soft
	Bowel sounds present	Bowel sounds present	Bowel sounds present
	Fundus firm, location WNL	Fundus firm, location WNL	Fundus firm, location WNL
	Lochia WNL	Lochia WNL	Lochia WNL
	Hemor./Varicosities(-)	Hemor./Varicosities(-)	Hemor./Varicosities(-)
	Urine clear, yellow	Urine clear, yellow	Urine clear, yellow
	Voiding Q.S.	Voiding Q.S.	Voiding Q.S.
	Intake sufficient	Intake sufficient	Intake sufficient
	Pain level:coping	Pain level:coping	Pain level:coping
	Incision clean & dry	Incision clean & dry	Incision clean & dry
	Staples intact	Staples intact	Staples intact
	Reflexes WNL	Reflexes WNL	Reflexes WNL
	VS Q8h	***VS Q8h***	***VS Q8h***
	Reassessed Q8h	Reassessed Q8h	Reassessed Q8h
	Assumed Care Initials	Assumed Care Initials	Assumed Care Initials
	Time assumed care	Time assumed care	Time assumed care
SAFETY	Call light in reach	Call light in reach	Call light in reach
	Side rail position______	Side rail position______	Side rail position______
	Bed in low position	Bed in low position	Bed in low position
	Fall risk score______	Fall risk score______	Fall risk score______
	If >or=to 50 Fall protocol initiated	If >or=to 50 Fall protocol initiated	If >or=to 50 Fall protocol initiated
	Reassessed for fall risk	Reassessed for fall risk	Reassessed for fall risk
	Nursing Rounds Q2h	Nursing Rounds Q2h	Nursing Rounds Q2h
	Isolation(other than BSI)______	Isolation(other than BSI)______	Isolation(other than BSI)______
	Pt./visitors instructed on precautions	Pt./visitors instructed on precautions	Pt./visitors instructed on precautions
	Date:	Date:	Date:

Key : Users Initials = Met, U = Unmet, [ ] = N/A

*Any unmet must have a reason documented in progress note

*Circled initials = Change in assessment requiring documentation

* A Physician's order is required for anything bolded & in italics

ADDRESSOGRAPH

CESAREAN BIRTH CLINICAL PATH
UNIVERSITY COMMUNITY HOSPITAL TAMPA, FLORIDA
10/09/95 Rev Average Length of Stay 3 Days Page 5 of 7

APPENDIX I. Cesarean Birth Clinical Path cont.

	Post-op Day 2 Hospital day:	Post-op Day 3 Hospital day:	Post-op Day 4 Hospital day:
ACTIVITY	***OOB ad lib***	***OOB ad lib***	***OOB ad lib***
DIET	***Regular***	***Regular***	***Regular***
TESTS			
TREAT-MENT	***IV discontinued when criteria met*** Massage Therapy	***IV discontinued when criteria met*** Massage Therapy	***IV discontinued when criteria met***
RESPIR-ATORY THERAPY	See MAR for Respiratory medication 'treatment 'ordered & R.T. log for treatments performed.	See MAR for Respiratory medication 'treatment 'ordered & R.T. log for treatments performed.	See MAR for Respiratory medication 'treatment 'ordered & R.T. log for treatments performed.
MEDI-CATIONS	SAM packet @ bedside Patient achieved pain relief with SAM Patient achieved pain relief with narcotics PRN ***Rhogam (if indicated)*** ***Rubella (if indicated)***	SAM packet @ bedside Patient achieved pain relief with SAM Patient achieved pain relief with narcotics PRN ***Rhogam (if indicated)*** ***Rubella (if indicated)***	SAM packet @ bedside Patient achieved pain relief with SAM Patient achieved pain relief with narcotics PRN ***Rhogam (if indicated)*** ***Rubella (if indicated)***
CLINICAL CONSULTS	Lactation Specialist if breast feeding	Lactation Specialist if breast feeding Pediatrician has examined baby	Lactation Specialist if breast feeding
	Date:	Date:	Date:

Key : Users Initials = Met, U = Unmet, [ ] = N/A

***Any unmet must have a reason documented in progress note**

***Circled initials = Change in assessment requiring documentation**

*** A Physician's order is required for anything bolded & in italics**

ADDRESSOGRAPH

CESAREAN BIRTH CLINICAL PATH
UNIVERSITY COMMUNITY HOSPITAL TAMPA, FLORIDA
10/09/95 Rev Average Length of Stay 3 Days Page 6 of 7

	Post-op Day 2 Hospital day:	Post-op Day 3 Hospital day:	Post-op Day 4 Hospital day:
PSYCHO-SOCIAL	Support systems present Bonding with newborn	Support systems present Bonding with newborn	Support systems present Bonding with newborn
SOCIAL WORK SERVICES			
TEACHING	Given Food & Drug Interaction Sheet Videos: Infant CPR Breast Feeding Diaper Delirium Aware signs/symptoms to report to Dr. after discharge for self or baby Pt./SO verbalizes understanding of instruction	Discharge Pamphlets at bedside Newborn Care: Infant feeding Diaper change Cord care Given Food & Drug Interaction Sheet Videos: Infant CPR Breast Feeding Diaper Delirium Aware signs/symptoms to report to Dr. after discharge for self or baby Pt./SO verbalizes understanding of instruction	Discharge Pamphlets at bedside Newborn Care: Infant feeding Diaper change Cord care Given Food & Drug Interaction Sheet Videos: Infant CPR Breast Feeding Diaper Delirium Pt./SO verbalizes understanding of instruction
DIS-CHARGE PLANNING	Assess home & family support system Birth Certificate complete	Assess home & family support system Birth Certificate complete	Assess home & family notified for post-hospital care needs Birth Certificate complete
	Date:	Date:	Date:

Key : Users Initials = Met, U = Unmet, = N/A

*Any unmet must have a reason documented in progress note

*Circled initials = Change in assessment requiring documentation

* A Physician's order is required for anything bolded & in italics

ADDRESSOGRAPH

CESAREAN BIRTH CLINICAL PATH

UNIVERSITY COMMUNITY HOSPITAL TAMPA, FLORIDA

10/09/95 Rev Average Length of Stay 3 Days Page 7 of 7

APPENDIX I. Normal Newborn Clinical Path

PATIENT PROBLEM LIST		Delivery Date________	Delivery Time________	Apgars____/____
A. Potential for alteration in breathing	D Potential for hypoglycemia	Mother Blood Type____	HBsAG ________	RPR__________
B. Potential for unstable thermoregulation	E Potential for hyperbilirubinemia	Baby Blood Type & Coombs_______	Breast_________	Bottle_________
C Potential for alteration of nutrition	F Potential for complication of circumcision	Sex___	Pediatrician Notified (Y)	
		Name of person taking call		

LEGEND

Br 1 = Good latch, audible swallow
Br 2 = Needs assistance * (unmet)
Br 3 = No latch * (unmet)

Cardio WNL=R 120-160, reg, no murmur
Resp WNL=R 40-60, unlabored
Abd WNL=Soft, non-distended

TEMP KEY
S = Skin to Skin
C = Open Crib

	Path suspended/resumed	Path suspended/resumed	Path suspended/resumed
	Day of Birth: 0-2h old / 3-6h old	7 - 24 h old	> 24 h old
NURSING ASSESS-MENT	Newborn admission assessment completed	Problem list reprioritized________	Problem list reprioritized________
	Problem list prioritized________	**_Notify Dr. if:_**	**_Notify Dr. if:_**
	Maintain under radiant warmer or skin to skin until temp WNL (97.7-99)	**_* No VOID in 12hr_**	**_* No VOID in 12hr_**
	B/P X 1 on admissi Time/Initial /	**_*No 2nd VOID in 24hr_**	**_*No 2nd VOID in 24hr_**
	arm & leg B/P in arm__________ B/P in leg__________	**_* No STOOL in 48hr or prior to discharge_**	**_* No STOOL in 48hr or prior to discharge_**
	Time/Initials / / / /	**_TPR Q8h_**	**_TPR Q8h_**
	Temp Q1h X 4 T T T T	T_____ P_______ R_______	T_____ P_______ R_______
	Pulse Q1h X 4 P P P P	**_TPR Q8h_**	**_TPR Q8h_**
	Resp Q1h X 4 R R R R	T_____ P_______ R_______	T_____ P_______ R_______
	TPR Q2h X 1 Time/Init / T P R		**_TPR Q8h_** T_____ P_______ R_______
	_Wt in lbs._________ **_Wt in kg._**________	**_Wt in lbs_**______________	**_Wt in lbs_**______________
	_Length_________ **_in._** __________ **_cm._**	**_Wt in kg_**______________	**_Wt in kg_**______________
	_Head_________ **_in._** __________ **_cm._**		
	_Chest_________ **_in._** __________ **_cm._**		
	_Abdomen_________ **_in._** __________ **_cm._**		
		Assessment Time:	Assessment Time:
	Resp status WNL	Resp status WNL	Resp status WNL
	Cardiovascular status WNL	Cardiovascular status WNL	Cardiovascular status WNL
	Color pink	Color pink	Color pink
	Skin intact	Skin intact	Skin intact
	Fontanelle soft & flat	Fontanelle soft & flat	Fontanelle soft & flat
	Abdomen WNL	Abdomen WNL	Abdomen WNL
	Reflexes WNL	Reflexes WNL	Reflexes WNL
	Recorded void	Recorded void	Recorded void
	Recorded stool	Recorded stool	Recorded stool
	Chemstrip protocol Time Value	**_Chemstrip protocol_** Time Value	**_Chemstrip protocol_** Time Value
	Assumed Care Initials	Assumed Care Initials	Assumed Care Initials
	Time Assumed Care	Time Assumed Care	Time Assumed Care
SAFETY	I.D. bracelet X 2	I.D. bracelet X 2	I.D. bracelet X 2
	Bulb syringe at bedside	Bulb syringe at bedside	Bulb syringe at bedside
		Fastened in car seat at D/C by Mom/SO	Fastened in car seat at D/C by Mom/SO
	Date:	Date:	Date:

Key: Users Initials = Met U = Unmet ☐ = N/A
***Any unmet must have a reason documented in progress note**
*** Circled initial = Change in assessment reqiring documentation**
*** A Physician's order is required for anything bolded & in italics**

ADDRESSOGRAPH

NORMAL NEWBORN CLINICAL PATH
UNIVERSITY COMMUNITY HOSPITAL TAMPA, FLORIDA
Rev. 10/09/95 Page 1 of 4

APPENDIX I. Normal Newborn Clinical Path cont.

	Day of Birth / 0-2h old / 3-6h old	7 - 24 h old (Time)	> 24 h old (Time)
DIET	***Br/Bottle 10-20cc 1st feed then as tol.*** Formula type______ Time cc/Length Initial Time cc/Length Initial	***Br/Bottle as tol.*** Formula type______ Time cc/Length Initial Time cc/Length Initial Time cc/Length Initial	***Br/Bottle as tol.*** Formula type______ Time cc/Length Initial Time cc/Length Initial Time cc/Length Initial
TEST	***Type, Rh, Coombs if Rh(-) & O mothers*** ***Cord bili if coombs (+) infants*** ***Heel stick RPR if mom has (+)RPR*** ***Hepatitis protocol if mom HBsAG (+) or unknown***	***Bili as ordered*** ***Metabolic screen pre-D/C***	***Bili as ordered*** ***Metabolic screen pre-D/C***
TREAT-MENT	***Bath on admission (when temp. stable)*** ***Cord care QDiaper change*** ***Pediatrician visit***	***Cord care QDiaper change*** Circ ck. per protocol Cord clamp removed pre D/C ***Pediatrician visit***	***Cord care QDiaper change*** Circ ck. per protocol Cord clamp removed pre D/C ***Pediatrician visit***
CLINICAL CONSULTS		***Consult Lactation Consultant PRN***	***Consult Lactation Consultant PRN***
PSYCHO-SOCIAL			
SOCIAL WORK SERVICE			
DIS-CHARGE PLANN-ING		Parent(s) given copy of infant H&P for pediatrician	Parent(s) given copy of infant H&P for pediatrician
	Date:	Date:	Date:

Key: Users Initials = Met U = Unmet ☐ = N/A
***Any unmet must have a reason documented in progress note**
*** Circled initial = Change in assessment reqiring documentation**
*** A Physician's order is required for anything bolded & in italics**

ADDRESSOGRAPH

NORMAL NEWBORN CLINICAL PATH
UNIVERSITY COMMUNITY HOSPITAL TAMPA, FLORIDA
Rev. 10/09/95 Page 2 of 4

	Path suspended/resumed > 24 h old	Path suspended/resumed > 24 h old	Path suspended/resumed > 24 h old
NURSING ASSESS-MENT	Problem list reprioritized________ Time Initial ***TPR Q8h*** T______ P_______ R_______ ***TPR Q8h*** T______ P_______ R_______ ***TPR Q8h*** T______ P_______ R_______ ***Wt in lbs***________________ ***Wt in kg***________________ Resp status WNL Cardiovascular status WNL Color pink Skin intact Fontanelle soft & flat Abdomen WNL Reflexes WNL Recorded void Recorded stool ***Notify Dr. if:*** *** No STOOL in 48hr or prior to discharge*** Assumed Care Initials Time Assumed Care	Problem list reprioritized________ Time Initial ***TPR Q8h*** T______ P_______ R_______ ***TPR Q8h*** T______ P_______ R_______ ***TPR Q8h*** T______ P_______ R_______ ***Wt in lbs***________________ ***Wt in kg***________________ Resp status WNL Cardiovascular status WNL Color pink Skin intact Fontanelle soft & flat Abdomen WNL Reflexes WNL Recorded void Recorded stool ***Notify Dr. if:*** *** No STOOL in 48hr or prior to discharge*** Assumed Care Initials Time Assumed Care	Problem list reprioritized________ Time Initial ***TPR Q8h*** T______ P_______ R_______ ***TPR Q8h*** T______ P_______ R_______ ***TPR Q8h*** T______ P_______ R_______ ***Wt in lbs***________________ ***Wt in kg***________________ Resp status WNL Cardiovascular status WNL Color pink Skin intact Fontanelle soft & flat Abdomen WNL Reflexes WNL Recorded void Recorded stool ***Notify Dr. if:*** *** No STOOL in 48hr or prior to discharge*** Assumed Care Initials Time Assumed Care
SAFETY	I.D. bracelet X 2 Bulb syringe at bedside Fastened in car seat at D/C by Mom/S/O	I.D. bracelet X 2 Bulb syringe at bedside Fastened in car seat at D/C by Mom/SO	I.D. bracelet X 2 Bulb syringe at bedside Fastened in car seat at D/C by Mom/SO
	Parent(s) given copy of infant H&P for pediatrician	Parent(s) given copy of infant H&P for pediatrician	Parent(s) given copy of infant H&P for pediatrician
	Date:	Date:	Date:

Key: Users Initials = Met U = Unmet [ ] = N/A
***Any unmet must have a reason documented in progress note**
*** Circled initial = Change in assessment reqiring documentation**
*** A Physician's order is required for anything bolded & in italics**

ADDRESSOGRAPH

NORMAL NEWBORN CLINICAL PATH
UNIVERSITY COMMUNITY HOSPITAL TAMPA, FLORIDA
Rev 10/09/95 Page 3 of 4

APPENDIX I. Normal Newborn Clinical Path cont.

	> 24 h old Time	> 24 h old Time	> 24 h old Time
DIET	***Br/Bottle as tol.*** Formula type______ Time / cc/Length / Initial; Time / cc/Length / Initial; Time / cc/Length / Initial	***Br/Bottle as tol.*** Formula type______ Time / cc/Length / Initial; Time / cc/Length / Initial; Time / cc/Length / Initial	***Br/Bottle as tol.*** Formula type______ Time / cc/Length / Initial; Time / cc/Length / Initial; Time / cc/Length / Initial
TEST	***Bili as ordered*** ***Metabolic screen pre-D/C***	***Bili as ordered*** ***Metabolic screen pre-D/C***	***Bili as ordered*** ***Metabolic screen pre-D/C***
TREAT-MENT	***Cord care QDiaper change*** Circ ck. per protocol Cord clamp removed pre D/C ***Pediatrician visit***	***Cord care QDiaper change*** Circ ck. per protocol Cord clamp removed pre D/C ***Pediatrician visit***	***Cord care QDiaper change*** Circ ck. per protocol Cord clamp removed pre D/C ***Pediatrician visit***
CLINICAL CONSULTS	***Consult Lactation Consultant PRN***	***Consult Lactation Consultant PRN***	***Consult Lactation Consultant PRN***
PSYCHO-SOCIAL			
SOCIAL WORK SERVICE			
DIS-CHARGE PLANN-ING			
	Date:	Date:	Date:

Key: Users Initials = Met U = Unmet ☐ = N/A

*Any unmet must have a reason documented in progress note

* Circled initial = Change in assessment reqiring documentation

* A Physician's order is required for anything bolded & in italics

NORMAL NEWBORN CLINICAL PATH

UNIVERSITY COMMUNITY HOSPITAL TAMPA, FLORIDA

Rev 10/09/95 Page 4 of 4

ADDRESSOGRAPH

ST. MARY'S HEALTH CENTER
St. Louis, Missouri

PRE-NATAL CARE PATHWAYS ™

PT. LABEL

PRENATAL EDUCATION CLINICAL PATHWAY

INITIAL VISIT AND ORIENTATION: ________ SOCIAL SERVICE: ________ DIETICIAN: ________

I. EARLY PREGNANCY (WEEKS 1-20) *(initial and date after education given)*

Fetal Growth and Development ________

Maternal Changes ________

Lifestyle: Exercise / Stress / Nutrition ________
Drugs, OTC, Tobacco, Alcohol ________
STD's ________

Psycho / Social Adjustments:
Acceptance ________
FOB Involved / Accepts ________
BFA ________

Testing: Labs ________ Ultrasound ________

Possible Complications:
a. Threatened AB ________
b. Diabetes ________
c. ________ ________

Introduction to Breastfeeding ________
and Childbirth Preparation ________

Dietary Follow Up ________

II. MID PREGNANCY (WEEKS 21-27) *(initial and date after education given)*

Fetal Growth and Development ________

Maternal Changes ________

Daily Fetal Movement ________

Possible Complications:
a. Preterm Labor Prevention ________
b. PIH Symptoms ________
c. ________ ________

Breast or Bottle Feeding ________

Birth Plan Initiated ________

Childbirth Preparation ________
____

Dietary Follow Up ________

III. LATE PREGNANCY (WEEKS 28-40) *(initial and date after education given)*

Fetal Growth and Development ________

Fetal Evaluation:
Daily Movement ________ NST's ________
Kick Counts ________ BPP's ________

Maternal Changes ________

Possible Complications:
a. Preterm Labor Prevention ________
b. PIH Symptoms ________
c. ________ ________

Breastfeeding Preparation:
Nipple Assessment ________

Dietary Follow Up ________

Childbirth Preparation:
S/S of Labor; Labor Process ________
Pain Management: NCB, Meds, Epidural ________
C/Section; VBAC ________
Birth Plan Complete ________
Review Hospital Policies ________

Parenting Preparation:
Pediatrician ________ Childcare ________
Siblings ________ Immunizations ________
Car Seat/Safety ________

Post-Partum:
P.P. Care/Check-Up ________
Emotional Changes ________
B.C. Options ________
Safe Sex/STD's ________

SIGNATURE: ________ ________ ________

11/94

APPENDIX J. Information Sheet

ST. MARY'S HEALTH CENTER
St. Louis, Missouri

INFORMATION SHEET

PT. LABEL

NAME: ______________________________

ADDRESS: ______________________________

PHONE NUMBER: (________) ______________ MARITAL STATUS: ______________

SIGNIFICANT OTHER: ______________________ RELATIONSHIP: ______________

PHONE NUMBER: (________) ______________

EDUCATION LEVEL: ______________ OCCUPATION: ______________

EDC: ________ GRAVIDA: ________ PARA: ________ AB: ________ BLOOD TYPE: ________ RUBELLA TITRE: ________

HIV: ________ HEP B SAg: ________

PEDIATRICIAN: ______________________________

HISTORY/COMPLICATIONS: ______________________________

____

____

____

SIGNATURE: ______________________ DATE: ______________

CLASS ATTENDANCE LIST

PREGNANCY:	DATE ________	INITIAL ________		PREPARED CHILDBIRTH:	DATE ________	INITIAL ________
INFANT CARE:	DATE ________	INITIAL ________				
INFANT FEEDING:	DATE ________	INITIAL ________		PRENATAL BREASTFEEDING	DATE ________	INITIAL ________
PARENTING:	DATE ________	INITIAL ________		OTHER:	DATE ________	INITIAL ________
WOMEN'S HEALTH:	DATE ________	INITIAL ________			DATE ________	INITIAL ________

NOTES

APPENDIX J. Vaginal Delivery Care Pathways

ST. MARY'S HEALTH CENTER
St. Louis, Missouri

VAGINAL DELIVERY CARE PATHWAYS™

PT. LABEL

D = DAY SHIFT
E = EVE SHIFT
N = NOC SHIFT

N/A = (cross through and initial)
COMPLETED = (initial)
TO BE COMPLETED = (circle in red, initial)

NURSING PARAMETERS	NSG DX	1 hour OBRR	N	D	E	2-12 HRS p̄ DELIVERY	N	D	E	13-24 HRS AFTER DELIVERY	N	D	E	25-36 HRS DISCHARGE p̄ DELIVERY	N	D	E	OUTCOMES WRITE IN DATE OF COMPLETION	HOSP	PP
ASSESSMENT																				
VITAL SIGNS		VS q̄ 15'				VS AT ADMIT +q̄ 4°				VS BID				VS BID				VSS		
FUNDUS/LOCHIA		FUNDUS/LOCHIA CHECKS q̄ 15				FUNDUS/LOCHIA CHECKS & ADMIT +q̄ 4°				FUNDUS/LOCHIA CHECK BID				FUNDUS/LOCHIA CHECK BID				FUNDUS FIRM s̄ EXCESSIVE LOCHIA RUBRA		
IV THERAPY		VIV SITE				VIV SITE				DC IV										
CIRCULATORY						CHECK HOMAN'S SIGN				CHECK HOMAN'S SIGN				CHECK HOMAN'S SIGN BID				NEGATIVE HOMAN'S SIGN		
TREATMENTS																				
ICE TO PERINEUM		ICE TO PERINEUM AS ORDERED				ICE TO PERINEUM AS ORDERED				ICE TO PERINEUM AS ORDERED								PERINEUM INTACT		
SITZ BATH										SITZ BATH AS ORDERED				SITZ BATH				UTILIZING SITZ BATH		
BREAST CARE						USE OF BRA				WEARING BRA				WEARING BRA				PROPER BREAST SUPPORT		
MEDICATIONS																				
ANALGESIC	5	ANALGESIC AS ORDERED				ANALGESIC PRN q̄ 3-4°				ANALGESIC PRN q̄ 3-4°				ANALGESIC PRN q̄ 3-4°				PAIN RELIEVED & PO ANALGESIC		
PITOCIN		PITOCIN INFUSION AS ORDERED				DC PITOCIN PER ORDER														
STOOL SOFTENER										BEGIN STOOL SOFTENER AS ORDERED				TEACHING RE: DC PAIN MEDS				VERBALIZES UNDERSTANDING OF HOME PRN MEDS		
TESTS										RHOGAM								RHOGAM GIVEN		
						CBC												CBC WNL		
NUTRITION	13	NPO x̄ ICE				DIET AS TOLERATED				DIET AS TOLERATED				DIET AS TOLERATED				TOLERATING DIET NO N/V		
ELIMINATION																				
VOID	15	ATTEMPT TO VOID				ATTEMPT TO VOID				VOIDING s̄ DIFFICULTY				VOIDING s̄ DIFFICULTY				VOIDING s̄ DIFFICULTY		
BM	14									CHECK FOR BM				CHECK FOR BM				VERBALIZES UNDERSTANDING OF NORMAL BOWEL FUNCTION RESUMPTION		
ACTIVITY	19	TRANSFER VIA W/C TO MOTHER/BABY UNIT				AMBULATE c̄ ASSIST x 2				UP AD LIB				UP AD LIB				TOLERATES ACTIVITY PROGRESSION		
TEACHING																				
PERI CARE/ HYGIENE	4	PERI CARE				PERI CARE: USE OF SPRAY, TUCKS, FOAM				PERI CARE				PERI CARE				MAINTAIN PROPER HYGIENE		
FUNDAL MASSAGE		FUNDAL MASSAGE																		
INITIAL INFANT CARE	4	ATTEMPT 1st BREAST FEEDING																REFER TO NEWBORN PATHWAY UNDER TEACHING AND FEEDING PARAMETERS		
		TEACH/REVIEW: USE OF BULB SYRINGE																		
		TEACH/REVIEW: INFANT HANDLING																		
DISCHARGE PLANNING														SCHEDULE pp VISIT				VERBALIZED FLU APPT. DATE/TIME		
PSYCH/SOCIAL																				
MATERNAL/INFANT BONDING	24	ASSESS BONDING BEHAVIOR				ASSESS BONDING BEHAVIOR				ASSESS BONDING BEHAVIOR				ASSESS BONDING BEHAVIOR				POSITIVE BONDING & EMOTIONAL BEHAVIORS OBSERVED		
	24	ASSESS EMOTIONAL STATUS				ASSESS EMOTIONAL STATUS				ASSESS EMOTIONAL STATUS				ASSESS EMOTIONAL STATUS				SOCIAL SERVICE REFERRAL AS NECESSARY		

KEYS TO NURSING DIAGNOSIS (NSG DX) CODES

- 4 LACK OF KNOWLEDGE
- 5 ALTERATION IN COMFORT
- 13 ALTERATION NUTRITION
- 14 ALTERATION IN BOWEL ELIMINATION
- 15 ALTERATION IN URINARY ELIMINATION
- 19 ACTIVITY INTOLERANCE
- 24 ALTERATION IN COPING

SIGNATURES ____________ ____________ ____________ ____________ ____________

7/95

"The CARE PATHWAYS™ are guidelines of suggestion for providing coordinated patient care. The pathways are not intended to replace well-reasoned, sound clinical judgement."

APPENDIX J. Cesarean Section Care Pathways

ST. MARY'S HEALTH CENTER
St. Louis, Missouri

CESAREAN SECTION CARE PATHWAYS®

PT. LABEL

D = DAY SHIFT | N/A = (cross through and initial)
E = EVE SHIFT | COMPLETED = (initial)
N = NOC SHIFT | TO BE COMPLETED = (circle in red, initial)

NURSING PARAMETERS	NSG DX	2° DBRR DATE	DOS DATE	POD 1 DATE	POD 2 DATE	DISCHARGE DATE	OUTCOMES WRITE IN DATE OF COMPLETION	HOSP	PP
ASSESSMENT									
VITAL SIGNS		VS	VS q̄ 1° x 2, q̄ 4° x 24° (RESP q̄ 1° x 24 IF ON DURAMORPH PROTOCOL)	VS	VS	VS BID	VSS		
FUNDUS/LOCHIA		FUNDUS/LOCHIA CHECK	FUNDUS/LOCHIA q̄ 1° x 2, THAN q̄ 4° x 24 HRS	CHECK: FUNDUS/LOCHIA BID	CHECK BID: FUNDUS	CHECK BID: FUNDUS	FUNDUS FIRM s̄ EXCESSIVE LOCHIA SEROSA		
DSG/INCISION/ STAPLES	22	DSG CHECK q̄ 15' x 4, q̄ 30' x 2	DSG CHECK q̄ 2 HRS	REMOVE DSG	LOCHIA	LOCHIA			
				CHECK INCISION/ STAPLES	INCISION	INCISION	INCISION HEALING s̄ REDNESS OR DRAINAGE		
					STAPLES	DC STAPLES			
			CHECK HOMAN'S SIGN q̄ SHIFT	HOMAN'S BID	HOMAN'S BID	HOMAN'S BID	NEGATIVE HOMAN'S SIGN		
IV THERAPY		VIV SITE	VIV SITE	VIV SITE	DC IV				
	12	INITIATE I/O	MAINTAIN I/O	DC I/O					
TREATMENTS									
TC & DB	4	INITIATE/ASSIST TC & DB	TC & DB q̄ 2° x 24	DC TC & DB					
			AUSCULTATE LUNGS				LUNGS CLEAR		
			USE OF BRA	WEARING BRA	WEARING BRA	WEARING BRA	PROPER BREAST SUPPORT		
MEDICATIONS									
PAIN MEDS	5	INITIATE DURAMORPH PROTOCOL, PCA PUMP OR IM MEDS	CONTINUE PAIN CONTROL MEASURES	DC PREVIOUS PAIN CONTROL MEASURE					
				BEGIN PO PAIN MEDS PRN	PO PAIN MED PRN	PO PAIN MED PRN	PAIN RELIEVED & PO MEDS		
TESTS					RHOGAM		RHOGAM GIVEN		
				CBC			CBC WNL		
NUTRITION	13	NPO	NPO → CLEAR LIQUIDS	CLEAR LIQUIDS → DAT	DAT	DAT	TOLERATING DIET		
ELIMINATION	15	FOLEY CATHETER	FOLEY CATHETER	DC FOLEY	VOIDING WNL				
			CHECK BOWEL SOUNDS q̄ SHIFT	CHECK BOWEL SOUNDS			NORMAL BOWEL FUNCTION		
	14			CHECK FLATUS	CHECK FOR BM/FLATUS	CHECK FOR BM/FLATUS			
ACTIVITY	19	BR	BR OR UP c̄ ASSIST	UP c̄ ASSIST	UP AD LIB	UP AD LIB	TOLERATES ACTIVITY PROGRESSION		
TEACHING									
PERI CARE/ HYGIENE		PERI CARE	PERI CARE q̄ SHIFT	SELF PERI CARE	SELF PERI CARE	SELF PERI CARE	MAINTAIN PROPER HYGIENE		
INITIAL INFANT CARE	4	ATTEMPT 1st BREAST FEEDING							
	4	TEACH/REVIEW: USE OF BULB SYRINGE							
	4	TEACH/REVIEW: INFANT HANDLING					REFER TO NEWBORN PATHWAY UNDER TEACHING & FEEDING PARAMETERS		
DISCHARGE PLANNING						SCHEDULE PP VISIT	VERBALIZED F/U APPT DATE/TIME		
PSYCH/SOCIAL									
MATERNAL/INFANT BONDING	24	ASSESS BONDING BEHAVIOR	ASSESS BONDING BEHAVIOR	ASSESS BONDING BEHAVIOR	ASSESS BONDING BEHAVIOR	ASSESS BONDING BEHAVIOR	POSITIVE BONDING & EMOTIONAL BEHAVIORS OBSERVED		
	24	ASSESS EMOTIONAL STATUS	ASSESS EMOTIONAL STATUS	ASSESS EMOTIONAL STATUS	ASSESS EMOTIONAL STATUS	ASSESS EMOTIONAL STATUS	SOCIAL SERVICE REFERRAL AS NECESSARY		

KEYS TO NURSING DIAGNOSIS (NSG DX) CODES

- 4 LACK OF KNOWLEDGE
- 5 ALTERATION IN COMFORT
- 12 ALTERATION IN FLUID VOLUME
- 13 ALTERATION NUTRITION
- 14 ALTERATION IN BOWEL ELIMINATION
- 15 ALTERATION IN URINARY ELIMINATION
- 19 ACTIVITY INTOLERANCE
- 24 ALTERATION IN COPING

SIGNATURES

7/95

"The CARE PATHWAYS™ are guidelines of suggestion for providing coordinated patient care. The pathways are not intended to replace well-reasoned, sound clinical judgement."

ST. MARY'S HEALTH CENTER
St. Louis, Missouri

UNCOMPLICATED NEWBORN CARE PATHWAYS®

PT. LABEL

ADM. DATE__________ D = DAY SHIFT
DISC. DATE__________ E = EVE SHIFT
PATH START DATE__________ N = NOC SHIFT

DRG 391 PATH # 24

N/A = (cross through and initial)
COMPLETED = (initial)
TO BE COMPLETED = (circle in red, initial)

NURSING PARAMETERS	1-3° $\bar{p}$ DELIVERY	N	D	E	3-24° $\bar{p}$ DELIVERY	N	D	E	24-48° $\bar{p}$ DELIVERY (DISCHARGE)	N	D	E	OUTCOMES — WRITE IN DATE OF COMPLETION	HOSP	PP
ASSESSMENT															
VITAL SIGNS	VITAL SIGNS $\bar{q}$ 15min x 1hr				VITAL SIGNS $\bar{q}$ 4hr x 2 days				VITAL SIGNS $\bar{q}$ 4°				VITAL SIGNS MEDICALLY ACCEPTABLE		
	VITAL SIGNS 1hr x 4hrs				CHECK COLOR				CHECK COLOR				COLOR PINK		
	HCT @ 1hr of age														
	CHEMSTRIP @ 1hr of age				FOLLOW CHEMSTRIPS AS NECESSARY OR WHEN ORDERED								CHEMSTRIP & HCT COMPLETED & MEDICALLY ACCEPTABLE		
HEAD TO TO ASSEMENT	PHYSICAL ASSEMENT COMPLETED				CHECK RESP EFFORT $\bar{c}$ VITAL SIGNS				CHECK RESP EFFORT						
	BATHED (axillary temp 98°)				CHART PHYSICIAN VISIT - RENOTIFY IF NEEDED								BATH GIVEN		
	REMOVE FROM RADIANT WARMER (axillary temp 98°)				CORD CARE $\bar{c}$ TRIPLE DYE x 1				CORD CARE $\bar{c}$ BETADINE $\bar{q}$ 4°						
	NOTIFY PHYSICIAN'S OFFICE, EXCHANGE OR IN PERSON				CORD CARE CLEANSE $\bar{c}$ BETADINE $\bar{c}$ EACH DIAPER CHANGE								MD EXAMINATION COMPLETED		
TRANSFER TO MOTHER-BABY UNIT	REPORT, TRANSFER TO MOTHER-BABY UNIT														
NUTRITION															
					TEACH/REVIEW: ENGORGEMENT/ESTABLISHING SUPPLY				TEACH/REVIEW: ENGORGEMENT/ESTABLISHING SUPPLY						
BREAST	ATTEMPT 1st FEEDING				OBSERVE/ASSIST $\bar{c}$ FEEDING				OBSERVE/ASSIST $\bar{c}$ FEEDING				ABLE TO BREAST FEED ON DEMAND $\bar{c}$ NO SUPPLEMENT		
	TEACH/REVIEW: USE OF BULB SYRINGE				TEACH POSITIONS				TEACH POSITIONS				LATCHES ON & NURSES $\bar{s}$ PROBLEM		
					FEEDING CUES				FEEDING CUES						
					BREAST/NIPPLE CARE				BREAST/NIPPLE CARE				LACTATION FOLLOW UP IF NEEDED; VERBALIZES KNOWLEDGE OF CONTACT INFO		
					BREAKING SUCTION				BREAKING SUCTION						
					BURPING				BURPING						
					FREQUENCY & LENGTH OF FEEDING				FREQUENCY & LENGTH OF FEEDING						
					NUTRITIVE SUCK				NUTRITIVE SUCK						
					PATTERNS OF ELIMINATION				PATTERNS OF ELIMINATION						
					OBSERVE FEEDING				OBSERVE FEEDING						
BOTTLE	TEACH/REVIEW: USE OF BULB SYRINGE				INFANT CARE PAMPHLET				INFANT CARE PAMPHLET						
	ASSIST $\bar{c}$ 1st FEEDING				FREQUENCY/AMT OF FEEDING				FREQUENCY/AMT OF FEEDING				NIPPLE WELL $\bar{s}$ PROBLEMS		
					TEACH/REVIEW: FORMULA PREP				TEACH/REVIEW: FORMULA PREP				TOLERATES FORMULA FEEDINGS		
					BOTTLE CARE				BOTTLE CARE						
					BURPING				BURPING				MOTHER VERBALIZES UNDERSTANDING OF FORMULA FEEDING		
					HOME FEEDING SCHEDULE				HOME FEEDING SCHEDULE						
MEDICATIONS/ IMMUNIZATIONS															
	GIVE ILOTYCIN O.U. GIVE 1mg VIT K IM				GIVE IMMUNIZATION RECORD & BOOKLET TO PARENT(S)				GIVE IMMUNIZATION RECORD & BOOKLET TO PARENT(S)				BABY HAS RECEIVED ILOTYCIN BABY HAS RECEIVED VIT K		
	GIVE INFORMATIONAL PAMPHLET TO PARENT(S) ON HEPB VACCINE				IF ORDERED, GIVE HEPB VACCINE IM $\bar{p}$ OBTAINING PARENTAL PERMISSION				IF ORDERED, GIVE HEPB VACCINE IM $\bar{p}$ OBTAINING PARENTAL PERMISSION				BABY HAS RECEIVED FIRST HEP VACCINE IF ORDERED & E $\bar{c}$ PARENTAL PERMISSION		
TREATMENTS															
	OBTAIN CIRC PERMIT				OBTAIN CIRC PERMIT				OBTAIN CIRC PERMIT						
					ASSESS FOR BLEEDING $\bar{q}$ hr x 2-3 hrs				ASSESS FOR BLEEDING $\bar{q}$ hr x 2-3 hrs				CIRC CLEAN, DRY $\bar{s}$ SIGNS OF INFECTION OR BLEEDING		
					IF PLASTIBELL USED, GIVE PRINTED INFO TO PARENT(S)				IF PLASTIBELL USED, GIVE PRINTED INFO TO PARENT(S)				PLASTIBELL INFO GIVEN TO PARENT(S)		
					KEEP AREA CLEAN				KEEP AREA CLEAN						
					TEACH CARE TO PARENT(S)				TEACH CARE TO PARENT(S)						
					OBSERVE PARENT(S) GIVE CIRC CARE				OBSERVE PARENT(S) GIVE CIRC CARE				PARENT(S) ABLE TO RETURN DEMONSTRATE CIRC CARE		

7/95 "The CARE PATHWAYS™ are guidelines of suggestion for providing coordinated patient care. The pathways are not intended to replace well-reasoned, sound clinical judgement."

ST. MARY'S HEALTH CENTER
St. Louis, Missouri

UNCOMPLICATED NEWBORN CARE PATHWAYS©

(continued)

PT. LABEL

ADM. DATE______________ D = DAY SHIFT
DISC. DATE______________ E = EVE SHIFT
PATH START DATE______________ N = NOC SHIFT

DRG 391 PATH # 24

N/A = (cross through and initial)
COMPLETED = (initial)
TO BE COMPLETED = (circle in red, initial)

	1-3° p̄ DELIVERY	N	D	E	3-24° p̄ DELIVERY	N	D	E	24-48° p̄ DELIVERY DISCHARGE	N	D	E	OUTCOMES WRITE IN DATE OF COMPLETION	HOSP	PP
TESTS	GIVE PARENT(S) PAMPHLET ON METABOLIC SCREENING				EXPLAIN METABOLIC SCREENING & RESULTS				OBTAIN METABOLIC SCREENING				METABOLIC SCREENING COMPLETED		
													METABOLIC SCREENING RELEASE FORM SIGNED BY MOTHER		
													PARENT(S) VERBALIZE UNDERSTANDING OF NEED TO RETURN FOR TESTING		
ELIMINATION	NOTE VOIDINGS AND RECORD				RECORD VOIDINGS				RECORD VOIDINGS				VOIDINGS s̄ DIFFICULTY		
	NOTE BM AND RECORD				RECORD BMs				RECORD BMs				STOOLING s̄ DIFFICULTY		
					INSTRUCT CARE OF DIAPER AREA c̄ PARENT(S)				INSTRUCT CARE OF DIAPER AREA c̄ PARENT(S)						
TEACHING	INFANT CARE BOOKLET GIVE TO PARENT(S)				INFANT CARE (bathing, diapering, cord care, genital care)				INFANT CARE (bathing, diapering, cord care, genital care)				PARENT(S) DEMONSTRATES USE OF BULB SYRINGE, CORD CARE, CAPABILITY AT BEDSIDE		
	ORIENT PARENT(S) TO NURSERY				INFANT SAFETY (car seats, immunizations, metabolic screening)				INFANT SAFETY (car seats, immunizations, metabolic screening)				USES PROPER HYGIENE BEFORE BREAST FEEDING		
	INFANT POSITIONING				SIGNS/SYMPTOMS OF ILLNESS				SIGNS/SYMPTOMS OF ILLNESS				VERBALIZES UNDERSTANDING OF BABY CARE		
	HANDWASHING														
	INFANT IDENTIFICATION & SECURITY														
DISCHARGE PLANNING	ASSESS DISCHARGE NEEDS				REVIEW HOME PREPAREDNESS				REVIEW HOME PREPAREDNESS				DISCHARGE HOME c̄ FAMILY		
					CAR SEAT, CRIB, BABY CLOTHES & SUPPLIES				CAR SEAT, CRIB, BABY CLOTHES & SUPPLIES				APPOINTMENTS & REFERRALS MADE		
					W/C REFERRAL IF NEEDED				W/C REFERRAL IF NEEDED						
					FINAL D.C. TEACHING				FINAL D.C. TEACHING						
					DEAR DR. LETTER, IF NEEDED				DEAR DR. LETTER, IF NEEDED						
					PICTURE TAKEN				PICTURE TAKEN						
					METABOLIC SCREENING DONE				METABOLIC SCREENING DONE						
					CIRCUMCISION IF INDICATED				CIRCUMCISION IF INDICATED						
					FINAL BABY IDENTIFICATION				FINAL BABY IDENTIFICATION						
					SCHEDULE PP VISIT/HOME HEALTH				SCHEDULE PP VISIT/HOME HEALTH				VERBALIZES FLU APPT. TIME/DATE		
	SIGNATURES				SIGNATURES				SIGNATURES				SIGNATURES		

7/95 "The CARE PATHWAYS™ are guidelines of suggestion for providing coordinated patient care. The pathways are not intended to replace well-reasoned, sound clinical judgement."

ST. MARY'S HEALTH CENTER
St. Louis, Missouri

POST PARTUM HOME VISIT

PT. LABEL

INFANT ASSESSMENT

VITAL SIGNS: ____________________

FEEDING: ____________________

____

____

ELIMINATION: ____________________

COLOR: ____________________

ACTIVITY: ____________________

CORD CARE/CIRCUMCISION: ____________________

FUTURE INFANT NEEDS: PEDIATRIC FOLLOW-UP: ____________________

IMMUNIZATIONS: ____________________

MATERNAL ASSESSMENT

VITAL SIGNS: ____________________

BONDING/BEHAVIOR: ____________________

INCISION/EPISIOTOMY: ____________________

BREAST/NIPPLE: ____________________

ELIMINATION: ____________________

ADL'S: ____________________

MEDICATIONS: ____________________

HOME ENVIRONMENT/SAFETY

ASSESS NURSERY: ____________________

FORMULA PREPARATION AREA: ____________________

SAFETY: CAR SEAT: ____________________

PUMPKIN SEAT: ____________________

CRIB: ____________________

POTENTIAL HAZARDS *(electric cords, blind & drapery cords, burns, windows, toys)*: ____________________

____

REFERRALS

____

____

____

SIGNATURE: ____________________ DATE: ____________________

APPENDIX J.

Developed by: Susie Anderson RN,BSN
Susan Hoffstetter RN, BSN
Kathy Pimmel RN, BSN
Mary Jane Soehlke RN, BSN
Ron Tompkins RN, MA, MSN

APPENDIX K. Normal Spontaneous Vaginal Delivery MAP

Beth Israel Medical Center

MULTIDISCIPLINARY ACTION PLAN

DAY OF DELIVERY

MD/CNM: ______________________________

DIAGNOSIS: NORMAL SPONTANEOUS VAGINAL DELIVERY

RN/MD REVIEW: ______________________________

DATES: ______________________________

MAP DOES NOT REPLACE MD ORDERS

		VARIANCE
HISTORY/PHYSICAL EXAM/TESTS/ PROCEDURES/ TREATMENTS:	Ice to perineum PRN x24 hours. Vital signs Q12H. Call MD/CNM if T >100.4 or unable to void within 8H.	
MEDICATION:	IV D5LR + 10 units Pitocin/L x2. Dibucaine ointment and Tucks per rectum at bedside PRN for discomfort. Pain Medication ______________. Sleep Medication ______________. Stool Softener ______________. Rhogam, if needed.	
ACTIVITY:	Out of bed with assistance first time, then ad lib.	
NUTRITION:	Regular diet.	
CONSULTS:	VNS as indicated in discharge planning section. Social Work prn. Lactation Consultant prn. HIV Counselor prn.	
BREASTFEEDING: **- OR -**	IF BREASTFEEDING INSTRUCT PATIENT ABOUT: 1. Frequency and duration of feedings. 2. Offering breast in response to hunger cues. 3. Alternating breasts and burping infant. 4. Importance of draining first breast before offering second. 5. Risks of limiting length of feedings and bottles use. 6. Use of pillows to aid positioning. 7. Clutch and transitional positions. 8. Correct head, neck, and body alignment. 9. Repositioning for proper latch on and comfort.	
BOTTLEFEEDING:	IF BOTTLEFEEDING INSTRUCT PATIENT ABOUT: 1. Correct positioning of infant. 2. Frequency and amount of feedings. 3. Choice and preparation of formula. 4. Burping of infant.	
SOCIAL WORK:	Consult with RN and MD/CNM to screen for hi-risk psychosocial and discharge planning needs. Where appropriate initiate psychosocial assessment and discharge plan.	
DISCHARGE PLANNING:	Determine individual patient needs. Initiate proper referrals and consults as needed. Refer to HHIC for home health care assessment.	
PATIENT VARIANCE: (on admission)		

DATE/SHIFT	INITIALS	PRINT NAME/TITLE	SIGNATURE/TITLE

APPENDIX K. Normal Spontaneous Vaginal Delivery MAP cont.

Beth Israel Medical Center

MULTIDISCIPLINARY ACTION PLAN

DAY 1 OF 2

MD/CNM: ______________________

DIAGNOSIS: NORMAL SPONTANEOUS VAGINAL DELIVERY

DATES: ______________________

MAP DOES NOT REPLACE MD ORDERS

PATIENT PROBLEM	EXPECTED PATIENT OUTCOME/ DISCHARGE OUTCOME	NURSING INTERVENTIONS	ASSESSMENT/INTERVENTION/OUTCOME SHIFT:	SHIFT:
1. Alternation in body systems R/T post-partum period	1A. Vital signs within normal limits. B. Fundus firm at midline within 24 hours. C. Lochia scant to moderate rubra. D. Patient without signs or symptoms of post-partum complications (i.e. infection, phlebitis, bleeding, and breast problems).	1A. Vital signs Q12H and PRN. B. Palpate fundus for height and consistency Q12H and PRN. C. Observe lochia for color, odor and amt. D. Assess perineum for intactness, swelling, redness, odor, bleeding, and hemorrhoids. E. Assess for bladder distention, measure and record first void, question patient re: frequency and amount of void. F. Asses for phlebitis re: redness, swelling, pain, and +/- Homan's sign. G. Assess for: - prior surgery, symmetry, and fullness - nipple trauma and breast inflammation.		
2. Alteration in comfort related to post-partum period	2A. Patient will experience minimum discomfort. B. Patient will verbalize relief of pain after interventions implemented.	2A. <u>FOR PERINEAL/RECTAL PAIN</u>: - Provide ice packs for first 24° prn. - Provide dibucaine, tucks, and Sitz bath (prn) upon admission. B. <u>FOR UTERINE CRAMPS:</u> - Administer pain med prn. C. <u>FOR BREAST DISCOMFORT</u>: - Assess breasts for engorgement and inflammation. - Instruct patient on how to prevent engorgement. - Apply cool compress to reduce tissue swelling. - Refer to lactation staff if problem persists for 1 shift. D. <u>FOR NIPPLE PAIN</u> - Determine cause of pain. - Develop care plan to resolve cause of pain. E. Assess for pain relief (i.e. perineal, uterine, breast, nipple).		
3. Knowledge deficit R/T self-care	3A. Patient states she knows who to call if F/U needed and when post partum checkup is scheduled. B. Patient verbalizes understanding of written and verbal instructions on selfcare activities and breastfeeding.	3A. Review discharge plan and date with patient and/or significant other. B. Follow breastfeeding or bottle feeding teaching plan. C. Provide written and verbal instructions about: - Diet and exercise. - Contraception. - Sexual activity and return of menstruation and ovulation. - Medications. - Signs of complications. D. Provide information about postpartum checkup appointment. E. Provide information about support groups and community services if applicable.		
4. Alteration in family process R/T addition of new family member	4A. Parent(s) will demonstrate good coping skills, acceptance and understanding of role and responsibility as parent(s). B. Demonstrates positive Parenting behaviors.	4A. Assess parenting behaviors. B. Include significant others in teaching and discharge planning. C. Discuss the difference between postpartum blues and depression, and how support system, hormones, rest, and nutrition influence the problem.		

APPENDIX K. Normal Spontaneous Vaginal Delivery MAP cont.

Beth Israel Medical Center
MULTIDISCIPLINARY ACTION PLAN
DAY 2 OF 2

MD/CNM: ______________________________
DIAGNOSIS: NORMAL SPONTANEOUS VAGINAL DELIVERY
DATES: ______________________________

MAP DOES NOT REPLACE MD ORDERS

PATIENT PROBLEM	EXPECTED PATIENT OUTCOME/ DISCHARGE OUTCOME	NURSING INTERVENTIONS	ASSESSMENT/INTERVENTION/OUTCOME SHIFT:	SHIFT:
1. Alternation in body systems R/T post-partum period	1A. Vital signs within normal limits. B. Fundus firm at midline within 24 hours. C. Lochia scant to moderate rubra. D. Patient without signs or symptoms of post-partum complications (i.e. infection, phlebitis, bleeding, and breast problems).	1A. Vital signs Q12H and PRN. B. Palpate fundus for height and consistency Q12H and PRN. C. Observe lochia for color, odor, and amount. D. Assess perineum for intactness, swelling, redness, odor, bleeding, and hemorrhoids. E. Assess for bladder distention, measure and record first void, question patient re: frequency and amount of void. F. Asses for phlebitis re: redness, swelling, pain, and +/- Homan's sign. G. Assess for: - prior surgery, symmetry, and fullness. - nipple trauma and breast inflammation.		
2. Alteration in comfort related to post-partum period	2A. Patient will experience minimum discomfort. B. Patient will verbalize relief of pain after interventions implemented.	2A. FOR PERINEAL/RECTAL PAIN: - Provide ice packs for first 24° PRN. - Provide dibucaine, tucks, and Sitz bath (prn) upon admission. B. FOR UTERINE CRAMPS: - Administer pain med prn. C. FOR BREAST DISCOMFORT: - Assess breasts for engorgement and inflammation. - Instruct patient on how to prevent engorgement. - Apply cool compress to reduce tissue swelling. - Refer to lactation staff if problem persists for 1 shift. D. FOR NIPPLE PAIN - Determine cause of pain. - Develop care plan to resolve cause of pain. E. Assess for pain relief (i.e. perineal, uterine, breast, nipple).		
3. Knowledge deficit R/T self-care	3A. Patient states she knows who to call if F/U needed and when post partum checkup is scheduled. B. Patient verbalizes understanding of written and verbal instructions on selfcare activities and breastfeeding.	3A. Follow breastfeeding or bottle feeding teaching plan. B. Provide written and verbal instructions about: - Diet and exercise. - Contraception. - Sexual activity and return of menstruation and ovulation. - Medications. - Signs of complications. C. Provide information about postpartum checkup appointment. D. Provide information about support groups and community services if applicable.		
4. Alteration in family process R/T addition of new family member	4A. Parent(s) will demonstrate good coping skills, acceptance and understanding of role and responsibility as parent(s). B. Demonstrates positive Parenting behaviors.	4A. Assess parenting behaviors. B. Include significant others in teaching and discharge planning. C. Answer all questions pertaining to parenting and discharge.		

APPENDIX L. The Laboring Patient Clincial Pathway

KQC:

- **Mom identifies individual learning needs.**
- **Mom verbalizes & demonstrates effective infant feeding processes as observed by RN.**

KPV:

- **Indicated on pathway with an "*".**

THE LABORING PATIENT

DEFINITION:

MONTEVIDEO UNITS: Equal number of contractions per 10 minutes multiplied by the contraction pressure.

OUTCOMES	ADMISSION ---> 2ND STAGE
PAIN	___ Pt. demonstrates adequate pain relief.
KNOWLEDGE	___ Pt. understands labor process
FAMILY PROCESS	___ Pt's. support person is identified; individual customs and ethnic background recognized.
PROGRESSION OF LABOR	___ Labor pattern established: External: 2-5 contractions in 10 minutes lasting at least 40 seconds OR Internal: > 200 Montevideo units in 10 minutes. ___ Primip with cerv. chg. > 1.2 cm/hr. in active labor ___ Multip with cerv. chg. > 1.5 cm/hr. in active labor ___ Prolonged latent phase is not > 20 hr. (nullip); > 14 hr. (multip) ___ Essential primip with 2nd stage < 2 hr., or 3 hr. with epidural ___ Multip with 2nd stage < 1 hr., or 2 hr. with epidural ___ Has adequate descent of the presenting part.
FETAL WELLBEING	___ Initial reassuring 20" external monitor strip ___ Ongoing reassuring fetal heart pattern

June 3, 1994

Fairview Health Systems, Minneapolis, MN.

APPENDIX L. Patient Progress

PATIENT PROGRESS
RECORD/LABORING
PATIENT

V = Variance
A = Action plan

DATE	TIME	

DATE	
RN	
MD	
SOCIAL WORKER	
WOMANKIND	
PASTORAL CARE	
CONSULTS	

June 3, 1994

ADMIT DATE/TIME______ ROOM NO.:__________	ADMIT STATUS: ☐ OP ☐ IP	DISCHARGE STATUS ☐Delivered ☐Undelivered ☐Transfer

NURSING ADMISSION DATA BASE SECTION A

NAME__________ DOB__________ AGE________ MARITAL STATUS__________
SPK/SPNK/AGENCY/CONTACT__________ PHONE__________ BABY'S LAST NAME__________
F.O.B. INVOLVED ☐YES ☐NO SUPPORT PERSON__________
MD/CNM__________ CLINIC__________ BABY DOCTOR__________

PAST OB HISTORY	G	T	PT	A	L	LMP	EDD/DATE	EDD/US	GEST

C/S PIH PPH PTL PREGNANCY LOSS OTHER:

DELIVERY HX

SIBLING HEALTH - NORMAL, "ABNORMALITIES":

PRESENT OB HISTORY: INFERTILITY BLEEDING PIH ANEMIA VERSION VBAC
CTX: Onset/Frequency:__________ Labor start date__________ Time__________
MEMBRANES: Intact Ruptured Date________ Time________ COLOR: Clear____ Odor______ Meconium: ☐Thin ☐Moderate ☐Thick/Particulate
OTHER__________
PTL (Tocolytics/Dates)__________
DIABETES (Type/Control)__________ Height________ Weight__________
HOME CARE AGENCY__________ REASON__________
Allergies__________ Band On______
Alcohol Consumption__________ Tobacco__________ Chemicals Used__________ Date Last Used______ Toxicology Screen_
FEEDING: Breast Bottle Previous Problems__________
CIRCUMCISION: ☐Yes ☐No PPTL: ☐Yes ☐No Prenatal Education: ☐Yes ☐No PHN/HH Agency__________

Special Requests:__________
Are you now or have you ever been in a relationship where you have been abused physically, emotionally, or sexually? ☐Yes ☐No ☐Not asked

LABS	ANTENATAL TESTING			MEDICATIONS THIS PREGNANCY			
Blood type/Rh:		Date	Result	Medication	Dose	Freq.	Last Dose
Rh immune globulin:	Amnio						
Rubella: ☐Immune	CVS						
☐Not Immune	US						
Hepatitis B:							
HIV:	BPP			Meds brought to hospital ☐Yes ☐No			
STD's: gonorrhea/herpes/chlamydia/syphilis				Disposition:__________			
Beta Strep:	NST						
Sickle Cell:	CST						

ORIENTATION TO ROOM: (Call Light, Bed, TV/Radio, Smoking Policy, Visiting Hours) ☐Yes ☐No

Initials/Signatures	

NURSING ADMISSION DATA BASE

FAIRVIEW RIDGES
Clinical Pathway

LABORING PATIENT - POSTPARTUM

PROBLEM/FOCUS	3RD/4TH STAGE --> 12H Date_______Time_______to Date_____Time______
PAIN	___ ___ Pt. states pain relief is adequate
PHYSIOLOGICAL CHANGES	___ Delivery of viable infant ___ Pt. delivers placenta within 30" ___ ___ ___ Emptying bladder ___ ___ ___ Uterus involuting ___ ___ ___ Moderate or minimal lochia (< 500 cc total blood loss) ___ ___ ___ VS WNL ___ ___ ___ Perineum intact ___ ___ ___ Hydration maintained
KNOWLEDGE	*Pt. identifies individual learning needs: ___ ___ Pt. verbalizes understanding of physiologic changes ___ ___ Pt. verbalizes comfort with infant
FAMILY PROCESS	___ ___ ___ Positive family interactions ___ ___ ___ Active involvement by support person ___ ___ ___ Demonstrates positive infant bonding
INTERVENTIONS	
TESTS	___ Rh studies as appropriate
TREATMENTS	___ ___ IV access maintained as appropriate ___ ___ Perineal ice pack ___ ___ Perineal hygiene instruction ___ ___ Topical preparation for: ☐Episiotomy ☐Hemorrhoids ___ If unable to void, cath per MD order
MEDICATIONS	___ Discuss oral pain med availability ___ Oxytocin prn ___ Stool softener
NUTRITION	___ ___ Diet as tolerated ___ ___ Fluids encouraged
SAFETY	___ Pt instructed on use of nurse call light, bed controls, need for BR assist. 1st time up, no smoking policy.
ACTIVITY/ HYGIENE	___ ___ Up as tolerated with assist ___ Shower ___ ___ Encourage rest
TEACHING	Formulate teaching plan using: ___ CCTV with schedule review ___ Folder/literature review ___ ___ Promote good handwashing ___ Instruct on emptying bladder ___ ___ Assisted with baby's nutrition as per baby pathway.*
DISCHARGE COORDINATION/ PLANNING	___ Review data base for abuse assessment Ask this question if not asked on admission: Are you now or have you ever been in a relationship where you have been abused physcially, emotionally or sexually? ☐ Yes ☐ No ___ Assess for risk factors ___ Referral as appropriate: ☐Social Service ☐Fairview Home Health ☐Chaplain ☐Public Health Referral to:_________(County) ☐WomanKind ☐Other:_______________ • Anticiated discharge: Date_________Time_____________

APPENDIX L. Patient Progress

PATIENT PROGRESS RECORD/LABORING PATIENT

V = Variance
A = Action plan

DATE	TIME	

DATE				
RN				
MD				
SOCIAL WORKER				
WOMANKIND				
PASTORAL CARE				
CONSULTS				

June 3, 1994

FAIRVIEW RIDGES
Clinical Pathway

LABORING PATIENT - POSTPARTUM

TIMEFRAME: 4th Stage Labor --> Discharge from Hospital

Key Quality Characteristics:
- Mom identifies individual learning needs.
- Mom verbalizes and demonstrates effective infant feeding process as observed by RN.

Key Process Variables: Indicated on pathway with an "*".

DATE	12-24 HR Date______ Time______ to Date________ Time________
PAIN	___ ___ Pt. states pain relief is adequate
PHYSIOLOGICAL CHANGES	___ ___ ___ Emptying bladder ___ ___ ___ Uterus involuting ___ ___ ___ Moderate or minimal lochia (< 500 cc total blood loss) ___ ___ ___ VS WNL ___ ___ ___ Perineum intact ___ ___ ___ Hydration maintained
KNOWLEDGE	*Baseline educational needs identified by pt's. nurse ___ ___ Pt. learning about infant cares ___ ___ Pt. demonstrates ability to do self cares
INTERVENTIONS	
TESTS	• Hb as appropriate_____
TREATMENTS	___ ___ Topical preparation for: ☐Episiotomy ☐Hemorrhoids ___ Instruction sitz ___ Positioning instructions • If unable to void, cath per MD order
MEDICATIONS	___ ___ Pain meds ___Take home meds ___Oxytocin prn ___Rh immune globulin & MR as appropriate ___Stool softener
NUTRITION	___ ___ Diet as tolerated
SAFETY	
ACTIVITY/ HYGIENE	___ ___Up ad lib without assist. ___Encourage rest ___Shower
TEACHING	•Reinforce plan ___ ___ CCTV being observed ___Instruction sheet(s) reviewed ___Breastfeeding handout reviewed •Information/demonstration basic infant care as appropriate: ___diapering ___burping ___jaundice ___cord care ___feeding ___circumcision care
DISCHARGE COORDINATION/ PLANNING	___ Discharge plan developed and initiated (specify):
PHYSICIAN ASSESSMENT	Date/Time:__________________ ___VSS ___Normal lochia ___Epis. intact ___Fundus firm ___Voiding ___Other:________________ ___Discharge meds Signature:____________________

34-2468 DEVELOPED BY: FRH/FSH/FRMC; DATE DEVELOPED: 8/93; DATE REVISED: June 3, 1994

APPENDIX L. Patient Progress

PATIENT PROGRESS
RECORD

V = Variance
A = Action plan

DATE	TIME	

FAIRVIEW RIDGES
Clinical Pathway

LABORING PATIENT - POSTPARTUM

PROBLEM/FOCUS	24 Hrs + Date_____ Time_____
PAIN	___ ___ ___ Pt. states pain relief is adequate
PHYSIOLOGICAL CHANGES POST DELIVERY	___ ___ ___ Emptying bladder ___ ___ ___ Fundus firm ___ ___ ___ Moderate or minimal lochia ___ ___ ___ VSS ___ ___ ___ Perineum clean & intact
KNOWLEDGE	___ ___ ___ Reinforcement teaching needs identified
FAMILY PROCESS	___ ___ ___ Positive family interactions ___ ___ ___ Active involvement by support person with cares of mom & infant ___ ___ ___ Demonstrates positive infant bonding
INTERVENTIONS	
MEDICATIONS	___ ___ ___ Pain meds ___ Rh immune globulin or MR if unable to give in 24 hours
ACTIVITY/ HYGIENE	___ ___ ___ Shower/sitz
TEACHING	• Reinforcement teaching on: ___ ___ ___ ____________ ___ ___ ___ ____________ ___ ___ ___ ____________
DISCHARGE COORDINATION/ PLANNING	• Continued assessment of needs & referral as appropriate:____________ ____________

PROBLEM/FOCUS	AT DISCHARGE DATE__________ TIME__________
PAIN	___ Pt. able to manage discomfort with comfort measures & oral pain meds ___ Pt. able to manage ADL and care of infant or have assistance at home
KNOWLEDGE	• Pt. states/demonstrates knowledge of: ___ basic postpartum hygiene/care ___ basic infant care & feedings
FAMILY PROCESS	___ Pt. identifies and utilizes support systems/person(s)
PHYSIOLOGIC CHANGES POST DELIVERY	___ ___ ___ Emptying bladder ___ ___ ___ Moderate or minimal lochia ___ ___ ___ VSS ___ ___ ___ No signs of infection
PHYSICIAN ASSESSMENT	Date/time:____________ ___ VSS ___ Normal lochia ___ Epis. intact ___ Fundus firm ___ Voiding ___ Other:____________ Discharge meds:____________ Signature:____________

8

APPENDIX L. Patient Progress Record

PATIENT PROGRESS RECORD

V = Variance
A = Action plan

DATE	TIME	

APPENDIX L. Newborn Baby Clinical Pathway

FAIRVIEW RIDGES
Clinical Pathway

NEWBORN BABY

PROBLEM/FOCUS	Birth ---> 12h Date:____ to Date:___ Time:____ to Time:___	12-24 Hours Date:____ to Date:___ Time:____ to Time:___
Newborn Stabilization	___ ___Assessments & any tests done are WNL. ___ ___TPR is stabilized - WNL. ___ ___*Newborn able to latch & suck	___ ___Newborn able to latch & suck ___ ___TPR is stabilized - WNL
Potential for bleeding from circumcision		___ ___No excess bleeding
INTERVENTIONS		
Assessments and Vital Signs	• Physical & gestational age assessments.	• Assessments & VS
Tests/Procedures	___ Initial glucose screening on LGA, SGA, IDM & symptomatic babies. ___ Lab/x-rays if indicated	___ Lab/x-rays if indicated
Activity/Hygiene	___ Initial bath after T. regulated. ___ Parents instructed on good handwashing	
Medications	• Vit. K. & Erythromycin	
Safety/Security	___ Parents instructed on infant safety: transport per crib, bulb syringe, position change. Security: ID bands, baby not left unattended. ___ Car seat safety.	___ Newborn photo ID
Nutrition/ Teaching	___ ___ Breastfed baby given opportunity to nurse with assistance. ___ Bottle fed baby has first feed with assist or by nurse.	___ ___ Baby feeding 2-4h or as tolerated & mother aware to request assist when needed ___ Circ. care instructions
Discharge Coordination/ Planning		___ Family - infant bonding observed/assessed Anticipated discharge: Date _______________ Time _______________
Physician assessment		___ Circumcision as applicable Date/Time____________ Method____________ Analgesic____________ ___ Reportable infant signs discussed with parent(s)

Fairview Health Systems, Minneapolis, MN.

APPENDIX L. Newborn Baby Clinical Pathway cont.

PATIENT PROGRESS RECORD

V = Variance
A = Action plan

DATE	TIME	

APPENDIX L. Newborn Baby Clinical Pathway cont.

FAIRVIEW RIDGES
Clinical Pathway

NEWBORN BABY

TIMEFRAME: Birth ---> discharge from hospital
Key Quality Characteristics:
- **Mom identifies individual learning needs.**
- **Mom verbalizes and demonstrates effective infant feeding process as observed by RN**

Key Process Variables: Indicated on pathway with a "*".

PROBLEM/FOCUS	24 Hours + Date:____ Time:_____ to discharge	BY DISCHARGE Date:______ Time:________
Newborn Stabilization	___ ___ ___ Baby able to latch, suck, swallow with feedings. ___ ___ ___ VSS ___ ___ ___ Voiding and stooling in adequate amounts.	• Infant discharged with ___ VSS ___ Voiding & stooling ___ Able to latch, suck, swallow w/feedings ___ Minimal regurgitation ___ No clinical signs of infection.
Potential for bleeding from circumcision	___ ___ ___ No excess bleeding	___ ___ ___ No excess bleeding
INTERVENTIONS		
Assessments and Vital Signs	___ ___ ___ Assess for jaundice	
Tests/Procedures		• Metabolic screen: - >24°______ - <24°______
Safety/Security		___ ID bands matched at discharge ___ Car seat safety discussed
Nutrition/ Teaching and Discharge Planning	• Continued assessment of needs • Reinforcement assistance/teaching with: ___ ___ ___ ___ ___ ___ ____________ ___ ___ ___ ___ ___ ___ ____________ ___ ___ ___ ___ ___ ___ ____________	___ Complimentary formula pack given & preparation procedures discussed ___ Referral as appropriate:____________ ____________________________
Physician Assessment	___ Circumcision as applicable Date/time______________ Method______________ Analgesic______________ ___ Reportable infant signs discussed with parent(s) Noteworthy information:	___ Circumcision as applicable Date/time______________ Method______________ Analgesic______________ ___ Reportable infant signs discussed with parent(s) Noteworthy information:

APPENDIX M. Vaginal Birth Clinical Map

UNIVERSITY of ILLINOIS at CHICAGO MEDICAL CENTER
DEPARTMENT of NURSING
PARENT CHILD HEALTH DIVISION

CLINICAL MAP

DRG ______________ Case Manager ______________________ Ext_______

Case Type ***NSVD: INTRAPARTUM*** ____________________ Expected LOS ***2 DAYS***

Attending Physician/Resident __________________ Primary Resident/Midwife__________________

Patient Problems/Nursing Diagnoses

1. Potential for infection R/T multiple vaginal exams and/or prolonged rupture of membranes 2. Potential for fluid volume deficit R/T limitation of oral intake and diaphoresis

3. Pain R/T uterine contractions and cervical dilatation 4. Altered pattern of urinary elimination R/T pressure of presenting part and to anesthesia

5. Anxiety R/T unknown surroundings & procedures, absent childbirth education, fatigue or excitement 6. Potential for Fetal Injury R/T uteroplacental insufficiency

CATEGORY	*OUTCOME*	*Admission - 1 Hour* / /	*1 Hour - Delivery* / /
ASSESSMENT FOCUS	- VS WNL - Maternal-fetal well-being will be maintained throughout antepartum course - No S/S of infection - Minimal discomfort	VS taken in triage and labor room Evaluate fetus by EFM for minimum 30 minutes Systems review per admission assessment. OB Data base initiated Evaluate risk, monitor per protocol. Evaluate pts decision/obtain consent for: Newborn circumcision	If membranes intact, temp Q 4 hrs. If ROM, temp Q 1 hr. P, RR, BP Q 1 hr. EFM/Auscultation per policy OB Database Systems review Q shift Assess patient for risks, consider intermittent FHT auscultation: - 1st Stage (latent phase), Q 60 min each hour - 1st Stage (>4 cm, active labor, transition), Q 30 min each hour - 2nd Stage (pushing), Q 15 min each hour

APPENDIX M. Vaginal Birth Clinical Map cont.

CATEGORY	*OUTCOME*	*Admission - 1 Hour* / /	*1 Hour - Delivery* / /
LAB TESTS	- Lab results WNL - If not WNL, appropriate follow-up initiated.	Pts with prenatal care at UIH & C: CBC with diff RPR Type and Screen Pts ***not*** registered at UIH & C: Type and Screen CBC with Diff RPR HBSAG Urine toxicology screen Cervical cultures GBBS culture	Lab results normal_____ Lab results abnormal, reported to MD/CNM_____
DIAGNOSTIC TESTING		Pts ***not*** registered at UIH & C, ultrasound for fetal presentation Ultrasound for fetal presentation, as ordered Nitrazine/ferning test as indicated	Scalp pH as ordered
ACTIVITY/POSITIONING	- Labor progresses within expected timeframes for each stage	May ambulate, if: - Fetal well-being established via EFM - Membranes intact; or if ROM, presenting part well applied to cervix - MD/CNM order	May ambulate on 4th floor only; to return to L & D every 30-60 minutes or if ROM occurs Position as appropriate for stage of labor: LL Sims Right side Squatting Semifowlers Sitting
TREATMENTS	- Pain within tolerable limits - FHR pattern remains reassuring throughout labor	Effleurage Warm packs to back/ cold cloths to neck forehead Shower Epidural, per MD with patient discussion O_2 per reservoir type mask, as indicated by fetal status LL/RL position	--> --> --> --> --> Amnioinfusion for variable decels and/or thick meconium per MD order
MEDS/IVS	- Hydration, glucose & energy levels maintained during labor - Pain relief effective	IV fluids for : - non-reassuring FHR pattern - maternal fever - inability to tolerate PO hydration - pain management	--> IV Narcotics per MD order
DIET	- No risk of aspiration for patients with possibility of C-section - Energy levels maintained	NPO except for clear liquids per MD/CNM order Ice chips	Strict NPO, if potential C-section

APPENDIX M. Vaginal Birth Clinical Map cont.

CATEGORY	OUTCOME	Admission - 1 Hour / /	1 Hour - Delivery / /
PSYCHOSOCIAL/ SPIRITUAL NEEDS		Introduce self as primary caregiver, orient to environment, determine religious preferences Explain all procedures Encourage participation of significant other Determine level of childbirth preparation Identify potential risk factors for maternal-infant attachment Be sensitive and accommodate as possible cultural differences and needs	 ---> ---> Provide appropriate coaching through L&D experience
REFERRALS/CONSULTS	- Referrals made within 24 - 48 hrs of identified need	Identify factors that may create need for referrals/consultations: Lactation consultant Social services Anesthesia	Initiate referrals/consultations as indicated
PATIENT/FAMILY EDUCATION	- Patient will care for self independently. - Patient can identify warning signs of illness for self.	Discuss with patient and labor coach: the labor process dilatation, comfort techniques and non-pharmaceutical interventions to decrease pain	Initiate self-assessment of learning needs by 3rd hour. Initiate breastfeeding at delivery, if appropriate.
DISCHARGE PLANNING	- Special discharge needs identified	Inform patient of discharge at 48 hrs.	Discuss time and day of discharge (48 hrs post delivery)
SIGNATURE *Day* *Eve* *Noc* *** CIRCLE INTERVENTION, IF NOT COMPLETED WITHIN SPECIFIED TIME FRAME*		____________________ ____________________ ____________________	____________________ ____________________ ____________________

APPENDIX M. Vaginal Birth/Postpartum Clinical Map

UNIVERSITY of ILLINOIS at CHICAGO MEDICAL CENTER
DEPARTMENT of NURSING
PARENT CHILD HEALTH DIVISION

CLINICAL MAP

DRG ______________ Case Manager __________________ Ext ______

Case Type ***NSVD: POSTPARTUM with REACTIVE RPR*** Expected LOS ***2 DAYS***

Attending Physician/Resident __________________ Primary Resident/Midwife__________________

Patient Problems/Nursing Diagnoses

1. Potential for infection R/T multiple vaginal exams and/or prolonged rupture of membranes 2. Potential for fluid volume deficit R/T blood loss

3. Pain R/T episiotomy repair and contracting uterus 4. Altered pattern of urinary elimination R/T trauma, overdistension, and/or anesthesia

5. Knowledge deficit R/T self care after delivery 6. Potential for Ineffective Breastfeeding

CATEGORY	*OUTCOME*	*DELIVERY - 3° PP* / /	*PP ADM - 6° PP* / /	*7 - 12 HRS PP* / /	*12 - 24 HRS PP* / /	*24 - 48 HRS PP* / /
ASSESSMENT FOCUS	- VS WNL - No S/S of infection - No S/S of excessive bleeding - Normal involution process - Minimal discomfort - Pt will void by 6 hours PP - Pt will be demonstrate self care	VS Q 15min x 4, Q 30min x2, then Q 1 hr x 1 Assess: Fundus with VS Lochia with VS Perineum with VS Bladder for distension Time of first void:_____ Nipples, if breastfeeding Pain	VS upon transfer & within 2 hrs thereafter. ------------------------> ------------------------> ------------------------> ------------------------> ------------------------> ------------------------> ------------------------> Maternal - infant attachment behaviors	VS Q shift 8 point PP assessment Q shift ------------------------> ------------------------>	------------------------> ------------------------> ------------------------> ------------------------>	------------------------> ------------------------> ------------------------> ------------------------>
LAB TESTS	- Lab results WNL - If not WNL, appropriate follow-up initiated		Check results: Blood type & Rh_____ Rubella__________ RPR__________ HBSAG__________ ***Report abnormal values to OB and Pediatric services***	CBC (within 8 - 12 hrs PP) If PPTL to be done, record on Pre-Op Checklist: PP H/H____ PAP Smear results____ If RPR reactive, screen for: Chlamydia Gonorrhea HIV (if patient consents)	CBC results: Normal,____ Abnormal, notify MD or CNM___	CBC (AM of Discharge)
DIAGNOSTIC TESTING		If PPD (+) and no current CXR, obtain CXR.				

APPENDIX M. Vaginal Birth/Postpartum Clinical Map cont.

CATEGORY	OUTCOME	DELIVERY - 3° PP / /	PP ADM - 6° PP / /	7 - 12 HRS PP / /	12 - 24 HRS PP / /	24 - 48 HRS PP / /
ACTIVITY/POSITIONING	- Resumption of normal activity within safe limits	Assist to BR for 1st void.	Encourage/observe patient to perform care for self and infant.	Independent in care of self and infant with RN as resource Instruct pt on Kegel exercises. Provide handout.	----------------------------> Encourage patient to perform Kegel exercises.	----------------------------> ---------------------------->
TREATMENTS	- Discomfort within tolerable level for patient	Ice pack to perineum	----------------------------> Tucks for hemorrhoids PRN	----------------------------> ---------------------------->	----------------------------> ----------------------------> Sitz bath TID	 ----------------------------> ---------------------------->
MEDS/IVS	- Pain/discomfort within tolerable level for patient	IV D/C'd unless other wise indicated. Pain meds PRN	Tucks/dermoplast PRN	----------------------------> Prenatal vitamins with iron as ordered If 1°, 2°, or early latent Syphilis, ***Benzathine penicillin G 2.4 million units IM once*** (1.2 million units in each buttock) If Late latent or late latent of unknown duration Syphilis, ***Benzathine penicillin G 7.2 million units total administered as 3 doses*** of 2.4 million units IM given 1 week apart for 3 consecutive weeks	----------------------------> ----------------------------> If infant Rh (+) and Mom Rh (-), administer RhoGam	----------------------------> ----------------------------> If mom not Rubella immune, administer Rubella vaccine
DIET	- Tolerates full diet	General diet	---------------------------->	---------------------------->	---------------------------->	---------------------------->
PSYCHOSOCIAL/ SPIRITUAL NEEDS	- Evidence of attachment between mother, infant and significant other - Verbalizes satisfaction with birth process within context of cultural/spiritual beliefs	Assess patients coping mechanisms, support system, and evidence of attachment to infant Provide opportunities for maternal infant attachment to occur.	----------------------------> Provide pt with info re: normal feelings/emotions which can occur post-partum	----------------------------> ---------------------------->	----------------------------> ---------------------------->	---------------------------->

APPENDIX M. Vaginal Birth/Postpartum Clinical Map cont.

CATEGORY	OUTCOME	DELIVERY - 3° PP / /	PP ADM - 6° PP / /	7 - 12 HRS PP / /	12 - 24 HRS PP / /	24 - 48 HRS PP / /
REFERRALS/CONSULTS	- Referrals made within 24 - 48 hrs of identified need	Lactation consultant/CNM PRN.	-------------------------->	---------------------------	-------------------------> WIC Form completed. BOH/VNA referral completed.	
PATIENT/FAMILY EDUCATION	- Patient will care for self independently. - Patient can identify warning signs of illness for self.	Initiate mother care teaching plan. Identify priority areas for learning. Provide Mother-Baby Pamphlet.	Encourage participation in/teach priority self care needs	----------------------------> Provide education re:syphilis/treatment/complications	---------------------------> Reinforce syphilis education	---------------------------> --------------------------->
DISCHARGE PLANNING	- All follow-up appointments made - Pt feels prepared to care for self at home	Discharge notification letter provided(identifies time/date of discharge)				Verbalizes F/U Appointments: Family Planning/Gyn (4-6 wks)____ Dermatology (1 wk x 2) ____
SIGNATURE *Day* *Eve* *Noc* *** CIRCLE INTERVENTION, IF NOT COMPLETED WITHIN SPECIFIED TIME FRAME*		____ ____ ____	____ ____ ____	____ ____ ____	____ ____ ____	____ ____ ____

E9

INTEGRATED CLINICAL PATHWAY

VAGINAL DELIVERY W/ & W/O TUBAL LIGATION
DRG #372 & 373
Mothers OB/GYN Physician: ________________
Family Physician: ________________
Baby's Physician: ________________
Primary RN: ________________
Date Reviewed by MD/RN/Patient: ____________
Advance Directive: Yes_____ No_____

MEDICAL HISTORY

Admit Date	Transfer Date:	Transfer To:	Allergies:

Present Problem: ________________

Past History: ________________

Surgical & Special Procedures: ________________

ABO/Rh: Maternal ________ Newborn ________
Rubella: Immune ________ Non-Immune ________
HBsAg: Negative ________ Positive ________

Multi Disciplinary Consults:

Date	Consultant	Reason	First Visit	Signed Off

DISCHARGE PLANNING

Discharge Destination	Date/Time	Initial	Community Services	Date	Initial	Equipment	Date	Initial
Home w/________			Childbirth Education			Home Oxygen		
			Parenting Education			Home IV Therapy: ____		
Other: ________			Lactation Consultant					
			WIC/Baby Care			Home Phototherapy		
			Social Services			Apnea Monitor		
			MWH/Perinatal Connections			Breast Pump		
			Business Office			Terb. Pump		
			Grief Follow-up			HUAM ________		
			VNA/CHN			Insulin Pump		
			LSS/CSS/SSS			Home Blood Glucose		
			Support Group ________			Monitor: ________		
						Papa Pager		
			Other: ________			O2 Sat		
						Diabetic Supplies		
						BP Machine: ________		
						Other : ________		

Initials/Signature:
____/________ ____/________ ____/________
____/________ ____/________

47 OFF PATHWAY ☐ YES
DATE ____/____/____

02/94 CHART FORM

APPENDIX N. Integrated Vaginal Birth Clinical Pathway cont.

DAY/DATE	First Stage of Labor Admit Date __________ Time ________	Second & Third Stage of Labor Date ________ Delivery Time __________
CONSULTS	Resident to complete H and P Maternal/infant physician notified of admission	Notify appropriate personnel of impending birth
LABS X-RAY OTHER	CBC without diff. Type & Rh Antibody HBSAG - if not on history Urine dipstick for protein & ketones	Cord blood gases prn
TREATMENTS	Enema prn No routine prep Clip prn Fetal monitor to document reactivity	Forceps/Vacuum extraction
MEDICATIONS/ IVs	IV/hep lock prn Analgesics/sedatives Oxytocin Epidural	IV/hep lock prn Oxytocin IM or IV Epidural Local/pudendal
NUTRITION	Ice chips Popsicles Clear liquids	Ice chips
ACTIVITY/PT SAFETY	As patient desires unless contraindicated	Position for delivery
DISCHARGE PLANNING	Review/initiate data base	
NURSING DX/ INTERDISCI-PLINARY FOCUS	Anxiety Fetal tissue perfusion Fluid volume Potential for infection Comfort Knowledge	Anxiety Fetal tissue perfusion: resolved Potential: postpartum hemorrhage Potential for infection Comfort Fluid volume
KEY NURSING ACTIVITIES/ TEACHING	Assessment within 30 min. of admission TPR & BP q 4 hrs (early labor) P, R & BP q 1 hr (active labor) Assess FHR/UA q 15 min if high risk Assess FHR/UA q 30 min if low risk Assist to void q 2 hrs/straight cath prn Cervical exam prn I&O Implement coping/relaxation techniques Institute Advance Directive Policy Review clinical pathway & unit routines Whirlpool prn	Prep for delivery P, R & BP q 30 min Assess FHR/UA q 15 min of low risk Assess FHR/UA q 5 min if high risk Assist to void q 2 hrs/straight cath prn Cervical exam prn I&O Implement coping/relaxation techniques Assess fundus, lochia
KEY PATIENT OUTCOMES	TPR & BP WNL Reassuring fetal heart rate & contraction pattern Able to urinate without difficulty Bladder is emptied Fluid volume deficit is prevented Labor is progressing Pain and anxiety are reduced to a manageable level Verbalizes understanding of admission process Verbalizes understanding of Advance Directives, clinical pathway, & unit routines Verbalizes understanding of labor process/coping strategies	TPR & BP WNL Reasurring FHR and contraction pattern until delivery Bladder is emptied Fluid volume deficit is prevented Pain and anxiety is reduced to a manageable level Baby and placenta delivered vaginally Moderate amount rubra lochia Fundus firm at midline at umbilicus or below
INITIALS/ SIGNATURE/ TIME	____/________________/______ ____/________________/______ ____/________________/______ ____/________________/______ ____/________________/______	____/________________/______ ____/________________/______ ____/________________/______ ____/________________/______ ____/________________/______

APPENDIX N. Integrated Vaginal Birth Clinical Pathway cont.

Recovery/Immediate Postpartum Date ____________________	First Postpartum Day Date ____________________	Special Orders
	Lactation consultant Business office	
	Blood profile Rhogam screening Rubella titer	
	Catheterize prn Whirlpool Tucks __________	
DC Epidural unless anticipating tubal Analgesics DC IV/Hep lock Maintain IV if anticipating tubal	Analgesics Stool softener Maintain IV if anticipating tubal Prenatal vitamins prn @ bedside DC IV after tolerates liquids	
Diet ______________ as tolerated NPO for 8 hrs prior to tubal	Diet ____________________ as tolerates NPO for 8hrs prior to tubal	
Activity as tolerated Transfer to post partum care (2-4 hrs) Shower prior to tubal ID band on prior to OR	Activity as tolerated ID band on prior to OR Shower prior to tubal	
	Review data base Interventions/referral as needed	
Anxiety: resolved Comfort Potential: postpartum hemorrhage Family process Knowledge Effective breast feeding Potential for infection	Comfort Potential: postpartum hemorrhage: resolved Family process Knowledge Effective breast feeding Potential for infection	
Assessments, VS q 15 min x 4, q 30 min x 2, q 1 hr x 2 then assessments q shift and VS qid Assessments upon transfer of care, then per shift if assessments WNL Assist with personal hygiene, pericare, ice to perineum Assist with breast/bottle feeding Initiate family education Complete infant security sheet Promote family interaction Obtain permit for tubal (Title 19 permits obtained 30 days prior to tubal) Tubal recovery: Assessments/VS q 15 min x 5, q 30 min x 2, q 1hr x 2 then assessments q shift and VS QID	PP assessments q shift VS qid Tubal Recovery: Assessments/VS q 15 min x 5, q 30 min x 2, q 1 hr x 2 then assessments q shift and VS QID Assist with first shower as needed Whirlpool prn Continue education Assist with personal hygiene, peri care as needed Weigh Discuss parental adjustment and emotional needs/support & coping strategies Provide learning materials and initiate teaching based on learning needs assessment Obtain permit for tubal	
Vital signs WNL Moderate rubra lochia, odorless Fundus firm at midline at U or below Able to urinte without difficulty Pain is reduced to a manageable level Verbalizes, demonstrates knowledge of self & newborn care Expressess feelings regarding L&D experience Interacts appropriately with infant Exhibits basic feeding skills Fluid volume deficit is prevented Laporoscopy incision clean, dry, intact	VS WNL Moderate rubra lochia, odorless Fundus firm at midline at U or below Able to urinate without difficulty Pain is reduced to a manageable level Verbalizes, demonstrates knowledge of self & newborn care Expresses feelings regarding L&D experience Initiate positive bonding behavior Exhibits skills necessary for infant feeding Verbalizes understanding of adjustments/coping strategies Tolerates ADLS without assistance Laporoscopy incision clean, dry, intact	Key 1. Initialed in Red=Ordered 2. Black Line=Not Ordered 3. Circled in Black= Exception
______/______________/______ ______/______________/______ ______/______________/______ ______/______________/______ ______/______________/______	______/______________/______ ______/______________/______ ______/______________/______ ______/______________/______ ______/______________/______	

APPENDIX N. Integrated Vaginal Birth Clinical Pathway cont.

Second Postpartum Day Date______________	Extra Day Date: ________	
Lactation consultant		
Catheterize prn Whirlpool Tucks		
Home meds Analgesics Rubella Rhogam Stool softener Prenatal vitamins prn @ bedside		**Special Orders**
Diet ______________ as tolerates		
Activity as tolerated		
Complete intervention/referral		
Comfort: resolved Family process: resolved Knowledge: resolved Effective breast feeding: resolved Potential for infection: resolved		
PP assessments q shift VS qid Whirlpool prn Complete teaching--identify unmet needs & refer Discharge per security SOP		
VS WNL Moderate rubra lochia, odorless Fundus firm at midline Learning needs met according to database or appropriate referrals made Demonstrates appropriate bonding behaviors Verbalizes understanding of PP adjustments Understands need for physician follow-up Demonstrates basic techniques for infant feeding Laporoscopy incision clean, dry, intact		**Key** 1. Initialed in Red=Ordered 2. Black Line=Not Ordered 3. Circled in Black= Exception
____/____________/____ ____/____________/____ ____/____________/____ ____/____________/____ ____/____________/____	____/____________/____ ____/____________/____ ____/____________/____ ____/____________/____ ____/____________/____	

APPENDIX N. Integrated Cesarean Birth Clinical Pathway

INTEGRATED CLINICAL PATHWAY

C-SECTION
DRG #370 & 371
Mothers OB/GYN Physician: ________________
Family Physician: ________________
Baby's Physician: ________________
Primary RN: ________________
Date Reviewed by MD/RN/Patient: ________________
Advance Directive: Yes______ No______

MEDICAL HISTORY

Admit Date	Transfer Date:	Transfer To:	Allergies:

Present Problem: ________________

Past History: ________________

Surgical & Special Procedures: ________________

ABO/Rh: Maternal ________ Newborn ________
Rubella: Immune ________ Non-Immune ________
HBsAg: Negative ________ Positive ________

Multi Disciplinary Consults:

Date	Consultant	Reason	First Visit	Signed Off

DISCHARGE PLANNING

Discharge Destination	Date/Time	Initial	Community Services	Date	Initial	Equipment	Date	Initial
Home w/________			Childbirth Education			Home Oxygen		
			Parenting Education			Home IV Therapy: ____		
Other:________			Lactation Consultant					
			WIC/Baby Care			Home Phototherapy		
			Social Services			Apnea Monitor		
			MWH/Perinatal Connections			Breast Pump		
			Business Office			Terb. Pump		
			Grief Follow-up			HUAM ________		
			VNA/CHN			Insulin Pump		
			LSS/CSS/SSS			Home Blood Glucose Monitor: ______		
			Support Group ________			Papa Pager		
						O2 Sat		
			Other: ________			Diabetic Supplies		
						BP Machine:______		
						Other : ______		

Initials/Signature:
____/________ ____/________ ____/________
____/________ ____/________

81 **OFF PATHWAY** ☐ **YES**
DATE ____/____/____

02/94 CHART FORM

APPENDIX N. Integrated Cesarean Birth Clinical Pathway cont.

DAY/DATE	Admission Date: _______ Delivery Time: _____	RECOVERY/DELIVERY DAY DATE:_____
CONSULTS	Notify physician of admission Notify pediatrician, ICN, MDA, CRNA	
LABS	CBC w/o diff Type & screen HBsAG if not on history Cord blood gases prn Urine dipstick for protein & ketones	
TREATMENTS	EFM strip to document reactivity Foley catheter	Volurex prn Oxygen 8-10L per face mask prn
MEDICATIONS/ IVs	IV Bicitra 30 cc PO Oxytocin per anesthesia	IV Analgesics Antiemetics PCA pump
NUTRITION	NPO	As tolerated
ACTIVITY/ SAFETY	As tolerated	Spinal anesthesia - gradually allow pt to sit up if BP stable, no sign of dizziness and sensation is returning to legs Bed rails up Activity as tolerated -- OOB minimum 1x/shift
DISCHARGE PLANNING	Review database Complete infant security sheet	Begin needs & learning assessment
NURSING DX/ INTERDISCI-PLINARY FOCUS	Anxiety Knowledge Fetal Tissue Perfusion	Fluid volume Comfort Knowledge Potential: PP hemorrhage Potential post op ileus Anxiety Effective breast feeding Potential for infection/injury Family process Potential post op atelectisis
KEY NURSING ACTIVITIES/ TEACHING	Institute advance directive & infant security policy Review data base, clinical pathway & unit routine Facilitate participation in decision making Answer questions & explain treatment procedures Facilitate involvement of support person(s) Provide emotional support - encourage verbalization of feeling about cesarean delivery Obtain informed consent Obtain vital signs Complete admission assessment Instrument, sponge & needle count completed and correct Knee strap & ground pad on	Assessments/VS/TCDB: q 15 min x 5, q 30 min x 2, q 1 hr x 2, then q 4 hrs until 0800 1st POD EKG, O2 sat monitor until stable Observe/document blood loss I & O Medicate as needed for pain - ensure effective use of PCA pump Assist with breast feeding/bottle feeding Assist with personal hygiene Promote family interaction Transfer to PP room if applicable Post anesthetic recovery score with VS until score of 9 Initiate family education Assist with infant cares
KEY PATIENT OUTCOMES	Verbalizes understanding of cesarean delivery, unit routines - clinical pathway, routine procedures, advance directive & infant security Verbalizes understanding of options & participates in decision making Demonstrates appropriate coping behavior Anxiety is reduced to manageable level Reassuring fetal heart rate pattern TPR & BP / Assessments WNL Instrument, sponge, needle count correct	Fluid volume deficit is prevented - absence of significant bleeding Verbalize feelings regarding the cesarean birth experience Pain is reduced to manageable level Effective breast feeding is initiated TPR & BP/Assessments WNL & stable Infection/Injury is prevented Interacts appropriately w/newborn O_2 sats above 95% Benign arrhythmia Orientated to time and place Satisfactory airway and respiratory function No signs/symptoms of ileus, atelectasis
INITIALS/ SIGNATURE/ TIME	____/__________/____ ____/__________/____ ____/__________/____ ____/__________/____ ____/__________/____	____/__________/____ ____/__________/____ ____/__________/____ ____/__________/____ ____/__________/____

1st POD Date:________________	2nd POD Date: ________________	Special Orders
Lactation consultant	Lactation consultant Business office	
Blood profile 1st POD Rhogam screening if indicated Rubella titer if not on history		
Seabrook pad prn Volurex prn	Seabrook pad prn	
Antiemetics Sedative Rubella/Rhogam if indicated Analgesics Stool softener/laxative/fleets DC IV/PCA a.m. of 1st PO day ________________ Prenatal vitamins prn at bedside	Sedative Analgesics Stool softener/laxative/fleets Rubella/Rhogam if indicated Prenatal vitamins prn at bedside	
Diet ________________ as tolerated	Diet __________ as tolerates	
Activity as tolerated - OOB, ambulate minimum of once per shift until ambulating independently Up w/assistance until ambulating independently Weight 1st POD	Activity as tolerated	
Review database-interventions/referrals as needed Continue needs & learning assessment	Continue intervention /referral as needed	
Anxiety Comfort Knowledge Potential for infection/Injury Potential postpartum hemorrhage Potential post op atelectisis Family process Potential post op ileus Effective breast feeding Fluid volume	Comfort Potential for infection/injury Potential: postpartum hemorrhage: resolved Family process Knowledge Effective breast feeding Anxiety	
VS until 0800 1st post-op day then qid x 48 hrs post op Assessments w/VS until 0800 1st post op day then assessments q shift Assist with personal hygiene Assist with breast/bottle feeding Assist with infant cares Promote family interaction TCDB with assessments until ambulatory Intake and output x 24 hrs after foley removed Provide learning materials & initiate teaching based on learning needs assessment DC foley am of 1st PO day __________ DC dressing ___________ DC staples, clips ______ yes ______ no ______ 2" tape ______ 2 steri strips	PP assessments q shift VS qid Continue education Assist with personal hygiene, as needed Discuss parental adjustment and emotional needs/ support & coping strategies Assist with newborn cares Assist with breast/bottle feeding Promote family interaction DC staples, clips _____ yes _____ no _____ 2" tape _____ 2 steri strips	
TPR & BP/assessment WNL Pain is reduced to a manageable level Begins to verbalize, demonstrate knowledge of self & newborn care Expresses feelings regarding birth experience Interacts appropriately with infant Exhibits skills necessary for infant feeding Exhibits basic feeding skills Fluid volume deficit is prevented No signs/symptoms of ileus, atelectasis Infection/injury is prevented Able to urinate without difficulty	TPR & BP/assessments WNL Pain is reduced to a manageable level Verbalizes, demonstrates knowledge of self & newborn care Expresses feelings regarding birth experience Initiates positive bonding behavior Exhibits skills necessary for infant feeding Verbalizes understanding of adjustments/coping strategies Tolerates ADLS without assistance Infection/injury is prevented Able to urinate without difficulty	**Key** 1. Initialed in Red=Ordered 2. Black Line=Not Ordered 3. Circled in Black= Exception
_____/_____________________/_____ _____/_____________________/_____ _____/_____________________/_____ _____/_____________________/_____ _____/_____________________/_____	_____/_____________________/_____ _____/_____________________/_____ _____/_____________________/_____ _____/_____________________/_____ _____/_____________________/_____	

3rd POD Date: ________________	DAY ____ DATE: __________	
Lactation consultant		
Home meds Analgesics Stool softener/laxative/fleets Prenatal vitamins prn at bedside		
Diet _________ as tolerates		
Activity as tolerated		
Complete intervention/referral		**Special Orders**
Comfort: resolved Anxiety: resolved Family process: resolved Knowledge: resolved Effective breast feeding: resolved		
PP assessments q shift VS BID Complete teaching - identify unmet needs & refer Discharge per security SOP Assess ability to care for self and baby - make referrals as needed DC staples, clips ____ yes ____ no ____ 2" tape ____ 2 steri strips		
TPR & BP/assessments WNL Learning needs met according to database or appropriate referrals made Demonstrates appropriate bonding behaviors Verbalizes understanding of PP adjustments - has identified coping strategies Understands need for physician follow-up Demonstrates techniques for infant feeding and newborn cares and self cares Infection/injury is prevented Pain is reduced to a manageable level Able to urinate without difficulty		
____/____________/____ ____/____________/____ ____/____________/____ ____/____________/____ ____/____________/____	____/____________/____ ____/____________/____ ____/____________/____ ____/____________/____ ____/____________/____	Key 1. Initialed in Red=Ordered 2. Black Line=Not Ordered 3. Circled in Black=Exception

E5

INTEGRATED CLINICAL PATHWAY

NORMAL NEWBORN
DRG #391
Mothers OB/GYN Physician: ____________
Family Physician: ____________
Baby's Physician: ____________
Date Reviewed by MD/RN/Patient: ____________
Advance Directive: Yes_____ No_____

MEDICAL HISTORY

Admit Date	Transfer Date:	Transfer To:	Allergies:

Present Problem: ____________

ABO/Rh: Maternal ________ Newborn ________
Rubella: Immune ________ Non-Immune ________
HBsAg: Negative ________ Positive ________

Past History: ____________

Surgical & Special Procedures: ____________

Multi Disciplinary Consults:

Date	Consultant	Reason	First Visit	Signed Off

DISCHARGE PLANNING

Discharge Destination	Date/Time	Initial	Community Services	Date	Initial	Equipment	Date	Initial
Home w/______			Childbirth Education			Home Oxygen		
Other:______			Parenting Education			Home IV Therapy: ____		
			Lactation Consultant					
			WIC/Baby Care			Home Phototherapy		
			Social Services			Apnea Monitor		
			MWH/Perinatal Connections			Breast Pump		
			Business Office			Terb. Pump		
			Grief Follow-up			HUAM ______		
			VNA/CHN			Insulin Pump		
			LSS/CSS/SSS			Home Blood Glucose Monitor: ______		
			Support Group ______			Papa Pager		
			Other: ______			O2 Sat		
						Diabetic Supplies		
						BP Machine:______		
						Other : ______		

Initials/Signature:
____/____________ ____/____________ ____/____________
____/____________ ____/____________ ____/____________

41 OFF PATHWAY ☐ YES
DATE ____/____/____

03/94 CHART FORM

APPENDIX N. Integrated Normal Newborn Clinical Pathway cont.

DAY/DATE	DATE OF BIRTH: ____________ TIME: ______	DAY 1 DATE:__________
CONSULTS	Notify physician of admission	
LABS/ TREATMENTS	Cord blood: 1) Blood type, Rh, coombs if mom Rh neg 2) VDRL Rh pos infant with Rh neg mom: heelstick CBC & retic Bilirubin if jaundiced Prior to phototherapy: CBC with diff, cord blood type, RH & coombs Chemstrips Triple dye to cord	Bilirubin if jaundiced Prior to phototherapy: CBC with diff, cord blood type, Rh & coombs Discharge <48 hrs: PKU, T4 by 2 weeks
MEDICATIONS/ IVs	Erythromycin Aquamephyton	
NUTRITION	Breast ___ Formula ___ Supplement ___ NPO 2 hrs. prior to circumcision	Breast ___ Formula ___ Supplement ___ NPO 2 hrs. prior to circumcision
ACTIVITY/ SAFETY	Complete safety & security SOP Screen visitors for infection Position on side, back Keep bulb syringe in crib	Screen visitors for infections Position on side, back Keep bulb syringe in crib
DISCHARGE PLANNING	Identify parents learning needs Review Perinatal Data Base	Referrals as appropriate Discharge <48 hrs: return check up in 2-4 days
NURSING DX/ INTERDISCI-PLINARY FOCUS	Thermoregulation Breathing pattern Nutrition Infection Parents knowledge Family process Injury	Thermoregulation: resolved Nutrition Parents knowledge Family process Infection Injury
KEY NURSING ACTIVITIES/ TEACHING	Dry, warm blankets, tactile stim., suction, apgars Weight TPR q 30 min x 3, q 1 hr x 1, q 2 hr x 2, then q 4 hrs x 24hrs BP RA and 1 Leg on admit BP at completion of transition vitals Physical/gestational age assessments Monitor urine, stools--change diapers prn Sponge bath Begin feedings at breast or with bottle Initiate newborn teaching Observe circumcision q 15 min x 2, q 30 min x 1, q 1 hr x 1 Verify arm/leg band q 24 hrs Notify Physician within 1 hr of any problems	TPR q 4 hr x 24 hrs - then TPR 0800; temp 1600, 2400 Physical assessment q shift Weigh daily in late p.m. Breast/bottle feed Cleanse umbilical cord with alcohol every diaper change & bath Bathe prn Remove cord clamp Monitor urine, stools--change diaper prn Educate parents about newborn cares Observe circumcision q 15 min x 2, q 30 min x 1, q 1 hr x 1 Verify arm/leg band q 24 hrs Notify Physician of any problems Document/assess circumcision q shift
KEY PATIENT OUTCOMES	Able to adapt to extrauterine environment TPR & BP within normal range (97-99.8° F, P 120-160 R 30-60) Lung sounds clear Physical and behavioral characteristics WNL Measurements and weight WNL Signs & symptoms of infection are absent Initiates and sustains suck/swallow Parents interact appropriately with newborn Parents begin to verbalize knowledge of newborn cares Arm/leg band present	TPR stable within normal range (97-99.8°F; P120 - 160; R, 30 - 60) Signs infection/injury are absent Consumes 15-30 ml formula or nurses at breast 10 min/feeding Parents verbalize & begin to demonstrate safe, appropriate newborn care activities & behaviors Weight remains within 10% of birthweight Voiding and stooling within 24 hrs of age Arm/leg band present
INITIALS/ SIGNATURE/ TIME	____/______________/____ ____/______________/____ ____/______________/____ ____/______________/____ ____/______________/____	____/______________/____ ____/______________/____ ____/______________/____ ____/______________/____ ____/______________/____

APPENDIX N. Integrated Normal Newborn Clinical Pathway cont.

DAY 2 DATE: ________	DAY 3 DATE: ________	Special Orders
Bilirubin if jaundiced Prior to phototherapy: CBC with diff, cord blood type, Rh & coombs Galactosemia at discharge PKU, T4 at discharge	Bilirubin if jaundiced Prior to phototherapy: CBC w/diff, cord blood type, Rh & coombs Galactosemia at discharge PKU, T4 at discharge	
Hepatitis B IM prior to discharge	Hepatitis B IM prior to discharge	
Breast ___ Formula ___ Supplement ___ NPO 2 hrs prior to circumcision	Breast ___ Formula ___ Supplement ___ NPO 2 hrs prior to circumcision	
Screen visitors for infection Position on side, back Keep bulb syringe in crib	Screen visitors for infection Position on side, back Keep bulb syringe in crib	
Return check up Referrals Discharge	Return check up Referrals Discharge	
Nutrition: resolved Infection: resolved Parents knowledge: resolved Family process: resolved Injury: resolved	Nutrition: resolved Infection: resolved Parents knowledge: resolved	
TPR at 0800; temp 1600, 2400 Physical assessment q shift Weigh daily in late p.m. Cleanse umbilical cord w/ alcohol q diaper change & bath Monitor stools, urine--change diapers prn Bathe prn Observe circumcision q 15 min x 2, q 30 min x 1, q 1 hr x 1 Educate parents about newborn cares Verify arm/leg band q 24 hrs Notify physician of any problems Document/assess circumcision q shift	TPR at 0800; temp 1600, 2400 Physical assessment q shift Weigh daily in late p.m. Cleanse umbilical cord w/alcohol q diaper change & bath Monitor stools, urine--change diapers prn Bathe prn Observe circumcision q 15 min x 2, q 30 min x 1, q 1 hr x 1 Educate parents about newborn cares Verify arm/leg band q 24 hrs Notify physician of any problems Document/assess circumcision q shift	
Signs infection/injury are absent Consumes 15-30 ml formula or nurses at breast 10 min/feeding Parents demonstrate safe, appropriate newborn care activities & behaviors TPR stable within normal range (97-99.8°F; P 120-160; R 30-60) Weight remains within 10% of birthweight Voiding and stooling Arm/leg band present	Signs infection/injury are absent Consumes 15-30 ml formula or nurses at breast 10 min/feeding Parents demonstrate safe, appropriate newborn care activities & behaviors TPR stable within normal limits (97-99.8° F; P 1220-160; R 30-60) Weight remains within 10% of birthweight Arm/leg band present	Key 1. Initialed in Red=Ordered 2. Black Line=Not Ordered 3. Circled in Black=Exception
___/___________/___ ___/___________/___ ___/___________/___ ___/___________/___ ___/___________/___	___/___________/___ ___/___________/___ ___/___________/___ ___/___________/___ ___/___________/___	

APPENDIX N. Integrated Normal Newborn Clinical Pathway cont.

DAY 4 DATE: ____________	DAY ___ DATE: _________	
Bilirubin in jaundiced Prior phototherapy: CBC w/diff, cord blood type, Rh & coombs Galactosemia at discharge PKU, T4 at discharge		
Hepatitis B IM prior to discharge		**Special Orders**
Breast ____ Formula ____ Supplement ____ NPO 2 hrs prior to circumcision		
Screen visitors for infection Position on side, back Keep bulb syringe in crib		
Return check up Referrals Discharge		
Nutrition: resolved Infection: resolved Parents knowledge: resolved Family process: resolved Injury:resolved		
TPR at 0800; temp 1600, 2400 Physical assessment q shift Weigh daily in late p.m. Cleanse umbilical cord w/alcohol q diaper change & bath Monitor stools, urine--change diapers prn Bathe prn Observe circumcision q 15 min x 2, q 30 min x 1, q 1 hr x 1 Educate parents about newborn cares Verify aarm/leg band present Notify physician of any problems Document/assess circumcision q shift		
Signs of infection/injury are absent Consumes 15-30 ml formula or nurses at breast 10 min/feeding Parents demonstrate safe, appropriate newborn care activities & behaviors TPR stable within normal limits (97 - 99.8°F; P 120-160; R 30-60) Weight remains within 10% of birth weight Arm/leg band present		**Key** 1. Initialed in Red=Ordered 2. Black Line=Not Ordered 3. Circled in Black= Exception
____/____________/____	____/____________/____	
____/____________/____	____/____________/____	
____/____________/____	____/____________/____	
____/____________/____	____/____________/____	
____/____________/____	____/____________/____	

APPENDIX N. Integrated Preterm Labor Clinical Pathway

INTEGRATED CLINICAL PATHWAY

DRG #379 PRETERM LABOR
Mother's OB/GYN Physician: ____________
Family Physician: ____________
Baby's Physician: ____________
Primary RN: ____________
Date Reviewed by MD/RN/Patient: ______
Advance Directive: Yes_____ No_____

MEDICAL HISTORY

Admit Date	Transfer Date:	Transfer To:	Allergies:

Present Problem: ____________

Past History: ____________

Surgical & Special Procedures: ____________

ABO/Rh: Maternal ______ Newborn ______
Rubella: Immune ______ Non-Immune ______
HBsAg: Negative ______ Positive ______

Multi Disciplinary Consults:

Date	Consultant	Reason	First Visit	Signed Off

DISCHARGE PLANNING

Discharge Destination	Date/Time	Initial	Community Services	Date	Initial	Equipment	Date	Initial
Home w/________			Childbirth Education			Home Oxygen		
			Parenting Education			Home IV Therapy: _____		
Other:________			Lactation Consultant					
			WIC/Baby Care			Home Phototherapy		
			Social Services			Apnea Monitor		
			MWH/Perinatal Connections			Breast Pump		
			Business Office			Terb. Pump		
			Grief Follow-up			HUAM ________		
			VNA/CHN			Insulin Pump		
			LSS/CSS/SSS			Home Blood Glucose Monitor: ________		
			Support Group ________			Papa Pager		
						O2 Sat		
			Other: ________			Diabetic Supplies		
						BP Machine:________		
						Other : ________		

Initials/Signature:
____/________ ____/________ ____/________
____/________ ____/________ ____/________

42 OFF PATHWAY ☐ YES
DATE ____/____/____

APPENDIX N. Integrated Preterm Labor Clinical Pathway cont.

DAY/DATE	STABILIZATION STAGE DATE(S):____________________	TRANSITION DATE(S):____________________
CONSULTS		
DIAGNOSTIC PROCEDURES	CBC, Na, K, Glucose if on IV Betamimetics Repeat glucose, NA, K q 12 hrs during infusion of terbutaline UA, C&S Amniotic Fluid 1. Gram stain 2. C&S 3. L/S ratio MgSO4 level if indicated Ultra Sound Exam 1. Assessment of presenting part 2. Gestational age 3. Multiple gestation 4. AFV 5. Doppler flow studies	Check on results of cultures & report results Repeat any lab work if indicated
TREATMENTS	Continuous EFM for FHR pattern & contx status Hydrate with po or IV fluids Left lateral bed rest position	Continue hydration either po or IV Continue left lateral bedrest EFM per Dr. order
MEDICATIONS/ IVs	Follow routine orders for administration of IV Tocolytics for suppression of preterm labor Antibiotics if UTI present	Continue antibiotics if UTI If ordered, begin T-pump therapy
NUTRITION	Diet as tolerates	Diet as tolerates
ACTIVITY/ SAFETY	Bedrest with possible BRPs Assist to BR	Bedrest w/BRPs
DISCHARGE PLANNING	Assess family needs Assess pts knowledge level regarding preterm labor Complete data base	Reevaluate family needs--referrals--social worker Begin planning for possible home tx w/ T-pump Reinforce preterm labor teaching
NURSING DX/ INTERDISCI-PLINARY FOCUS	Anxiety Comfort Anticipatory grieving Knowledge	Knowledge Family process Anxiety Comfort Anticipatory grieving
KEY NURSING ACTIVITIES/ TEACHING	Monitor VS q 15 min until infusion maintenance rate is obtained & has remained unchanged x 1 hr; VS thereafter at a minimum of q 2 hrs Assess lung sound q 2 hrs during tocolytic infusion Monitor FHR & EFM Explain use of tocolytic agents, side effects & expected outomes Assess for medication intolerence Monitor I&O; use of foley catheter Explain risk factors for preterm labor	If Dr. orders, Terbutaline pump, set up pump & place on pt Begin pt teaching R/T Terbutaline pump therapy Routine VS including lung sounds & reflexes FHR per EFM as ordered by physician Monitor I&O Teach pt to recognize s/s of PTL Teach pt to palpate for uterine contractions Reinforce teaching R/T preterm labor
KEY PATIENT OUTCOMES	Pt has <4 ctx/hr & no cervical change Pt will be free from medication intolerance Complies with activity restrictions VS will be w/in parameters on standing orders FHR remains reactive Pt will verbalize understanding of s/s PTL Pt will have adequate fluid intake & output	Pt has <4 ctx/hr & no cervical change FHR remains reactive BP & resp. remain w/in normal limits, pulse <120 Pt will verbalize understanding of use of Terbutaline pump Pt will have adequate fluid intake & output Pt will demonstrate proper uterine palpation
INITIALS/ SIGNATURE/ TIME	___/__________/___ ___/__________/___ ___/__________/___ ___/__________/___ ___/__________/___	___/__________/___ ___/__________/___ ___/__________/___ ___/__________/___ ___/__________/___

APPENDIX N. Integrated Preterm Labor Clinical Pathway cont.

MAINTENANCE DATE(S): ______	DAY ______ DATE: ______	Special Orders
Heparin lock		
Discharge teaching done regarding T-pump Reinforce PTL teaching		
Knowledge: resolved Comfort: resolved Anticipatory grieving: resolved Anxiety: resolved Family process: resolved		
Pt discharged understanding s/s of PTL, use of Terbutaline pump & self care & when to notify healthcare provider		
Pt discharged understanding s/s of PTL, use of Terbutaline pump & self care & when to notify healthcare provider		
___/___/___ ___/___/___ ___/___/___ ___/___/___ ___/___/___	___/___/___ ___/___/___ ___/___/___ ___/___/___ ___/___/___	Key 1. Initialed in Red=Ordered 2. Black Line=Not Ordered 3. Circled in Black= Exception

DAY ____ DATE: ____________	DAY ___ DATE: _________	
		Special Orders
		Key 1. Initialed in Red=Ordered 2. Black Line=Not Ordered 3. Circled in Black= Exception
____/____________/____	____/____________/____	
____/____________/____	____/____________/____	
____/____________/____	____/____________/____	
____/____________/____	____/____________/____	
____/____________/____	____/____________/____	

APPENDIX O. Newborn Clinical Path

NEWBORN CLINICAL PATH

Birthdate ________ **Time** ________	1st 4 hours ______to ______ Day 0 ________	4-12 hours ______to ______	12-24 hours ______to ______	Day 1 ____________	Day 2 ____________ Day 3 ____________
Tests/ Treatments/ Consults	__Cord Gases __Accucheck __Repeat accucheck __Lab glucose __Dr. notified of birth	__Cord care __Group/Rh____ __DAT________		__Neonatal screen before dismissal . . . . __Circumcision type ____________ size ____________	. . . . >
Assessment & Monitoring	Capillary Hct ________ Venous Hct ________ Gestational age______wks __Initial BPs; Hourly VS __Wt:____# ________oz	__VS/assess every shift	__Initial Dr. exam __VS/assess every shift . . . . __Documented void & stool	__Physician dismissal exam . . . . > Wt: ______#______oz.	. . . . > Day 2 Wt: ______#______oz. Day 3 Wt: ______#______oz.
Medications	__Aquamephyton IM __Erythromycin OD __Triple dye to cord	__Hepatitis B vaccine __HBIG			
Activity/Safety	__Stabilet probe __Initial bath ________ __Complete slick sheet & bracelets __Attach security sensor	__Open crib at__		__Photo taken before dismissal . . . . __Cord clamp off __ID & dismissal	. . . . > . . . . >
Nutrition **Breast**	__To breast within first hour	__Functional assessment of infant at breast	. . . . >	__Lactation rounds __Consult if needed, inpatient/outpatient	__≥ 8 BAS in 24 hrs
Formula ________ **(type)**	__Feed as soon as awake & stable	__Feed every 2-4 hrs. 1/2-1 oz. . .	. . . .	. . . . >	__Feed every 2-4 hrs. 2-3 oz.
Discharge Planning	__Assessment of data base & home care situation. __Consult social service if indicated.	__Determine if infant car seat available. __Complete hearing screening	__Assist in obtaining car seat PRN __Consult audiologist if at risk	__Home Health referral if indicated __Repeat neonatal screen __________	
Teaching/ Mother Response (See Code)	__Positioning ______ __Bulb syringe ______ __Baby guidelines handout given	__Cord care ___ __Diapering ____ __Sibling relations __Bottle feeding_ __Breastfeeding_ __Burping _____	. . . . >	__Signs & symptoms to report__________ __Follow-up appointment with doctor __Circumcision care __Bath demonstration __Rectal/axillary temp __Formula preparation	____________ ____________ ____________ ____________ ____________ ____________
Outcomes			#1, 2 & 5	#3, 4, 6	. . . . >
Signatures:					

Mother Response:
A. Verbalizes understanding.
B. Demonstrates understanding by return demonstrations and questioning.
C. Demonstrates understanding but needs reinforcement and/or practice.
D. Shows limited understanding, further teaching needed.
E. Recall limited.

PATIENT IDENTIFICATION

St. Joseph Medical Center
Wichita, Kansas 67218
The Family Birthplace

NEWBORN CLINICAL PATH
P-1378 10/93

APPENDIX O. Newborn Clinical Path cont.

START DATE/ INITIALS	PROBLEMS/NEEDS	OUTCOME CRITERIA	MET DATE/ INITIALS
	1. Potential for impaired gas exchange.	Respiratory rate remains between 30 to 60 per minute, no signs of respiratory distress.	
	2. Potential alteration in body temperature.	Skin and axillary temperature between 36.5 ° C to 37.0° C (97.4° F-98.6° F).	
	3. Effective feeding pattern.	a. Baby latches on and suckles effectively with more than 6 feedings in first 24 hours then ≥ 8 BAS every 24 hours. b. Baby able to initiate and sustain suck and swallow coordination with normal color and respiratory effort.	
	4. Potential for infection, related to immune system.	Newborn is free from signs of infection, no drainage or odor to umbilical cord, skin lesions.	
	5. Urinary and bowel elimination.	a. Meconium is passed within 24 hrs after birth and beginning of normal stool cycle is evident. b. Baby voids within first 24 hours.	
	6. Hypoglycemia	Blood glucose >40, asymptomatic.	
	7.		

NEWBORN DEPARTURE SUMMARY	Y	N
PULSE: 90 <P> 200 in past 24 hours?		
RESP: 30 <Resp> 60 in past 24 hours?		
BP: 50 <SBP> 90 and 30 <DBP> 50 in past 24 hrs?		
T: 97.4° F <T> 98.6° F axillary temp in past 24 hrs?		
Lab/EKGs/chest x-rays with abnormal findings in past 24 hrs List abnormal findings:		
Blood Sugar: < 40 or > 120 in last 24 hours?		
Newborn demonstrates inability to tolerate oral intake?		
Caregiver unable to provide adequate feeding/nutrition or medications?		
Parenteral fluids/drugs received after midnight the day of dismissal? (except antibiotics or IV/heparin to keep vein open)		
Bleeding at circumcision site (if circumcised)?		
Skin: Dry and intact __Other ____________ Cord Stump: Dry ____or Clamped ____ Level of Consciousness: __Appropriate for age __Other __ Bowel/Bladder Function: __Appropriate for age __Other __ Activity Level: Appropriate for age _ Other ________ Physician notified of abnormal findings? How?________		

Departure Date: ____________

Time: ____________

To Home: [ ]

Other: ____________

____

Address

____

City Phone

Carried by ____________

Accompanied by ____________

Personal belongings sent [ ]

Directed to cashier [ ]

Discharge Nurse:

____

PATIENT IDENTIFICATION

St. Joseph Medical Center
Wichita, Kansas 67218
The Family Birthplace

NEWBORN CLINICAL PATH
P-1378 10/93

APPENDIX P. Family Focused Childbirth Care Path

FAMILY FOCUSED CHILDBIRTH CARE PATH						
	PRENATAL PERIOD	EARLY LABOR	ACTIVE LABOR/BIRTH	0 - 4 HOURS AFTER BIRTH	1 st DAY AFTER BIRTH	HOME FOLLOW-UP
MEDICAL AND NURSING CARE	Your prenatal blood tests will be done You will see the doctor every month. As you get closer to your due date, you may see the doctor more frequently. During prenatal visits, your doctor or nurse will listen to your baby's heart rate, check your weight, blood pressure, and urine, and measure your baby's growth. You may have an ultrasound or other prenatal tests as your doctor decides is appropriate. Ask your doctor and nurse about prenatal diet, activity level, warning signs of pregnancy complications and when to call or come to the labor and birth unit.	Your labor nurse will check your blood pressure, pulse, respirations, and temperature, and your progress of labor. A fetal monitor will be used to observe your baby's heart rate and response to labor contractions. Your nurse will feel your abdomen to check strength and frequency of contractions. Your doctor will be notified of your admission and collaborate with your nurse about your plan of care. If your bag of waters has not ruptured, you will be encouraged to walk as you feel comfortable. Your nurse will help you with strategies to minimize discomfort.	As labor progresses, your baby's heart rate, your contractions, blood pressure, temperature, pulse and respirations will be closely monitored by your nurse. Your doctor may visit and will be in close contact with your nurse about your progression in labor and how you and your baby are doing. You will have an IV. If you feel up to walking or sitting in the chair, you will be able to do so. Your nurse will help you to manage discomforts of labor. If you want an epidural or other form of pain relief, your nurse will make arrangements after talking with your doctor. Your doctor may prescribe medication to maintain regular contractions and insure steady progress of your labor.	You and your baby will be closely observed by your doctor and nurse. If you are breastfeeding, you will be encouraged to feed your baby. After one or two hours, you will be transferred to a room on the family focused care unit. Your baby will be with you in your room as much as you prefer. The first few times you get up to the bathroom, your nurse will assist you. Your nurse will massage your uterus and check your vaginal bleeding. Your IV may be discontinued. You will be given something to eat. You may have visitors as you feel appropriate. You will be encouraged to rest.	You and your baby will continue to be closely observed by your nurse. Your blood pressure, temperature, pulse respirations, uterine firmness and vaginal bleeding will be checked regularly. Your doctor and your baby's doctor will visit. If you want your baby boy circumcised, your doctor will do this before your baby goes home. Your nurse will help you with breastfeeding or formula feeding. Your baby will have blood drawn for PKU test. You can have visitors as you feel appropriate. You will have a regular diet.. Let your nurse know what we can do for you. If you need pain medication, it will be available.	Some insurance companies cover and arrange for home visits by a profession nurse. If that option is not offerred, you can obtain homecare for a fee. Home visits are available through St. John's Mercy's homecare services department. If you would like a home visit, ask your doctor or nurse. Feel free to call the family focused care unit with any questions you may have after you go home 569-6287. Your doctor and your baby's doctor will give you their phone numbers so you can call if you need to talk to them.

St. John's Mercy Medical Center, St. Louis, MO.

APPENDIX P. Family Focused Childbirth Care Path cont.

FAMILY FOCUSED CHILDBIRTH CARE PATH						
	PRENATAL PERIOD	**EARLY LABOR**	**ACTIVE LABOR/BIRTH**	**0 - 4 HOURS AFTER BIRTH**	**1 st DAY AFTER BIRTH**	**HOME FOLLOW-UP**
FAMILY TEACHING	Call the Baby-Line 961-BABY to register for classes. Classes are available for childbirth preparation/Lamaze, infant care, breastfeeding, sibling preparation, grandparenting, cesarean birth, and prenatal exercise. If you are planning on an epidural for labor pain relief, call 569-2688 to register for anesthesia classes. Call your insurance company to find out about how long you can stay in the hospital after birth, precertification and copayments, and if a home visit will be provided after birth and the homecare agency's name. Plan to bring a car seat to the hospital for your baby's trip home. Begin preparing baby's room and gathering clothes and equipment.	Your labor nurse will explain how the fetal monitor works to observe your baby's response to labor and frequency of your labor contractions. Your nurse will help you and your labor coach with early labor breathing techniques and positioning.	Your labor nurse will keep you updated on the progress of your labor and your baby's well-being. Your nurse will explain options for pain relief measures during labor. If you desire epidural anesthesia, your nurse will assist you in frequent position changes and collaborate with your doctor on dosage adjustment. Your nurse will explain all necessary medical and nursing procedures to you and your support persons. You can have family and friends visit as you feel appropriate.	After birth you will be encouraged to hold and feed your baby. Your labor nurse will assist you with newborn feeding and holding positions. You will be given instructions on how to care for your stitches and vaginal discharge when you go home. Your nurse will begin teaching about newborn care.	Your nurse will continue to teach you how to care for yourself and your newborn after you go home. You will be provided information about breastfeeding, formula feeding, cord care, circumcision care, newborn awake and sleeping patterns, how to tell when your baby is hungry, how to comfort the crying baby, diapering, how to tell if your baby is getting enough to eat, what to do if the baby is choking or spitting up feedings, and how to bath your baby. Your nurse will answer your questions or concerns. You will be given information about your diet and activity level, warning signs of complications and when to call the doctor, and when to schedule your and your baby's first doctors visit.	During the home visit, your nurse will check your stitches, your vaginal bleeding, your breasts, blood pressure, temperature, pulse, and respirations, and ask about your urination and bowel movements. Your baby's cord and circumcision will also be checked. Your nurse may observe a breastfeeding or formula feeding session and ask about your baby's urination and bowel movements. Any questions about your care or baby care will be answered.

St. John's Mercy Medical Center, St. Louis, MO.

APPENDIX P. Family Focused Childbirth Care Path:Scheduled Cesarean Birth

FAMILY FOCUSED CHILDBIRTH CARE PATH: SCHEDULED CESAREAN BIRTH					
	ADMISSION/ BIRTH PROCESS	**0 - 4 HOURS AFTER BIRTH**	**1 st DAY AFTER BIRTH**	**2 nd DAY AFTER BIRTH**	**HOME FOLLOW-UP**
MEDICAL AND NURSING CARE	The day before your planned cesarean birth, you will come to the hospital for preadmission laboratory tests. You will have the opportunity to talk with someone from the anesthesia department about anesthesia during surgery and after birth. Your doctor will tell you what time to come to the labor and delivery unit the morning of your cesarean birth. Your labor nurse will interview you about your pregnancy and medical history. An external fetal monitor will be used to check your baby's well-being. You will have an IV. A catheter will be placed in your bladder. Your abdomen will be shaved. You will be asked to remove your jewelry and/or dentures. Your valuables will be given to family members. A support person of your choice can be present during surgery if you are having epidural anesthesia.	After birth you and your support person will be able to see and hold your baby. After surgery is completed, your will be transferred to the recovery room. You will be closely observed by your doctor and nurse. Your blood pressure, pulse, respirations, temperature, and incision dressing will be checked frequently. Your nurse will massage your uterus and observe vaginal bleeding. You will still have an IV. Your doctor will prescribe medications for pain relief. If you are uncomfortable, ask your nurse for pain medication. You may have ice chips and sips of water. If you are breastfeeding, your nurse will assist you in positioning your baby for feeding. Your family and friends may visit. After approximately 2 hours, you will be transferred to a room on the family focused care unit. You and your baby will continue to be closely observed.	The first day after cesarean birth is one of rest and recovery. Your vital signs, incision and vaginal bleeding will continue to be closely observed by your doctor and nurse. Your baby will be with you in the room as much as you prefer. Your nurse will help you with breast or formula feeding your baby. You will be given a liquid diet such as jello, broth, soda, etc. Your IV may be discontinued. The catheter in your bladder will be removed. Your nurse will assist you to the bathroom. You will be encouraged to sit in the chair and take short walks to prevent gas pain and speed the recovery process. If you are uncomfortable, ask your nurse for pain medication your doctor has prescribed. Your doctor and your baby's doctor will visit. Family and friends may visit as you desire. You will be encouraged to rest and get to know your new baby.	Your nurse and doctor will continue to monitor your recovery. You will be able to do more today. You will be encouraged to sit in the chair and take short walks. If you need assistance, your nurse is available. If you are uncomfortable, ask your nurse for pain medication your doctor has prescribed. Your nurse will listen to your abdomen for bowel activity. Your baby will be with you in the room as much as you prefer. Your nurse will continue to help you with breast or formula feeding if needed. If you want your baby boy circumcised, your doctor will do this before your baby goes home. Your doctor and your baby's doctor will visit. Your baby will have blood drawn for PKU. Your family and friends may visit you as you desire. Be sure to let your nurse know what we can do to make your stay as comfortable as possible.	Some insurance companies cover and arrange for home visits by a professional nurse. If that option is not offered, you can obtain homecare for a fee. Home visits are available through St. John's Mercy homecare services department. If you would like a home visit, ask your doctor or nurse. Feel free to call the family focused care unit with any questions you may have after you go home @ 569-6287. If you have questions about breast feeding, call 961-2229 to arrange to speak with a lactation consultant. Your doctor and your baby's doctor will give you their phone numbers so you can call them if you need to ask questions.

St. John's Mercy Medical Center, St. Louis, MO.

APPENDIX P. Family Focused Childbirth Care Path:Scheduled Cesarean Birth cont.

FAMILY FOCUSED CHILDBIRTH CARE PATH: SCHEDULED CESAREAN BIRTH					
	ADMISSION/ BIRTH PROCESS	**0 - 4 HOURS AFTER BIRTH**	**1 st DAY AFTER BIRTH**	**2 nd DAY AFTER BIRTH**	**HOME FOLLOW-UP**
FAMILY TEACHING	Your labor nurse will explain how the fetal monitor works to observe your baby before surgery. Your nurse will discuss all procedures before they are done such as inserting your IV, placing the catheter in your bladder, and shaving your abdomen. Someone from the anesthesia department and your doctor will be present to answer any additional questions your and your family member may have. Your support person will be given clothes to wear during the surgery. Your family members and friends will be shown to the family waiting room and notified when to visit you after surgery is completed.	After birth, your nurse will assist you in getting to know your new baby. If you are breastfeeding, you will be given information and tips for success. Your baby will be with you as much as you desire. Your nurse will teach you how to massage your uterus. Your nurse will discuss your diet and activity level for the next few days. Information will be provided to family and friends about visiting hours.	Your nurse will begin teaching you how to care for yourself and your baby after you go home. You will be provided with information about breast and formula feeding, cord care, circumcision care, newborn awake and sleeping patterns, how to tell if the baby is hungry, how to comfort the crying baby, how to know if the baby is getting enough to eat, what to do if the baby is choking or spitting up feedings, how to bathe your baby. Your nurse will answer your questions or concerns. You will be given information about your diet and activity level, expected vaginal bleeding, incision care, breast care, and pain relief measures.	Your nurse will continue to teach you how to care for yourself and your baby after you go home. Feel free to ask any questions or seek clarification. Your doctor and your baby's doctor will visit and be available to answer your questions as well. You will be given information about warning signs of complications and when to call the doctor and when to schedule your and your new baby's first doctor's visit.	During the home visit, your nurse will check your incision, vaginal bleeding, breasts, and blood pressure, temperature, pulse and respirations. She will ask about your diet, urination and bowel movements Your baby's cord and circumcision will be checked. Your nurse may observe a breastfeeding or formula feeding session and ask about your baby's urination and bowel movements. Questions about your care or baby care will be answered.

St. John's Mercy Medical Center, St. Louis, MO.

APPENDIX P. Family Focused Childbirth Care Path: Vaginal Birth

FAMILY FOCUSED CHILDBIRTH CARE PATH: VAGINAL BIRTH					
	EARLY LABOR	**ACTIVE LABOR/BIRTH**	**0 - 4 HOURS AFTER BIRTH**	**1 st DAY AFTER BIRTH**	**HOME FOLLOW-UP**
MEDICAL AND NURSING CARE	Your labor nurse will check your blood pressure, pulse, respirations, and temperature, and your progress of labor. A fetal monitor will be used to observe your baby's heart rate and response to labor contractions. Your nurse will feel your abdomen to check strength and frequency of contractions. Your doctor will be notified of your admission and collaborate with your nurse about your plan of care. If your bag of waters has not ruptured, you will be encouraged to walk as you feel comfortable. Your nurse will help you with strategies to minimize discomfort.	As labor progresses, your baby's heart rate, your contractions, blood pressure, temperature, pulse and respirations will be closely monitored by your nurse. Your doctor may visit and will be in close contact with your nurse about your progression in labor and how you and your baby are doing. You will have an IV. If you feel up to walking or sitting in the chair, you will be able to do so. Your nurse will help you to manage discomforts of labor. If you want an epidural or other form of pain relief, your nurse will make arrangements after talking with your doctor. Your doctor may prescribe medication to maintain regular contractions and insure steady progress of your labor. You may have visitors as you feel appropriate.	You and your baby will be closely observed by your doctor and nurse. If you are breastfeeding, you will be encouraged to feed your baby. After one or two hours, you will be transferred to a room on the family focused care unit. Your baby will be with you in your room as much as you prefer. The first few times you get up to the bathroom, your nurse will assist you. Your nurse will massage your uterus and check your vaginal bleeding. Your IV may be discontinued. You will be given something to eat. You may have visitors as you feel appropriate. You will be encouraged to rest.	You and your baby will continue to be closely observed by your nurse. Your blood pressure, temperature, pulse, respirations, uterine firmness and vaginal bleeding will be checked regularly. Your doctor and your baby's doctor will visit. If you want your baby boy circumcised, your doctor will do this before your baby goes home. Your nurse will help you with breastfeeding or formula feeding. Your baby will have blood drawn for PKU test. You can have visitors as you feel appropriate. You will have a regular diet. Let your nurse know what we can do for you. If you need pain medication, it will be available.	Some insurance companies cover and arrange for home visits by a profession nurse. If that option is not offerred, you can obtain homecare for a fee. Home visits are available through St. John's Mercy's homecare services. . If you would like a home visit, ask your doctor or nurse. Feel free to call the family focused care unit with any questions you may have after you go home @569-6287. Your doctor and your baby's doctor will give you their phone numbers so you can call if you need to talk to them.

St. John's Mercy Medical Center, St. Louis, MO.

APPENDIX P. Family Focused Childbirth Care Path: Vaginal Birth cont.

FAMILY FOCUSED CHILDBIRTH CARE PATH: VAGINAL BIRTH					
	EARLY LABOR	**ACTIVE LABOR/BIRTH**	**0 - 4 HOURS AFTER BIRTH**	**1 st DAY AFTER BIRTH**	**HOME FOLLOW-UP**
FAMILY TEACHING	Your labor nurse will explain how the fetal monitor works to observe your baby's response to labor and frequency of your labor contractions. Your nurse will help you and your labor coach with early labor breathing techniques and positioning.	Your labor nurse will keep you updated on the progress of your labor and your baby's well-being. Your nurse will explain options for pain relief measures during labor. If you desire epidural anesthesia, your nurse will assist you in frequent position changes and collaborate with your doctor on dosage adjustment. Your nurse will explain all necessary medical and nursing procedures to you and your support persons. You can have family and friends visit as you feel appropriate. A support person of your choice is welcome to be with you at birth. If you would like addtional support persons/family members present,tell your nurse and doctor.	After birth you will be encouraged to hold and feed your baby. Your labor nurse will assist you with newborn feeding and holding positions. You will be given instructions on how to care for your stitches and vaginal discharge when you go home. Your nurse will begin teaching about newborn care.	Your nurse will continue to teach you how to care for yourself and your newborn after you go home. You will be provided information about breastfeeding, formula feeding, cord care, circumcision care, newborn awake and sleeping patterns, how to tell when your baby is hungry, how to comfort the crying baby, diapering, how to tell if your baby is getting enough to eat, what to do if the baby is choking or spitting up feedings, and how to bath your baby your diet activity level, warning signs of complications when to call the doctor, when to schedule your and your baby's first doctors visit, and any other questions or concerns you may have.	During the home visit, your nurse will check your stitches, vaginal bleeding, breasts, blood pressure, temperature, pulse, respirations, ask about your urination and bowel movements and ask about your baby's urination and bowel movements. Your baby's cord and circumcision will also be checked. Your nurse may observe a breastfeeding or formula feeding session. Any questions about your care or baby care will be answered.

St. John's Mercy Medical Center, St. Louis, MO.

APPENDIX P. Family Focused Childbirth Care Path:Cesarean Birth

FAMILY FOCUSED CHILDBIRTH CARE PATH: CESAREAN BIRTH				
	0 - 4 HOURS AFTER BIRTH	**1 st DAY AFTER BIRTH**	**2 nd DAY AFTER BIRTH**	**HOME FOLLOW-UP**
MEDICAL AND NURSING CARE	After birth you and your support person will be able to see and hold your baby. After surgery is completed, your will be transferred to the recovery room. You will be closely observed by your doctor and nurse. Your blood pressure, pulse, respirations, temperature, and incision dressing will be checked frequently. Your nurse will massage your uterus and observe vaginal bleeding. You will still have an IV. If you are uncomfortable, ask your nurse for pain medication. You may have ice chips and sips of water. If you are breastfeeding, your nurse will assist you in positioning your baby for feeding. Your family and friends may visit as you desire. After approximately 2 hours, you will be transferred to a room on the family focused care unit.	The first day after cesarean birth is one of rest and recovery. Your vital signs, incision and vaginal bleeding will continue to be closely observed by your doctor and nurse. Your baby will be with you in the room as much as you prefer. Your nurse will help you with breast or formula feeding. You will be given a liquid diet such as jello, broth, soda, etc. Your IV may be discontinued. The catheter in your bladder will be removed. Your nurse will assist you to the bathroom. You will be encouraged to sit in the chair and take short walks to prevent gas pain and speed the recovery process. If you are uncomfortable, ask your nurse for pain medication. Your doctor and your baby's doctor will visit. Your family and friends may visit as you desire. You will be encouraged to rest and get to know your new baby.	Your nurse and doctor will continue to monitor your recovery. You will be able to do more today. You will be encouraged to sit in the chair and take short walks. If you need assistance, your nurse is available. If you are uncomfortable, ask your nurse for pain medication. Your nurse will listen to your abdomen for bowel activity. Your baby will be with you in the room as much as you prefer. Your nurse will continue to help you with breast or formula feeding if needed. If you want your baby boy circumcised, your doctor will do this before your baby goes home. Your doctor and your baby's doctor will visit. Your baby will have blood drawn for PKU. Your family and friends may visit you as you desire. Be sure to let your nurse know what we can do to make your stay as comfortable as possible.	Some insurance companies cover and arrange for home visits by a professional nurse. If that option is not offered, you can obtain homecare for a fee. Home visits are available through St. John's Mercy homecare services department. If you would like a home visit, ask your doctor or nurse. Feel free to call the family focused care unit with any questions you may have after you go home @ 569-6287. If you have questions about breast feeding, call 961-2229 to arrange to speak with a lactation consultant. Your doctor and your baby's doctor will give you their phone numbers so you can call them if you need to ask questions.

St. John's Mercy Medical Center, St. Louis, MO.

APPENDIX P. Family Focused Childbirth Care Path:Cesarean Birth cont.

FAMILY FOCUSED CHILDBIRTH CARE PATH: CESAREAN BIRTH				
	0 - 4 HOURS AFTER BIRTH	**1 st DAY AFTER BIRTH**	**2 nd DAY AFTER BIRTH**	**HOME FOLLOW-UP**
FAMILY TEACHING	After birth, your nurse will assist you in getting to know your new baby. If you are breastfeeding, you will be given information and tips for success. Your baby will be with you as much as you desire. Your nurse will teach you how to massage your uterus. Your nurse will discuss your diet and activity level for the next few days. Information will be provided to family and friends about visiting hours.	Your nurse will begin teaching you how to care for yourself and your baby after you go home. You will be provided with information about breast and formula feeding, cord care, circumcision care, newborn awake and sleeping patterns, how to tell if the baby is hungry, how to comfort the crying baby, how to know if the baby is getting enough to eat, what to do if the baby is choking or spitting up feedings, how to bathe your baby. your diet activity level, expected vaginal bleeding, incision care, breast care, and pain relief measures. Your nurse will answer your questions or concerns.	Your nurse will continue to teach you how to care for yourself and your baby after you go home. Feel free to ask any questions or seek clarification. Your doctor and your baby's doctor will visit and be available to answer your questions as well. You will be encouraged to rest. You will be given information about warning signs of complications, when to call the doctor, and when to schedule your and your new baby's first doctor's visit.	During the home visit, your nurse will check your incision, vaginal bleeding, breasts, blood pressure, temperature, pulse, and respirations. ask about your diet, urination and bowel movements ask about your baby's diet, urination and bowel movements. Your baby's cord and circumcision will be checked. Your nurse may observe a breastfeeding or formula feeding session. Questions about your care or baby care will be answered.

St. John's Mercy Medical Center, St. Louis, MO.

APPENDIX Q. Maternal Confidence Scale

MATERNAL CONFIDENCE SCALE

Please indicate the extent to which you agree or disagree with each statement by circling the appropriate number between 1 and 5.

1 = strongly disagree
2 = disagree
3 = uncertain
4 = agree
5 = strongly agree

	Strongly Disagree				Strongly Agree
1. I do not feel confident about my mothering role.	1	2	3	4	5
2. I can generally tell what my baby needs at this time.	1	2	3	4	5
3. When my baby cries I usually feel irritated.	1	2	3	4	5
4. I consider myself a "motherly" person.	1	2	3	4	5
5. I feel very close to my baby now.	1	2	3	4	5
6. My adjustment to feeding my baby was very easy.	1	2	3	4	5
7. I know what to do to care for my baby.	1	2	3	4	5
8. I have very little self-confidence regarding child care.	1	2	3	4	5

Bradley, C. F. (1983). Psychological consequences of intervention in the birth process. *Canadian Journal of Behavior Science, 15*(4). 422–438.

APPENDIX R. Satisfaction with Nursing Care

SATISFACTION WITH NURSING CARE

We are interested in how you felt about the nursing care that you received from the nurses who visited you during the first 5 days postpartum.

1. How many visits did a nurse make to your home after you left the hospital?
   _____ visits

2. How did you feel about this number of home visits? (Please circle)
   (1) just right
   (2) too many
   (3) too few

We are interested in how you felt about the visiting nursing care that you received during the first 5 days postpartum. Please use the following code to answer the questions below:

1 = strongly disagree
2 = disagree
3 = uncertain
4 = agree
5 = strongly agree

	Strongly Disagree				Strongly Agree
1. The nurses made me feel that they understood me and my concerns.	1	2	3	4	5
2. The nurses gave me the information I wanted.	1	2	3	4	5
3. The nurses reassured me when I needed it.	1	2	3	4	5
4. The nurses made me feel that they respected me as a person.	1	2	3	4	5
5. The nurses did not spend enough time with me.	1	2	3	4	5
6. The nurses gave me time to discuss my concerns/problems without rushing me.	1	2	3	4	5
7. The nurses made me feel that I could ask them anything about my experience.	1	2	3	4	5

APPENDIX R. Satisfaction with Nursing Care cont.

1 = strongly disagree 2 = disagree 3 = uncertain 4 = agree 5 = strongly agree

	Strongly Disagree				Strongly Agree
8. The nurses sensed when I needed reassurance.	1	2	3	4	5
9. The nurses explained things in terms I could understand.	1	2	3	4	5
10. The nurses listened carefully to what I had to say.	1	2	3	4	5
11. The nurses shared their thoughts about my condition, problem, or concern with me.	1	2	3	4	5
12. The nurses helped me to talk about topics that are uncomfortable for me to discuss.	1	2	3	4	5
13. The nurses felt positively towards me.	1	2	3	4	5
14. The nurses seemed concerned with me as a person as well as a patient.	1	2	3	4	5
15. The nurses described the kind of help that they could provide for me.	1	2	3	4	5
16. When I was upset, the nurses encourage me to talk about it.	1	2	3	4	5
17. Sometimes the nurses knew how I felt without me saying anything.	1	2	3	4	5
18. The nurses helped me sort out my concerns and look at them one at a time.	1	2	3	4	5
19. I had confidence in the nurses assigned to my care.	1	2	3	4	5
20. The information given me by the nurses was useful.	1	2	3	4	5
21. I enjoyed participating in the maternity study.	1	2	3	4	5
22. The care that I received helped me deal with my situation at home.	1	2	3	4	5
23. I would recommend similar care to my friends.	1	2	3	4	5
24. Overall, I was very satisfied with the care that I received.	1	2	3	4	5
25. If I have another baby, I would want the same type of maternity care.	1	2	3	4	5

APPENDIX R. Satisfaction with Nursing Care cont.

26. What did you like about the early discharge?
27. What did you dislike about the early discharge?
28. How would you improve it?

Bradley, C. F., Carty, E.M., & Hall, W. A. (1989). An evaluation of early postpartum discharge from a tertiary maternity hospital. Final report, School of Nursing, University of British Columbia, Vancouver, British Columbia, Canada.

APPENDIX S. Loyola University Medical Center Perinatal Network: Acutely ILL Neonatal Transport Collaborative Carepath

COLLABORATIVE CAREPATH: **ACUTELY ILL NEONATAL TRANSPORT**

Patient: ____________________	Date/Time of Birth: ____________________
Neonatologist/Pediatrician: ____________________	Infant Apgars: ______________
Referring Obstetrician: ____________________	Gestational Age: ______________
Referral Hospital Phone #: ____________________	Maternal Gravida/Parity: ___________

Date: Time:	TRANSFER **ACCEPTED** (TIME_____) UNTIL TEAM ARRIVES	TEAM **ARRIVAL** (TIME_______)	TEAM **DEPARTURE** (TIME________)	DISCHARGE OUTCOMES
Care Unit:	LEVEL II NURSERY			Safe transport.
Consults/Physicians:	Neonatology/Pediatrician Written transfer order			Follow-up for return transport criteria.
Tests: **(Check all that were done)**	_CBC _Blood Cultures _Blood Type/Coomb _Blood Gases _Glucose (serum) _Newborn Screen (PKU, etc.) _Mother's Maiden Name:__________ _Mother's Social Security #:__________ _Urine CIE _Urine Toxicology _Surface Cultures _CXR _X-ray post tube/line placement OTHER: ____________________			Values available at time of transfer, except cultures.
Treatment/ Procedures: **(Check all that were done)**	_Resuscitation:_O2 _Bag/ Mask _Compressions _Medications _Intubation Tube size ____ Cm at lip line _____ _Surfactant Time________ Type____________ _Umbilical Line _Chest Tube _Lumbar Puncture		Complete newborn identification verification.	Infant stable for transport post treatment intervention and identification.
Activity:	**Skin Care:** Utilize pectin based barriers under any/all tape (i.e. E.T., Umbilical lines, NG, etc.). Use of bowel bag (Vi-drape) for abdominal defects.			Skin integrity will be maintained.
Nutrition:	Intake: IV fluid__________________ Rate___________ enteric (type)__________________ Output: Urine: Mother desires: _ Breast/ _ Bottle Stool: Blood: Other:		TOTALS: Intake: Output:	Promote optimal maintenance of hydration/ nutrition.

APPENDIX S. Loyola University Medical Center Perinatal Network: Acutely ILL Neonatal Transport Collaborative Carepath cont.

Medications: (Check or write meds given)	_EES _Vitamin K Antibiotics (Dosage/time): Ampicillin ________ Gentamicin ________ Other Meds: ____________________		Medications ordered but not administered: ____________ ____________	Endorsement of medication plan.
Assessment & Monitoring:	Evaluate: skin color ___________ need for NG ___________ cardio/respiratory monitoring __ V/S with dinamap B/P ______ Invasive B/P monitoring _____ Pulse oximetry _________ Anomalies/defects _________ Glucose screen (most recent level ________) time: ___			Stabilization for a safe transport.
Expected Outcomes: (Check all that were done)	Items to prepare for transport: _XEROX CHART: * _**Baby Chart** _**Mother's delivery record** _X-Ray copies _Labelled cord blood _Mother's blood (pilot tubes) _Parent/Guardian available for consents _Referral Hospital "Release of information" consent _Referral Hospital "procedure" consent(s) _Will fax unavailable items LUMC NICU FAX: 216-4125 Completion of appropriate consults; tests; procedures; skin care; nutritional evaluation; medication delivery; and assessment and monitoring	Referral center obtains transport consent. Transfer to Level III care initiated.	Endorsements completed.	Stabilization for safe transport.
Psychosocial & Educational Needs: Patient & Family <u>(Check all that were done)</u>	_Reason for transport. _Chaplain notified. _Infant baptized, per parent request. _Polaroid picture taken and given to parent. _Parents see infant prior to departure.	Transport pack given to parents by transport team.		Patient and family needs are met.
Discharge Plan:		Transport team member signs for "receiving patient"	Document transfer. Discharge from computer. Complete neonatal transport log and nursery log. Complete charting, include: transport team arrival time, infant's condition on team's arrival and departure, and time of team departure with infant.	Safe transport and appropriate documentation completed.

REFERRAL HOSPITAL R.N. (INITIALS) ____________________ (____) **TRANSFER HOSPITAL R.N. (INITIALS)** ____________________ (____)

REFERRAL HOSPITAL R.N. (INITIALS) ____________________ (____) **TRANSFER HOSPITAL R.N. (INITIALS)** ____________________ (____)

6/1/94 CCAINT.

APPENDIX S. Loyola University Medical Center Perinatal Network: Neonatal Return Collaborative Carepath

COLLABORATIVE CAREPATH: **NEONATAL RETURN TRANSPORT**

Patient: ____________ Gestational age @ Birth:________ DOL:______ Date: ________

Birthweight:____________ Current Weight:__________ Diagnosis:____________ Current Condition:________

Accepting Neonatologist/Pediatrician: ____________ Referring Neonatologist:______________

Accepting Hospital:____________________ Accepting Hospital Phone #: ____________

Date: Time:	TRANSFER TIME AGREED UPON (TIME_____)	TIME TEAM ARRIVED AT LEVEL II (TIME___)	DISCHARGE OUTCOMES
Care Unit:	LEVEL III NURSERY	LEVEL II NURSERY	Safe transport.
Communication:	Nurse verifies consent for transfer. Nurse to Nurse report. Parent notification of tentative transfer time. Parent given Level II phone number.	Infant identification process completed.	Return transport and infant identification safely completed.
Tests: (Check all that are done)	_Newborn Screen (PKU, etc.) Date:______ _Hearing Screen Date:______ _Pass/_Fail _Eye Exam Date:______ Follow-up:________ _Last Hematocrit Date:______ Result:________ _Drug Levels ____________ _Other pertinent Labs (i.e. toxicology screen, blood cultures, blood gases, etc.) ________________ ____________________		Values available and endorsed at time of transfer, except newborn screen.
Treatment/ Procedures: (Check those applicable)	Environment: _Open Crib _Isolette (bed temperature ___) _Warmer Respiratory Support: _None _02____% _NC____L flow _Hood _CPAP +___ _Other: (Circumcision,etc.)__________ ____________		Infant stable for transport post treatment intervention and identification.
Medications: (list current medications)	MEDICATION DOSE ROUTE FREQUENCY LAST DOSE ________ ____ ______ ______ ______ ________ ____ ______ ______ ______ ________ ____ ______ ______ ______ ________ ____ ______ ______ ______ If antibiotic, list day of treatment_____/anticipated length of treatment______ _Immunization card provided to referral hospital		Endorsement of medication plan.
Activity: (Check those applicable)	_Reflux precautions. _Kangaroo care. _Apnea and bradycardia status. _Other:______________ ______________		Outlined activities will be maintained.

APPENDIX S. Loyola University Medical Center Perinatal Network: Neonatal Return Collaborative Carepath cont.

Nutrition:	**Intake:** IV fluid__________ Rate______ IV lock in place, Last flushed:__________ Milk used:________ Route: _CNG _intermittent _ng _po/ng _po _ad lib Feeding amount:________ Feeding frequency: q______ Last feeding time:________ Feeding issues: Emesis Reflux Residuals Other:________ Breast: _Mom pumping _Attempted at breast _Breastfeeding well _Breastmilk supply brought with patient **Output:** Last Void: __________ Last Stool:__________ Problems:__________ Other:__________		Promote optimal maintenance of hydration/ nutrition.
Assessment & Monitoring:	Head circumference:______ Abdominal circumference:______ Chest circumference:______ Length:________ V/S frequency:______ Last V/S: T___ P___ R___ B/P___ Pulse oximeter: _None _Continuous _Intermittent Pulse oximetry 02 Saturation range: ____ to ____ Other:__________		Stabilization for a safe transport.
Expected Outcomes:	Transfer Summary (history) prepared. _Brought with infant _To be faxed	Transfer Summary endorsed. Level II admission documentation initiated.	Hospitalization history endorsed for safe transition of care.
Psychosocial & Educational Needs: Patient & Family <u>(Check those applicable)</u>	Parent contact history endorsed. Parent competencies achieved: _bath _temperature taking _diapering _feeding _CPR _Other:________ ________	Parent involvement and competencies endorsed to Level II. Personal belongings accepted by Level II.	Patient and family needs are met. Orientate parents to unit.
Discharge Plan:	Pediatrician identified ______ Neonatal Follow-up Clinic Appointment ________ Ophthalmology Follow-up Appointment ________ Other Follow-up needs: ________ ________	Infant admitted to Level II for ongoing care and discharge planning.	Safe transport and appropriate documentation completed.

REFERRAL HOSPITAL R.N. (INITIALS) ____________ (____)

TRANSFER HOSPITAL R.N. (INITIALS) ____________ (____)

REFERRAL HOSPITAL R.N. (INITIALS) ____________ (____)

TRANSFER HOSPITAL R.N. (INITIALS) ____________ (____)

REFERRAL HOSPITAL M.D. ____________

6/1 ccrt

INDEX

Note: Page numbers in italics represent figures; those followed by "t" represent tables; those followed by "d" represent displays.

G